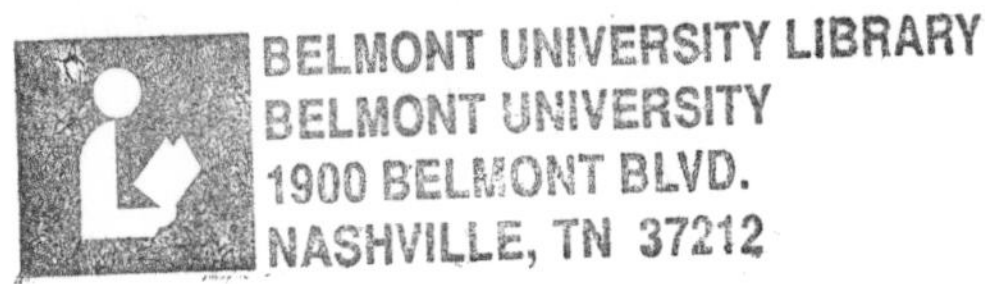

PHYSICAL THERAPY IN
ARTHRITIS

PHYSICAL THERAPY IN ARTHRITIS

Joan M. Walker, PhD, PT
Professor
School of Physiotherapy
Associate Professor
Department of Anatomy and Neurobiology
Dalhousie University
Halifax, Nova Scotia, Canada

Antoine Helewa, MSc(Clin Epid), PT
Professor
Department of Physical Therapy
Elborn College
University of Western Ontario
London, Ontario, Canada

W. B. SAUNDERS COMPANY
A Division of Harcourt Brace & Company
Philadelphia, London, Toronto, Montreal, Sydney, Tokyo

W. B. SAUNDERS COMPANY
A Division of Harcourt Brace & Company

The Curtis Center
Independence Square West
Philadelphia, Pennsylvania 19106

Library of Congress Cataloging-in-Publication Data

Physical therapy in arthritis / Joan M. Walker, Antoine Helewa. — 1st ed.
p. ; cm.
Includes bibliographical references and index.
ISBN 0-7216-4999-8
1. Arthritis—Physical therapy. 2. Arthritis. I. Walker, Joan M. II. Helewa, Antoine.
[DNLM: 1. Arthritis—rehabilitation. 2. Physical Therapy—methods. WE 344 P577 1996]
RC933.P465 1996
616.7'22062—dc20
DNLM/DLC 95-41652

PHYSICAL THERAPY IN ARTHRITIS ISBN 0-7216-4999-8

Printed in the United States of America.

Last digit is the print number: 9 8 7 6 5 4 3 2 1

With love and appreciation
to
our parents and families

CONTRIBUTORS

ALAN COVERT, MD, FRCP
Assistant Professor, Department of Pathology, Faculty of Medicine, Dalhousie University; Associate Pathologist, Queen Elizabeth II Health Science Center, Victoria General Site, Halifax, Nova Scotia, Canada
Diagnosis and Management of Arthritic Conditions

CHARLES H. GOLDSMITH, MSc, PhD
Professor of Biostatistics, McMaster University, Department of Clinical Epidemiology and Biostatistics; Head of Biostatistics, Father Sean O'Sullivan Research Centre, St. Joseph's Hospital, Hamilton, Ontario, Canada
Methodological Principles for Physical Therapy Research in Arthritis—How to Critically Appraise the Literature

BARBARA HANES, BSc(OT)
Occupational Therapy Services, Community Services Department, Homes for the Aged Division, Corporation of Metropolitan Toronto, Toronto, Ontario, Canada
Orthotics, Splinting, and Lifestyle Factors

DONNA J. HAWLEY, RN, MN, EdD
Professor and Director, Graduate Nursing Program, School of Nursing, Wichita State University, Wichita, Kansas
Psychological Distress and Clinical Outcomes

ANTOINE HELEWA, MSc(Clin Epid), PT
Professor, Department of Physical Therapy, Faculty of Applied Health Sciences; Professor, Department of Epidemiology, Faculty of Medicine, University of Western Ontario, London, Ontario, Canada
Epidemiology and Economics of Arthritis; Assessment of Joint Disease; Physical Therapy Management of Patients with Rheumatoid Arthritis and Other Inflammatory Conditions; Methodological Principles for Physical Therapy Research in Arthritis—How to Critically Appraise the Literature

JOHN VERRIER JONES, BCh, FRCP, FRCPC
Retired. Former Professor and Head, Division of Rheumatology, Department of Medicine, Dalhousie University, Halifax, Nova Scotia, Canada
Diagnosis and Management of Arthritic Conditions

MARY ANN KEENAN, MD
Professor, Department of Orthopaedic Surgery; Professor, Department of Physical Medicine and Rehabilitation, Temple University School of Medicine; Chairman, Department of Orthopaedic Surgery, Albert Einstein Medical Center, MossRehab Hospital, Philadelphia, Pennsylvania
Surgical Interventions

MARION A. MINOR, PhD, PT
Assistant Professor, University of Missouri, Columbia, Missouri
Cardiovascular Health and Physical Fitness for the Client with Multiple Joint Involvement

CAROLEE MONCUR, PhD, PT
Professor, Division of Physical Therapy; Adjunct Professor, Division of Rheumatology; Adjunct Professor, Department of Bioengineering, University of Utah, Salt Lake City, Utah
Physical Therapy Management of the Patient with Osteoarthritis

IRA RICHTERMAN, MD
Chief Resident, Department of Orthopaedic Surgery, Albert Einstein Medical Center, Philadelphia, Pennsylvania
Surgical Inverventions

ELAINE SMITH, MSW
Social Worker, Arthritis Orthopaedic Program, Hugh MacMillan Rehabilitation Centre, Toronto, Ontario, Canada
Physical Therapy Management of the Child and Adolescent with Juvenile Rheumatoid Arthritis

HUGH A. SMYTHE, MD, FRCP (C)
Professor, Department of Medicine, Faculty of Medicine, University of Toronto; Rheumatic Disease Unit, Wellesley Hospital, Toronto, Ontario, Canada
Pain and Tender Points: Fibrositis/Fibromyalgia and Related Syndromes; Assessment of Joint Disease

BARBARA STOKES, PT
Clinical Instructor, University of Ottawa; Director, The Arthritis Society, Consultation and Therapy Service, Eastern Region (Ontario Division), Ottawa, Ontario, Canada
Physical Therapy Management of Ankylosing Spondylitis; Community-Based Physical Therapy Management of Arthritis

JOAN M. WALKER, PhD, PT
Professor, School of Physiotherapy; Associate Professor, Department of Anatomy and Neurobiology, Dalhousie University, Halifax, Nova Scotia, Canada
The Historical Record: Paleopathology and Physical Therapy in Management of Arthritis; Epidemiology and Economics of Arthritis; Pathophysiology of Inflammation, Repair, and Immobility; Pharmacology and the Interaction with Physical Therapy; Methodological Principles for Physical Therapy Research in Arthritis—How to Critically Appraise the Literature

ANNE MARIE WHELAN, BSc(Pharm), PharmD
Associate Professor, College of Pharmacy, Dalhousie University; Consultant Pharmacist, Department of Family Medicine, Camp Hill Medical Center, Halifax, Nova Scotia, Canada
Pharmacology and the Interaction with Physical Therapy

F. VIRGINIA WRIGHT, MSc(Clin Epid), PT
Lecturer, Department of Physical Therapy, University of Toronto; Clinical Physical Therapist, Arthritis Orthopaedic Program; Research Physical Therapist, The Hugh MacMillan Rehabilitation Centre, Toronto, Ontario, Canada
Physical Therapy Management of the Child and Adolescent with Juvenile Rheumatoid Arthritis

FOREWORD

The philosopher Charles Pierce identified four general ways of knowing: the methods of *authority*, *intuition*, *tenacity*, and the method of *science*. In the first, *authority*, if an idea has the weight of tradition and public sanction behind it, it is so. For the second method, *intuition*, truth is based on the a priori assumption that the proposition agrees with reason or is self evident. According to the third, *tenacity*, one holds firmly to the truth, the truth that is known to be true because one holds firmly to it. Authority and intuition, and failing that tenacity, have been the historical mainstay for physical therapy management in arthritis. The foundation of physical therapy in arthritis, by and large, has been built on clinical experience, physiological principles, tradition, and common sense.

This tradition, as Walker and Helewa, so ably document in **Physical Therapy in Arthritis**, is changing. During the past two decades, arthritis, one of the most common sets of diagnoses encountered by physical therapists, has received unprecedented attention from the scientific community. Traditional treatment programs have come under close scrutiny, traditional assumptions have been examined empirically, and new management strategies have been developed and tested by a growing cadre of researchers in physical therapy and associated professions. The basis of arthritis management is shifting from traditional forms of 'knowing' to a scientifically, justified foundation. Gradually the method of *science*, with its emphasis on subjecting clinical beliefs to objective measurement and testing, has assumed a more prominent role in laying the foundation of physical therapy management of arthritis. In turn, the traditional methods of authority, intuition, and tenacity are receding in importance. The fruits of this changing tradition are before us in this impressive volume.

Walker and Helewa have organized and written a comprehensive review of the state-of-the-science in physical therapy management in arthritis. The range of topics included in this volume is unprecedented in existing arthritis and physical therapy literature; the approach is analytic and critical. From the paleopathological roots of arthritis, to a comprehensive review of contemporary management strategies, the authors present a scholarly update on contemporary arthritis management.

This volume documents the merging scientific basis for contemporary physical therapy management of arthritis. It also advances many of the pressing questions that need to be addressed by arthritis researchers. It fills an important void in the growing physical therapy and arthritis literature. It will serve as a valuable reference for the clinician and researcher alike, and is sure to become a standard text for physical therapy curricula for years to come.

ALAN M. JETTE, PT, MPH, PhD
Chief Research Scientist
New England Research Institute
Professor of Social & Behavioral Sciences
Boston University School of Public Health
Boston, Massachusetts

PREFACE

The need for a textbook focused on physical therapy management in arthritis is derived from the large number of individuals, from children to senior citizens, whose quality of life is impaired by arthritis. The latest survey by the United States Public Health Service listed about 31,000,000 people with these disorders.

Recent years have seen a marked growth of physical therapy in arthritis. Clinical and basic investigations have expanded and more capable people have been attracted to the field. There is now optimism that much can be done to control many of the arthritic disorders through judicious pharmacologic and physical management.

This volume is the first textbook to provide a comprehensive approach to physical therapy management of arthritis, written largely by physical therapists but also including contributions from other health professionals. All of the authors are recognized in North America for their clinical research and educational skills and expertise. We have directed this textbook to the clinician, but also, in recognition of the importance of well prepared graduates, to physical therapy educators and students. The essential component of rheumatology in the entry-level curriculum has lacked a foundation reference. The editors hope that other health care workers in related fields will find the text a useful resource and addition to their libraries.

Initial chapters examine the historical record of arthritis, physical therapy involvement in care of patients with arthritis, epidemiology and economics of arthritis. Middle chapters cover pathophysiology of inflammation, immobility and repair, medical and surgical management, psychosocial issues, pharmacology, orthotics and life style factors to establish a firm foundation for physical therapy management. Subsequent chapters then focus on the physical assessment and management of common arthritis disorders, such as pain amplification syndromes, juvenile arthritis, inflammatory arthritis in adults, osteoarthritis and ankylosing spondylitis.

The editors believe that the textbook presents innovative approaches to the assessment, and to the management of the young and adult patient with arthritis. Uniquely, and we believe appropriately, one chapter focuses on cardiovascular health and physical fitness for the client with multiple joint involvement. The text also addresses the increasingly important area of community-based health care in management of the client with arthritis.

The important area of evaluation of the quality of the growing literature in arthritis, essential to the provision of evidence-based care, is contained in the final chapter. The approach advocated will provide students and graduates with a critical, planned method to review the literature that may be used in fields other than arthritis.

Treatment chapters include case studies, as well as identification of problem issues or research questions. We feel that this textbook will fill a void in the literature, contribute to further research in arthritis by physical therapists, contribute to the delivery of evidence-based care, improve the quality of care, and ultimately improve the quality of the lives of individuals with arthritis.

Many individuals have contributed to this textbook. We have been inspired by patients, students, and colleagues. Particularly, we recognize the valuable contributions of research assistants at our universities, Noreen Delorey, Janice Palmer, Jane Farrell, and Lisa Wilson. We have been assisted by the computer skills of Pat Darling, and by the reference staff of the Kellogg Health Sciences Library, Dalhousie University. We are also grateful for the encouragement of Margaret Biblis, Senior Editor at W.B. Saunders Company, and for the work of Berta Steiner and the staff of Bermedica Production, Ltd.

JOAN M. WALKER
ANTOINE HELEWA

CONTENTS

CHAPTER 1

The Historical Record: Paleopathology and Physical Therapy in Management of Arthritis

Joan M. Walker, PhD, PT

Prevalence rates in the United States for self-reported rheumatic diseases are rare in the under-18-year age group and increasingly common in the 65-year and older age groups[1] (Table 1-1). A population-based survey revealed that individuals with chronic conditions reported more restriction of their mobility due to arthritis and rheumatism than other conditions (22% cf. 6.3% for cerebrovascular disease).[2]

Peyron and Altman[3] cited British studies which showed that 2.3% of men and 1.3% of women in the work force had to retire because of osteoarthritis (OA) or allied conditions; a loss of 4.7 million working days in 1974. In 1973 OA was the second leading cause of permanent incapacity in individuals older than 50 years. OA affects some 40 million Americans and is evident radiologically in greater than 80% of individuals aged 55 years and older.[4] Incidence and prevalence are discussed in Chapter 2. Arthritic conditions constitute a significant social and economic burden in today's societies.

PHYSICAL THERAPY IN ARTHRITIS, Joan M. Walker, PhD, PT, and Antoine Helewa, MSc(Clin Epid), PT, W.B. Saunders Company © 1996.

Paleopathological Record

Next to traumatic conditions, arthritis is the oldest and most widespread pathological condition reported in paleopathology (study of disease and trauma in extinct societies).[5] The fossilized remains of animals and people reveal their patterns of injury and disease, which are an expression of the stresses and strains to which they were exposed, in response to their environment and behavior.[6]

First recognized in dinosaurs, arthritis has been seen continuously throughout history. Distinction is not always made, or possible, between rheumatoid arthritis (RA) and osteoarthritis; reports of "chronic arthritis" are more prevalent in publications. In hominids, chronic arthritis has been observed from the time of Neanderthal man (e.g., the man of La Chapelle-aux-Saints).[4] Studies of skele-

Table 1-1. Prevalence Rates per 1000 Persons for Self-Reported Cases of Arthritis by Age, United States, 1983–1985

Age (Years)	<18	18–44	45–64	65–74	>75
Arthritis	2.3	52.4	279.5	459.7	507.7

Adapted from Lawrence RC, Hochberg MC, Kelsey JL, et al: Estimates of the prevalence of selected arthritic and musculoskeletal diseases in the United States. J Rheumatol 1989; 16:429.

tons from the Saxon and Roman period of early England have shown "changes consistent with OA" in at least half the specimens.[7]

Spondylitis (arthritis of the vertebral column) is known to be present in ancient Egyptian populations since 4000 B.C. Three of 12 Egyptian royal family mummies from 1570 B.C. to 324 A.D. had radiographic evidence of OA in the hips, knees, or spine.[8] Spondylitis also was common in Cro-Magnon and pre-Columbian American populations. In early humans, lumbar involvement was common, dorsal and cervical involvement rare with the exception of ancient Egyptians, in whom dorsal involvement was frequent.[4] By comparison, cervical involvement is common in modern populations. Differences in sites, time periods, and populations probably reflect changing habits and forces. The increased involvement of the cervical spine in modern populations may be a reflection of the more sedentary life styles and more time spent in sitting postures.

While numerous joints have been shown to be affected, hip joint involvement has been only observed in hominids, not in animals. Estimation of involvement of joints of the hand and foot is affected by the existence of these small bones over large time periods. As evidence of arthritis has been observed in all time periods, climates, and locales, as well as in dinosaurs and cave bears, the paleopathological record offers no support for climate, alcohol, or tobacco as causative factors.

In some Nubian (Egyptian) populations, arthritis involved some 10% of vertebrae while lipping was present in 50%. Variation in reported frequency of osteophytes (lipping) between early populations is thought to reflect differences in life span; the longer the life span, the higher the frequency, a reflection of a longer exposure to stress.[9]

Rothschild[7] noted that systemic population radiography did not reveal evidence of OA in weight-bearing bones of several types of dinosaurs (e.g., tyrannosaurs). Although an isolated occurrence in dinosaurs, OA affected up to 26% of Pleistocene kangaroos and marsupial oxen. OA also is relatively rare in Old World primates.[10]

Rothschild and Wood[11] reported OA "in only 0.8% of free-ranging animals but 4.8% of artificially restrained animals." This study suggests that colony-raised animals may not constitute an adequate model for the study of "natural" OA. Not only did the frequency of involvement differ significantly but also the site of involvement; shoulder and elbow joints were more affected in colony animals compared with knees in free-ranging animals. It was not considered that the longer life spans of colony animals gave an adequate explanation of these differences.

In the eighteenth century, William Heberden made the first reference to "hard knots, little peas" known now as Heberden's nodes frequently seen on digits of patients with OA. He also recognized that these were different from those seen in gout.[4] Of interest is the report that such nodes are visible on ceramic figures made by pre-Columbian Indians (ca. 200–650 A.D.). While Heberden distinguished between OA and gout, some confusion remained through the nineteenth and early twentieth centuries on the relationship between OA and rheumatoid arthritis. Sir William Osler also distinguished between OA and gout, describing at length a chronic disorder of joints termed "arthritis deformans." Some of the lesions he described now would be termed RA (e.g., involvement of synovial membrane); however, he also described new bone formation in spinal ligaments, now termed ankylosing spondylitis.[4]

Substantial developments in investigative tools in the fields of radiology, immunology, and genetics have vastly improved our ability to distinguish between the many different types of arthritis. We have, however, not advanced much in our ability to prevent or alter the course of many rheumatological conditions.

Hippocrates is credited with "convincing descriptions of gout."[12] The introduction of roentgen rays at the turn of this century allowed distinction between "atrophic" and "hypertrophic arthritis," then OA and RA. Increasingly, sophisticated laboratory methods of analysis nowadays permit distinction of many different forms of RA, such as crystal deposition diseases, and lupus erythematosus.

Dieppe and Rogers[12] (whose article is recommended for any reader interested in skeletal paleopathology of rheumatoid disorders) cautioned making a diagnosis of OA solely on evidence of osteophytes, since these alone may only reflect aging changes. Fusion or erosive spondyloarthritis may have been overdiagnosed as ankylosing spondylitis; some cases may be indicative of psoriatic arthropathy or Reiter's disease (Fig. 1-1).[12] In contrast to OA, RA has not been convincingly demonstrated in ancient skeletons and RA, of the severity seen today, is "believed to be uncommon, if present at all, in previous centuries." The inability to identify RA clearly, as compared with gout, in old art or literature, suggests it may be a disease of modern origin.[12]

Physical Therapy in Management of Arthritis, Past to Present

Use of massage and exercises for a curative effect dates from prehistoric times. The Chinese used these modalities as early as 3000 B.C. Early use also has been recorded by Hindus.[13] Hippocrates (460–360 B.C.) advocated the use of "friction" and Romans, such as Julius Caesar (100 B.C.) and Galen (131–201 A.D.), apparently valued massage for arthritis. Fuller in 1740[14] advocated "rubbing and chafing for cutaneous exercise," walking, and riding. He referred to scorbutic rheumatism

> in which cafe, the perfons afflicted are generally ftrong, unable to undergo any sorts of exercifes;

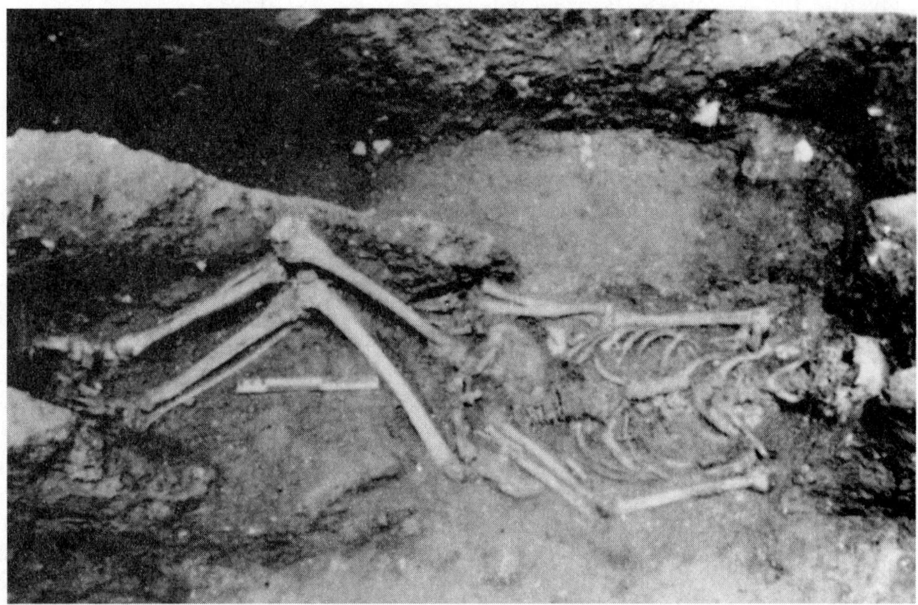

Figure 1-1. Medieval skeleton in situ. Note the flexed knees; this position was not a burial custom and suggests fixed flexion deformities antemortem. Subsequent examination showed an extensive, asymmetric sacroiliitis, spondylitis, and peripheral erosive arthropathy with bony proliferation. This picture is cautiously interpreted as a possible example of psoriatric or reactive spondyloarthropathy. (From Dieppe P, Rogers JM. Skeletal paleopathology of rheumatic disorders. In McCarty DJ, Koopman WJ [eds]: Arthritis and Allied Conditions, vol 1. Philadelphia, Lea & Febiger, 1993, p 11. With permission.)

> and therefore all sorts of exercifes which I shall hereafter mention will agree with them.[14, p 43]

He claimed that moderate exercise augmented the natural heat of the body and increased the velocity of the circulation.

Buchan,[15] writing on domestic medicine in 1803, recommended for obstinate fixed rheumatic pains

> a plafter of burgundy pitch worn for some time on the part affected to give great relief in rheumatic joints. The warm baths of Buxton or Matlock in Derbyshire are recommended for chronic or obstinate rheumatism. White mustard, a tablespoonful, taken twice a day. Cold bathing, especially in falt [salt] water often cures rheumatism and also recommend exercife and the wearing of flannel next to the fkin.[15, p 366]

Massage continued to be advocated through the nineteenth century. Roth[16] in 1851 stated that

> rheumatic pains of muscles are cured by pressure on the related nerves. This pressure, such as when given to the nervous accessorius willisii, can cure the most violent rheumatic pains of these parts. Acute rheumatic pains of intercostal muscles may disappear within a couple of hours by a kind of kneeling and rolling of the pectoral and other muscles combined with rotation of the arms. Rheumatic inflammation of the aponeurosis of the nates and left thigh, which occasioned at every movement the greatest pain, was cured in 6 days without medicines or bleedings, save only sawings on the suffering parts and longitudinal frictions of the skin towards the abdomen and back.[16, p 236]

Roth[16] also recognized the value of motion:

> limbs lamed by rheumatism are treated like the stiffness with this difference, that the supra abundant force of the parts adjacent to the diseased one must be diminished by the derivative movements, in order to increase the strength of the parts diseased. Stiffness of the limbs is treated according to the angles corresponding to the articulation in its healthy state, those stiffness that is caused by contractions of muscles and tendons are cured by frictions, combined with slow and extending movements.[16, p 254]

Osler[17] (1909) advocated "fresh air," a good diet, hydrotherapy, massage, and range-of-motion exercises; that salicylates may help; and that surgery could be employed to correct deformities. Few early medical textbooks, in describing the use of massage, hydrotherapy, and exercise, refer specifically to arthritis but more to "stiffness and lameness of limbs." One of the earliest detailed accounts of physiotherapy in the form of massage for the treatment of chronic rheumatism was given by Goodall-Copestake[16] in 1926.

> Deep massage can be borne and are very beneficial. Careful passive movements gradually increased. Hot air and other baths often beneficial combined with massage. For muscular rheumatism, rest and warmth are essential. Hot applications, hot air or Turkish baths and massage often affords great relief. . . . Time for treatment 15 to 40 minutes daily. For rheumatoid arthritis, massage forms part of the treatment in every stage of the disease except during acute attacks but it may begin as soon as the pain and swelling have subsided somewhat. Effleurage, frictions, muscle kneadings and passive movements to affected joints. The patient should be encouraged to perform active movements whether painful or not so as to keep up the nutrition of the muscles. Care should be taken not to force movements for fear of rupturing the tendons. If bony changes have occurred in the joints, deep friction should be avoided. The chief objective of treatment, then, is to maintain the strength of muscles. Passive movements must not be given until pain and swelling have subsided.[18, p 169]

While modern physical therapy only minimally uses massage, it is interesting that if used, it may be in the form of deep transverse frictions. Clients with arthritis obtain relief from general massage; however, there is no scientific evidence to support its use. Also, the modern university-prepared physical therapist is rarely a skilled practitioner in the art of massage.

It is rather remarkable, given the involvement of physical therapists in management of clients with arthritis, that since the earliest beginnings of the profession there have been so few textbooks devoted to this topic. There are references to treatments for arthritis and nonarticular manifestations that included myalgia, fibrositis, and lumbago. The first major paper in English, by a physiotherapist, was in 1953.[19] Forester described the conservative treatment of RA with special emphasis on changes needed when adrenocorticotropic hormone (ACTH) and cortisone therapy were used.[19] There was an emphasis on the prevention of deformity, relief of local symptoms, and the use of graduated exercise—a change from the earlier emphasis on the use of massage.

Although physical therapy (PT) was established as a unique profession at the turn of the century, even in the 1940s and 1950s, authors of PT texts rarely devoted even a single chapter to the management of patients with arthritis. This state existed despite the recommendation of the British Ministry of Health in 1928 that almost every case of chronic arthritis at some stage of the disease required physical treatment usually consisting of the application of heat in some form, either alone or together with massage and movement. It was stated that no scheme of treatment for chronic arthritis could be considered complete unless an extensive range of physical methods of treatment under skilled direction was available. Glover commented that "there appears to be a rapidly increasing demand for such treatment."[20]

Palmer[21] in 1942 continued to advocate use of effleurage, kneading, and petrissage in treatment of OA but noted that frictions should be avoided on the articular margins of joints, as they may cause pain and irritation. Movements should be active and performed within the limit of pain. Tidy[22] was one of the few authors to discuss treatment of different forms of arthritis (e.g., RA, Still's disease, OA, ankylopoietica, and infective arthritis). Amongst the modalities advocated were the use of evaporating lotions such as lead lotion or lead and opium lotion, faradism, radiant heat, and whirlpool baths. Forced movements were not advised; however, manipulation was recommended if stiffness did not respond to traditional therapy. Tidy also recommended massage for all forms of arthritis.[22]

Other modalities in use were histamine ionization or tincture of iodine in chronic cases "for a stronger effect on the circulation," constant current, and surged sinusoidal current to improve blood flow to the limbs.[23] Counterirritants used were galvanic current, ion transfer with vasodilators, high-frequency currents, and ultraviolet rays.[24] It is noteworthy, however, that bed rest was not advised for a patient with RA until swelling and pain had decreased, as "irreparable damage would be done."[25]

Generally, aims of therapy were to increase circulation and metabolism, prevent and relieve local arthritic changes, and correct faulty body mechanisms. The focus in textbooks was on the position of the patient (e.g., wing stoop high ride sitting), the movement or technique performed, but not on why the treatment was given. Cyriax[26] was one of the few authors of this time who attempted to identify the structure at fault and define a treatment related to that specific structure. He stated

> only when it is realized that arthritis and diffuse capsulitis are synonymous can a masseur understand the theory on which the treatment of non-specific arthritis is based. . . . The treatment of arthritis is the treatment of the capsule of the joint.[26, p 22]

Cyriax advocated massage to the capsule, mobilization of the joint to strengthen the capsule, exercises, and splinting as required. He considered massage the best treatment for effusion, and also recommended the use of resisted faradism to obtain full extension of the knee, and gait reeducation.[26]

At the middle of this century the rationale given for physical therapy intervention in arthritis was:

> general or systemic physical measures may serve as part of constitutional therapy for increase of circulation and metabolism. . . . Physical measures locally applied serve to prevent and relieve local arthritic changes.[27, p 462]

The practice of massage has been a commonly applied form of therapy in all population groups, ancient and modern. Evidence also exists for the application of orthotic principles across population groups. A report describes an Aleut "midwife" whose fingers had become "crooked and flexed with arthritis; she straightened them by binding them to wooden sticks and thus continued her practice until her death."[28]

Despite the numerous medical textbooks on arthritis and specific forms of arthritis, contribution to the literature by physical therapists was meager until about the 1970s. There currently are only two textbooks in English on PT in arthritis authored by physical therapists; both were published in the 1980s.[29,30] The establishment of the Association of Rheumatology Health Professionals (ARHP), formerly the Arthritis Health Professions Association, and a section of the American College of Rheumatology (ACR), provided a venue for health professionals interested in this area to interact. While there has been significant growth in physical therapists' involvement in arthritis research that is impacting on PT management, much more needs to be achieved. Worldwide, few PTs are known for research publications in the field of arthritis; Helewa, Jette, Moncur, Minor, Guccione, and Banwell are noteworthy among these few.

The Arthritis Society in Canada has provided direct physiotherapy and social work services in most Canadian provinces since the early 1950s. Because PTs and occupational therapists (OTs) received combined training in the early days, only physiotherapy as a service was officially designated. PTs, however, also provided occupational therapy. At present, the two services are distinct in all the provinces where they are provided in Canada.

With a current major focus on fund-raising for research and education, the Arthritis Society in 1994 is active in direct care for clients with arthritis in only three provinces: Ontario, British Columbia, and Nova Scotia. A characteristic of the health service provided by the Society was home care. PTs traveled within about a 50-mile radius of an urban center. In some cases, as in Manitoba, a therapist would spend 2–3 days in one away-from-base community. Outreach clinics are provided today to remote communities by traveling clinics. Whereas Ontario's programs are funded by the provincial government, in Nova Scotia a fee is charged for service (Helewa, personal communication). Both the Arthritis Society in Canada and the Arthritis Foundation in the United States play a significant role in the continuing education of therapists involved in arthritis care.

Attitudes and Beliefs

In addition to understanding the pathophysiology of arthritis, a therapist should recognize that clients may differ in their attitudes and beliefs about health and effective health care. Arthritis through the ages has been associated with a rich variety of "folk" remedies, such as the wearing of copper bracelets or the following of a special diet.[31] If such remedies *do no harm* or do not serve as substitutes to modern evidence-based care, it may be wise for the therapist not to interfere with such practices.

Logan[32] suggested that some of the problems encountered when modern health care workers attempt to bring Western-style health care to indigenous groups can be averted if practitioners attempt to understand and appreciate attitudes and beliefs of different ethnic groups. There is a need to determine where such beliefs may impede delivery of care and compliance with prescribed therapy, and to work out a system of delivery that is sensitive to an individual's philosophy of health. Consideration of such factors is as important in large urban cities of the Western world as it is for the health care worker in "third world" countries, given the ease of mobility in modern populations.

If folk remedies *do no harm* or do not serve as a substitute to modern evidence-based care, it may be wise not to interfere with such practices.

Logan[32] observed that it can be inappropriate to employ a medicine (or therapy) known locally to be hot (or cold). Local beliefs, as in Guatemala, regarding the interplay between beliefs about the natural world and its elements (temperature) may make the therapy not only ineffective but harmful. Logan reported symptoms and diseases recognized by natives and their response to prescribed treatments (acceptance or rejection). Rheumatism is one recognized disease for which natives accept the prescribed treatment of aspirin and Vicks VapoRub (data from Guatemala and New York–based Puerto Rican patients who display similar behavioral patterns in response to treatment of specific disorders). Certain drugs, however, are rejected because they are perceived as being harmful to "the natural order." This behavior may impede the management of arthritis, as drug therapy is an important component of modern programs.

Therapists working with multicultural populations of clients with arthritis should be cognizant of differences in attitudes and beliefs about health and health care. No studies were located that described the impact of such attitudes and beliefs on delivery of health care by physical therapists. Therapeutic programs need to be constructed that are sensitive to, and compatible with, an individual's attitudes and beliefs (i.e., culture friendly), or compliance is unlikely.

Physical Therapy Today

Modern management of the client with arthritis generally requires a client-centered team approach. Members, with varying roles at different stages of the disease, include physicians, physical and occupational therapists, social workers, nutritionists, orthotists, orthopedic surgeons and, most importantly, the client. Especially in children, family members and school teachers should be included. Other team members may be vocational counselors, pharmacists, registered nurses, psychologists, and recreational therapists.

This interdisciplinary team interacts to develop therapy goals and plans. It is part of a multidisciplinary approach to care, in which effort is made to "unify individual treatments into a comprehensive plan."[33] The role of the PT extends from the client (in hospital, clinic, or home) to the family and the public.

The community has numerous organizations that can assist both the client and the therapy team in the provision of resources (see Appendix I). The community can play a major role in facilitating the independence and mobility of the client with arthritis (e.g., provision of parking spots for the physically challenged, ramp access to buildings, and assistance with yard work and snow removal). Employers also have a responsibility and positive role to play in workplace modifications, and in expanding employment options, such as permitting work pacing and job sharing.

No one health care provider can be expert and knowledgeable on all aspects of care; however, knowledge of *who* to contact or refer to, and *when* is critical to evidence-based management. Banwell[33] has identified the roles and responsibilities of the major health disciplines involved in the management of the client with arthritis, noting that these roles and responsibilities often overlap.

The past decade has seen considerable development in identification of arthritis curricula content for entry-level PT programs. Jette and Becker[34] in 1980 surveyed programs in Canada and the United States; 31% indicated their curricula were inadequate. Moncur[35,36] has developed PT competencies in rheumatology, reporting competencies statements for seven domains: basic knowledge; patient evaluation; design of the PT plan of care; implementation of the PT plan; patient compliance; patient, family, and community education; and research activation (see Appendix II). Questions Moncur posed from this study remain valid today.

The most important advance in the last decade in physical therapy management of arthritis patients is the recognition that passive therapies are of limited use and at best serve only as adjuncts to active therapies. It also is recognized that a major consequence of arthritis is poor cardiopulmonary performance, often leading to serious endurance deficits and serious pathological sequelae, and that physical fitness programs which respect the integrity of joints improve therapeutic outcomes.

References

1. Lawrence RC, Hochberg MC, Kelsey JL, et al: Estimates of the prevalence of selected arthritic and musculoskeletal diseases in the United States. J Rheumatol 1989; 16:427–441.
2. Kelsey JL: Epidemiology of Musculoskeletal Disorders. New York, Oxford University Press, 1982.
3. Peyron JG, Altman RD: The epidemiology of osteoarthritis. In Moskowitz RW, Howell DS, Goldberg VM, Mankin HJ (eds): Osteoarthritis. Diagnosis and Medical/Surgical Management. Philadelphia, WB Saunders Co, 1992, pp 15–37.
4. Fife RS: A short history of osteoarthritis. In Moskowitz RW, Howell DS, Goldberg VM, Mankin HJ (eds): Osteoarthritis. Diagnosis and Medical/Surgical Management. Philadelphia, WB Saunders Co, 1992, pp 11–14.
5. Ackerknecht EH: Paleopathology. In Landy D (ed): Culture, Disease, and Healing. Studies in Medical Anthropology. New York, Macmillan Publishing Co, Inc, 1977, pp 71–77.
6. Wells C: Bones, Bodies, and Disease: Evidence of Disease and Abnormality in Early Man. London, Thomas & Hudson, 1964, p 17.
7. Rothschild BM: Skeletal paleopathology of rheumatic diseases: the subhomo connection. In McCarty DJ, Koopman WJ (eds): Arthritis and Allied Conditions, 12th edition. Philadelphia, Lea & Febiger, 1993, pp 3–8.
8. Braunstein EM, White SJ, Russell W, et al: Paleoradiographic evaluation of Egyptian royal mummies. Skeletal Radiol 1988; 17:348–351.
9. Armelagos GL: Disease in Ancient Nubia. In Landy D (ed): Culture, Disease, and Healing. Studies in Medical Anthropology. New York, Macmillan Publishing Co, Inc, 1977, pp 77–83.
10. Jurmain R: Trauma, degenerative disease, and other pathologies among Gombe chimpanzees. Am J Phys Anthropol 1989; 80:229–237.
11. Rothschild BM, Wood RJ: Osteoarthritis, calcium pyrophosphate deposition disease and osseous infection in Old World primates. Am J Phys Anthropol 1992; 87(3):341–347.
12. Dieppe P, Rogers JM: Skeletal paleopathology of rheumatic diseases. In McCarthy DJ, Koopman WJ (eds): Arthritis and Allied Conditions, 12th edition. Philadelphia, Lea & Febiger, 1993, pp 9–16.
13. Tod EM: Massage and Medical Gymnastics, 4th edition. London, JMA Churchill Ltd, 1951, p 1.
14. Fuller F: Medicina Gymnaftica: or, every man his own phyfician. A treatise concerning the power of exercise with refpect to the animal oeconomy, and the great neceffity of it in the cure of several diftempers. 7th edition. London, E Curll 1740.
15. Buchan W: Domestic Medicine, 18th edition. London, A Strahan, 1803.
16. Roth M: The Prevention and Cure of Many Chronic Diseases by Movements. London, John Churchill, 1851, p 254.

17. Osler W: The Principles and Practice of Medicine, 7th edition. New York, D. Appleton & Co, 1909.
18. Goodall-Copestake BM: The Theory and Practice of Massage, 4th edition. London, AK Lewis & Co Ltd, 1926, p 169.
19. Forester AL: The use of physiotherapy in the treatment of rheumatoid arthritis with special reference to its use combined with A.C.T.H. and cortisone. Fellowship Thesis for the Chartered Society of Physiotherapy, London, England, 1953.
20. Glover JA: A report on chronic arthritis with special reference to the provision of treatment. Ministry of Health, London, His Majesty's Stationery Office, 1928.
21. Palmer MD: Lessons on Massage, 6th edition. London, Bailliere, Tindall & Cox, 1942, p 42.
22. Tidy NM: Massage and Remedial Exercise, 7th edition. Bristol, Wright, 1947, p 112.
23. Clayton EB: Electrotherapy with Direct and Low Frequency Currents. London, Balliere, Tindall & Cox, 1947, pp 137–139.
24. Journal of the American Medical Association: Editorial. The treatment of arthritis. JAMA 1947; 135(3):288–289.
25. Solomon WM: Physical treatment of arthritis. JAMA 1948; 137(2):128–130.
26. Cyriax J: Massage, Manipulation and Local Anaesthesia. London, Hamish Hamilton Medical Books, 1943.
27. Kovacs R: Electrotherapy and Light Therapy with Essentials of Hydrotherapy and Mechanotherapy, 6th edition. London, Henry Kimpton, 1949.
28. Laughlin WS: Acquisition of anatomical knowledge. In Landy D (ed): Culture, Disease, and Healing. Studies in Medical Anthropology. New York, Macmillan Publishing Co, Inc, 1977, p 258.
29. Banwell BF, Gall V (eds): Physical Therapy Management of Arthritis. Clinics in Physical Therapy. New York, Churchill Livingstone, 1988.
30. Hyde S: Physiotherapy in Rheumatology. London, Blackwell Scientific Publications, 1980.
31. Jarvis DC: Arthritis and Folk Medicine. New York, Holt, Rhinehart & Winston, 1960.
32. Logan MH: Humoral medicine in Guatemala. In Landy D (ed): Culture, Disease, and Healing. Studies in Medical Anthropology. New York, Macmillan Publishing Co, Inc, 1977, pp 487–495.
33. Banwell BF: Comprehensive care. In Banwell BF, Gall V (eds): Physical Therapy Management of Arthritis. New York, Churchill Livingstone, 1988, pp 17–28.
34. Jette AM, Becker MJ: Nursing, occupational therapy and physical therapy preparation in rheumatology in the United States and Canada. J Allied Health 1980; 9:268–275.
35. Moncur C: Physical therapy competencies in rheumatology. Phys Ther 1985; 65:1365–1372.
36. Moncur C: Perceptions of physical therapy competencies in rheumatology. Physical therapists versus rheumatologists. Phys Ther 1987; 67(3):331–339.

CHAPTER 2

Epidemiology and Economics of Arthritis

Antoine Helewa, MSc(Clin Epid), PT
Joan M. Walker, PhD, PT

Epidemiology is the study of the distribution and determinants of health-related states and events in populations, and the application of this study to the control of health problems.[1] Epidemiology has a broad mandate, and involves a variety of disciplines including clinical, public health, and laboratory science. Most epidemiological applications in arthritis have focused on the more elementary descriptions of disease occurrence; however, increasingly, clinical epidemiology methods are being used as a strategy to evaluate health delivery programs under the rubric of "health services research," using experimental investigative techniques. In this chapter the focus will be on the frequency and distribution of the various forms of arthritis and their socioeconomic impact. The chapter will end with a discussion of the politics of arthritis.

Is There an Epidemic of Arthritis?

In the past two decades the field of arthritis has received more attention than in previous decades. This can be attributed to a changing image of the field of arthritis and people with arthritis: from an affliction of old age with significant psychosomatic overtones, to a disease that respects no age, gender, or geographic boundaries. Even though it affects older individuals more than any other age group, the politicization of the young elderly and not-so-young elderly has helped focus attention on the disease as a major health problem. Furthermore, the overall costs of physical and mental disabilities is receiving greater attention from legislators and health insurers. Due to the high prevalence of people with arthritis among the disabled, the field of arthritis has not escaped that scrutiny. Are we seeing more people affected by arthritis on our streets, or is that an illusion?

Political activity by seniors has helped to focus attention on arthritis as a major health problem.

A recent ground-breaking study by the National Arthritis Data Workgroup (NADW) outlined the

PHYSICAL THERAPY IN ARTHRITIS, Joan M. Walker, PhD, PT, and Antoine Helewa, MSc(Clin Epid), PT, W.B. Saunders Company © 1996.

scope of arthritis in the United States.[2] They estimated that 38 million Americans—15% of the population, or one in seven people—were affected by arthritis in 1990. In 1994, they projected that this figure will have grown to nearly 40 million. More significant is the projection by the NADW that, by the year 2020, the number of Americans with arthritis will increase by more than 57% (59.4 million Americans) from the 1990 estimate, affecting about 18.2% of the population, or one in five persons.

Is there a looming epidemic of arthritis? Where will these additional people with arthritis come from? Since arthritis affects the elderly more than any other age group, the increase in the number of elderly individuals can contribute to that increase. More significantly, by the year 2020, a large number of the elderly will be from the "baby boom generation," further swelling the number of those affected. This generation and its preoccupation with fitness and healthy life styles may be at higher risk of developing osteoarthritis. This could be due to impact loading during weight-bearing exercises, a lifetime of jogging and running, leading to a high prevalence of sports injuries. This in turn could predispose joints to the onset of early osteoarthritis. Can a similar case be made for inflammatory arthritis?

With aging of the "baby boom generation," by the year 2020 more seniors will have arthritis.

Recent studies have suggested that the incidence of rheumatoid arthritis (RA) is decreasing, probably due to the increased use of oral contraceptives among women. However, true cause-and-effect associations have not been shown.[3–7] Another report indicates that RA is becoming less severe in successive generations of patients, who are decreasingly likely to become seropositive, develop subcutaneous nodules, or develop erosive forms of arthritis.[8]

Prevalence and Incidence of Arthritis

Prevalence is the proportion of cases identified in a population at a given point in time (*point prevalence*) or during a specified interval (*period prevalence*). Point prevalence is determined in a single survey and period prevalence is determined in one or more surveys.[9] Incidence is defined as the rate of occurrence of new cases of a disease during a given period, in a defined population at risk.[10] Incidence is a more specific and sensitive indicator of disease risk acquisition than is prevalence. Studies of incidence, however, are more demanding than prevalence studies because larger populations are required, and definitions of disease on first diagnosis may be difficult.[9]

In a report by Statistics Canada, based on a 1981 self-report survey of the health of Canadians, 16% (3.5 million) of the population of Canada was estimated to have arthritis; rheumatism; or back, limb, and joint disorders.[11,12] In 85%, the duration of the disorder was greater than 1 year. More women (18.8%) than men (13.2%) reported these complaints. The prevalence among those 65 years of age and over was almost 50%, while among those 15–64 years of age, it was 17%; in the pediatric age group, the prevalence was 1.3%. This still represented a total of 74,000 children with arthritis or rheumatism. These findings are in agreement with a limited survey in southern Ontario (Canada), which revealed that 16% of the adult population had arthritic or rheumatic complaints.[13] In contrast, in 1984 32.6% of the U.S. population were estimated to have joint swelling, tenderness, limitation of motion, or pain on motion, as observed by a physician in a formal musculoskeletal examination, and 29.7% had musculoskeletal symptoms.[14] The wide variation reported is likely explained on the basis of marked differences in survey methodology. It is likely that the detailed physical examination carried out by physicians in the U.S. survey may have detected articular abnormalities in subjects who were otherwise asymptomatic. Similarly, including all subjects with musculoskeletal symptoms in the Canadian reports may lead to an overestimation of important disease.[12] Another distinction between the Canadian and U.S. surveys is that the former dealt with the existence of symptoms today (*point prevalence*), while the U.S. data refer to the presence of disease on most days, for at least 2 weeks at any time (*lifetime prevalence*).

More recently, the results of a 1990 Ontario Health Survey (OHS)(Canada) based on household interviews showed that musculoskeletal disorders (MSD) are a leading cause of morbidity in the population. MSD ranked first in prevalence as the cause of chronic health problems, long-term disabilities, and consultations with a health professional, and ranked second for restricted activity days and use of medications.[15] The rate of overall MSD reported in this study (22%), as well as arthritis and rheumatism (15%), was remarkably similar to rates reported elsewhere, based on self-reported conditions.[12,13]

Inflammatory Arthritis

In inflammatory arthritis, epidemiologists have great difficulty in assessing the frequency or natural history of these diseases. Differences in reported incidence and prevalence arise from differences in the interpretation of existing criteria for diagnosis or severity. While classic advanced RA, which represents a small part of the disease spectrum, can be reliably diagnosed, definition of RA during its earliest stages is difficult, since the disease may follow a variable course for months or years before becoming typical.[9] For example, using American Rheumatism Association (ARA) criteria for definite RA, rheumatologists achieved a sensitivity (true-positives) of 71% and a specificity (true-negatives) of 91%.[16] These criteria have been since revised twice, in 1966 and more recently in 1987.[17,18] The new 1987 criteria have a 91–94% sensitivity, and an 89% specificity (Table 2-1). Therefore, to obtain reliable estimates of disease patterns, the diagnosis must be established accurately and the population studied must be representative.

Several epidemiologic studies of RA and related connective tissue diseases[9,19] show that similarities in the patterns of occurrence are more striking than the discrepancies. On the whole, these tend to be disorders of women, with onset most often during the childbearing ages and tend to affect blacks more frequently than whites.[20] The ratio seems to vary with age: under age 60, women predominate by a ratio of 5:1. After age 60, the sex ratio approximates equality, suggesting that males may have a protective factor that may be lost at older ages.

All races seem capable of developing RA.[9] Prevalence estimates for ARA criteria of definite RA are remarkably constant at 1% in white populations.[21] Using the same criteria, another report showed RA's prevalence in major reported surveys for the average adult (age 15 and older) has ranged from a low of 0.1% in a rural South African black community,[22] to 3.0% among Finnish whites.[23] Climate itself does not seem to be a factor.[9]

In 1972, a survey showed that a larger proportion of single and divorced women, compared to married women, had RA, leading to speculations that the disability influences marital status.[24] RA has also been associated with lower income and lower educational levels.[25,26] Overall, the familial aggregation of RA is weak, and a putative susceptibility gene must have a low penetrance.[27]

The natural history of RA is variable. Essentially, investigators agree that a high serum rheumatoid factor and early bony erosions indicate a poor prognosis.[21] Other factors associated with worse disease are female sex, white race, two or more swollen upper extremity joints, Raynaud-like phenomena, and malaise or weakness.[28–30] Because of the systemic nature of RA, reported mortality tends to be high.[31] Factors that are strongly associated with early mortality are high rheumatoid factor titre, high joint counts, and a worse ARA functional class (see Chapter 8).[32–34]

Connective tissue diseases tend to be disorders of women, with onset most often in the childbearing ages. These diseases affect all ethnic groups and climate does *not* seem to be a factor.

Juvenile Arthritis

Juvenile arthritis, or juvenile rheumatoid arthritis (JRA), is one of a large group of connective tissue disorders that occur in children and adolescents. Incidence and prevalence estimates for JRA vary considerably, due in part to use of two different sets of criteria: ARA criteria versus more rigid European criteria,[35] heterogeneity of JRA subtypes, and lengthy periods of remission that complicate inclusion decisions in prevalence studies.[36] Annual incidence estimates from European-, American-, and Canadian-based studies vary from 2.6–12.0 per 100,000 children.[35] Prevalence estimates vary from 0.16 per 1,000 children[37] to 1.13 per 1,000 children.[38] Considerable variation also exists in the estimates of distribution of the three JRA subtypes. Ansell[39] reported an onset distribution of 65% pauciarticular, 14% polyarticular, and 21% systemic in a tertiary care incidence survey, while Cassidy and Petty[35] reported classification of 50% pauciarticular, 40% polyarticular, and 10% systemic onset types. In the pauciarticular and polyarticular subtypes the female-to-male ratio is 3:1, however incidence is equal in the sexes in the systemic subtype.[35]

Table 2-1. The 1987 Revised Criteria for the Classification of Rheumatoid Arthritis (RA)*†

Criterion	Definition
1. Morning stiffness.	Morning stiffness in and around the joints, lasting at least 1 hour before maximal improvement.
2. Arthritis of three or more joint areas.	At least three joint areas simultaneously have had soft tissue swelling or fluid (not bony overgrowth alone) observed by a physician. The 14 possible areas are right or left PIP, MCP, wrist, elbow, knee, ankle, and MTP joints.
3. Arthritis of hand joints.	At least one area swollen (as defined above) in a wrist, MCP, or PIP joint.
4. Symmetric arthritis.	Simultaneous involvement of the same joint areas (as defined in 2) on both sides of the body (bilateral involvement of PIPs, MCPs, or MTPs is acceptable without absolute symmetry).
5. Rheumatoid nodules.	Subcutaneous nodules, over bony prominences, or extensor surfaces, or in juxta-articular regions, observed by a physician.
6. Serum rheumatoid factor.	Demonstration of abnormal amounts of serum rheumatoid factor by any method for which the result has been positive in <5% of normal control subjects.
7. Radiographic changes.	Radiographic changes typical of rheumatoid arthritis on posteroanterior hand and wrist radiographs, which must include erosions or unequivocal bony decalcification localized in or most marked adjacent to the involved joints (osteoarthritis changes alone do not qualify).

*Adapted from Arnett FC, Edworthy SM, Bloch DA, et al: The American Rheumatism Association 1987 revised criteria for the classification of rheumatoid arthritis. Arthritis Rheum 1988; 31(3): 315–324.

†For classification purposes, a patient shall be said to have rheumatoid arthritis if he/she has satisfied at least four of these seven criteria. Criteria 1 through 4 must have been present for at least 6 weeks. Patients with two clinical diagnoses are not excluded. Designation as classic, definite, or probable rheumatoid arthritis is not to be made.

Spondyloarthropathies

Ankylosing spondylitis (AS), representing the spectrum of the seronegative forms of arthritis, has a variable prevalence, ranging from a virtual absence in Australian aborigines[40] or black Africans,[41] to a 10% diagnosed frequency of sacroiliitis in adult male Haida Indians.[42] The most frequently reported prevalence is 1 per 1,000 population, based on surveys of hospital and clinical records, with a sex ratio of three males to one female.[43,44] Criteria for diagnosis of AS were proposed at the Rome symposium[45] and later revised at a New York symposium[46] (Table 2-2). A fair degree of variation can be seen in the interpretation of symptoms of pain and stiffness in the dorsal and lumbar spine.[47] A high degree of variation also was seen in the interpretations of radiographic sacroiliitis,[21,48] especially unilateral and milder bilateral changes in films of persons aged 50 or younger. However, certain manifestations of back pain may be more characteristic of AS than of osteoarthritis (e.g., insidious development, symptoms persisting longer than 3 months, morning stiffness, and relief with mild exercise).[49]

Reiter's syndrome bears a close clinical relationship to AS, with nearly half the patients eventually developing spinal involvement.[20] Although once considered rare, it is perhaps the leading cause of arthritis among young adult males. It is reported in epidemic occurrences, such as after

Table 2-2. Ankylosing Spondylitis Population Survey Criteria*

Rome Symposium, 1961[40]	New York Symposium, 1966[41]
Clinical Criteria	
1. Low back pain and stiffness for more than 3 months that is not relieved by rest.	Pain at the dorsolumbar junction or in the lumbar spine by history or at present.
2. Pain and stiffness in the thoracic region.	
3. Limited motion in the lumbar spine.	Limitation of motion of the lumbar spine in all three planes: anterior flexion, lateral flexion, and extension.
4. Limited chest expansion.	Limitation of chest expansion to 1 inch (2.5 cm) or less, measured at the level of the fourth intercostal space.
5. Iritis or its sequelae (history or evidence).	
Radiographic Criteria	
Bilateral sacroiliac changes characteristic of ankylosing spondylitis.	Grade 3 to 4 bilateral sacroiliitis.
Definite Ankylosing Spondylitis	
Positive roentgenogram and one or more clinical criteria, or Four of the five clinical criteria.	Grade 3 to 4 bilateral sacroiliitis and one or more clinical criteria, or Grade 3 or 4 unilateral or grade 2 bilateral sacroiliitis either with limitation of back movement in all planes, or with both other clinical criteria.
Probable Ankylosing Spondylitis	
	Grade 3 to 4 bilateral sacroiliitis with no clinical criteria.

*Adapted from Masi AT, Medsger TA: Epidemiology of the rheumatic diseases. In McCarty DJ (ed): Arthritis and Allied Conditions, 11th edition, Philadelphia, Lea & Febiger, 1989.

bacillary dysentery. Development of the disease may be triggered by the encounter of a genetically susceptible (HLA-B27) host with some triggering environmental insult, such as an infectious agent.[20]

Epidemiologic studies show that 20% of patients with seronegative polyarthritis have psoriasis; but only 1.2% of patients with seropositive arthritis also have psoriasis.[50,51] The prevalence of polyarthritis among individuals with psoriasis is about 7%.[52] Various population studies of this syndrome show conflicting results. A statistical analysis of radiographic changes showed that erosions and mutilation of the distal and proximal interphalangeal joints were the best criteria to distinguish patients with seronegative arthritis and psoriasis from those with seronegative arthritis without psoriasis.[53] This strong association between seronegativity and psoriasis suggests that the presence of psoriasis leads to a more severe form of arthritis.

Osteoarthritis

Population studies of osteoarthritis (OA) show that its frequency, as expected, increases steadily with age, especially as observed in roentgenographic surveys, in which articular alterations are found in many asymptomatic individuals.[20] However, only 30% of those with radiographic evidence complain of pain in affected sites. Prevalence varies from 4% among those aged 18–24 years, to 85% among those aged 75–79 years, with an average of 37% overall.[54] It is more frequent in men below age 54 years, but the sex ratio is reversed thereafter.[55] Moderate or severe involvement (overall 9%) is more prevalent in women (11%) than in men (6%) after adjusting for age.[54] No racial or urban-rural difference was found.

Epidemiologic surveys show a strong association between OA and wear and tear, prolonged immobilization, continuous pressure, impact loading, anatomic abnormalities, and previous inflammatory joint injury, among others.[56,57] Repetitive use of the hands in industry was associated with radiographic evidence of OA in certain joints,[58] but no association was found between long-distance running and clinical evidence of OA in the lower extremities,[59,60] although women runners had more sclerosis and spur formations in their knees.[60] There is a suggestion in the literature that body weight is positively associated with OA of the knees; however, a cause-and-effect relationship between OA and obesity has not been clearly identified.[9]

Socioeconomic Impact of Arthritis

Chronic diseases produce significant economic, social, and psychological problems as a result of their biological effects. It seems reasonable to turn our attention to these problems as we seek ways to improve the overall well-being of patients with these conditions.[61] As the mean age of the population increases in the next decades, the prevalence of these chronic diseases also will increase.

Most studies that attempt to measure the socioeconomic impact of arthritis have been concerned with the costs of RA. According to Meenan,

> This is an appropriate condition to study for a number of reasons. First, it is a chronic illness which, once established, usually lasts for the balance of a lifetime. Second, this illness generally produces significant sociomedical effects as a result of progressive physical impairment. Third, it exemplifies the epidemiologic trend in chronic disease.[61, p 549]

Patients with RA incur health care costs three times greater than those of an age- and sex-matched population, and incur hospitalization costs twice as high.[62] The indirect costs of RA disability are significantly higher than those in a matched population.[63,64] A recent study showed that the value of expected lifetime costs of RA, on a per capita basis, amounted to $20,412 U.S. Of these, per capita direct costs to the patients amounted to $4,398.[65] Figure 2-1 shows the percentage distribution of direct costs of RA, and Figure 2-2 shows the total costs of RA by age and sex per case.[65] It is interesting to note that the total cost of RA for young males is very high, and overall, the costs to males up to age 59 is considerably higher than the costs for females (Fig. 2-2). This is probably due to sex differences in earning levels, and potential loss of income.

In another study, the ambulatory care costs for 940 RA patients were on average $1,092 per annum across the entire group.[66] Medications accounted for 40% of outpatient costs, which included gold and steroid injections, while laboratory tests and physician visits amounted to 20% each. When inpatient and miscellaneous costs were added, the total annual costs rose to $2,532 per individual in 1982 U.S. dollars. Outpatient and inpatient costs (excluding miscellaneous costs) were equal and together they averaged $2,005, or more than twice the per-capita health expenditures of $770 for the general population over 19 years of age in 1981.[67]

A Canadian study showed that the average cost of hospitalization in a rheumatic disease unit for an RA patient, in 1985 dollars, was about $3,000 Canadian (about $2,200 U.S.) for an average stay of 16 days. This is considerably less than the average per diem cost of $6,600 for hospitalization at that hospital in 1985.[68]

The most frequent psychosocial impacts of RA are changes in marital and employment status, and leisure activities.[61] Eighteen percent of individuals who had ever married were divorced or separated, compared to a U.S. average of 11%.[69] Fifty-nine percent had stopped working completely, while others changed their occupation or worked fewer hours per week.[61] A substantial number (85%) reported a change in their recreational activities.

Apart from gender, the sociodemographic risk factors are similar for musculoskeletal disability and nonmusculoskeletal causes of disability.[70] Musculoskeletal disability is independently associated with increasing age, not being married, less years of schooling, lower income, and not being employed. Noteworthy in this study is the association between disability and an educational level of grade 8 or less, and lower income. Other studies also have shown a strong association between these factors and reported joint symptoms in the population.[14,71,72]

The clinician should recognize that RA has a psychosocial impact and may result in changes in marital and employment status, and leisure activities.

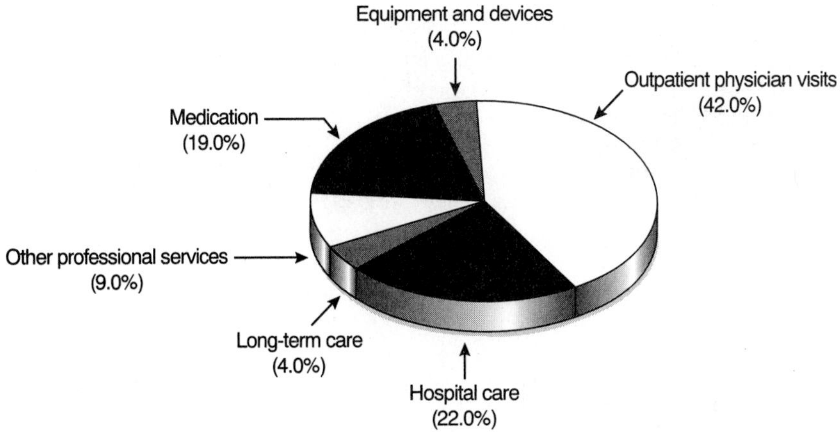

Figure 2-1. Percentage distribution of direct costs of RA by component, averaged over the entire incidence cohort with initial onset of RA in 1977. (Data from Stone CE: Lifetime economic costs of rheumatoid arthritis. J Rheumatol 1984; 11:819–827. With permission.)

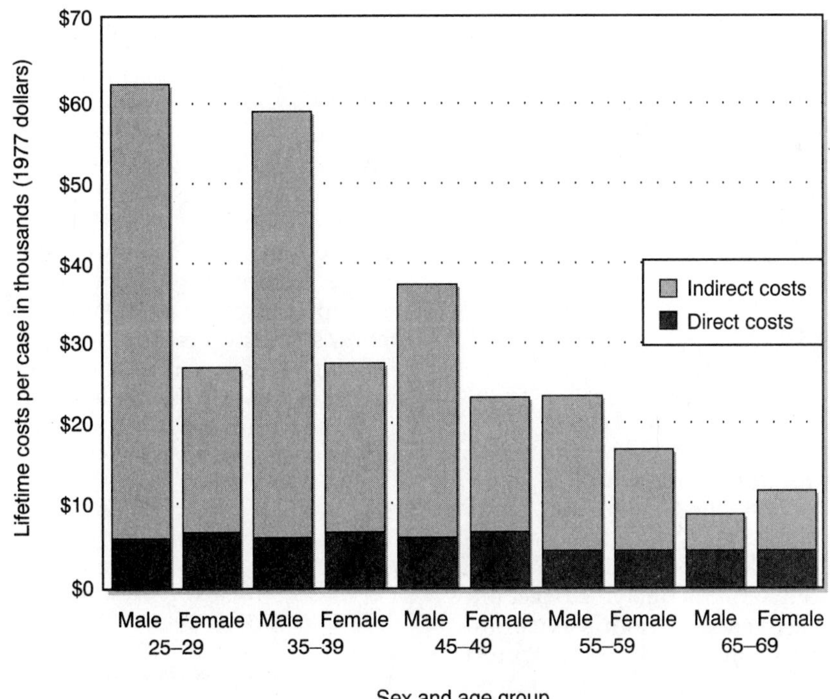

Figure 2-2. Total cost of RA per case by age and sex. (Data from Stone CE: Lifetime economic costs of rheumatoid arthritis. J Rheumatol 1984; 11:819–827. With permission.)

Overall, the economic impact of musculoskeletal disability in the United States represents about 1% of the gross national product, and even in Canada, according to StatsCan data, arthritis is responsible for the loss of more than $1.4 billion in wages annually, and nearly $150 million in tax revenues.[73]

Politics of Arthritis

Compared to heart disease, cancer, or acquired immunodeficiency syndrome (AIDS), arthritis and politics do not mix. Generally, people with arthritis are not among the movers and shakers in society, especially as arthritis seems to affect those who are socioeconomically disadvantaged. This situation is changing due to the changing demographics of people with arthritis. *The increase in the number of elderly individuals in our society who are becoming more politicized will help empower people with arthritis.* Although those with arthritis are largely elderly, they also are well represented in all age groups. Another factor that may contribute to this change is the high cost of disability. Political and community leaders are becoming more aware of the burden of chronic illness on society, especially the burden resulting from musculoskeletal disability (MSD). This increased awareness manifests itself in many ways. Chief among these is the impact of MSD on the workplace in terms of absenteeism and therefore compensation costs; low back pain and repetitive injury syndromes lead the way.

While the elderly to date have not been vocal in this arena, leaders in the field of arthritis are becoming more determined in recruiting elderly celebrities to their cause, and these celebrities are more forthright in joining fundraising campaigns or in lobbying politicians. Rosalind Russell and the late Henry Fonda, among others, have been very effective in the fight for arthritis in the United States.

On balance, individuals of all ages are striving for a better quality of life. Those with arthritis are striving for improved services, increased accountability, and cost-effectiveness. Health service providers will no longer be masters of their own turf. Public representation on health service agencies will increase to ensure that care providers are more sensitive and responsive to the needs of their clients. These societal trends have been evolving for at least two decades, and the demand for improved services and quality of life will accelerate, sweeping in its path care providers, politicians, and society's leaders alike.

Publicly recognized individuals can be very effective in promoting arthritis as a worthy funding cause and important health problem in today's societies.

Effects on Physical Therapy Practice

These developments are already having an impact on how physical therapy is generally practiced. On the one hand, individualized management will no longer be cost-effective as the ranks of people with arthritis swell. On the other hand, the voices asking for greater accountability and improved communications will place even heavier demands on overburdened services. Physical therapists must become innovative in the manner with which their services are delivered to satisfy these opposing challenges. Recent health care reports in North America have highlighted the importance of community rehabilitation delivery systems for patients with chronic disabilities to enhance their integration in their own homes or place of work. This will require physical therapists to introduce innovative service delivery mechanisms that provide for periodic monitoring or follow-up of these unrelenting diseases. Greater reliance on information technology through computer-aided management, and the creation of other support systems such as self-help groups, will greatly enhance physical therapy's effectiveness, and possibly reduce health care costs. Experiments using these models are already underway in the United States, Canada, and the United Kingdom. The results of these experiments are eagerly awaited.

References

1. Thomas CL (ed): Taber's Cyclopedic Medical Dictionary, 15th edition. Philadelphia, FA Davis Co, 1993.
2. National Arthritis Data Workgroup: Arthritis prevalence and activity limitations. US Morbidity and Mortality Weekly Report 1994; 4:433–438.
3. Linos A, Worthing JW, O'Fallon WM, et al: The epidemiology of rheumatoid arthritis in Rochester, Minnesota: a study of incidence, prevalence, and mortality. Am J Epidemiol 1980; 111:87–98.

4. Wingrave SJ, Kay CR: Reduction in incidence of rheumatoid arthritis associated with oral contraceptives. Lancet 1978; 1:569–571.
5. Del Junco DJ, Annegers JF, Luthra HS, et al: Do oral contraceptives prevent rheumatoid arthritis? JAMA 1985; 254:1938–1941.
6. Vandenbroucke JP, Witteman JCM, Valkenburg HA, et al: Noncontraceptive hormones and rheumatoid arthritis in perimenopausal and postmenopausal women. JAMA 1986; 255:1299–1303.
7. Liang MH, Stoker V, Larson M, et al: Oestrogen-use, menopausal status, and relationship to rheumatoid arthritis. Ann Rheum Dis 1984; 43:115–116.
8. Silman A, Davies P, Currey HLF, et al: Is rheumatoid arthritis becoming less severe? J Chronic Dis 1983; 36:891–897.
9. Masi AT, Medsger TA: Epidemiology of the rheumatic diseases. In McCarty DJ (ed): Arthritis and Allied Conditions, 11th edition, pp 16–54. Philadelphia, Lea & Febiger, 1989.
10. Dorn HF: Methods of measuring incidence and prevalence of disease. Am J Public Health 1951; 41: 271–278.
11. Health and Welfare Canada, Statistics Canada: The Health of Canadians. Report of the Canada Health Survey. Ottawa: Ministry of Supply and Services, 1981.
12. Lee P, Helewa A, Smythe HA, et al: Epidemiology of musculoskeletal disorders (complaints) and related disability in Canada. J Rheumatol 1985; 12:1169–1173.
13. Spitzer WO, Harth M, Goldsmith CH, et al: The arthritic complaint in primary care: prevalence, related disability, and cost. J Rheumatol 1976; 3:88–99.
14. Cunningham LS, Kelsey JL: Epidemiology of musculoskeletal impairments and associated disability. Am J Public Health 1984; 74:574–579.
15. Badley EM, Rasooly I, Webster GK: Relative importance of musculoskeletal disorders as a cause of chronic health problems, disability and health care utilization: findings from the 1990 Ontario Health Survey. J Rheumatol 1994; 21:505–514.
16. Ropes MW, Bennett GA, Cobb S: 1958 revision of diagnostic criteria for rheumatoid arthritis. Arthritis Rheum 1959; 2:16–20.
17. Bennett PH, Burch TA: New York symposium on population studies in the rheumatic diseases: new diagnostic criteria. Bull Rheum Dis 1967; 17:453.
18. Arnett FC, Edworthy SM, Bloch DA, et al: The American Rheumatism Association 1987 revised criteria for the classification of rheumatoid arthritis. Arthritis Rheum 1988; 31:315–324.
19. Lawrence JS: Rheumatism in Populations. London, William Heinemann Medical Books Ltd, 1977.
20. Rodnan GP, Schumacher HR: Primer on the Rheumatic Diseases. Arthritis Foundation, 1983.
21. Hochberg MC: Adult and juvenile rheumatoid arthritis: current epidemiologic concepts. Epidemiol Rev 1981; 3:27–44.
22. Beighton P, Solomon L, Valkenburg HA: Rheumatoid arthritis in a rural South African Negro population. Ann Rheum Dis 1975; 34:136–141.
23. Laine VAI: Rheumatic complaints in an urban population in Finland. Acta Rheum Scand 1962; 8:81–88.
24. Medsger AR, Robinson H: Comparative study of divorce in rheumatoid arthritis and other rheumatic diseases. J Chronic Dis 1972; 25:269–275.
25. National Center for Health Statistics: Public Health Service Publication No 1000, Series 11, No 17. Washington, DC, United States Government Printing Office, 1966.
26. Pincus T, Callahan LF: Taking mortality in rheumatoid arthritis seriously—predictive markers, socioeconomic status and comorbidity. J Rheumatol 1986; 13:841–845.
27. Del Junco DJ, Luthra HS, Annegers JF, et al: The familial aggregation of rheumatoid arthritis and its relationship to the HLA-DR4 association. Am J Epidemiol 1984; 119:813–829.
28. Masi AT, Maldonada-Cocco JA, Kaplan SB, et al: Prospective study of the early course of rheumatoid arthritis in young adults: comparison of patients with and without rheumatoid factor positivity at entry and identification of variables correlating with outcome. Semin Arthritis Rheum 1976; 5:299–326.
29. Feigenbaum SL, Masi AT, Kaplan SB: Prognosis in rheumatoid arthritis: a longitudinal study of newly diagnosed younger adult patients. Am J Med 1979; 66:377–384.
30. Josipovic D: Prognostic indicators in early rheumatoid arthritis. Clin Exp Rheumatol 1987; 5(Suppl 2): 26.
31. Abruzzo JL: Rheumatoid arthritis and mortality. Arthritis Rheum 1982; 25:1020–1023.
32. Mitchell DM, Spitz PW, Young DY, et al: Survival, prognosis and causes of death in rheumatoid arthritis. Arthritis Rheum 1986; 29:706–714.
33. Allebeck P, Rodvall Y, Allander E: Mortality in rheumatoid arthritis, particularly as regards drug use. Scand J Rheumatol 1985; 14:102–108.
34. Vandenbroucke JP, Hazevoet HM, Cats A: Survival and cause of death in rheumatoid arthritis: a 25-year prospective follow-up. J Rheumatol 1984; 11:158–161.
35. Cassidy JT, Petty RE: Juvenile rheumatoid arthritis. In Cassidy JT (ed): Textbook of Rheumatology. New York, Churchill Livingstone Inc, 1990, pp 113–219.
36. Hochberg MC: Adult and juvenile rheumatoid arthritis: current epidemiological concepts. Epidemiol Rev 1981; 3:27–44.
37. Gewanter L, Roghmann KJ, Baum J: The prevalence of juvenile arthritis. Arthritis Rheum 1983; 26:599–603.
38. Towner SR, Michet CJ, O'Fallon WM, et al: The epidemiology of juvenile arthritis in Rochester, Minnesota 1960–1979. Arthritis Rheum 1983; 26: 1208–1213.

39. Ansell BM: Chronic arthritis in childhood. Ann Rheum Dis 1978; 37:107–120.
40. Cleland LG, Hay JAR, Milazzo SC: Absence of HL-A 27 and of ankylosing spondylitis in central Australian aboriginals. Scand J Rheumatol 1975; 8:30.
41. Solomon L, Beighton P, Valkenburg HA, et al: Rheumatic disorders in South African Negro. Part 1. Rheumatoid arthritis and ankylosing spondylitis. S Afr Med J 1975; 49:1292–1296.
42. Gofton JP, Chalmers A, Price GE, et al: HL-A 27 and ankylosing spondylitis in B.C. Indians. J Rheumatol 1975; 2:314–318.
43. Carter ET, McKenna CH, Brian DD, et al: Epidemiology of ankylosing spondylitis in Rochester, Minnesota: 1935–1973. Arthritis Rheum 1979; 22:365–370.
44. Masi AT: Epidemiology of B-27 associated diseases. Ann Rheum Dis 1979; 38:131–134.
45. Kellgren JH, Jeffrey MR, Ball J: The Epidemiology of Chronic Rheumatism. Oxford, Blackwell Scientific Publications, 1963.
46. Bennett PH, Wood PH: Proceedings of the Third International Symposium on Population Studies of the Rheumatic Diseases. Amsterdam, Excerpta Medica, 1968.
47. Moll JMH, Wright V: New York clinical criteria for ankylosing spondylitis: a statistical evaluation. Ann Rheum Dis 1973; 32:354–363.
48. Hollingsworth PN, Cheah PS, Dawkins RL, et al: Observer variation in grading sacroiliac radiographs in HLA-B27 positive individuals. J Rheumatol 1983; 10:247–254.
49. Calin A, Porta J, Fries JF, et al: Clinical history as a screening test for ankylosing spondylitis. JAMA 1977; 237:2613–2614.
50. Taylor KB, Truelove SC: Immunological reactions in gastrointestinal disease. Gut 1962; 3:277–288.
51. Palumbo PJ, Ward KE, Sauer WG, et al: Musculoskeletal manifestations of inflammatory bowel disease-ulcerative and granulomatous colitis and ulcerative proctitis. Proc Mayo Clin 1973; 48:411–416.
52. Dekker-Saeys BJ, Meuwissen SGM, Van Den Berg-Loonen EM, et al: Ankylosing spondylitis and inflammatory bowel disease. II. Prevalence of peripheral arthritis, sacroiliitis and ankylosing spondylitis in patients suffering from inflammatory bowel disease. Ann Rheum Dis 1978; 37:33–35.
53. Strober W, James SP: The immunologic basis of inflammatory bowel disease. J Clin Immunol 1986; 6: 415–432.
54. National Centre for Health Statistics: Public Health Service, Publication No 1000, Series 11 No 15, Washington, DC, US Government Printing Office, 1966.
55. Kelsey JL: Epidemiology of Musculoskeletal Diseases. New York, Oxford University Press, 1982.
56. Peyron JG: Osteoarthritis: the epidemiologic viewpoint. Clin Orthop 1986; 213:13–19.
57. Acheson RM: Heberdeen oration 1981: Epidemiology and the arthritides. Ann Rheum Dis 1982; 41: 325–334.
58. Hadler NM, Gillings DB, Imbus HR, et al: Hand structure and function in an industrial setting: influence of three patterns of stereotyped, repetitive usage. Arthritis Rheum 1978; 21:210–220.
59. Panush RS, Schmidt C, Caldwell JR, et al: Is running associated with degenerative joint disease. JAMA 1986; 225:1152–1154.
60. Lane NE, Bloch DA, Jones HH, et al: Long distance running, bone density, and osteoarthritis. JAMA 1986; 255:1147–1151.
61. Meenan RF, Yelin EH, Nevitt M, et al: The impact of chronic disease: a socio medical profile of rheumatoid arthritis. Arthritis Rheum 1981; 24:544–549.
62. Yelin E: From social theory to social policy: social class and the epidemiology of disability among persons with rheumatoid arthritis (thesis). University of California, Berkeley, 1979.
63. Kelsey J, Pastides J, Bisbee G: Musculoskeletal Disorders: Their Frequency of Occurrence and Their Impact on the Population of the U.S. New York, Prodist, 1978.
64. Yelin E, Nevitt M, Epstein W: Toward an epidemiology of work disability. Milbank Mem Fund Q 1980; 58:384–415.
65. Stone CE: Lifetime economic costs of rheumatoid arthritis. J Rheumatol 1984; 11:819–827.
66. Lubeck DP, Spitz PW, Fries JF, et al: A multicentre study of annual health service utilization and costs in rheumatoid arthritis. Arthritis Rheum 1986; 29: 488–493.
67. National Centre for Health Statistics: Health, United States 1983. Public Health Service, Washington, DC, US Government Printing Office, USDHHS publication No (PHS) 84–1232, 1983.
68. Helewa A, Bombardier C, Goldsmith CH, et al: Cost-effectiveness of inpatient and intensive outpatient treatment of rheumatoid arthritis. A randomized, controlled trial. Arthritis Rheum 1989; 32:1505–1514.
69. US Bureau of the Census: Statistical abstract of the United States, 1977. Washington DC, US Government Printing Office, 1977, p 75.
70. Badley EM, Ibanez D: Socioeconomic risk factors and musculoskeletal disability. J Rheumatol 1994; 21:515–522.
71. Pincus T, Callahan LF, Burkhauser RV: Most chronic diseases are reported more frequently by individuals with fewer than 12 years of formal education in the age 18–64 United States population. J Chronic Dis 1987; 40:865–874.
72. La Vecchia C, Negri E, Pagano R, et al: Education prevalence of disease, and frequency of health care utilisation. The 1983 Italian National Health Survey. J Epidemiol Community Health 1987; 41:161–165.
73. Gordon DA, Inman RD: Musculoskeletal disability and rheumatology. J Rheumatol 1994; 21:387.

CHAPTER 3

Pathophysiology of Inflammation, Repair, and Immobility

Joan M. Walker, PhD, PT

The different forms of arthritis may involve many joints in the human body in addition to often having systemic effects. All tissues within a joint may be involved in the pathological process (Fig. 3-1). In most forms of arthritis, the involvement of freely movable (diarthroses) joints produces the greatest dysfunction. Not all joints have sliding surfaces and are capable of function. A brief overview of the different types of joints, their tissues, and structures is given, then the pathophysiology of inflammation, highlights of specific conditions, immobilization, and repair are reviewed.

PHYSICAL THERAPY IN ARTHRITIS, Joan M. Walker, PhD, PT, and Antoine Helewa, MSc(Clin Epid), PT, W.B. Saunders Company © 1996.

Types of Joints

Joints may be classified by their degree of motion as being fibrous (fixed or synarthroses), cartilaginous (slightly movable, amphiarthroses), or synovial (movable, diarthroses). Fibrous joints include fixed joints (sutures), as well as those allowing minimal movement (between tibia and fibula, syndesmosis) and the junction between teeth and their sockets (gomphoses). Cartilaginous joints include symphyses and primary cartilaginous joints

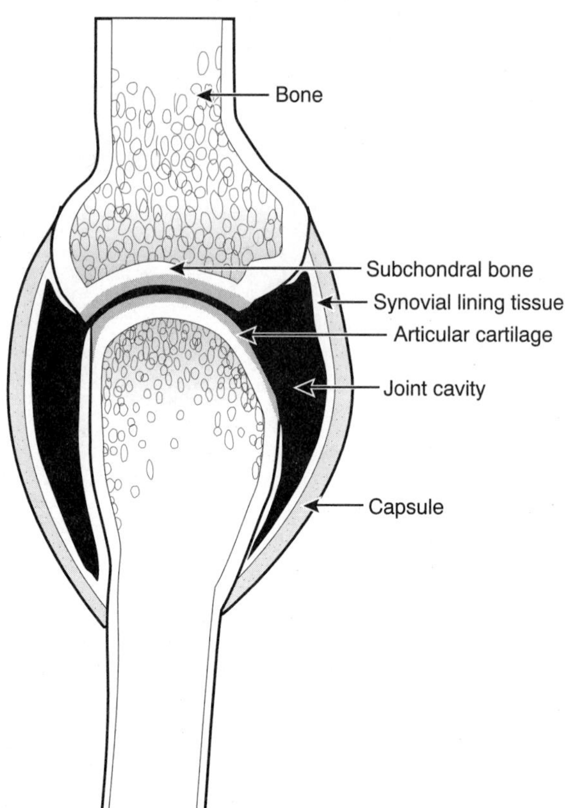

Figure 3-1. Features of a typical synovial joint. The extent of the synovial joint cavity is exaggerated to show features more clearly.

(synchondroarthroses). Mechanically, joints are perhaps better described as one of two major groups: (1) none or minimal motion, fibrous and cartilaginous, nonsynovial; or (2) movable, synovial.

Synovial joints are distinguished by hyaline cartilage-covered surfaces that are in contact but not intimately bound together. There is a potential joint space for the lubricating fluid (synovial). Some joints are a mixture of types; for example, the sacroiliac joint is synovial in its anterior half, complete with fibrous capsule and lined by a synovial lining tissue but it is amphiarthrosis in its posterior half where the two surfaces are united by a strong interosseous ligament. The intravertebral joint (IVJ) between an intravertebral disk and the inferior and superior surfaces of adjacent vertebrae is classified as an amphiarthrosis; it does not possess a synovial lining tissue. While each IVJ unit permits only minimal motion, thus fitting the slightly movable classification, collectively IVJs contribute to a considerable range of motion in all planes.

The type and amount of motion, as well as the static and dynamic stability are dependent on the shape of the articulating surfaces, the supporting connective tissue structures; that is, ligaments, fibrous capsule, and bulk of adjacent limb muscles. All these tissues may be affected by inflammatory or degenerative processes.

Components of a Diarthrodial Joint

A diarthrodial joint is a load-bearing unit that consists of two or more skeletal surfaces, the subchondral bone covered with hyaline (articular) cartilage (HAC), and united by a fibrous capsule. The fibrous capsule is lined by synovial tissues that cover all intra-articular structures except for the central load-bearing portion of disks, menisci, and articular cartilage.

Fibrous ligaments reinforce the capsule and may blend with the capsule or be separate from it. Some ligaments are intra-articular but are extrasynovial (e.g., cruciate ligaments of the knee joint). Joint surfaces are lubricated by synovial fluid (SF). Surface adaptation may be enhanced by intra-articular structures such as menisci (knee), labra (hip, glenohumeral), or disks (radiocarpal).

Subchondral Bone

HAC overlies and is intimately bound to the subchondral bone plate (SBP), a specialized layer at the articulating surface. The SBP in long bones covers the expanded articular end or epiphysis, which is separated in growth from the bone shaft (diaphysis) by the growth plate (physis). Bone is a highly vascular, constantly changing connective tissue. Cells (osteophytes, osteoclasts, osteoblasts) are embedded in the fibrous and the amorphous organic matrix permeated by bone salts.

While the exterior bone shaft shell is compact bone, the articulating ends are characterized by cancellous or trabecular bone (spongy) that is more deformable than cortical bone. The organization of SBP differs from the underlying bone in that the haversian systems "appear to run parallel to the joint rather than the long axis of the bone."[1, p 188] In the knee, SBP is formed by a meshwork of fine trabeculae (<0.2 mm in diameter) and in a density of fewer than two trabeculae per millimeter of bone. While SBP is stiffer than HAC, it is more resilient than the underlying bone, some ten times that of the bone shaft.[2]

The greater resilience of SBP assists in load transmission and is also a factor in the health of HAC. SBP undergoes significant deformation when a load is imposed on the joint surfaces and is the major site of deformation under loading. Thickening or increased stiffness limits the ability of SBP to disperse loads, leading to load concentration and cumulative damage, such as microfractures. Radin[3–5] theorizes that either the calcified layer of HAC or SBP is the initial locus of pathological changes leading to osteoarthritis.

In mature bone, organic material forms about 30–50% of its weight, water about 20% of its weight, and mineral salts 60–70% of the dry weight. Collagen (Type I) forms 90–95% of the organic matrix.[6] Branches of epiphyseal nutrient arteries pass towards the subchondral bone plate where they anastomose to form a series of arcades, off which a series of end-arterial loops occur. The latter may enter the calcified layer of HAC before returning to connect with venous sinusoids of the epiphyses. Nutrient vessels are accompanied by fine medullated and nonmedullated nerve fibers. The articular surfaces (when small, termed "articular facets") of dry bone are smooth and lack small vascular foramina typical of bone surfaces. The calcification of the zone of HAC in contact with SBP means that no effective interchange of nutrients occurs between the two layers. In pathology, however, such as osteoarthritis where there may be vertical splitting of HAC extending into the SBP, the vascular SBP is then a source of blood vessels and new cells. This provides the avascular HAC a means to attempt repair.

It is important to note that, throughout life, bone is constantly remodeling itself. While osteoblasts make new bone, osteoclasts remove old bone. A potent stimulus for remodeling is change in the individual's level of physical activity. Radin et al.[7] demonstrated in rabbits a 150% increase in the number of labeled secondary osteons in tibial SBP compared with controls when subjected to repetitive impulse loading.

Hyaline Articular Cartilage

HAC covering the subchondral bone plate functions to distribute and transmit loads and shear forces to the underlying bone, protects the underlying bone, and permits synovial joints to have a wide range of almost frictionless movement. HAC is aneural, largely avascular, and only sparsely cellular; it is up to 80% water.[8]

Chondrocytes are responsible for the synthesis of the proteoglycans and collagen fibers that comprise the cartilage matrix. Cartilage cells are embedded in the finely textured matrix in small zones that conform to cell shape. Chondrocytes are surrounded by a thin pericellular matrix, and the two are termed a "chondron." The mature chondrocyte has small rounded surface projections, round or oval nuclei. Multinucleated cells are common. The cell cytoplasm contains Golgi apparatus, mitochondria, granular endoplasmic reticulum, a few fat goblets, pigment granules, and glycogen deposits. In immature cartilage, both Golgi apparatus and granular reticulum are particularly prominent, indicative of their ability to synthesize matrix components.[6]

A potent stimulus for remodeling is change in an individual's level of physical activity.

While chondrocytes in the superficial layers are flattened, those in the deeper layers are more rounded. There is a higher cell density at the articular surface that progressively decreases to be about one half to one third of the superficial layer in the mid to deep zones.[9,10] HAC is characterized by having relatively sparsely distributed cells and abundant extracellular matrix. This matrix confers to the tissue its specialized loading and mechanical properties. The elastic modulus of the matrix allows some deformation under loading that assists in gradual load distribution. The creep characteristic prevents instantaneous compression on load application. The extracellular matrix is composed of collagens (mainly Type II), proteoglycans (PG) (in large groups called aggregates), nonprotein proteoglycans (NCP), and H_2O, between 60 and 80%. Water content is greater in the superficial layers.

Proteoglycans

The proteoglycans and glycosaminoglycans (GAGs) are hydrophilic (water-loving) and play an important role in regulating the movement of water within the matrix, thereby influencing the mechanical and lubricant properties of cartilage.[11] Large protein aggregates are groupings of collagen protein monomers and are termed "aggrecans" (Fig. 3-2). An aggrecan is bound at intervals with a single central filament of hyaluronate and is stabilized by link proteins. Aggrecans have three globular domains with chondroitin sulfate (CS-4, -6) and keratin sulfate (KS) regions. CS and KS are polysaccharides that consist of sugar residues.

A feature of chondroitin sulfate and keratin sulfate is that their repeating units of GAGs contain closely packed, negatively charged groups so that when these chains are linked to the aggrecan core protein they stand out like bristles on a brush. The strongly repellant forces of thousands of negatively charged groups means that the protein aggregate occupies a greater volume of solution in vitro. In vivo, the protein aggregates are constrained by the collagen network. It is this feature that gives articular cartilage its elastic properties; the elastic forces are balanced by the tensile forces of the collagen network. When cartilage is com-

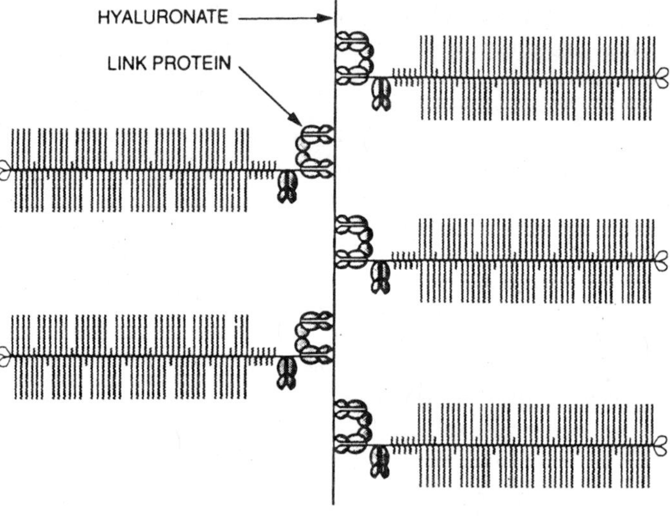

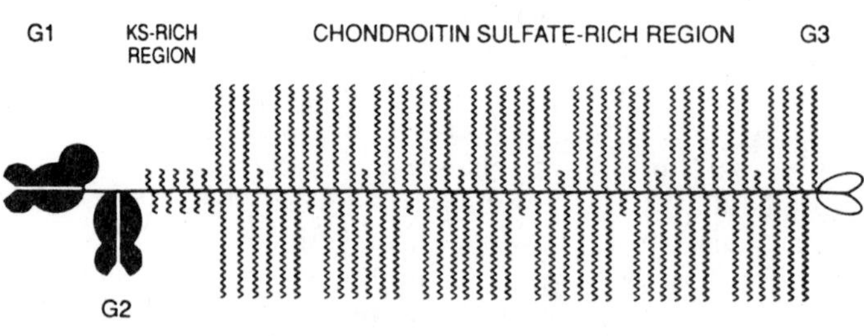

Figure 3-2. Cartilage proteoglycan aggregate, several monomers (*bottom*) bound by link proteins to a central hyaluronate core. (From Rosenburg L: Structure and function of cartilage proteoglycans. In McCarty DJ, Koopman WJ [eds]: Arthritis and Allied Conditions, 12th edition, vol 1, p 230. Philadelphia, Lea & Febiger, 1993. With permission.)

pressed, interstitial fluid will be extruded from unloaded regions of the cartilage. With relief of pressure, the aggregate will expand (like a sponge) until it is limited by the collagen fiber network; simultaneously, cartilage will imbibe water and the volume of cartilage will increase.

The other two proteoglycans are dermatan sulfate proteoglycans (DSPG, DSPG-1, biglycan; DSPG-2, decorin). These are multifunctional micromolecules that tend to be most concentrated near the articular surface.[9] They are bound to extracellular matrix macromolecules and regulate or modulate their biological properties.[12] DSPGs inhibit processes involved in tissue development and repair. They may bind to the surface of collagen fibers and inhibit the formation of new collagen fibrils or bind to fibronectin inhibiting cell adhesion, thrombin activity, and clot formation. Their activity could explain why lesions of articular cartilage do not heal well or repair spontaneously.

Figure 3-3 (left) shows the typical two-layered arrangement of HAC. There is an uncalcified superficial layer and a deeper calcified cartilage layer that is bound and merges with the subchondral bone. The junction between the uncalcified and calcified layers is called the tidemark. Within the uncalcified cartilage, there is a superficial or gliding zone, a middle transitional, and a deep or radial zone. Each zone is relatively unique with regard to cell number, cell shape, orientation, collagen fiber arrangement, and nutrition.

The tidemark is the boundary of a metabolically active zone between the calcified and noncalcified layers. Variations in the subchondral bone volume are thought to influence the tidemark region and the changes that lead to osteoarthritis.[13] Because of the calcifying activities in the tidemark region, the tidemark slowly advances in the direction of the noncalcified cartilage during life. The number of tidemarks increases with aging, and in

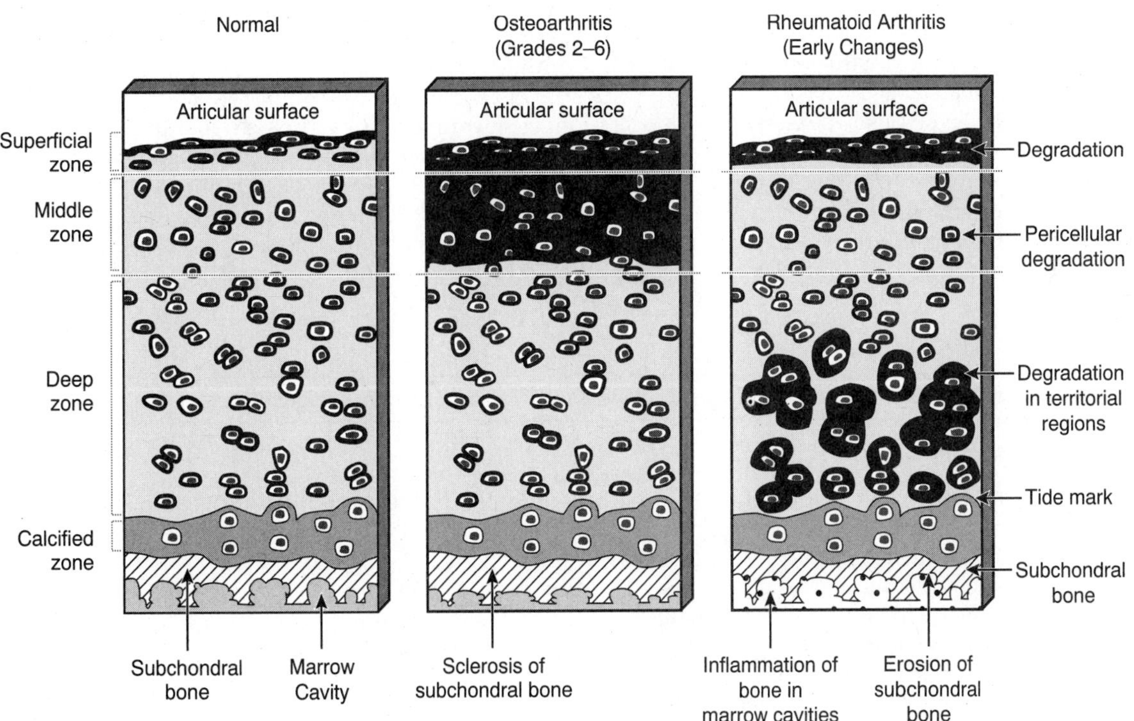

Figure 3-3. Diagrammatic representation of zones of normal cartilage (*left*) and sites of degradation of Type II collagen in rheumatoid and osteoarthritic femoral cartilages showing sites of damage. Pericellular degradation is normally seen throughout healthy cartilage. (From Poole AR: Cartilage in health and disease. In McCarty DJ, Koopman WJ [eds]: Arthritis and Allied Conditions, 12th edition, vol 1, p 305. Philadelphia, Lea & Febiger, 1993. With permission.)

pathological conditions such as osteoarthritis. The calcified zone tends to become thinner with age.[14]

The difference in orientation of cells within the articular cartilage is shown in Figure 3-3. In the calcified zones, the cells are heavily encrusted with hydroxyapatites (crystals of calcium salts) and are surrounded with calcified matrix in mature cartilage. These cells are considered to be relatively metabolically inactive.[15] Different regions can be distinguished within the matrix. The cells are surrounded by a thin layer of pericellular matrix (Fig. 3-3). Outside of that is the life-sustaining interterritorial matrix; adjacent and surrounding that is the territorial matrix. The latter has a high concentration of keratin sulphate,[16] which may enable the interterritorial matrix to better resist compressive deformation.[17]

Bundles of collagen fibers in the superficial zone of HAC lie in parallel to the joint cavity, whereas in the transitional zone they are more randomly dispersed. In the radial zone, fibers have an arcade-type pattern with radial rows in the deepest regions. The fibers in the radial zone are also coarser than those in the superficial zone. The fibers in the calcified zone are thicker and orientated perpendicular to the surface.[18]

The calcified layer also possesses antiangiogenic (blood vessel formation) molecules.[19] These molecules appear to confirm the ability to inhibit vascular invasion and prevent ossification, which occurs in cartilage of the growth plate. Therefore, the calcified cartilage persists and is a transitional zone between the softer uncalcified articular cartilage and the harder subchondral bone. Articular cartilage is bathed by synovial fluid and it is via synovial fluid that cartilage receives nutrients and extrudes its waste products.

It is important to note that in the healthy joint there is no real joint space. The joint space is a potential space and the amount of synovial fluid present is minimal, about a few drops or milliliters in a healthy joint.

Collagen

As has been recounted, articular cartilage, bone, fibrous capsule, tendon, and ligaments are all comprised of a high proportion of collagen constituting the extracellular matrix of these tissues. Articular cartilage differs from bone, capsule, tendon, and ligament in that it is chiefly composed of Type II collagen as opposed to Type I in the other tissues (Table 3-1). The collagen family is now recognized to have at least 15 types of collagen, which are labeled from I to XV.[20] The various types of collagen are strands of α-chains that are comprised of amino acids.

Each collagen is comprised of three polypeptides forming a triple helix structure. Type I has two identical polypeptide chains and one that is slightly different; every third amino acid is glycine. Type II, in comparison, has three identical helix chains, and contains more hydroxylysin and excessive glycosylation.[21,22] The collagen of HAC and

Table 3-1. Location of the Various Types of Collagen in Healthy Human Articular Tissues*

Type	Location
I	Fibrous capsule, synovial lining tissues, tendons, menisci, annulus fibrosus, periosteum, perichondrium, bone matrix
II	Hyaline cartilage, nucleus pulposus, fibrous capsule†
III	Perichondrium, periosteum, synovial lining tissues, tendons†
IV	Basement membranes (endothelial)
V	Perichondrium, periosteum, endosteal layer bone trabeculae
VI	Hyaline articular cartilage,† ligaments,† ?synovium
VIII	Endothelial basement membrane
X	Hypertrophic cartilage (growth plate)
XI	Hyaline articular cartilage†
XII	Tendon

*Data from Lane and Weiss,[18] Fleischmajor et al,[20] Prockop et al,[22] and Poole.[70]

†Small amounts.

fibrocartilage is 50–90% Type II collagen. Type II is a fibrillar type of collagen found in the tissue as fibrils several thousand molecules in diameter that are packed into bundles to form large fibers. HAC also contains fiber-associated Type IX (5–20%) and two types of short-chained collagen, Type VI, also found in ligaments, and some Type X, which is principally found in the hydrotropic cartilage of the growth plate.

The metabolic turnover of collagen is continuous through growth to maturity when the collagen fibers become more metabolically stable and have half-lives of weeks or months.[22] Collagen turnover is increased in conditions of malnutrition, starvation, Paget's disease, hypoparathyroidism, and metastatic diseases of bone. The degradation of collagen under these conditions or diseases provides the body with a source of amino acids.

Collagen synthesis is a multistep process with intracellular and extracellular events. Collagen achieves maturity in the extracellular matrix. Several factors are important in collagen formation. There is increased glucose transport, mediated by a group of glucose-transport proteins that have distinct tissue distributions in HAC and synovial cells. A connective tissue activating protein (CTAP-III) is involved.[21] Amino acids also are transported into the cells. Insulin-like growth factors (IGF-I and IGF-II) stimulate connective tissue replication and extracellular matrix synthesis; that is, the synthesis of proteoglycans. A type of bone morphogenic protein, osteogen, is present and can induce the formation of both bone and cartilage. It is theorized that osteogen may be involved in bone and cartilage repair. Insulin-like growth factors also may have a role in cartilage metabolism.[21]

Fibrous Capsule

The fibrous capsule is a type of regular white connective tissue similar to that of tendons and ligaments. The capsule consists mainly of parallel bundles of collagen (Type I, II) with cells sparsely distributed. The fiber diameter varies from 150–1,500 mm; a few elastic fibers may be present. Collagen and elastin are the fibrous proteins that constitute some 90% of the dry weight tissue, water forms about 70%, and organic solids are mainly collagen and small proteins; a small portion is proteoglycan. Compared with hyaline cartilage, about 30% is hyaluronic acid, 40% chondroitin sulphate, and 20% dermatan sulphate.[1]

The orientation of the fiber bundles reflects the tissue's functional role. This is particularly evident in tendons and ligaments. In the fibrous capsule, the collagen bundles lie both in parallel and as interlacing bundles. The localized thickening of strongly parallel fibers are the real joint ligaments; those that stand apart from the capsule are often termed accessory ligaments. The capsule can be reinforced and/or replaced by tendons and expansions from tendons of the surrounding muscles. The thickness and attachment of the fibrous capsule varies according to the joint. It may be thin and redundant as in the shoulder joint or thick and dense as in the hip and the knee. The extent of redundancy in the fibrous capsule and its associated synovial tissue, or lack thereof, has important consequences to the mobility of the joint, especially when involved in an inflammatory process. The redundancy permits full range of motion (Fig. 3-4).

Ligaments

Ligaments have a distinct parallel orientation of their fiber bundles. They have few blood vessels within their substance. Close to the insertion into bone, the tissue becomes mineralized and calcified and the collagen fibers penetrate the cortical osseous tissue. This arrangement of progressive stiffening decreases the likelihood of avulsion injuries. As with tendons, the cells (fibroblasts, often termed fibrocytes when old and inactive) are elongated and sparsely distributed. The presence of fibroblasts on the external surface of both ligaments and tendons affords a pool of cells from which repair and regeneration can arise.

Tendons

Tendons bridge muscle and bone. They may have a single or multiple attachment. They are formed by longitudinally arranged Type I collagen bundles interspersed with a reticular network of Type III collagen. Blood vessels tend to be associated with the exterior aspect of the tendon. They have a specialized insertion into bone (Sharpey's perforated fibers) where fibers are continuous with the outer bony lamina. Similar to ligaments, tendon tissue becomes calcified close to the bony attachment.

Tendons may be encased in a vascular sheath of discontinuous collagen fibers lined with mesenchymal cells that resemble synovium. This is particularly true of long tendons that traverse multiple joints, as in the wrist and hand and ankle-foot region. Hyaluronic acid secreted by the lining cells may enhance the gliding function of the

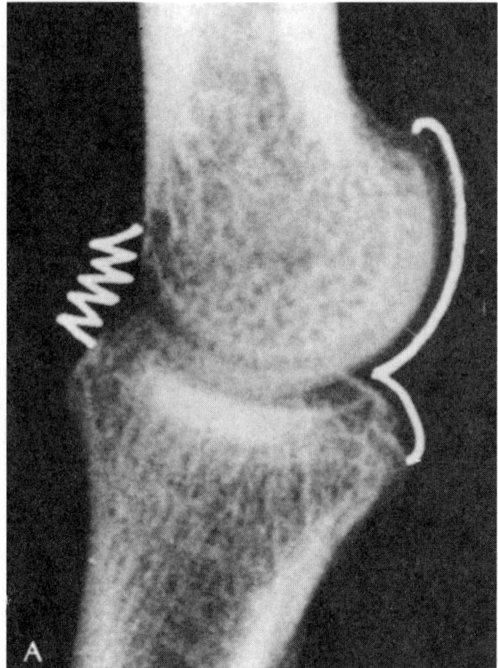

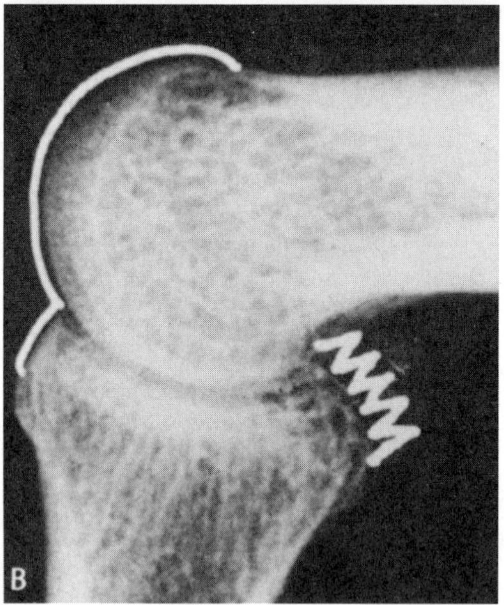

Figure 3-4. Lateral views of an interphalangeal joint in extension (*A*) and flexion (*B*). Redundant synovium (shown schematically) gathers above the superior margin in extension and below the inferior margin in flexion. (From Simkin PA: Synovial physiology. In McCarty DJ, Koopman WJ [eds]: Arthritis and Allied Conditions, 12th edition, vol 1, p 200. Philadelphia, Lea & Febiger, 1993. With permission.)

sheaths.[23] The fibroblasts of both ligaments and tendons are known to synthesize metalloproteinases and cholinase inhibitors, as well as a latent form of cholinase.[24] These have implications in the breakdown and repair of the structures.

Bursae

Bursae are closed sacs lined by mesenchymal cells that are similar to synovial cells. Deep bursae may have communications with the joint cavity (e.g., subacromial bursa at the shoulder joint). Bursae facilitate gliding and provide a low-friction movement of one tissue over another. In life, bursae may develop in response to stress. Similar to tendon sheaths, there is a high potential for resolution of bursal inflammation to involve fibrosis, thickening, and adhesions, which may seriously impair motion.

Synovial Lining Tissue

Synovial lining tissue (SLT, synovium) borders the joint cavity and covers all intra-articular structures except for the central load-bearing portions of the joint. As there is no clearly defined membrane, the term "synovial membrane" is now considered inappropriate.[25,26] Immediately adjacent to the joint space is synovial intima layer. Beneath this layer is the subintimal tissue, which merges on its external surface with the fibrous capsule of the joint or the fibrous outer coating of the tendon sheath or bursae. SLT is a critical tissue in arthritis pathology. Since it is vascular, SLT is invariably involved in the inflammatory reaction and release of substances that can degrade articular cartilage. Resolution of inflammation may result in thickening and adhesions that interfere with cartilage nutrition and joint mobility.

The intimal layer consists of cells one to three deep that are set in the matrix. This layer is not a continuous layer so that both synoviocytes and the matrix may come in contact with the joint fluid. Between the cells in the intimal layer, there are collagen fibers (Type I) and some electron dense amorphous material that includes hyaluronate. There is no basement membrane, and cell processes (thin branching filaments) appear to provide a supportive membrane for the cells.

The subsynovial layer is a vascular connective tissue framework consisting of fibrous, areolar, and fatty tissues. The predominance of any one of these tissues varies by site and within the joint. Few blood vessels and only nonmedullated nerve fibers penetrate into the synovial lining tissues. In the subsynovial layer, there is a rich plexus of blood vessels and lymphatics. The former are believed to be responsible for the transfer of nutrients to the synovial cavity and the formation of synovial fluid, the latter for removal of waste products of HAC. In the intima, capillaries are of the fenestrated variety that facilitates the movement of solutes and water into the tissues; in subsynovial tissues they are a continuous variety.[27] Vascularity varies both between joints and within the joint. Fibrous synovial surfaces are the least vascular.[28] Blood sacs from the deeper lymphatic plexus penetrate the intima but do not reach the surface, as do capillaries.[29]

Synovial Lining Cells

While the two main types are Type A and Type B, cells with features of both are quite common and are termed AB lining cells. It is believed that the two major types of cells do not represent two distinct cell lines but are functional variants of a single cell line.[30]

Type A cells with prominent Golgi complexes, many vacuoles and vesicles, filopodia, and small amounts of rough endoplasmic reticula appear to be equipped for phagocytosis and may be termed surface macrophages.[31] These cells have the capacity for endocytosis and are thought to synthesize and secrete hyaluronic acid into the joint fluid.

Type B cells essentially are the converse of Type A cells, with prominent nucleoli and long cytoplasmic processes. They are equipped for protein secretion and are hypothesized to be responsible for polypeptide secretion due to their abundant rough endoplasmic reticulum. They also have the capacity to secrete enzymes that can degrade cartilage. Type B cells may be primarily involved in synthesizing and releasing neutrophils or neutral proteinases that can degrade cartilage. Cholinase can digest the collagenous lattice within the articular matrix. Other enzymes produced are gelatinase and strombolycin.[32]

The Type A cells are believed to release cytokines such as interleukin-1 and prostaglandin E_2. Interleukin-1 is an inflammatory mediator that can cause chondrocytes to decrease matrix synthesis and absorb the surrounding matrix. Cytokines may play a major role in perpetuation of synovitis.[33] It is believed that synovial cells also are activated by proteoglycans released from the enzymatically digested cartilage. Synoviocytes may influence the immune response by presenting other targets for immune leukocytes or influence immune leukocytes by expressing cell membrane molecules that affect immune responses.[33]

Tissue cavitation may stimulate fibroblasts and macrophages to differentiate into synovial lining cells, and the environment, composed of synovial fluid, cells, and matrix, is necessary to maintain the differentiated state of these cells.[33] Mitotic cells have not been reported in the intima of the synovium. It is believed that intimal cell replacement or regeneration is derived from cells in the subintimal layer.[30,34,35]

Synovial lining tissues play an important role in the function of the healthy joint and are a significant factor in the pathology of arthritis. Synovial lining tissues normally function to provide low adherence to the surfaces, a low-friction lining, biological lubricants, deformable packing, and blood supply for the chondrocytes. These tissues also control volume and composition of synovial fluid-transporting nutrients into the joint space and removing metabolic waste; they may have an antimicrobial effect.[31,36]

Synovial Fluid

Synovial fluid (SF) has a concentration of electrolytes and small molecules similar to blood plasma.[37] It is now recognized that while vessel endothelium pore size limits the passage of protein (out of capillaries), the tissue space that must be traversed to reach the synovial cavity (i.e., the synovial interstitium) is a critical control of the passage of small solutes. It is no longer correct to term SF a "dialysate." Synovial lining cells are responsible for secretion of hyaluronate into SF (Fig. 3-5). A knee joint normally has less than 4 ml of SF. The fluid is usually clear to pale yellow in color, of a transparent clarity, with high viscosity, and does not display spontaneous clotting. Normal synovial fluid is almost acellular. SF has a number of molecules with lubricating properties, mainly glycoproteins,[38] and the clearance rates are dependent upon the molecular size.

SF volume is dependent on conditions in the lining interstitium, the forces acting on it, and the permeability of the tissue surface to water and solutes. Hyaluronic acid, a nonsulfated GAG, exists in synovial fluid in a higher concentration than in other connective tissue interstitial fluids. Hyaluronic acid is in fluid as a complex with protein and appears to be synthesized by synovial lining cells. Some 60% of the protein in synovial fluid is al-

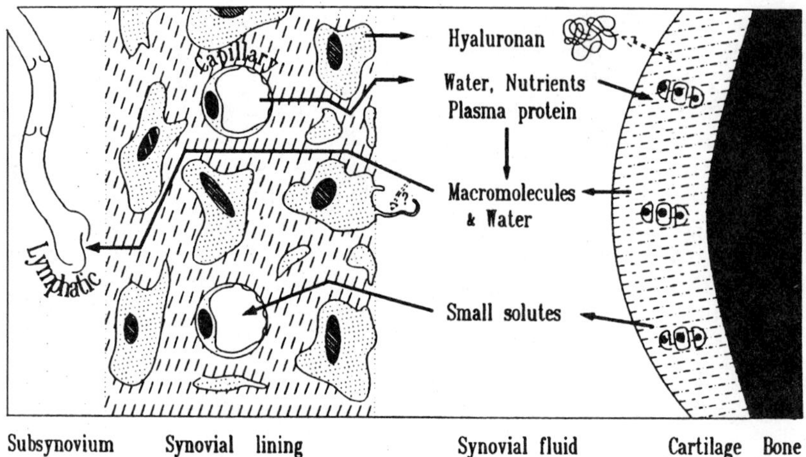

Figure 3-5. Diagram depicting synovial transport pathways (not drawn to scale). (From Levick JR: Synovial fluid determinants of volume turnover and material concentration. In Kuettner K, et al [eds]: Articular Cartilage and Osteoarthritis, p 530. New York, Raven Press, 1992. With permission.)

bumin, a small molecule that is responsible for the synovial fluid's colloid or osmotic pressure.[25]

Hyaluronate is responsible for the high viscosity of synovial fluid. Small molecules, such as lactose, carbon dioxide, and inorganic pyrophosphate, are produced by the joint tissues and diffused into the synovial fluid; glucose enters synovial fluid via a facilitated diffusion. There is little lipid in synovial fluid. All plasma proteins can cross the vascular endothelium, traverse the synovial interstitium, and enter synovial fluid. The major mechanism is a size-selective process of passive diffusion. In healthy tissue, small molecules such as albumin enter easily, while large molecules such as fibrinogen are largely excluded.[36] Protein passage from synovial fluid to the bloodstream is largely dominated by lymph flow.[39] The interstitium or tissue space of the synovial lining appears to be the important factor in the transsynovial exchange of small molecules into the synovial fluid. Because of capillary infiltration and lymphatic absorption, synovial fluid is constantly turning over. Fluid turnover rates, and thus the concentration of macromolecules, may be increased 100–300% in arthritis.[39]

Lubrication

As joints exist to provide motion within the constraints of the surrounding soft tissues, an effective lubrication system is vital. Healthy human synovial joints have a remarkable ability to permit reciprocal movements, within a wide range of loads and speeds while maintaining stability. Their low frictional resistance gives a remarkable slipperiness to human joints. The type of loading is an important factor in the mechanism of joint lubrication. Human joints may be subject to a steady or static, as well as dynamic loading; the latter may be very transient, as in jumping. Loading can vary from a very light load, as in the swing phase of gait, to a very high load; for example, heel contact in gait when the load may be three to five times body weight.[40] These high loads tend to occur for only very brief periods (<0.15 second), while low loads may occur for longer periods. Joint surfaces can tolerate higher dynamic than static forces.

The body-support interface can play a major role in damping joint forces[41] and can be an important factor in management of clients with arthritis. Radin et al[42] demonstrated negative changes similar to osteoarthritis in articular cartilage of weight-bearing joints in sheep that walked for long distances on concrete floors. Those that walked on wood chips did not show similar effects. Similarly, Light et al[43] demonstrated that variation in shoe heel construction can decrease the impact of walking on hard surfaces, by inference reducing joint loading. Joint forces have an enormous potential to promote degenerative changes in joint tissues that initially are subclinical and may not produce symptoms for years. The repetitive impulsive loading of a variety of activities undertaken in adolescence and young adulthood has potential consequences in later life. Consider that a runner or jogger, doing 20 miles per week over 30 years, delivers some 50 million shock waves through their bodies, across joint surfaces.[44] Workers in factories or warehouses may spend years standing and moving on unyielding concrete floors.

Critical variables in the joint lubrication mechanisms appear to be the surface compliance or elasticity (adjusts to loading), roughness (prevents immediate total contact), the low coefficient of friction (facilitates lubrication, especially of synovial tissues), the viscosity and protein lubricants of synovial fluid, the velocity of the rolling or sliding motion (maintains a fluid film between surfaces), the permeability of the surface (blocks large molecules), and the joint surface contour (prevents total contact of surfaces and assists in maintaining a fluid film). Lubrication of joint surfaces appears optimal when a film of fluid is maintained on the surfaces.

Surface compliance (yielding, conforming) is an important variable because the harder the surface, the higher the friction. If the surface is compliant under loading, more of the joint surface is brought into contact. With higher loads, because of surface compliance, joint surfaces become more congruent and stability of the joint is increased. It is believed that surface roughness produces points of contact between the surfaces, and in unloaded "dips" fluid is trapped when the joint is loaded, thus providing a fluid film between the surfaces.[27] Some investigators, however, consider cartilage surface roughness detected by electron microscopy to represent artifacts.[45] Pathological changes as seen in rheumatoid arthritis (RA) and osteoarthritis (OA) alter these factors, limit the ability to maintain a fluid film, and enhance the potential for boundary lubrication and surface wear.

The remarkable slipperiness of human joints is measured by the coefficient of friction (COF). The COF is the shear force needed to make one surface slide on another divided by the normal force pressing them together. The lower the COF, the lower the resistance to sliding. The theorized COF for cartilage on cartilage, between 0.02 and 0.001,[46,47] is lower than that of a skate on ice (0.03).

It is believed that fluid film mechanisms can operate in healthy joints under most conditions. In this situation the two joint surfaces are separated by a very thin layer of fluid. A number of mechanisms are proposed to explain the ability of a fluid film to exist. A fluid film can be generated when the cartilage is compressed by high loads; fluid will be extruded, especially on surfaces ahead of the load. Even when the load is high, as long as motion is occurring, a fluid film is still theoretically present to separate the two joint surfaces (hydrostatic mechanism). Elastic deformation of the surfaces (elastrohydrodynamic mechanism) can assist in maintaining a small fluid film.

When an individual stands for long periods, as, for instance, on guard duty, a condition is created where the fluid film would not be maintained; cartilage, however, may weep in the noncontact areas just ahead of the load, providing a fluid film in those areas. Boundary lubrication is theorized to operate with pools in the roughened dips of the cartilage that are not in full contact as the surfaces are separated by a thin layer of large molecules adsorbed onto the surface. These molecules are theorized to be hyaluronic acid protein complexes which, because of their size, cannot penetrate cartilage ("boosted" lubricant mechanism). Under this condition, friction will increase with a greater contact area of the surface cartilage. SF contains a lubricant (glycoprotein) that can reduce the friction and wear once the motion is recommenced and the fluid film restored. In boundary lubrication, the coefficient of friction is theorized to be from 0.1–0.5 independent of the speed of sliding or the load.[40] For further detail of theorized lubrication mechanisms, see Unsworth, 1993[40]; Unsworth, 1991[48]; McCutchen, 1978[49]; and Dintenfass, 1963.[50]

It is important to recognize that arthritic changes, regardless of the specific name, significantly alter the variables that should ensure the existence of a fluid film to lubricate joint surfaces and slippery structures, such as tendon sheaths and bursae. Such changes promote early contact of a greater area of the load-bearing surfaces and enhance their wear. Disruption of the surfaces then permits ingress and egress of substances that can maintain and enhance the pathological changes.

Inflammation and Repair

The typical protective reaction of most body tissues to injury, pathologic insult, and microbes is one of inflammation. The classic inflammatory process, as seen in wound repair, is characterized by redness, swelling, heat, and pain. The process involves increased vascular permeability, vasodilation, cell proliferation, neovascularization, and fibroplasia. In this review of inflammation and repair in arthritis, the models will be RA and OA; changes specific to other forms of arthritis will follow.

The inflammatory reaction is initiated by antigen-antibody complexes and represents the body's efforts to restore tissue integrity and function; it is an attempt to heal. The ability of a tissue to exhibit the classic inflammatory response is strongly related to its vascularity. Hence, in arthritis, synovial lining tissues invariably demonstrate a degree of inflammation, while hyaline articular cartilage, being avascular, does not demonstrate the typical inflammatory response. Similarly, strongly fibrous, less vascular structures such as tendons and ligaments demonstrate a poor inflammatory response.

Healing with restoration of the original tissue is dependent on the intrinsic ability of the tissue to regenerate and the complexity of the tissue. When regeneration does not occur, there is replacement by fibrous tissue, which organizes into a firm scar and frequently lacks the characteristics of the original tissue. Hyaline articular cartilage has a very limited and imperfect repair mechanism, particularly where the defect only involves HAC; that is, does not extend into the subchondral bone plate.[24,51] Mitotic figures have been rarely observed in healthy HAC,[52–54] although hypertrophic cells and cell clusters have been observed in osteoarthritic cartilage.[55] This indicates an attempt by local chondrocytes to reconstitute the extracellular matrix and repair the defect.

In ligaments and tendons, which are poorly vascularized, healing times are long.[56] Healing is complicated by the need to reconstitute the typical compact, precise arrangement of collagen bundles on which their function depends. An inflammatory process involving these structures results in extensive fibrosis due to the action of the fibroblasts laying down scar tissue. Extensibility, tensile strength, and loading characteristics of this scar tissue are compromised by the random organization of fibers, and by cross-linking of new fibrils. Scar tissue may stretch over time, lengthening the overall structure and decreasing joint stability.

In comparison, bone retains a high regenerative capacity throughout the life span. The periosteum is a source of stem cells, and most parts of the skeleton are well vascularized. Healing times are long, passing through a collagenous phase (callus), through differentiation into cartilage and eventually bone. Bone's regenerative capacity means this tissue also is very responsive to altered loading (stress). With progressive damage to articular cartilage and exposure of collagen fibers there is altered loading on the subchondral bone that responds by remodeling. Remodeling is evident in osteoarthritis when thickening (sclerosis) of trabeculae occurs, and in the formation of osteophytes (excess bone formation [i.e., Heberden's nodes in the hand]) at joint margins. These changes in bone, exclusive of osteophytes, eventually occur in RA. Exposure of subchondral bone allows joint debris to be compressed into medullary spaces forming debris cysts. Such cysts may be "walled off" by sclerosed bone. These bony changes are enhanced by degradation of articular cartilage or detachment of cartilage secondary to its splitting.

Tissue damage leads to extravasation of plasma, initiation of intrinsic and extrinsic coagulation (wounds), complement cascade, and release of important mediators of repair (Fig. 3-6).[57] Inflammatory mediators include histamine, bradykinin, substance P, prostaglandins, and leukotrienes.[31] A major source of prostaglandins in human tissues is polyunsaturated fatty acids including arachidonic acid. Effusion is common when inflammatory processes involve joint tissues. Damaged tissues, particularly SLT, are infiltrated with leukocytes; there is an influx of neutrophils via increased blood flow and time-related chemoattractants. Neutrophils can cause further damage secondary to release of proteolytic enzymes and oxygen free radicals. Platelets release protease inhibitors that serve to limit tissue damage. Platelets release serotonin and cytokines including the transforming growth factor alpha (TGF-α), TGF-beta (TGF-β), and the platelet-derived growth factor (PDGF). Cytokines are peptide growth factors secreted by a variety of inflammatory cells and have multiple biologic activities that regulate a variety of cell types. Cytokines are believed responsible for many features of RA, including RA systemic effects as a result of transport from inflamed synovium into the general circulation.[58]

Neutrophils and macrophages arrive to remove cellular and matrix debris. Neutrophils release TGF-β, that acts as a monocyte, a fibroblast chemoattractor, and activates fibroblast differentiation from stem mesenchymal cells. Mononuclear cells differentiate into macrophages, produce proinflammatory mediators such as interleukin-1(IL-1), tumor necrosis factor (TNF), matrix degrading enzyme (collagenase), and also can express cellular fibronectin, which will contribute to the initial repair of tissue matrix. Interleukin-1 is secreted by synoviocytes.[59] With TGF-α, interleukin-1 can increase the synthesis of proteases, such as metalloproteases (collagenase, stromelysin, serine proteases)

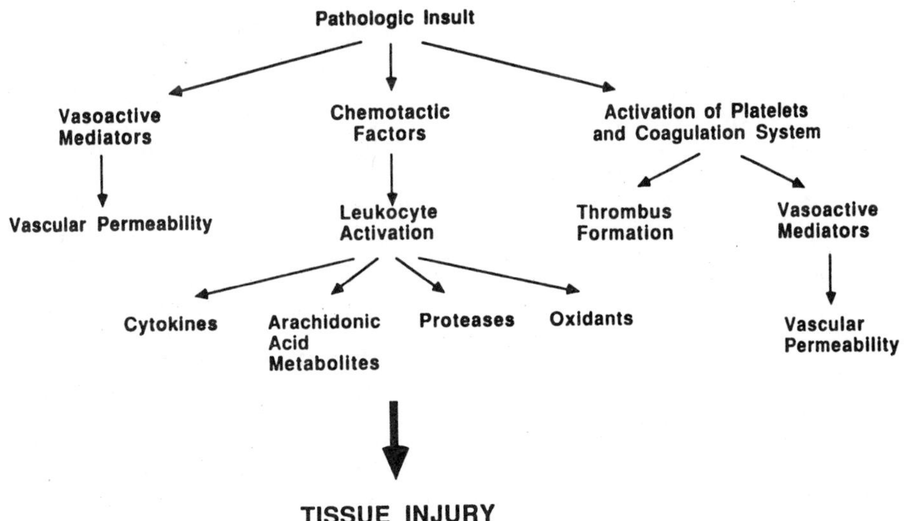

Figure 3-6. Mediators of the inflammatory response. (From Fantone JC: Basic concepts in inflammation. In Sports-Induced Inflammation: Clinical and Basic Science Concepts, p 26. Park Ridge, IL, American Academy of Orthopedic Surgeons, 1990. With permission.)

and plasminogen activators (PAs). Interleukin-1 also has been shown to favor synthesis of collagen Types I and III over Types II and IX.[25] Transforming growth factors are cytokines believed linked to the OA disease process and catabolism of HAC. The normal balance between matrix synthesis and degradation is upset in arthritis. The enzymatic processes involve both chondrocytes and synoviocytes; both can produce degradative enzymes. Matrix pH and physical factors, such as temperature, influence the enzymatic activity. Collagenase, for example, is more active at high joint temperatures (36° versus 33°C).[25] If cells are even mildly heated, they synthesize "heat shock proteins," which are found present in synovia of RA and OA joints. It is believed that the temperature of an inflamed joint can induce synthesis of these proteins.[60] Such data support the use of cold over heat in acutely inflamed joints.

Complement System

The complement system, a group of 20 plasma proteins, also is involved in the body's defense and immune systems. There are two pathways: the classic complement pathway, that may be activated by inflammatory mediators, immune complexes, and microbial products; and the alternate pathway, that may be activated by cell products, microbial products, and foreign substances such as x-ray contrast.[57] The results of activation of either pathway are similar—formation of a membrane attack complex, which can induce cell lysis.

Cell membrane phospholipids of injured cells and inflammatory cells may release arachidonic acid. Two enzyme pathways (lipoxygenase and cyclooxygenase) are critical in the conversion (oxygenation and hydrolysis) of arachidonic acid into other acids and metabolites (e.g., prostaglandins, thromboxane) (Fig. 3-7 and Table 3-2). Products of the lipoxygenase pathway are much more potent than those of the cyclooxygenase pathway.[61] Varieties of prostaglandins (I_2, E_2) enhance vascular permeability as they produce vasodilatation; effusion is increased. Nonsteroidal anti-inflammatory drugs (NSAIDs) act on this pathway to inhibit synthesis of prostaglandins and thromboxane. Prostaglandins of the E series and I_2, however, also inhibit inflammatory cell function (mast, neutrophil, macrophage) "secondary to their ability to activate adenylate cyclase and increase intracellular CAMP."[57] Although the main ability of prostaglandins is to influence vascular tone and permeability, PGE_2, produced by rheumatoid synovia, has been demonstrated to produce tissue injury via stimulation of bone resorption.[62] For further information on the complex cellular, molecular, and immune mechanisms affecting the inflammatory response

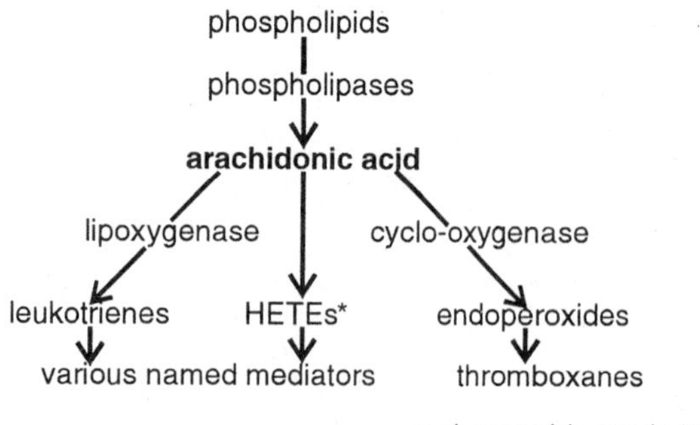

Figure 3-7. Steps in the production of inflammatory mediators, a simplistic version. HETEs = hydroxyeicosatetraenoic acids.[61]

the reader is referred to Fantone, 1990[57]; McCarty and Koopman, 1993[63]; and Kelley et al, 1993.[64]

As a result of matrix degradation, basic fibroblast growth factor and TGF-β, normally bound to matrix proteoglycans, are released. Such extracellular messenger proteins (termed cytokines or growth factors) are involved both in tissue degradation and synthesis. The degradative effects of IL-1 can be controlled by the insulin-like growth factor and TGF-β, which can stimulate collagen transcription and induce synthesis by connective tissue cells of tissue-inhibiting metalloproteases and plasminogen activator 1. Insulin-like growth factors (I and II) can stimulate chondrocyte mitotic activity, proteoglycan and collagen synthesis. Fibroblastic growth factors also can stimulate chondrocyte mitotic activity.

In acute inflammation tissues are infiltrated with polymorphonuclear leukocytes. In chronic inflammation, mononuclear cells, macrophages, and lymphocytes dominate the cellular infiltration. Neovascularization (angiogenesis) appears necessary to sustain chronic inflammation.[65] Angiogenesis is the primary vascular response in chronic inflammation and provides fresh monocytes and other inflammatory cells. Also seen in chronic inflammatory states is fibrosis, and potentially suppuration secondary to a bacterial infection (septic arthritis). The fibrosis phase may convert the proliferative fibrofatty connective tissue formed in the inflammatory process into adhesions that mature into strong scars, particularly if the part is immobilized. Such scars may result in significant joint contractures with consequent loss of mobility.

Cartilage Breakdown

Mechanisms of HAC breakdown involve multiple factors and imbalance between extracellular matrix degradation and synthesis. Radin[5] considers *repetitive impulsive loading* (RIL) to be a major factor. Other factors are stress deprivation (immobilization, bed rest, weightlessness), excessive loading (body weight, obesity), developmental etiologies (hip dysplasia, Perthes' disease, coxa valga),[66–69] joint surface incongruity, and joint instability (cruciate ligament trauma, generalized ligamentous laxity). Radin considers that the *type of load and manner of loading* is more important than the actual load on joint surfaces. RIL is detrimental to both HAC and subchondral bone (SCB). The more rapid the loading, the higher the tensile and shear rates and the greater the potential for damage. RIL produces microfractures (subclinical) in SCB, leading to cumulative damage.

It is thought that RIL activates the secondary ossification center, which gradually thins the articular cartilage layer and increases the shear forces in the deeper layers. The tidemark advances (duplicative tidemarks are seen in OA HAC), and the noncalcified layer thins. There is loss of proteoglycans, surface fibrillation, and vertical and horizontal splitting of HAC. Splitting and fibrillation of the cartilage surface produces articular debris in synovial fluid, which further irritates the synovial lining tissues and maintains the chronic inflammatory state. Although catabolic enzymatic activity may

Table 3-2. Sites and Effects of Arachidonic Acid Products

Site	Effect
Microvascular	Increase or decrease vessel permeability
Polymorphonuclear leukocytes Macrophages T-lymphocytes Platelets	Increase or decrease adherence to surfaces Alter response to other stimuli

contribute, Radin believes that RIL is a major culprit in production of osteoarthritis; cartilage is abraded, exposing the subchondral bone.

When collagen and proteoglycans of the extracellular matrix are broken down by the pathologic process in arthritis, their proteins or fragments may elicit an inflammatory immune response, triggering an inflammatory reaction.[70] Circulating antibodies to different types of collagens are increased in RA, psoriatic arthritis, and ankylosing spondylitis; the latter suggests an immune response to cartilage collagens.

In RA, free radicals, cytokines, neutral proteinase, and catabolic enzymes (derived from synoviocytes, chondrocytes, polymorphonuclear leukocytes) play a major role in articular cartilage breakdown; these substances also are involved in osteoarthritic HAC breakdown.[4,71,72] In osteoarthritic cartilage there is extensive damage to Type II collagen fibers, with eventual unwinding of the helix and the appearance of collagen fibrils.[9,22] This process appears to commence in the superficial layers and progresses to the deep layers. While cartilage proteoglycan loss can be reversed, loss of the structural integrity of cartilage and its collagen framework results in irreversible disintegration of the cartilage.[73] Repair is with fibrocartilaginous tissue in which Type I collagen, rather than the normal Type II, predominates and may facilitate calcification of repair tissue. It should be noted that Type II collagen appears to block deposit of hydroxyapatite crystals required for calcification.

Synovial Lining Tissue Changes

It is important to note that synovitis, inflammation of the synovial lining tissues, may result from a variety of stimuli and creates an environment that is hostile to articular cartilage. Such stimuli in arthritis include substances normally foreign to the joint space, such as cartilage wear particles, matrix molecules, immune complexes, hemosiderin (an iron blood corpuscle pigment), implant wear particles (i.e., from artificial ligaments), hydroxyapatite (released from bone matrix), and surgical chemical agents (ethylene oxide, glutaraldehyde).[74] Synovial intimal cells, absorptive by nature, take up such substances, which have been shown to persist indefinitely in the intimal layer. However, this process may cause the intimal cells to secrete substances that are harmful to articular cartilage, and provokes a chronic inflammatory reaction.

Vessels in the subsynovial layer become congested and dilated. Synovial villi proliferate and are larger. There is an increase in intimal cell size (hypertrophy) and number (hyperplasia), and in its matrix. Synovial lining tissues show fibroblastic proliferation and increased fibrosis. On its surface there is a fibrinous exudate. This inflammatory infiltrate may progress into a neovascular pannus that invades tendon sheaths and the joint, spreads over the joint surfaces, and destroys the articular cartilage.[65] This pannus is highly vascular and contains several cell types: macrophages, histocytes, mast cells, lymphocytes, and fibroblasts. Inflammatory cells may be infrequent directly adjacent to articular cartilage; however, cytokines and other mediators released by nonnuclear cells can affect cartilage from a distance.[75] Pannus is a characteristic feature of RA.

Joint effusion may accompany the synovitis, particularly in RA. The vascular changes allow transit into the joint space of substances not usually found there, such as large plasma proteins (e.g., fibrinogen), cells, enzymes, and inflammatory mediators. Proteinases may overwhelm proteinase inhibitors, permitting enzymes to have a destructive effect, especially on articular cartilage. The destructive effect may be enhanced by IL-1 and prostaglandin-E.[74] The enzymatically degraded cartilage releases proteoglycans that also may activate the synovial cells (termed "suicide" reaction, where cartilage hastens its own destruction). A vicious cycle develops with synovial intimal cells releasing more collagenase and proteinases, cytokines, and IL-1, which further weakens the cartilage and enhances mechanical damage. This process can lead to fibrous ankylosis, particularly in RA-like conditions.

The destruction and loss of articular cartilage occurs particularly in biomechanically vulnerable areas subjected to loading, and leads to subluxation or potential dislocation of the joint, seen more frequently in small joints of the hand and foot. In chronically inflamed synovial lining tissue of the joint capsule, especially in redundant folds and tendon sheaths, the fibrosis produces adhesions that may significantly limit both the normal gliding of tendons and the total joint range. As adhesion formation is aggravated by immobilization and rest, this supports use of gentle active assisted movement through range in the acutely inflamed joint.

Specific Joint Involvement

In RA the primary involvement and changes within synovium of small joints in the hand and foot stretches and weakens periarticular tissues. This produces mechanical imbalances that may progress to subluxation, dislocation, and severe deformity.

It should be noted, however, that a 1:1 relationship between dysfunction and deformity has not been demonstrated.

In RA, along with tenosynovitis, nodules may develop in sheaths producing "trigger fingers." Erosion of the extensor mechanism over proximal interphalangeal joints may cause a buttonhole (boutonnière) deformity and an inability to extend the digit. Contracture of intrinsic muscle tendons and/or erosion of the palmar or plantar plates may cause collateral ligaments to "bow string," producing "swan-neck" deformity of the digit(s) (Fig. 3-8).

Deformity in the hand or foot may be aggravated by the presence of mucous cysts associated with osteophytes (Heberden's nodes) and in gouty arthritis, urate crystal deposits (tophi). Pathological changes involving other tissues, such as calcification of finger tip pulp in scleroderma, or in the skin (psoriatic arthritis, systemic lupus erythematosus) contribute to the eventual deformity.

Particularly in RA, disease progression with resultant laxity of supporting structures and erosion of joint surfaces may lead to spinal subluxation (atlantoaxial) and neurologic symptoms due to excessive pressure on spinal nerves and the spinal cord.[75] Spondylolisthesis (slippage, commonly at L4–5) may occur in OA with potential stenosis of the spinal canal and neurological symptoms.

The previous chain of events affecting joint tissues in pathology of arthritis may be arrested at any point by intrinsic and extrinsic (e.g., drugs) factors.

Pathology in Specific Conditions

Rheumatoid Arthritis

Rheumatoid arthritis is a destructive chronic synovitis in multiple diarthrodial joints (polyarthritis) with a variety of systemic manifestations. In RA there is persistent immunologic activity with CD4(+)/CD29(+) memory T cells prominently involved.[76] Local production of immunoglobulin, autoantibody rheumatoid factor (RF) plays a role in tissue destruction. The rheumatoid synovium exhibits variable histopathology, infiltration of large numbers of mononuclear cells is characteristic, especially in the chronic phase. It is presumed that small lymphocytes differentiate into immunoglobulin (Ig)- and rheumatoid factor-secreting plasma cells.[76] Lymphoid follicles develop in synovial tis-

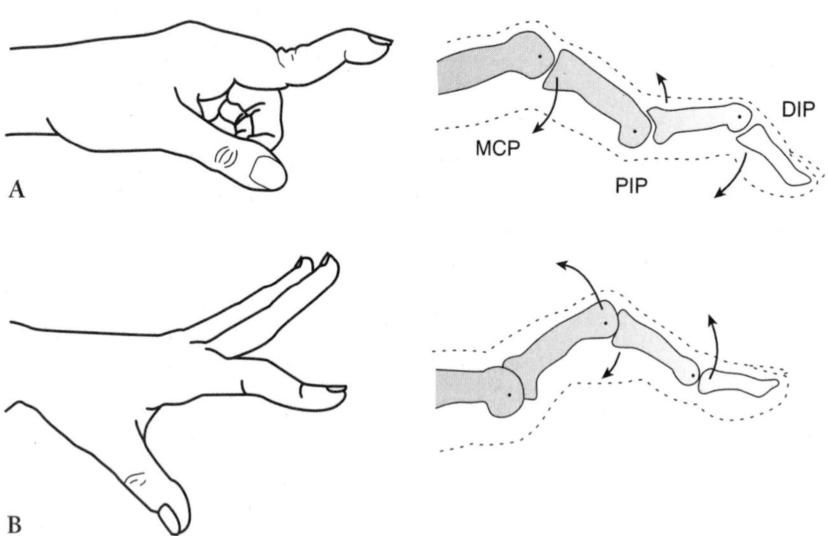

Figure 3-8. Diagrams to show the mechanism of boutonnière deformity (*A*) and swan-neck deformity (*B*).

sues and are one source of Ig and RF. Hypertrophy and hyperplasia are characteristic features of RA synovium, as well as microvascular abnormalities, especially of capillaries and postcapillary venules in the acute phase; neovascularization and pannus formation are prominent features. In RA, as with many inflammatory arthritis conditions, pathological changes are not restricted to those of the joint tissues given emphasis in this review. Changes are frequently seen in ocular tissues and in cardiopulmonary, skin, and the reticuloendothelial systems.

Psoriatic Arthritis

Synovial changes in psoriatic arthritis (PA) are not distinguishable from those in RA except that there is a greater tendency for bony ankylosis to occur, especially in interphalangeal and carpal joints.[77] There is a marked difference from RA in the pattern of joint involvement. Cellular infiltration is predominantly lymphocytic. TGF-α may be involved in the generalized abnormality of blood vessels and the abnormally fast keratinocyte growth rate (3 days versus 3 weeks).[77] Dystrophy (e.g., pitting) of nails may occur in 60–80% of patients with PA.[78,79]

Ankylosing Spondylitis

This form of arthritis involves specific areas of the body, primarily the spine, and appears to maximally involve the junction of ligaments to bone (enthesis). Enthesopathy involves vertebra in an ascending order with a process that commences around the sacroiliac joint. With inflammation at ligament junctions (enthesitis), bone becomes eroded and cartilage and cortical bone are replaced by fibrous and granulation tissues. New bone formation (syndesmophytes) causes ascending ossification of the inflamed tissues resulting in ossification of spinal ligaments, intervertebral disks, facet joint capsules, and ankylosis ("bamboo spine"). Typically there is a "squaring" off of the vertebral bodies. Changes may cause cauda equina symptoms as well as vertebrobasilar artery insufficiency.[80] Peripheral joints exhibit synovitis similar to other forms of inflammatory arthritis, differing only in distribution of joints affected, and in comparison to RA, in the absence of the RF and a frequently positive antigen HLA-B27.[81]

Infectious Arthritis

A number of microorganisms may produce an infectious process at a site distant to the primary infection and cause a suppurative (staphylococcal arthritis) or nonsuppurative inflammatory process (reactive arthritis). One form of nonsuppurative arthritis, Reiter's syndrome, is associated with other pathology (classically a syndrome of arthritis, ureteritis, and conjunctivitis) in less than 33% of patients.[76] About 60% of patients with Reiter's syndrome have subclinical inflammation of the terminal ileum and colon. Pathologic changes are similar to that in RA; however, enthesitis is more common. Bony erosions and pannus formation are uncommon, but will be seen with persistent inflammation.

Suppurative infectious arthritis in the absence of direct penetration of the joint by an object, or trauma, reflects failure in the body's extensive defense mechanisms. Under healthy conditions the joint cavity is highly protected from transmission of infectious agents. The initial site of infection is distant to the joint. Joint sepsis may result from agents such as gonococcal, staphylococcal, tuberculosis, hemophilus influenzal gram-positive bacteria (specially in young children), and salmonella species. Septic arthritis also is a grave and costly complication of patients with joint replacements.

The inflammatory process is similar to that of other forms of arthritis. Because of the tamponade (compression) of subsynovial vessels and resultant increase in intra-articular pressure, diffusion of solutes is slowed. This process may allow bacterial cells to remain dormant even in the presence of drugs.[82] Furthermore, while antibiotics may destroy the microorganisms, drug therapy does not remove microbial products. The persistence and retention of these products either within the joint cavity, embedded in joint crevasses, or in the articular cartilage, may cause persistent chronic inflammatory response (postinfectious synovitis), with further potential for irritation, damage, and dysfunction. While all joint tissues are vulnerable to damage from the infectious inflammatory process, articular cartilage is particularly vulnerable to the presence of pus, as chondrolysis is irreversible. Rupture of tendon sheaths may occur.

In an infant, the infectious agent may reach the joint space via small capillaries that cross the epiphyseal growth plate. This route is blocked in the older child and adult. Agents, however, may reach the joint via joint anastomoses, sideways extension into the subperiosteum and, in certain joints, from dependent synovial fold reflections (i.e., glenohumeral).

Bacterial infections may involve fibrocartilaginous midline joints that lack synovial lining tissue (symphysis pubis, sternomanubrium, sternoclavicular, posterior sacroiliac). When these joints are involved, osteomyelitis in adjacent bone may occur.[83] Bacteria, ticks (Lyme disease), and other microbial organisms in a joint can activate IL-I, TNF, and the complement resulting in aggravation of the inflammatory process due to production of chemotactic factors, mediators of inflammation, and other biologically active substances. The interested reader is referred to reviews for further detail.[63,64]

Hemophilic Arthritis

In hemophilia, repeated joint hemorrhages can produce severe articular cartilage damage, particularly in large peripheral joints such as the knee. The damage can be more severe than in OA.[84] Large amounts of hemosiderin, an iron-containing pigment, may be deposited as coarse aggregates in the synovium. These aggregates may persist indefinitely and act as an irritant promoting further disintegration of articular cartilage as a result of release of chondrolytic enzymes. The presence of plasmin (fibrinolysin) in synovial fluid in acute hemorrhages may enhance enzyme degradation. The contribution of interosseous bleeding to the development of often large cysts or cavities in the subchondral bone is not established.[85] Accelerated maturation and hypertrophy of adjacent epiphyses may result in stature reduction. (Growth disturbances, local and systemic, and premature closure of growth plates also may cause short stature in juvenile RA.) Repeated hemorrhages cause repetitive acute inflammatory episodes that are often associated with marked atrophy of muscles about the joint.

Gouty Arthritis

Crystal-induced inflammation with ensuing arthritis may be caused by various crystal deposits, such as monosodium urate monohydrate (MUM) in gout and calcium pyrophosphate dihydrate (CPPD). The presence of MUM or CPPD crystals in joint fluid may be "a result, as well as a cause, of joint inflammation,"[86, p 1821] since crystals may be released from enzymatic degradation of cartilage or mechanical disruption of its architecture.

In gout, the common lesion is that of joint degeneration with deposition of MUM or uric acid crystals from extracellular fluids in and around joint tissues. These tophaceous deposits can cause acute inflammatory episodes with severe destruction of articular structures. Single or multiple joints may be affected. Crystals, the end product of purine metabolism, may be deposited on and in articular cartilage, as well as subchondral bone.[84] Hyperuricemia (supersaturation of urate in serum), a biochemical abnormality, is a characteristic feature, where gout is the disease state.[87]

The tophaceous deposits (solid urate) may form in various soft tissues, such as the helix of the ear, olecranon, prepatellar bursa, and the Achilles tendon. Other features of gout may include ulceration of the tense skin overlying the tophi, renal disease, and crystals in the synovial fluid during quiescent periods (termed "intercritical"). Except for interphalangeal joints of the hand and foot, and carpal region, bony ankylosis is unusual.[88]

Neuropathic Arthritis

In neuropathic joint disease, arthritis, progressive and degenerative, develops secondary to sensory loss in a joint.[89] Sensory loss may result from diabetes mellitus with peripheral neuropathy, neurosyphilis, syringomyelia, paraplegia, and tabes dorsalis. Joint changes are similar to OA, but early effusion with later subluxation, para-articular debris, and bony fragmentation are considered diagnostic features. Compared with OA there is a greater degree of bony sclerosis, osteophytosis, and fragmentation of bone on radiographs.[90]

Effect of Unloading and Immobility

Articular cartilage, ligaments, and tendons are sensitive to abnormal loading. When unloaded, as in immobilization, there is rapid deterioration of biochemical and mechanical properties.

Ligaments

Ligaments show atrophy, decreased strength, and stiffness.[56,91] Loss of ligament strength appears exponential over time. While the loss may be minimal in the first few weeks, if immobilized for 6–9 weeks, ligaments are only 50% as strong and stiff as healthy ligaments. Bone resorption at the insertion sites further weakens the ligament.[92,93] Ligaments also tend to be less stiff, more resilient, after immobilization. The stiffness in a joint following immobilization is probably due to binding of nonligamentous periarticular tissues. Following immobilization, recovery of ligament properties is not homogeneous in all parts; the bony insertion area may recover in a few weeks, whereas recovery of ligament substance may take months.

Studies in animal models demonstrate that because the scar tissue formed in ligaments during immobilization is smaller in mass, materially weaker, and less viscous, ligaments are more vulnerable to repeat injury at comparable loads. Bray et al,[94] with a rabbit model of an anterior cruciate ligament–deficient knee, showed that short periods of immobilization may retard osteoarthritic changes associated with joint instability; this may relate to stability provided by immobilization. If instability is not corrected by immobilization, deterioration will continue. In ligaments, the short-term "benefit" of immobilization may not be worthwhile.[95]

It is pertinent to note that in arthritis, unlike isolated ligament injuries in sports, ligaments are not healthy prior to a period of immobilization. Inflamed joints, however, are subjected more to unloading and temporary immobilization for shorter time periods using removable splints. As rest is a basic principle of acute and chronic arthritis health management, the negative effects of immobilization on joint tissues produce a dilemma, to determine the balance between the period of rest to decrease inflammation yet not incur further functional loss. Anti-inflammatory drug therapy is an important component of treatment.

Articular Cartilage

When articular cartilage is unloaded by being deprived of mechanical stimuli (rest, non-weight bearing), synthesis activity by chondrocytes decreases.[96,97] Unloaded cartilage shows decreased thickness (atrophy), decreased hydration, decreased chondroitin sulfate, and decreased synthesis of GAGs.[98] Collagen synthesis, but not the total amount of collagen, may be enhanced. Effects of unloading on collagen may occur in all collagenous tissues. Fiber-fiber distances and lubrication between fibers is decreased. This hinders fiber-on-fiber gliding, and enhances cross-linking and adhesion formation. The collagen arrangement is more random. Fibers may be thicker, as fewer fibers are laid down without regard to the tissue's mechanical requirements.

When exposed to rigid immobilization, articular cartilage shows changes similar to that of osteoarthritis; cell necrosis may occur.[97,99,100] These changes presumably are related to interference with the chondrocytes' nutrition (pressure driven from synovial fluid through the cartilage matrix) due to absent or decreased amounts of cyclic compression and expansion of articular cartilage that occurs with intermittent loading.[101] While immobilization prevents joint motion and is associated with unloading of joint surfaces, some areas of the cartilage joint surface may be subjected to increased loading dependent on the position of immobilization.

If cartilage previously exposed to unloading is loaded, there may be "gross functional failure of matrix."[102] This appears to be related to a defect in the ability of proteoglycans to reform the hyaluronic acid–binding region of the aggregates. Unloaded cartilage is less stiff, the proteoglycan matrix is impaired and this may make articular cartilage more vulnerable to injuries if exposed to sudden, heavy loading. Such changes may be reversed by a gently graduated program; however, restoration of healthy structure and characteristics is uncertain.[103] It is important for therapists to recognize that following immobilization or unloading (rest), articular cartilage is less stiff and less capable of tolerating high loads; loads normally within the physiological capacity of healthy cartilage.

Bone

The response of bone to altered mechanical stimuli is important in arthritis. If mechanical stimuli are reduced by rest or immobilization, bone loss occurs, with a decrease in bone quantity but not the quality or composition of bone. Adaptive remodeling, the laying down of more bone, is stimulated by altered stress, a change in mechanical stimuli. Frost's mechanostat theory[104] postulates that remodeling is stimulated by decreased mechanical usage with concomitant net loss of bone, and is inhibited by increased mechanical usage with net increase in bone mass. Because the internal architecture of subchondral bone influences the load transfer to cortical bone, changes in bone associated with arthritis are important.

The changes in bone as a result of immobilization and decreased loading are significant and clear cut: increased resorption, and decreased trabeculae volume and bone mineral content. This mineral loss can be reversed; however, recovery is not as rapid.[105] The slower rate of reconstitution is more important in progressive arthritic conditions than in fractures occurring in a young adult.

Increased Loading

In osteoarthritis it is predicted that excessive mechanical loading (repetitive impulse loading) produces fatigue fractures, microscopic cracks in and around osteons that involve individual trabeculae and, over time, reduces the strength and stiffness of bone. If the damage is excessive, resorption exceeds deposition and failure occurs at the macroscopic level, such as crush fractures of vertebral bodies, and contour changes in joint surfaces. These changes in bone place greater stress on articular cartilage and are postulated to provoke osteoarthritis. Research has not yet established if such microcracks can trigger a cellular response to bring about repair of the damaged matrix.

Aging

The pathological changes in bone in the arthritides also may encompass changes associated with the natural decline in bone mass due to aging. This decline occurs at a greater rate in women than in men and may lead to osteoporosis. In osteoporosis there is reduced mineral mass, excessive resorption, increased bone porosity, more numerous and larger Haversian canals, and weaker and more brittle bone.[106,107] Moderate to severe arthritis, especially RA, enhances the osteoporotic process due to limited mobility and activity; the probability of fractures is further enhanced.

With aging there also is an increased risk of adult-onset diabetes. Insulin-dependent diabetes causes more marked osteopathic changes[108,109] with mechanical weakening of bone.[110,111] Bone mineral loss may be further aggravated by long-term corticosteroid therapy used in RA and juvenile RA, increasing the potential for stress fractures.

Pain Medication and Modulation

The mechanism(s) producing the sensation of pain, common in arthritic conditions, probably is not derived from cartilage damage, since articular cartilage is aneural. Pain sensation may be derived from increased pressure that results from abnormal motion, abnormal geometry, excessive loading, and distention of joint capsule tissues and other soft tissues related to the joint. Articular nerves contain both myelinated and unmyelinated fibers. Pain and vasomotor fibers are small in diameter. Unmyelinated nerve fibers are postganglionic sympathetic fibers that terminate in the walls of the many articular blood vessels found in subsynovial tissues.[112–116]

The articular nociceptive system, inactive in the healthy state, is activated by excessive levels of mechanical stress or deformation, and in the presence of inflammation when chemical irritants (prostaglandins, bradykinin, serotonin, histamine) accumulate in the tissues. If vascular permeability is decreased by fibrosis or acute inflammatory processes, the concentration of these chemical irritants increases.

In the presence of effusion or hemarthrosis, the synovial cavity is no longer a potential space and intra-articular pressures (IAP) may be supra-atmospheric (up to 33 mg Hg in RA knee).[37] Sustained synovitis with increased SF volume and pressure provokes tension and even pain. When an effusion forms rapidly, pain is more likely.[117] There is a critical effusion pressure, which in turn impairs and reduces synovial blood flow.[118,119]

The viscoelasticity of synovial cavity tissues influences the relationship between IAP and SF volume (compliance curve). At very small subatmospheric pressure the cavity tissues are at their most stretchable, neither collapsed nor distended. With increase in volume the stiffness of these tissues increases rapidly and linearly so that cavity walls are tense and stretched. If the increase in volume persists, as in chronic synovitis, stress relaxation occurs due to loss of tension in the cavity walls and the pressure, despite constant volume, will decrease. Thus a rapidly forming effusion (traumatic, infective, hemarthrotic) will be associated with more pain (and can be relieved by aspiration) than a slowly forming effusion.[120]

A patient with an effused joint will adopt a position where the cavity tissues are under the least tension (in the knee about 30–40 degrees of flexion) (Fig. 3-9).[121] Motion away from this position, in either direction, will increase IAP and potentially pain. Active motion, as displayed on Figure 3-9, is associated with higher IAPs. The greater the effusion (volume), the greater the sensitivity of pressure to the joint angle. Increased IAP in the knee has been shown to excite joint afferents strongly, probably through end organs in the capsule.[113] Firing of these afferents inhibits activation of muscles acting on the joint (quadriceps), contributing reflexly to disuse atrophy. Simultaneously, antagonists (hamstrings) may be stimulated to assist in maintenance of a loose-packed joint position that accommodates the effusion.[112]

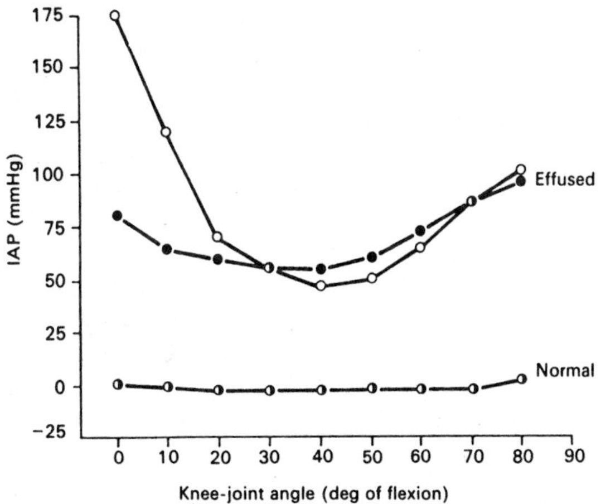

Figure 3-9. Intra-articular pressures (IAPs) recorded at a range of joint angles during active (o) and passive (●) positioning of the knee before and after injection of 10 ml of dextran into the joint (◑). Coincident IAPs shown for both active and passive positioning. Note that in the effused knee IAPs are lowest about 30–40 degrees. (From Baxendale RH, Ferrell WR, Wood L: Intraarticular pressures during active and passive movement of normal and distended human knee joints. J Physiol 1985; 369:179P. With permission.)

Elasticity and viscosity in particular contribute to total stiffness, a common and important symptom in arthritis. Different joint tissues appear to vary in their contribution to total stiffness from joint to joint. This symptom, that may be confused with pain, has not proven to be easily quantifiable by biomechanical devices. Work to date suggests that mechanical perception thresholds in patients with RA are normal.[122]

Several investigators suggest that a disease-related loss or alteration in joint or muscle proprioception is present in OA.[123–125] Function, such as gait, may be affected by changes in joint position sense which may result from small fluctuations in disease activity (i.e., effusion, intra-articular pressure changes) and not be due solely to the presence of pain.

Kidd et al[126] hypothesized that sensory nerve endings in synovial tissues also may, by releasing neuropeptides, modulate the response of synovial tissues to a variety of noxious stimuli, as may result from joint damage. This mechanism may selectively activate preganglionic sympathetic cells, which project to the opposite side, and is reflected in symmetrical joint involvement, common in RA. This projection to the contralateral side leads to recruitment of macrophages in the absence of a full inflammatory response.

In an acute inflammatory state, synovial inflammation is associated with increased blood flow and raised local temperature. In chronic inflammation with capsular fibrosis, however, there is reduced blood flow. Change in synovial plasma flow is correlated with variation in intra-articular temperature. Theoretically, a swollen but *cool* joint, indicative of reduced blood flow, is metabolically more impaired than a swollen hot joint (increased blood flow).

Modulation of Pain

Identification and removal of the cause(s) of arthritis is not yet achievable; therefore, therapy must be directed at relief of signs and symptoms, and prevention or delay of further damage. The interaction of increased IAP, tension, and pain strongly supports the approach that the most efficient modulation of pain is reduction and control of joint effusion.

Many modalities are in use to control pain (drugs, transcutaneous electrical nerve stimulation [TENS], thermal agents, acupuncture) and may be effective in accordance with the "gate theory."[127] Stimulation of large-diameter, myelinated fibers blocks the transmission of pain impulses from small-diameter, unmyelinated fibers at the synapse (presynaptic inhibition) and from reaching the dorsal gray column. Some modalities (i.e., cold) act to decrease the firing rate of muscle spindle afferents, thereby decreasing reflex muscle contractions, which decreases the tension on the effused joint tissues and lowers the pain threshold on motion. Management of abnormal mechanical deformation or stress by splinting also serves to decrease awareness of pain by limiting motion into areas of range where IAP is increased. Other mechanisms invoked by drug therapy are given in Chapter 9. The therapist and patient, however, must be aware that control and reduction of joint effusion is most likely to give long-lasting relief from pain.

Reduce and control effusion to decrease pain.

Restoration of Joint Surfaces

In considering the potential for restoration of joint surfaces, it is pertinent to distinguish between *repair*, "the replacement of damaged or lost cells and extracellular matrices with new cells and matrices," and *regeneration*, "a form of repair that produces new tissue that is structurally and functionally identical to the normal tissue."[128]

Bone is characterized by an ability to heal without fibrous tissue (scar) and, when healed, to regain its former strength and functional capabilities. Articular cartilage, however, is notorious for its limited potential for either repair or regeneration. Thus, arthritis, regardless of type, tends to be progressive once changes are initiated. Since articular cartilage is avascular, it is incapable of producing an inflammatory reaction, which is the typical tissue response to injury and the initial phase of a repair process. This may explain the failure to heal in partial thickness defects of articular cartilage.[129]

Healing of articular cartilage appears dependent on whether the defect penetrates the subchondral plate. Akeson et al.[130] stressed that a number of studies over the years have amply demonstrated that healing by articular cartilage only occurs in small-thickness defects (~$^1/_8$-inch diameter) and does not occur in large or full-thickness defects, with or without motion.

Unpublished data reported by Sokoloff[131] suggest that if the pressure on the joint surface can be relieved (i.e., surgically), resurfacing of the OA joint surface can occur. The regenerated surface, however, was fibrocartilaginous but apparently functionally adequate. Drug therapy may arrest or modify the enzymatic degradation of the joint surfaces that occurs in inflammatory arthritis (e.g., RA); however, it cannot reconstitute altered geometry and restoration is unlikely.

The type of training that best improves the ability of articular cartilage to withstand stress and that positively contributes to repair of articular cartilage is not established. Exercise is shown to increase blood flow and perfusion of soft tissues in the canine wrist and knee; however, effects on cartilage are unclear.[36] Such data support the use of only minimal activity to preserve range of motion in the acutely inflamed joint and also support the value of vigorous exercise in chronically inflamed joints. Increase in articular cartilage thickness, increased cell size, and improved anabolic processes of articular cartilage have been demonstrated following exercise training in animal models.[132–135] A species-specific effect may exist, since running exercise in rats has been shown to increase tendon collagen synthesis, but in mice there was a decrease in total collagen and in collagen tensile strength. A type-specific response also may exist, with flexor tendons responding to exercise differently from extensor tendons.[136]

While cells of healthy articular cartilage appear to have suppression or loss of the ability to replicate their DNA, when degeneration occurs, as in the early stages of OA, chondrocytes appear to recover their ability to divide.[137,138] Overall, repair by surviving cells seems absent when a cleft involves only articular cartilage, not subchondral bone. Salter et al[139] over the past two decades have demonstrated healing of full-thickness drill hole defects and free intra-articular periosteal grafts with continuous passive motion with hyaline-like tissue. Results have been less impressive in mature animals. It is not established how newly synthesized articular cartilage responds to normal loading over time. The evidence, however, is that physical signals such as motion and load are important in facilitating cartilage repair processes, however imperfect these may be. Data from animal studies also suggest that intermittent rather than continuous mechanical stress induces beneficial metabolic changes in chondrocytes and that absence of motion is detrimental.

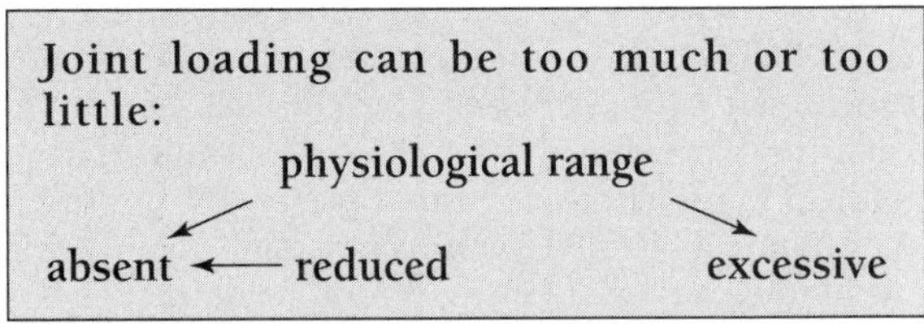

Bone, in comparison to articular cartilage, is a dynamic tissue that retains throughout life the capacity for regeneration. Remodeling is ensured because of penetration of blood vessels from underlying bone; however, this process also enhances further calcification of articular cartilage.[14] According to Wolff's law, as loads on bone change, remodeling reorients load-bearing trabeculae so that they are aligned with new trajectories of principal stress.[140] A program of graduated weight bearing/loading is important, since subchondral bone responds to cyclic loading by increased stiffness and strength.[141]

Conclusion

The structure and function of articular tissues, pathophysiology of inflammation, and repair and responses to unloading and loading have been reviewed. Musculoskeletal tissues are affected by inflammatory pathology, and not just locally—they may be also affected at a distance, in potential atrophy of muscle groups, and changes in joint range and position. In addition, systemic effects are often present that may influence the patient's response to therapy.

While no studies were located that report the effects of physical therapy intervention (i.e., stretching) at the cellular level, studies of the effects of unloading and loading can guide the therapist in selection of modality and intensity of use at different stages of the arthritic process. There is abundant evidence that, in form and function, cells of the musculoskeletal system respond to mechanical loading; loading may be the most controllable modality available. In time, it is hoped that the "physiologic window of stress" can be related to therapeutic exercise and functional activities. To date, margins of safety have not been defined.

References

1. Mankin HJ, Radin EL: Structure and function of joints. In McCarty DJ, Koopman WJ (eds): Arthritis and Allied Conditions, 12th edition, vol 1, pp 181–197. Philadelphia, Lea & Febiger, 1993.
2. Radin EL, Paul IL, Lowry YM: A comparison of the dynamic force transmitting properties of subchondral bone and articular cartilage. J Bone Joint Surg 1970; 52A:444–456.
3. Radin EL, Paul IL, Rose RM. Role of mechanical factors in pathogenesis of primary osteoarthritis. Lancet 1972; 1:519–522.
4. Radin EL: Osteoarthrosis. In Wright V, Radin EL (eds): Mechanics of Human Joints, pp 341–354. New York, Marcel Dekker Inc, 1993.
5. Radin EL. Mechanically induced periarticular and neuromuscular problems. In Wright V, Radin EL (eds): Mechanics of Human Joints, pp 355–370. New York, Marcel Dekker Inc, 1993.
6. Warwick R, Williams PL: Gray's Anatomy, 35th edition, pp 210–211. London, Longman, 1973.
7. Radin EL, Martin RB, Burr DB, et al: Effects of mechanical loading on the tissues of the rabbit knee. J Orthop Res 1984; 2:221–234.
8. Mankin HJ, Trasher AZ: Water content and binding in normal and osteoarthritic human cartilage. J Bone Joint Surg 1975; 57A:76–80.
9. Poole AR: Cartilage in health and disease. In McCarty DJ, Koopman WJ (eds): Arthritis and Allied Conditions, 12th edition, vol 1, pp 279–333. Philadelphia, Lea & Febiger, 1993.
10. Stockwell RA: Cell density of human articular and costal cartilage. J Anat 1967; 101:753–763.
11. Castor CW: Regulation of connective tissue metabolism. In McCarty DJ, Koopman WJ (eds): Arthritis and Allied Conditions, 12th edition, vol 1, pp 245–262. Philadelphia, Lea & Febiger, 1993.
12. Rosenberg L: Structure and function of cartilage proteoglycans. In McCarty DJ, Koopman WJ (eds): Arthritis and Allied Conditions, 12th edition, vol 1, pp 229–243. Philadelphia, Lea & Febiger, 1993.
13. Oettmeier R, Abendroth K, Oettmeier S: Analysis of the tidemark on human femoral heads. I. Histochemical, ultrastructural and microanalytical characterization of the normal structure of the intercartilaginous junction. Acta Morphol Hung 1989; 37(3–4):155–168.
14. Lane LB, Bullough PG: Age-related changes in the thickness of the calcified zone, the number of tidemarks in adult human articular cartilage. J Bone Joint Surg 1980; 62B(3):372–365.
15. Kenzora JE, Yosipovitch Z, Glimcher MJ: The calcified cartilage zone of adult articular cartilage: A viable functional entity. Orthop Trans 1978; 2:120–121.
16. Meachim G, Stockwell RA: The matrix. In Freeman MAR (ed): Adult Articular Cartilage, 2nd edition, pp 1–68. Tunbridge Wells, Pitman Medical, 1979.
17. Poole CA, Flint MH, Beaumont BW: Morphological and functional interrelationships of articular cartilage matrices. J Anat 1984; 138:113–138.
18. Lane JN, Weiss C: Current comment: review of articular cartilage collagen research. Arthritis Rheum 1975; 18(6):553–562.
19. Moses MA, Sudhalter J, Langer R: Identification of an inhibitor of neovasculization from cartilage. Science 1990; 248:1408–1410.
20. Fleischmajor R, Olsen BR, Kühn K: Structure, molecular biology and pathology of collagen. Ann NY Acad Sci 1990; 580:1–592.
21. Castor CW: Regulation of connective tissue metabolism. In McCarty DJ, Koopman WJ (eds): Arthritis and Allied Conditions, 12th edition, vol 1, pp 245–262. Philadelphia, Lea & Febiger, 1993.
22. Prockop DJ, Williams CJ, Vandenburg P: Collagen in normal and diseased connective tissue. In McCarty DJ, Koopman WJ (eds): Arthritis and Allied Conditions, 12th edition, vol 1, pp 213–227. Philadelphia, Lea & Febiger, 1993.
23. Swann DA: Macromolecules of synovial fluid. In Sokoloff L (ed): The Joints and Synovial Fluid, pp 407–435. New York, Academic Press, 1978.
24. Sledge CB: Biology of the joint. In Kelley WN, Harris ED, Ruddy S, Sledge CB (eds): Textbook of Rheumatology, 4th edition, vol 1, pp 1–21. Philadelphia, WB Saunders Co, 1993.
25. McCarty DJ: Synovial fluid. In McCarty DJ, Koopman WL (eds): Arthritis and Allied Conditions,

12th edition, vol 1, pp 63–84. Philadelphia, Lea & Febiger, 1993.
26. Andersen H: Development, morphology and histochemistry of the early synovial tissue in human fetuses. Acta Anat 1964; 58:90–115.
27. Ghadially FN: Fine structure of joints. In Sokoloff L (ed): The Joints and Synovial Fluid, pp 105–176. New York, Academic Press, 1978.
28. Knight AD, Levick JR: The effect of fluid pressure on the hydraulic conductance of the interstitium and fenestrated endothelium in the rabbit knee. J Physiol 1985; 360:311–332.
29. Davies DV: The lymphatics of the synovial membrane. J Anat 1946; 80:21–23.
30. Ghadially FN: Fine Structure of Synovial Joints. London, Butterworth, 1983.
31. Henderson B, Edwards JCW: The Synovial Lining in Health and Disease, p xv. London, Chapman and Hall, 1987.
32. Chapman WW, Swaim R, Froshsin H Jr, et al: Degradation of human articular cartilage by neutrophils and synovial fluid. Arthritis Rheum 1993; 36(1):51–58.
33. Fox RI, Kang H: Structure and function of synoviocytes. In McCarty DJ, Koopman WL (eds): Arthritis and Allied Conditions, 12th edition, vol 1, pp 263–278. Philadelphia, Lea & Febiger, 1993.
34. Barland P, Novikoff AB, Hamerman D: Electron microscopy of the human synovial membrane. J Cell Biol 1962; 14:207–220.
35. Ghadially FN, Roy S: Ultrastructure of Synovial Joints in Health and Disease. London, Butterworth, 1969.
36. Simkin PA: Synovial physiology. In McCarty DJ, Koopman WJ (eds): Arthritis and Allied Conditions, 12th edition, vol 1, pp 199–212. Philadelphia, Lea & Febiger, 1993.
37. Ropes NW, Bauer W: Synovial Fluid Changes in Joint Disease. Cambridge, Harvard University Press, 1953.
38. Swann DA, Slayter HS, Silver FH: The molecular structure of LGP-1, The boundary lubricant for articular cartilage. J Biochem 1981; 256:2921–2925.
39. Levick JR: Synovial fluid determinants of volume turnover and material concentration. In Kuettner K, et al (eds): Articular Cartilage and Osteoarthritis, pp 529–541. New York, Raven Press, 1992.
40. Unsworth A: Lubrication of human joints. In Wright V, Radin E (eds): Mechanics of Human Joints, pp 137–162. New York, Marcel Dekker Inc, 1993.
41. Bruggemann GP: Biomechanics in gymnastics. Med Sport Sci 1987; 45:142–176.
42. Radin EL, Orr RB, Kelman JL, et al: Effect of prolonged walking on concrete on the knees of sheep. J Biomech 1982; 15:487–492.
43. Light LH, McLellan GE, Klenerman L: Skeletal transients on heel strike in normal walking with different footwear. J Biomech 1980; 13:477–480.
44. Dickinson JA, Cook SD, Leinhart TM: The measurement of shockwaves following heel strike while running. J Biomech 1985; 18:415–422.
45. Clarke IC, Contini R, Kenedi RN: Friction and wear studies of articular cartilage: a scanning electron microscopy study. J Lubr Tech 1975; 97(3): 358–368.
46. Radin EL, Paul IL: A consolidated concept of joint lubrication. J Bone Joint Surg 1972; 54A:607–616.
47. Charnley J: How our joints are lubricated. Basel, Sandoz Pharma AG, Triangle, 1960; 4:175–179.
48. Unsworth A: Tribology of human and artificial joints. Proc Inst Mech Eng 1991; (H)205(3):163–172.
49. McCutchen CW: Lubrication of joints. In Sokoloff L (ed): The Joints and Synovial Fluid, vol 1, pp 437–483. New York, Academic Press Inc, 1978.
50. Dintenfass L: Lubrication and synovial joints: A theoretical analysis—a logical approach to the problems of joint movements and joint lubrication. J Bone Joint Surg 1963; 45A:1241–1256.
51. Landells JW: The reactions of injured human articular cartilage. J Bone Joint Surg 1957; 39B:548–562.
52. Stockwell RA, Meachim G: The chondrocytes. In Freeman MAR (ed): Adult Articular Cartilage, pp 69–145. London, Pitman Medical, 1979.
53. Hulth A, Lindberg L, Telhag H: Mitosis in human osteoarthritic cartilage. Clin Orthop 1972; 84:197–199.
54. Havdrup T, Telhag H: Mitosis of chondrocytes in normal adult joint cartilage. Clin Orthop 1980; 153:248–252.
55. Havdrup T, Telhag H: Scattered mitosis in adult joint cartilage after partial chondrectomy. Acta Orthop Scand 1978; 48:424–429.
56. Akeson WH, Woo SL-Y, Amiel D, et al: The chemical basis of tissue repair. The biology of ligaments. In Hunter LY, Funk FJ (eds): Rehabilitation of the Injured Knee, pp 93–148. St Louis, CV Mosby Co, 1984.
57. Fantone JC: Basic concepts in inflammation. In Leadbeater WB, Buckwalter JA, Gordon SL (eds): Sports-Induced Inflammation: Clinical and Basic Science Concepts, pp 23–54. Park Ridge, IL, American Academy of Orthopedic Surgeons, 1990.
58. Cush JJ, Lipsky PE: Reiter's syndrome and reactive arthritis. In McCarty DJ, Koopman WJ (eds): Arthritis and Allied Conditions, 12th edition, vol 1, pp 161–178. Philadelphia, Lea & Febiger, 1993.
59. Howell DS, Pelletier J-P: Etiopathogenesis of osteoarthritis. In McCarty DJ, Koopman WL (eds): Arthritis and Allied Conditions, 12th edition, vol 2, pp 1723–1734. Philadelphia, Lea & Febiger, 1993.
60. Evans CH, Brown TD: Role of physical and mechanical agents in degrading the matrix. In Woessner JF, Howell DS (eds): Joint Cartilage Degradation, p 199. New York, Marcel Dekker Inc, 1993.
61. Goetzl EJ, Goldstein IM: Arachidonic acid metabolites. In McCarty DJ, Koopman WJ (eds): Arthritis

and Allied Conditions, 12th edition, vol 1, pp 479–494. Philadelphia, Lea & Febiger, 1993.

62. Robinson DR, Tashjian AH Jr, Levine L: Prostaglandin-stimulated bone resorption by rheumatoid synovia. J Clin Invest 1975; 56:1181–1188.
63. McCarty DJ, Koopman WJ (eds): Arthritis and Allied Conditions, 12th edition, vols 1 and 2. Philadelphia, Lea & Febiger, 1993.
64. Kelley WN, Harris ED, Ruddy S, et al (eds): Textbook of Rheumatology, 4th edition, vols 1 and 2. Philadelphia, WB Saunders Co, 1993.
65. Folkman J, Brean H: Angiogenesis and inflammation. In Gallin JI, Goldstein IM, Snyderman R (eds): Inflammation: Basic Principles and Clinical Correlates, 2nd edition, pp 821–840. New York, Raven Press, 1992.
66. Salter RB: Textbook of Disorders and Injuries of the Musculoskeletal System. Baltimore, Williams & Wilkins, 1985.
67. Stulberg SD, Cordell LD, Harris WH, et al: Unrecognized childhood hip disease: a major cause of idiopathic osteoarthritis of the hip. In The Hip Society: The Hip, Proceedings of the Third Open Meeting of the Hip Society, pp 212–228. St Louis, CV Mosby Co, 1975.
68. Maquet P: Biomechanics of the Knee. Berlin, Springer-Verlag, 1976.
69. Smith BW: Recognizable patterns of human deformation. Identification and management of mechanical effects on morphogenesis. Major Probl Clin Pediatr 1981; 21:1–21.
70. Poole AR: Inflammatory mechanisms in soft tissues. In Leadbeater WB, Buckwalter JA, Gordon SL (eds): Sports-Induced Inflammation, pp 285–299. Park Ridge, IL, American Academy of Orthopedic Surgeons, 1990.
71. Brandt KD, Mankin HJ: Osteoarthritis and polychondritis. In Kelley WN, et al (eds): Textbook of Rheumatology, pp 1355–1373. Philadelphia, WB Saunders Co, 1993.
72. Krane SM: Mechanisms of tissue destruction in rheumatoid arthritis. In McCarty DJ, Koopman WJ (eds): Arthritis and Allied Conditions, 12th edition, vol 1, pp 763–780. Philadelphia, Lea & Febiger, 1993.
73. Harris ED Jr: Pathogenesis of rheumatoid arthritis. In Kelley WN, Harris ED, Ruddy S, et al (eds): Textbook of Rheumatology, 2nd edition, vol 1, pp 886–915. Philadelphia, WB Saunders Co, 1985.
74. Rodosky MW, Fu FH: Induction of synovial inflammation by matrix molecules, implant particles and chemical agents. In Leadbeater WB, Buckwalter JA, Gordon SL (eds): Sports-Induced Inflammation, pp 357–381. Park Ridge, IL, American Academy of Orthopedic Surgeons, 1990.
75. Lipson SJ: The cervical spine. In Kelley WN, et al (eds): Textbook of Rheumatology, 4th edition, pp 1798–1807. Philadelphia, WB Saunders Co, 1993.
76. Cush JJ, Lipsky PE: Cellular basis for rheumatoid inflammation. Clin Orthop 1991; 265:9–22.
77. Bennett RM: Psoriatic arthritis. In McCarty DJ, Koopman WJ (eds): Arthritis and Allied Conditions, 12th edition, vol 2, pp 1079–1094. Philadelphia, Lea & Febiger, 1993.
78. Wright V: Psoriatic arthritis: a comparative radiological study of rheumatoid arthritis associated with psoriasis. Ann Rheum Dis 1959; 20:123–132.
79. Scarpa R, Oriente P, Pucino A, et al: Psoriatic arthritis in psoriatic patients. Br J Rheumatol 1984; 23:246–250.
80. Hunter T: The spinal complications of ankylosing spondylitis. Semin Arthritis Rheum 1989; 19(3): 172–182.
81. Wollheim FA: Ankylosing spondylitis. In Kelley WN, et al (eds): Textbook of Rheumatology, 4th edition, vol 1, pp 943–960. Philadelphia, WB Saunders Co, 1993.
82. Schmid FR: Principles of diagnosis and treatment of bone and joint infections. In McCarty DJ, Koopman WJ (eds): Arthritis and Allied Conditions, 12th edition, vol 2, pp 1975–2001. Philadelphia, Lea & Febiger, 1993.
83. Ho G Jr: Bacterial arthritis. In McCarty DJ, Koopman WJ (eds): Arthritis and Allied Conditions, 12th edition, vol 2, pp 1457–1482. Philadelphia, Lea & Febiger, 1993.
84. Hough AJ: Pathology of osteoarthritis. In McCarty DJ, Koopman WJ (eds): Arthritis and Allied Conditions, 12th edition, vol 2, pp 1699–1722. Philadelphia, Lea & Febiger, 1993.
85. Weisman MH: Arthritis associated with hematologic disorders, storage diseases, disorders of lipid metabolism and disproteinemias. In McCarty DJ, Koopman WJ (eds): Arthritis and Allied Conditions, 12th edition, vol 2, pp 1457–1482. Philadelphia, Lea & Febiger, 1993.
86. Terkeltaub RA: Pathogenesis and treatment of crystal-induced inflammation. In McCarty DJ, Koopman WJ (eds): Arthritis and Allied Conditions, 12th edition, vol 2, pp 1819–1834. Philadelphia, Lea & Febiger, 1993.
87. Levinson DJ, Becker MA: Clinical gout and the pathogenesis of hyperuricema. In McCarty DJ, Koopman WJ (eds): Arthritis and Allied Conditions, 12th edition, vol 2, pp 1773–1806. Philadelphia, Lea & Febiger, 1993.
88. Good AE, Rapp R: Bony ankylosis: a rare manifestation of gout. J Rheumatol 1978; 5:335–337.
89. Ellman MH: Neuropathic joint disease (Charcot joints). In McCarty DJ, Koopman WJ (eds): Arthritis and Allied Conditions, 12th edition, vol 2, pp 1407–1426. Philadelphia, Lea & Febiger, 1993.
90. Resnik D, Niwayama G: Diagnosis of Bone and Joint Disorders with Emphasis on Articular Abnormalities. Philadelphia, WB Saunders Co, 1981.
91. Woo SL-Y, Matthews V, Akeson WH, et al: Connective tissue response to immobility. Correlative study of biomechanical and biochemical measurements of normal and immobilized knees. Arthritis Rheum 1974; 18(3):257–262.

92. Woo SL-Y, Gomez MA, Sykes TJ, et al: The biomechanical and morphological changes in the medial collateral ligament of the rabbit after immobilization and re-immobilization. J Bone Joint Surg 1987; 67A:1200–1211.
93. Noyes FR: Functional properties of knee ligaments and alterations induced by immobilization. The correlative biomechanical and histological study in primates. Clin Orthop 1977; 123:210–242.
94. Bray RC, Shrive NG, Frank CB, et al: The early effects of joint immobilization on medial collateral ligament healing in an ACL-deficient knee: a gross anatomic and biomechanical investigation in the adult rabbit model. J Orthop Res 1992; 10(2):157–166.
95. Frank CB: Ligament. In Zachazewski J, Magee D, Quillan W (eds): Athletic Injuries and Rehabilitation. Philadelphia, WB Saunders Co (in press).
96. Akeson WH, Eichelberger L, Roma N: Biochemical studies of articular cartilage. II. Values following the innervation of an extremity. J Bone Joint Surg 1958; 40A:153–162.
97. Akeson WH, Woo SL-Y, Amiel D, et al: The connective tissue response to immobility: biochemical changes in the periarticular connective tissue of immobilized rabbit knee. Clin Orthop 1973; 93: 356–362.
98. Caterson B, Lowther DA: Changes in the metabolism of the proteoglycans from sheep articular cartilage in response to mechanical forces. Biochem Biophys Acta 1978; 540:412–422.
99. Enneking WF, Horowitz M: The intra-articular effects of immobilization of the human knee. J Bone Joint Surg 1972; 54A:973–985.
100. Helminen HJ, Jurvelin J, Kuusela T, et al: Effects of immobilization for 6 weeks on rabbit knee articular surfaces as assessed by the semi-quantitative stereomicroscopic method. Acta Anat 1983; 115:327–335.
101. Stockwell RA: Structure and function of the chondrocyte under mechanical stress. In Helminen HJ, et al (eds): Joint Loading, pp 126–148. Bristol, Wright, 1987.
102. Palmoski MJ, Perricone E, Brandt KD: Development and reversal of proteoglycan, aggregation defect in normal canine knee cartilage after immobilization. Arthritis Rheum 1979; 22:508–517.
103. Tammi M, Paukkonen K, Kiviranta I, et al: Joint loading induced alterations in articular cartilage. In Helminen HJ, et al (eds): Joint Loading, pp 64–88. Bristol, Wright, 1987.
104. Frost HM: Bone "mass" and the "mechanostat": a proposal. Anat Rec 1987; 219:1–9.
105. Tuukkanen J, Wallmark B, Jalovaara P, et al: Changes induced in growing rat bone by immobilization and reimmobilization. Bone 1991; 12:113–118.
106. Martin RB, Burr DB: Structure, Function and Adaptation of Compact Bone. New York, Raven Press, 1989.
107. Nilas L, Christiansen C: Bone mass and its relationship to age and in menopause. J Clin Endocrinol Metab 1987; 65:697–702.
108. Hough FS: Alterations of bone and mineral metabolism in diabetes mellitus. Part II. Clinical Studies on 206 patients with Type I diabetes mellitus. S Afr Med J 1987; 72:120–126.
109. McNair P. Bone and mineral metabolism in human type I (insulin-dependent) diabetes mellitus. Dan Med Bull 1988; 35:109–121.
110. Einhorn TA, Boskey AL, Gundberg CM, et al: The mineral and mechanical properties of bone in chronic experimental diabetes. J Orthop Res 1988; 6:317–323.
111. Dixit PK, Stern AMK: Effect of insulin on the incorporation of citric and calcium into bones of alloxan-diabetic rats. Calcif Tissue Int 1979; 27:227–232.
112. Dee R: The innervation of joints. In Sokoloff L (ed): The Joints and Synovial Fluid, vol 1, pp 177–204. New York, Academic Press Inc, 1978.
113. Johansson H, Sjolander P: Neurophysiology. In Wright V, Radin E (eds): Mechanics of Human Joints, pp 243–292. Philadelphia, Marcel Dekker Inc, 1993.
114. Zimny ML: Mechanoreceptors in articular tissues. Am J Anat 1988; 182:16–32.
115. Wyke BD: The neurology of joints. Ann R Coll Surg Engl 1967; 41:25–50.
116. Wyke BD: The neurology of low back pain. In Jayson MIV (ed): The Lumbar Spine and Back Pain, pp 265–321. London, Pitman Medical, 1980.
117. Jayson MIV, Dixon A St J: Intra-articular pressure in rheumatoid arthritis of the knee. Ann Rheum Dis 1970; 29:401–408.
118. Knight AD, Levick JR: Time-dependence of the pressure-volume relationship in the synovial cavity of the rabbit knee. J Physiol 1983; 335:139–152.
119. Knight AD, Levick JR: Time-dependence of the pressure-volume relationship in the synovial cavity of the rabbit knee. J Physiol 1983; 335:139–152.
120. Levick JR: Synovial fluid and trans-synovial flow in stationary and moving normal joints. In Helminen HJ, et al (eds): Joint Loading, pp 149–186. Bristol, Wright, 1987.
121. Baxendale RH, Ferrel WR, Wood L: Intra-articular pressures during active and passive motion of normal and distended knee joints. J Physiol 1985; 369: 179P.
122. Helliwell PS: Joint stiffness. In Wright V, Radin E (eds): Mechanics of Human Joints, pp 203–218. New York, Marcel Dekker Inc, 1993.
123. Marks R, Wessel A, Quinney HA: Proprioceptive sensibility in women with normal and osteoarthritic knee joints. Clin Rheumatol 1993; 12:170–175.
124. Skinner HB, Barrack RL, Cook SD, et al: Joint position sense in total knee arthroplasty. J Orthop Res 1984; 1:276–283.

125. Stauffer RN, Chao EYS, Gyory AN: Biomechanical gait analysis of the diseased knee joint. Clin Orthop 1977; 126:246–255.
126. Kidd BL, Gibson SJ, O'Higgins F, et al: A neurogenic mechanism for symmetrical arthritis. Lancet 1989; 11:1128–1129.
127. Melzack R, Wall PD: Pain mechanisms: a new theory. Science 1965; 150:971–978.
128. Woo SL-Y, Buckwalter JD: Injury and Repair of the Musculoskeletal Tissues. Preface. Park Ridge, IL, American Academy of Orthopaedic Surgeons, 1988.
129. Mankin HJ: The articular cartilages, cartilage healing and osteoarthritis. In Cruess RL, Rennie WRJ (eds): Adult Orthopaedics, vol 1, p 207. New York, Churchill Livingstone, 1984.
130. Akeson WH, Amiel D, Woo SL-Y: Physiology and therapeutic value of passive motion. In Helminen HJ, et al: Joint Loading, pp 375–394. Bristol, Wright, 1987.
131. Sokoloff L: Loading and motion in relation to ageing and degeneration of joints: implications for prevention and treatment of osteoarthritis. In Helminen HJ, et al: Joint Loading, pp 412–424. Bristol, Wright, 1987.
132. Kiviranta I, Tammi M, Jurvelin J, et al: Moderate running exercise augments glycosaminoglycans and thickness of articular cartilage in the knee joint of young beagle dogs. J Orthop Res 1988; 6:188–195.
133. Tammi M, Saamanen A-M, Jauhiainen A, et al: Proteoglycan alterations in rabbit knee articular cartilage following physical exercise and immobilization. Connect Tiss Res 1983; 16:163–175.
134. Paukkonen K, Selkanaho K, Jurvelin J, et al: Cells and nuclei of articular cartilage chondrocytes in young rabbits enlarged after non-strenuous physical exercise. J Anat 1985; 142:13–20.
135. Holmdahl DE, Ingelmark BE: Der bau des gelenkknorpels unter verschiedenen funktionellen verhaltnissen. Experimentelle Untersuchung an wachsenden Kaninchen. Acta Anat (Basel) 1948; 6:309–375.
136. Woo SL-Y, Akeson WH: Response of tendons and ligaments to joint loading and movements. In Helminen HJ, et al (eds): Joint Loading, pp 287–315. Bristol, Wright, 1987.
137. Havdrup T, Telhag H: Scattered mitosis in adult joint cartilage after partial chondrectomy. Acta Orthop Scand 1978; 48:424–429.
138. Telhag H: Mitosis of chondrocytes in experimental *osteoarthritis* in rabbits. Clin Orthop 1972; 86:224–229.
139. Salter RB: Continuous Passive Motion (CPM): A Biological Concept for the Healing and the Generation of Articular Cartilage, Ligaments, and Tendons: From its Origination to Research to Clinical Applications. Baltimore, Williams & Wilkins, 1993.
140. Pugh J: Biomechanics of arthritis. In Winter D, Norman R, Wells R, et al (eds): Biomechanics IX-A, pp 135–139. Champaign IL, Human Kinetics, 1985.
141. Knets IV: Adaptation and remodelling of articular cartilage and bone tissue. In Helminen HJ, et al (eds): Joint Loading, pp 251–263. Bristol, Wright, 1987.

CHAPTER 4

Diagnosis and Management of Arthritic Conditions

John Verrier Jones, BCh, FRCP, FRCPC
Alan Covert, MD, FRCP

What is Arthritis?

The term **arthritis**, while strictly referring to any process of inflammation in a joint, is currently used to refer to any process by which a joint is damaged. There are two main processes involved in joint destruction: **inflammation** and **degeneration**. Inflammation may be either acute (typified by acute gouty arthritis) or chronic (rheumatoid arthritis). The process of joint degeneration is seen in **osteoarthritis**. This chapter will (1) describe the typical clinical presentation of some of the diseases representing inflammatory and degenerative joint destruction, (2) outline their pathological features, and outline some aspects of their medical management. Other related conditions, such as **systemic lupus erythematosus** and **scleroderma**, in which arthritis is not always the dominant feature, but which are often associated with joint problems, also will be considered in this chapter.

PHYSICAL THERAPY IN ARTHRITIS, Joan M. Walker, PhD, PT, and Antoine Helewa, MSc(Clin Epid), PT, W.B. Saunders Company © 1996.

Rheumatoid Arthritis

Rheumatoid arthritis (**RA**) is a chronic destructive inflammatory process involving tissues derived from the embryonic mesenchyme, but particularly focusing on diarthrodial (synovial) joints. Rheumatoid arthritis occurs in about 1% of the population of Canada and the United States, and appears equally distributed in whites and blacks. Throughout the world, all populations develop this disease[1]: some surveys report a lower prevalence (0.1%) in rural blacks in South Africa, while prevalence among Finns may be as high as 3%. Yakima and Chippewa Indians have an even higher prevalence. There is no particular relation to environmental factors, despite the widespread belief that RA and similar diseases are prevalent in a cold, damp climate. There is no direct evidence for an infectious etiology and there is no increased frequency of the disease in marital partners of affected subjects.

Age and Sex Distribution

The prevalence of RA increases with age, and may reach 5% above the age of 55. The overall ratio of females to males is 3:1. The female predominance is more marked under the age of 60.

Genetic Influence

When one member of the family has rheumatoid arthritis, the prevalence of RA shows a sixfold increase in siblings. The pattern of inheritance appears to be polygenic. There is a significant association with the HLA antigen DR4 with a relative risk (RR) of approximately 5.

Pathophysiology

The essence of the joint pathology of RA is a persistent **synovitis**—persistent inflammation of the synovial lining tissues.[2] The histologic pattern of the inflammation is characteristic but highly variable. The pattern of inflammation is characterized by exudation, inflammatory cell infiltration, and granulation tissue proliferation. The pattern is not unique to rheumatoid arthritis.

Early manifestations of the synovitis are hyperemia, edema, and an infiltration of lymphocytes around superficial capillaries and venules. Endothelial and synovial lining cells show swelling and other features of cell injury. Exudation of protein-rich fluid, fibrin, and inflammatory cells (particularly neutrophils) occurs into the joint space, which results in joint swelling. Synovial fluid analysis reflects this inflammatory exudation. Within a few weeks, small blood vessels proliferate and focal accumulation of T-lymphocytes is seen in the synovial stroma. Lymphocytes now form into clusters, and lymphoid follicles and plasma cells begin to appear. The inflammatory process in the rheumatoid synovium is accompanied by the deposition of immune complexes and rheumatoid factor in the synovial lining tissues and within the phagocytic cells of the synovium. The presence of immune complexes triggers activation of the complement system, which in turn amplifies the inflammatory response. Macrophages and dendritic cells develop in the rheumatoid synovium. These cells have large amounts of DR antigen on the surface, and one of their principal functions is to present antigen to cells of the immune system. The stimulated immune cells secrete cytokines and recruit other lymphocytes that participate in the process of tissue damage and antibody production.

As the synovial inflammation becomes chronic, the synovial lining and stromal cells proliferate, which leads to a thickened membrane (Fig. 4-1). This proliferative response to chronic inflammation is often referred to as a hyperplastic synovitis or proliferative synovitis. Both types of synovial lining cells (type A histiocyte-like and type B fibroblast-like) are involved in this proliferation.

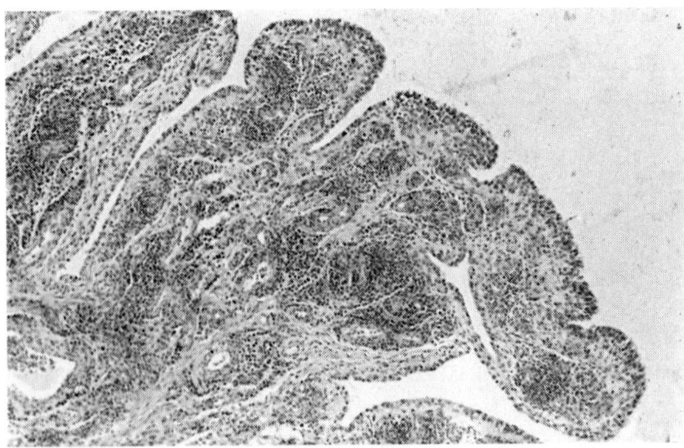

Figure 4-1. An example of chronic rheumatoid synovitis. The surface shows excessive folding and long finger-like processes referred to as villous hyperplasia. Villous hyperplasia is characteristic of chronic rheumatoid synovitis but not diagnostic.

The stromal proliferation (endothelial cells and fibroblasts) is similar to granulation tissue proliferation in response to inflammation at other sites and appears to be part of the process of organization of inflammatory debris, chiefly fibrin.

In the chronic stage of RA, the inflammatory tissue continues to liberate proteolytic enzymes, which directly attack articular cartilage and bone, together with the ligaments and tendons associated with the joint capsule. Bone erosions occur where the synovium attaches to bone, producing characteristic periarticular defects on radiographs. The articular cartilage is gradually destroyed by an inflammatory membrane referred to as **pannus**. It starts at the periphery of the articular surface (at the normal interface between synovium and articular cartilage) and gradually works toward the center. Joint ligaments are weakened by inflammation-induced collagenolysis (Fig. 4-2).

Bone erosion at the articular margin and articular cartilage destruction by pannus (Figs. 4-3 and 4-4) is mediated by powerful proteolytic enzymes released by inflammatory cells, particularly macrophages. These enzymes are able to break down proteoaminoglycans and collagen—the building blocks of the articular cartilage. Cytokines from inflammatory cells modulate chondrocytes in the articular cartilage to be more catabolic than in a physiologic state, contributing to the loss of cartilage.

As the cartilage and bone are damaged, the structure of the joint may begin to crumble and collapse, and the characteristic deformities of late RA develop. In some joints affected by RA, adhesions can form between opposite joint surfaces,

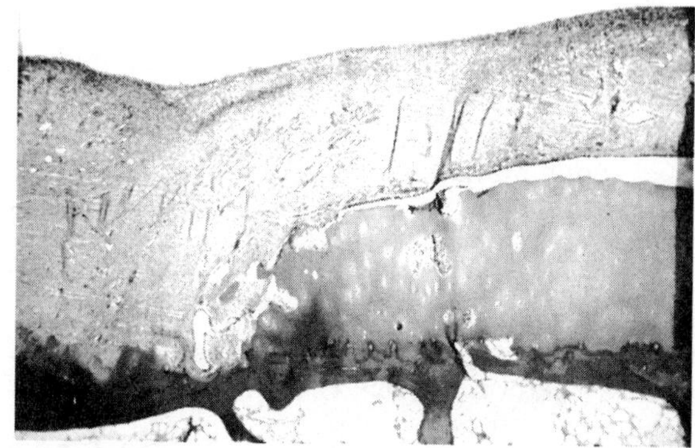

Figure 4-3. A medium-power histologic view in rheumatoid arthritis that demonstrates an inflammatory membrane (pannus) extending from the synovial lining tissues over the articular cartilage.

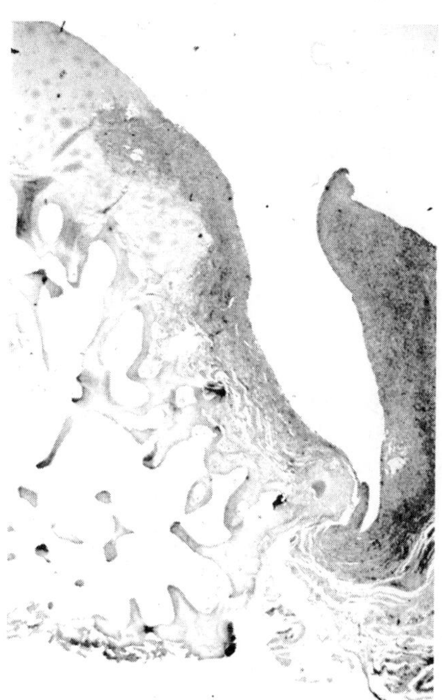

Figure 4-2. A low-power histologic view from the margin of a joint in rheumatoid arthritis. It demonstrates an active synovitis with early destruction of bone and articular cartilage near the attachment of the synovial lining tissues.

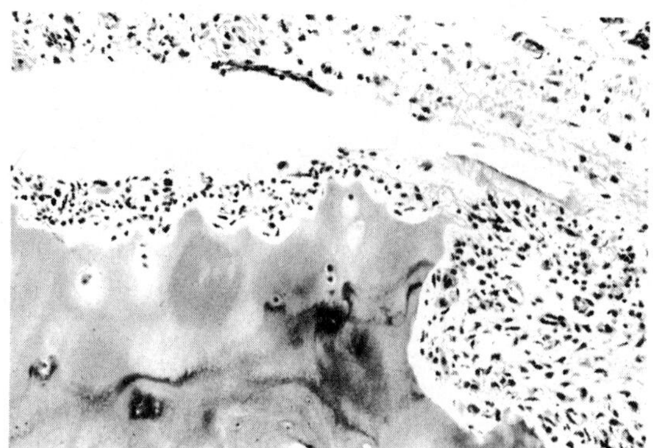

Figure 4-4. A high-power histologic view in rheumatoid arthritis that demonstrates an inflammatory membrane (pannus) actively destroying subjacent articular cartilage.

and fibrous tissue may develop, leading to fibrous ankylosis. This may be followed by bridging between the two joint surfaces with cartilage or bone. In extreme cases the bones may be completely fused (bony ankylosis). As the inflammatory process proceeds, the joint capsule and supporting ligaments can be damaged and destroyed by the enzymes produced, leading to contracture and eventual rupture of tendons. In the final stages, mechanical forces applied to the joint produce the extensive deformities that can be seen in end-stage rheumatoid arthritis.

Clinical Features

The diagnosis of RA is usually based on a typical clinical presentation.[2] The onset is frequently gradual. In the early stages the patient often complains of malaise and fatigue, and joint pain and swelling often begin in a symmetric distribution. The first joints to be involved are often the metacarpophalangeal (MCP) and proximal interphalangeal (PIP) joints in the hands (Fig. 4-5). The distal interphalangeal (DIP) joints are frequently spared. The wrists, elbows, and shoulders are often involved in the early stages.

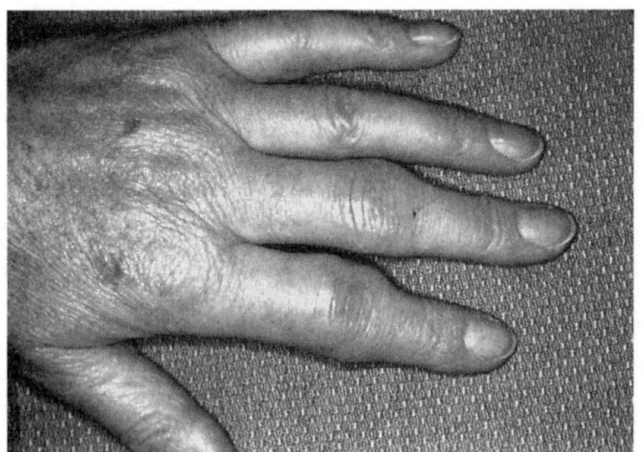

Figure 4-5. Soft tissue swelling occurs as an early finding in rheumatoid arthritis and usually appears as typical fusiform or spindle-shaped enlargement of proximal interphalangeal joints. The second and third fingers of this patient are most involved. These proximal interphalangeal joints are tender and have a limited range of motion. (Reprinted from the Clinical slide collection on the Rheumatic Diseases, copyright 1991, used by permission from the American College of Rheumatology.)

A frequent feature in early RA is stiffness after a period of immobility. This is particularly seen in the morning, after a night's sleep. On waking, patients will often complain of generalized stiffness, and of pain associated with any attempt to move their joints. This early morning stiffness may last for several hours, and is often relieved by taking a hot bath or shower. The duration of morning stiffness gives some indication of the severity of the inflammatory process, and in severe cases may last all day. A less severe form of stiffness may occur after any prolonged period of immobility, such as watching television or riding in a motor vehicle. This is sometimes described as "gelling."

Duration of morning stiffness gives an indication of the severity of the inflammatory process.

As the disease progresses, other joints may become involved. Commonly, the metatarsophalangeal (MTP) joints of the feet, the midtarsal joints, the ankles, and the knees may be affected. Involvement of the hip joint is usually found later in the disease, often several years from its onset. In advanced disease the upper cervical spine may be involved, sometimes with severe consequences. However, apart from this, involvement of the axial skeleton is unusual.

The American College of Rheumatology (formerly the American Rheumatism Association [ARA]) has established a provisional set of criteria for the diagnosis and classification of rheumatoid arthritis (see Table 2-2).[3] These criteria are helpful in comparative and epidemiologic studies but, since RA may develop in a serial or additive fashion, may not all be present initially in an individual patient.

Types of Onset

RA frequently has an insidious onset, often with periods of several months in which joint pain and stiffness develop gradually, followed by symptom-free periods lasting months or years. In some cases complete remission may occur in the early stages, but this becomes less frequent as the disease progresses. While the characteristic clinical course is chronic and progressive, some patients may have a fulminant course, rapidly developing severe disability and handicap.

The functional capacity of patients with RA is divided into four classes in the system developed by Steinbrocker et al (Table 4-1).[4] This is not particularly sensitive to change, and most teams working with RA now prefer to use one of the standardized instruments (such as HAQ, AIMS Appendix III) to assess functional ability and limitation.

Despite the fact that the major organs targeted by RA are diarthrodial joints, RA shows many systemic manifestations, and may involve the blood vessels, skin, heart, lungs, and peripheral nervous system.

Joint Manifestations of RA

As joints become progressively involved in RA, they may initially demonstrate pain, stiffness, and swelling. The swelling is frequently warm on palpation, but usually shows no signs of inflammation or discoloration. The initial swelling may be due to increased synovial fluid, and may be fluctuant. As joint involvement progresses, the synovial lining tissues will proliferate, and the joint swelling will be due in part to the accumulation of tender inflamed synovial lining tissues. In the final stages of the disease, joint destruction and deformity may occur, but there may be little residual evidence of inflammation and pain.

The initial manifestations of the RA are frequently in the smaller peripheral joints. As the disease progresses, inflammation may spread to the larger central joints, while the inflammation in the peripheral joints persists. The progress of the disease usually shows bilateral symmetry, but joints of the dominant side may be more severely involved in the upper limb and, in general, the degree of involvement of a particular set of joints may be related to the extent to which they are used. It has frequently been observed, that when RA develops in a patient with hemiparesis, the paretic side of the body may be almost completely spared from the pain and deformity of arthritis.

Hands

The small joints of the fingers are frequently the earliest to be involved in RA. The MCP and PIP joints of the index and middle fingers are commonly involved in the outset (Fig. 4-6). The initial joint changes may be pain, with tender swelling, and marked stiffness. Patients in the early stages may find it is difficult to flex the fingers, especially after a period of immobility, and it will become increasingly difficult to carry out activities of daily living that involve grasping and manipulating small objects (such as buttons or needles) and heavy objects (such as saucepans). At this stage in the disease, pressure on the joints may evoke tenderness, and pain will occur at the extremes of passive movement (**stress pain**).

As the disease progresses it is likely to involve all the fingers, as well as the thumb. Characteristic deformities develop in the rheumatoid hand, including boutonnière and swan-neck (see Fig. 3-8) deformities in the fingers, together with ulnar deviation and volar subluxation of the MCP joints. This will interfere significantly with all types of hand function, and in the final stages of RA, all power of pinch or grasp may be lost.

Wrists

The wrists are frequently involved in rheumatoid disease, and erosions may develop in all the

Table 4-1. Classification of Functional Capacity in RA*

Class I:	Complete functional capacity with ability to carry on all usual duties without handicaps.
Class II:	Functional capacity adequate to conduct normal activities despite handicap of discomfort or limited mobility of one or more joints.
Class III:	Functional capacity adequate to perform only a few or none of the duties of usual occupation or of self-care.
Class IV:	Largely or wholly incapacitated with patient bedridden or confined to wheelchair, permitting little or no self-care.

*From Steinbrocher O, Traeger CH, Batterman RC: Therapeutic criteria in rheumatoid arthritis. JAMA 1949; 140:659–662. With permission. Copyright 1949, American Medical Association.

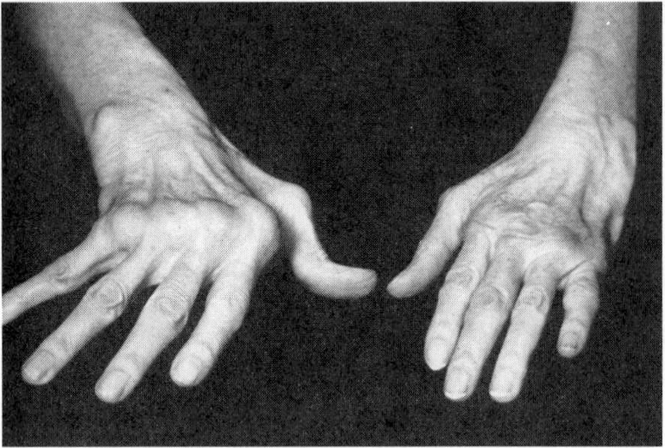

Figure 4-6. Rheumatoid arthritis. Ulnar deviation and subluxation of metacarpophalangeal joints have occurred in the patient's right hand. These joints also appear swollen. Muscle atrophy has developed in the dorsal musculature of both hands. (Reprinted from the Clinical slide collection on the Rheumatic Diseases, copyright 1991, used by permission from the American College of Rheumatology.)

carpal bones. In the process of grasping, there is a greater compression strain over the bones of the radial compartment of the wrist. Consequently, when the carpal bones are damaged by rheumatoid inflammation, the radial aspect of the carpus is likely to collapse first. This will produce radial deviation of the metacarpals. In later stages, the carpal bones may sublux towards the volar surface, and a step-like deformity will appear at the wrist. At this stage, there is increased friction as the extensor tendons run across the distal end of the radius, and stretching or rupture of the extensor tendons becomes a serious possibility.

The synovium of the flexor and extensor tendons also may become inflamed as these tendons run across the carpal bones, and this will increase the likelihood of tendon rupture. Inflammatory change in the flexor tendons may lead to compression of the median nerve as it runs under the flexor retinaculum of the wrist. The ischemia resulting from this may produce **carpal tunnel syndrome**, with pain, numbness, and tingling in the fingers supplied by the median nerve. This is often particularly troublesome at night, and the patient may be able to increase the circulation and obtain some relief by exercising the hands.

Elbows

When the elbows are involved in RA, the proliferating synovium may be felt as a bulge, filling in the notch under the medial and lateral epicondyles of the humerus, as well as the olecranon fossa. As the olecranon fossa becomes obliterated by synovium, extension of the elbow is limited, since the olecranon can no longer be driven home into its fossa. As inflammatory destruction of the elbow continues, the anterior margin of the articular surface of the proximal ulna becomes eroded and destroyed, allowing the olecranon to migrate in a cephalad direction. At the same time, the head of the radius may be eroded.

Shoulders

All components of the shoulder joint may be involved in RA, and in the early stages, glenohumeral involvement may limit abduction of the shoulder. Shoulder effusions may be found. The bursae that surround the shoulder joint, including the subdeltoid bursa and the subacromial bursa, may become inflamed and enlarged. As rheumatoid damage to the shoulder progresses, the tendons of the rotator cuff may become stretched or ruptured, allowing the head of the humerus to migrate upwards across the glenoid. This may progress until the humeral head impinges on the acromion. In the final stages, most glenohumeral movement will be lost, and the shoulder may be limited to a few degrees of abduction and flexion, associated with scapular rotation.

Feet

Involvement of the toes in RA frequently begins with synovitis of the metatarsophalangeal joints (MTP). The MTP joint of the great toe frequently develops a valgus deformity (hallux valgus), while the MTP joints of the remaining toes frequently develop hyperextension or dorsal subluxation. The interphalangeal joints of the toes remain flexed, producing the claw-toes or hammer-toe deformity (Fig. 4-7). Hyperextension of the MTP joints forces the head of the metatarsal against the sole of the foot, and this pressure, associated with walking, may lead to the formation of a callus under some or all of the MTP joints.

The midtarsal joints also may be involved and may lead to increasing pain on walking. Erosions may develop in the talocalcaneal joint, sometimes leading to fusion. The ankle joint may develop synovitis. This will produce tenderness over the medial and lateral joint line of the ankle as well as stress pain on flexion and extension of the ankle

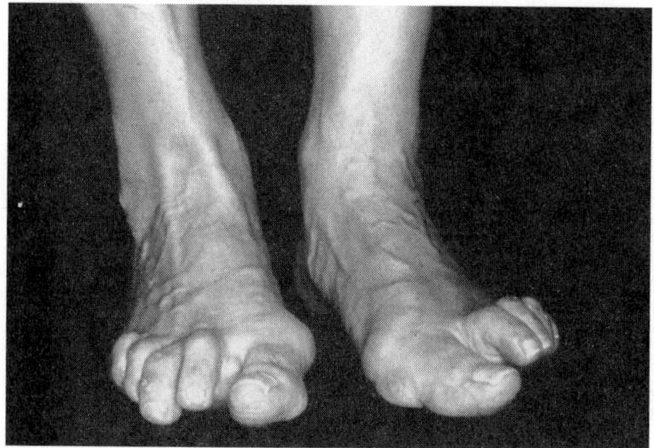

Figure 4-7. The most common foot deformities in rheumatoid arthritis are hallux valgus and hammer toes. The "cock-up" toe deformities in this patient are associated with subluxation of the metatarsophalangeal joints. Superimposed painful corns and bunions result primarily from irritation caused by faulty shoes. (Reprinted from the Clinical slide collection on the Rheumatic Diseases, copyright 1991, used by permission from the American College of Rheumatology.)

joint. As the disease progresses, the ankle frequently develops a valgus deformity.

Knees

In the early stages of RA of the knee, increased secretion of synovial fluid may lead to an effusion, which will produce pain at the extremes of flexion and extension, as well as a visible bulge. If pressure within the knee joint remains elevated, fluid may leak into the semimembranosus bursa, producing a Baker's cyst, which, in turn, may rupture, releasing fluid into the subcutaneous tissues of the calf. The characteristic clinical signs of a ruptured Baker's cyst include a sudden onset of severe calf pain, associated with inflammation and swelling. These symptoms may resemble those found with thrombophlebitis of calf veins. Treatment of this acute condition should focus on the avoidance of weight bearing. The extravasated synovial fluid will eventually be absorbed. If the ruptured Baker's cyst should recur, surgical synovectomy of the knee may be required.

As RA of the knee joint progresses, all three compartments (patellofemoral, medial, and lateral) may be involved. As the subchondral bone of the tibial plateau collapses, valgus or varus deformities of the knee may develop. In the later stages of rheumatoid damage, the knee may demonstrate lateral instability, due to weakness of the medial or lateral collateral ligaments, as well as anterior and posterior instability due to damage to the cruciate ligaments.

Hips

In advanced RA, inflammation of the hip joint may lead to pain and stiffness on all movements of the hip (Fig. 4-8). These symptoms will be particularly severe on weight bearing, and will be exacerbated on climbing stairs and hills. The pain may be referred anteriorly to the groin or posteriorly to the lower back and buttocks. Occasionally, hip pain may be referred downwards as far as the knee. With increasing damage to the hip joint, patients may develop an antalgic gait, and Trendelenburg's sign may become positive. Full extension of the hip may be limited by a flexion contracture, and this may be demonstrated by Thomas' test.

Temporomandibular Joints

Rheumatoid arthritis may involve the temporomandibular joint (TMJ) which, like the peripheral joints, is surrounded by synovial lining tissues. This may lead to increasing pain on chewing tough food, and can, in severe cases, even cause fusion

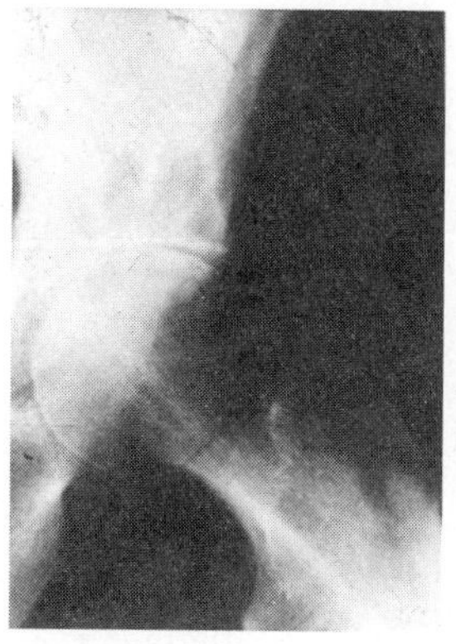
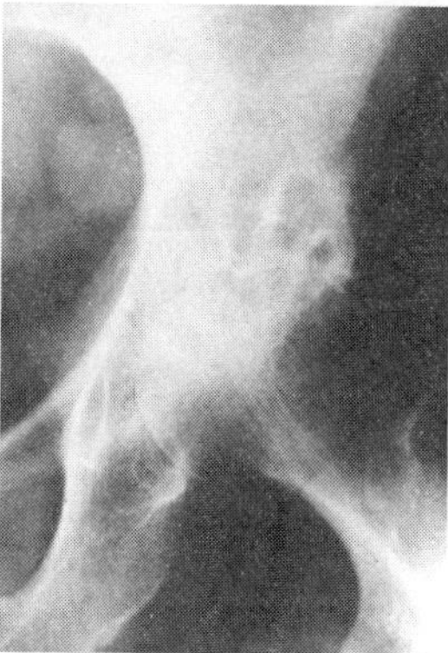

Figure 4-8. The roentgenogram on the left shows advanced joint space narrowing and osteopenia. The roentgenogram on the right reveals severe joint space narrowing, erosive change of adjacent bony margins, subchondral cysts, and osteopenia. Note the absence of reactive bone change. (Reprinted from Berens DL: Roentgen Diagnosis of Rheumatoid Arthritis. Springfield, IL, Charles C Thomas, 1969. With permission.)

or ankylosis of the jaw. When inflammation of the TMJ occurs before puberty, premature fusion of the epiphysis at the mandibular head may lead to impaired growth of the lower jaw (micrognathia). When this is severe, it may require corrective surgery.

Axial Skeleton

The upper cervical vertebrae, in particular C1 and C2, including the odontoid process may be involved in erosive destruction in RA. Subluxation between C1 and C2 may lead to pressure by the odontoid process on the cervical spinal cord, especially on neck flexion. This dangerous complication of RA may lead to neurological symptoms, such as numbness and tingling in the arms or legs, or significant weakness of the extremities. In severe cases, the pressure of the odontoid on the brain stem may cause tetraparesis. Patients found to have significant C1–C2 subluxation may require surgical fusion to immobilize the upper cervical vertebrae. While awaiting surgery, a rigid collar that limits neck flexion will be required. Subluxation also may be found in the lower cervical spine, leading to a "step deformity" of C5, C6, and C7.

Subluxation between C1 and C2 is a dangerous complication of RA and may lead to neurological symptoms, even tetraparesis.

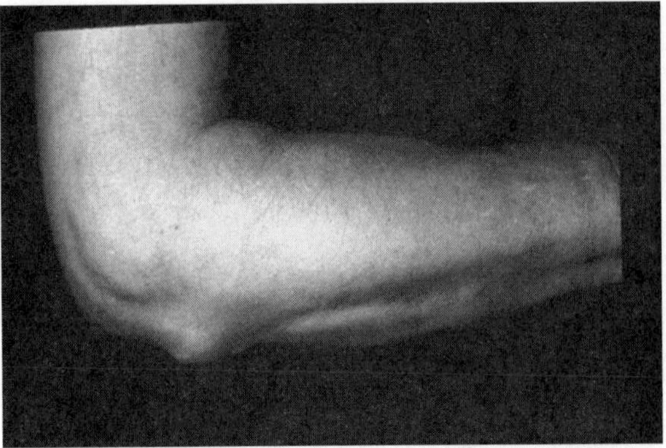

Figure 4-9. A large subcutaneous nodule is located on the extensor surface of the forearm near the elbow. Rheumatoid nodules may be fixed or moveable and are usually nontender. They occur most commonly at the elbow, but also may be found elsewhere, on the feet, fingers, occiput, heels, and buttocks. Nodules occur in about 20% of patients with rheumatoid arthritis and are usually associated with high titers of rheumatoid factor. They also may be seen in patients with other conditions, such as systemic lupus erythematosus and mixed connective tissue disease. (Reprinted from the Clinical slide collection on the Rheumatic Diseases, copyright 1991, used by permission from the American College of Rheumatology.)

Extra-articular Manifestations of Rheumatoid Arthritis

In the early stages of rheumatoid disease, lymphadenopathy, muscle pains and stiffness, fatigue, and fever are frequently seen.

Skin

Rheumatoid nodules, with a characteristic pathological appearance, are found in 25% of patients with RA (Fig. 4-9). They are frequently found in a subcutaneous location, where skin and subcutaneous tissues are subject to pressure. The commonest location is in the region of the olecranon process of the ulna. The nodules are firm and may be tethered either to the skin or to the periosteum, or may be freely mobile in the subcutaneous tissue. Nodules develop gradually and are usually not painful. Other sites at which they may be found include the MCP and PIP joints, and overlying the ischial tuberosities and the heels.

Vasculitis

Inflammation of small or medium size blood vessels may produce vasculitic lesions of the skin, particularly on the legs and fingers. In severe cases, ulcers may develop, particularly on the medial aspect of the ankle. Inflammation of blood vessels is usually associated with the deposition of antigen antibody complexes (immune complexes) in the blood vessel wall. When vasculitis occurs in the blood vessels supplying the peripheral nerves, nerve function may be lost, resulting in isolated areas of numbness and weakness (**mononeuritis multiplex**).

Pulmonary Manifestations

The pleural membranes may be inflamed in RA, leading occasionally to pleurisy, or more commonly to symptomless pleural thickening. Pleural effusions are found at times, and may lead to chest pain and breathlessness. Rheumatoid nodules may occur in the pleura.

The lung itself may be involved in RA, with interstitial fibrosis and pneumonitis. Rheumatoid nodules also may be found in the lung tissue. When RA develops in miners in association with pneumoconiosis, large nodules may be seen within the lungs (**Caplan's syndrome**). At times, these nodules may cavitate.

Cardiac Manifestations

Acute episodes of pericarditis are described in RA. These may lead to chest pain and breathlessness, and may be associated with a pericardial effusion. More commonly, a chronic, constrictive thickening of the pericardium is found in patients with longstanding RA, and this may lead to breathlessness and heart failure. Rheumatoid nodules are occasionally found in the myocardium and on the heart valves.

Sjögren's Syndrome

A chronic inflammatory condition affecting the lacrimal and salivary glands, leading to dryness of the eyes (**xerophthalmia**) or of the mouth (**xerostomia**) is found in up to 15% of patients with RA. Impairment of tear secretion may produce irritation of the eyes, particularly in a hot or smoky environment, and the presence of a sticky secretion on waking may cause discomfort. A simple measure of tear secretion is the Schirmer filter paper test. This may be readily carried out in an ambulatory setting: a sterilized strip of filter paper is folded at one end and allowed to hang from the lower eyelid. The length of paper wetted by tear secretion is measured after 5 minutes, and should be greater than or equal to 15 mm. While not particularly sensitive in mild cases, a reading of less than 5 mm makes the diagnosis of Sjögren's syndrome highly probable. Impaired tear secretion should be treated with the frequent use of artificial tears, to prevent the development of abrasions of the cornea.

Impaired salivary secretions may lead to increased dental caries and increased thirst. Some patients find it helpful to use a salivary replacement fluid such as Moistir.

Sjögren's syndrome may be complicated by enlargement of the salivary glands, and sometimes by secondary infection. Occasionally, in the late stages, lymphoid tumors may develop.

Ophthalmic Manifestations

Rheumatoid arthritis may be accompanied by inflammation of the sclera, which may be either superficial (**episcleritis**) or deep (**scleritis**). The lesions may be initially nodular but, as they develop, may lead to perforation of the sclera (**scleromalacia perforans**). This may be associated with bulging of vitreous onto the surface of the eye, and constitutes a rare but dangerous complication of RA.

Felty's Syndrome

Patients with chronic RA may develop an enlarged spleen, lymphadenopathy, anemia, and neutropenia, together with ulceration of the lower legs. The cause of this is not clear, but treatment with splenectomy may sometimes be helpful in reducing the incidence of infections.

Investigations

Laboratory Investigations

A number of laboratory tests may be helpful in the diagnosis and management of patients with RA.[5] In the initial stages, with mild, symmetrical swelling of small joints, it may be difficult to differentiate between rheumatoid arthritis and self-limiting postviral synovitis, such as may occur following infections with parvovirus or rubella. At this stage, a positive test for **rheumatoid factor**[6] may be helpful to confirm the diagnosis. Rheumatoid factor is an antibody (usually of IgM isotype) that reacts with antigenic determinants on the immunoglobulin molecule: it is thus an anti-antibody. It develops in any situation in which the immune system is subjected to a powerful and prolonged stimulus to antibody production. Rheumatoid factor may be found in the serum of patients with chronic infections, such as infectious endocarditis or malaria. It was first described in rheumatoid arthritis, and occurs in 85–95% of patients. It may, however, be absent in the first 1–2 years of the disease. Low levels are found in normal individuals in population surveys, and it is more common in the aged. As well as appearing in the serum, it also is synthesized by plasma cells in the synovial lining tissues of the inflamed rheumatoid joint, and may contribute to the persistence of inflammation in and around the joint.

In the early stages of RA it is common to find an elevated **erythrocyte sedimentation rate** (ESR), which is a nonspecific indicator of the presence of inflammation. An elevated level of **C-reactive protein** (CRP) has the same significance. As the disease progresses, it is common to find a progressive **normochromic normocytic anemia** and, especially in patients who have chronic gastrointestinal blood loss from nonsteroidal anti-inflammatory drugs (NSAIDs), an **iron-deficiency anemia** may develop, and may require treatment.

In the management of patients with rheumatoid disease, a number of drugs are used that may adversely affect the bone marrow or kidney. In following patients using these medications, it may be necessary to carry out blood and urine tests at regular intervals. These will be considered in more detail later in this chapter.

Radiological Investigations

The radiographic examination of affected joints may show no abnormality in the earliest stages of RA. After several months of inflammation, thinning of the bone may be seen in the vicinity of the synovium (**periarticular osteopenia**).[7] Later, as the inflammation persists, small erosive cysts known as **subchondral erosions** are seen, especially in the MCP and PIP joints of the hands and in the corresponding joints of the feet. These cystic changes correspond to the invasion of the subchondral bone by the rheumatoid synovium. With further progression of the disease, the cartilage is undermined and destroyed (see earlier under "Pathophysiology"), and the radiographs may show further destruction of the underlying bone (Fig. 4-10), together with the characteristic deformities described earlier under "Joint Manifestations." Radiographs may be useful in confirming the diagnosis of RA but are often negative in the first few months. They are also of value in determining the amount of joint destruction in chronic disease.

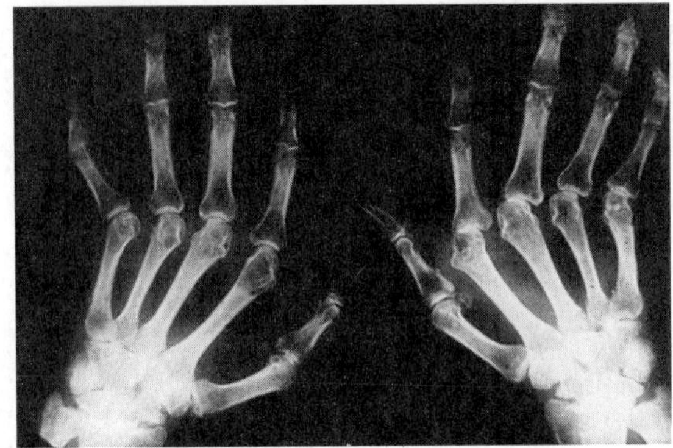

Figure 4-10. The metacarpophalangeal(MCP) joints demonstrate marked narrowing with subluxation and ulnar deviation. Erosions are seen in the metacarpal heads. The proximal interphalangeal (PIP) joints are narrowed, but there is no reactive bone change. Demineralization is present in bones adjacent to the MCP and PIP joints. The carpal spaces are narrowed and the carpal bones and the ulnar styloid processes also reveal erosions. (Reprinted from the Clinical slide collection on the Rheumatic Diseases, copyright 1991, used by permission from the American College of Rheumatology.)

General Management

Rheumatoid disease should be regarded as a systemic disorder, in which the joints are often the primary target organs. However, frequently, inflammation will involve the pericardium, pleura, and blood vessels, and less commonly, the eyes and lungs. This concept of a generalized inflammatory disease becomes important in considering the approach to patient management and life style modification.[8]

The general goals of management must include pain relief, the suppression of the inflammatory process, the maintenance of joint function, and preparation of the patient to cope with the responsibilities and pleasures of daily living. In an ideal setting, this is best achieved by a team approach to patient management. The ideal therapeutic team is likely to include a family physician, a rheumatologist, and members of the health professions with special skills in the care of arthritis, including physiotherapists, occupational therapists, pharmacists, social workers, dieticians, and nursing staff. While it rarely may be possible to assemble trained professionals in each of these fields, this should be the ultimate goal of any organized unit for the treatment of arthritis.

The therapeutic team should be in a position to meet to discuss the patient's immediate problems and short- and long-term requirements, and to propose and implement treatment tactics and strategies. In order to be able to plan and monitor treatment effectively, it will be necessary to begin with a detailed and, preferably, quantitative assessment of the patient's current status. This usefully may begin with a questionnaire to assess function and limitations. Two readily accessible, simple, and well-validated questionnaires are the Health Assessment Questionnaire (HAQ) and the Arthritis Impact Measurement Scales (AIMS) (see Appendix II). It has been repeatedly demonstrated that these measurement instruments, though subjective, show an excellent degree of validity and reproducibility. It also will be necessary, in examining the patient, to indicate the extent of joint involvement. Measures of this will include the painful joint count, the swollen joint count, and the grip strength. These, along with the patient's estimate of the duration of morning stiffness and such laboratory tests as the ESR and CRP, will give a useful assessment of the patient's status at the beginning of therapy.

A full assessment of the impact of the patient's impairment in activities of daily living will be necessary for all aspects of the patient's life. Each member of the therapeutic team will have their own responsibility in assessing components of the patient profile, and the best results will be obtained when this profile is completed at team meetings. Each team member then will be able to set realistic goals to be achieved either during a patient's hospital admission, or subsequently, during follow-up as an outpatient.

In most countries, the patient's first encounter with health professionals is likely to be with the family practitioner. It is vital that family practitioners become knowledgeable and experienced in the management of all types of arthritis, and particularly important that they should be able to make a diagnosis of inflammatory or degenerative joint disease. Once the diagnosis of arthritis is made, the family practitioner should be encouraged to refer the patient at once for appropriate care by a physiotherapist and/or an occupational therapist. The appropriate professional then will be in a position to determine the best management strategies for the early stages of rheumatoid arthritis. There is a strong impression, though no certain proof, that early and appropriate intervention in RA will improve the long-term outlook of this disease.

Medical Management

A detailed description of the clinical pharmacology of the many drugs used in the management of rheumatoid arthritis is presented in Chapter 9. In this section, we shall indicate the tactics and strategies for the use of these drugs in patients with RA.

Nonsteroidal Anti-inflammatory Drugs

NSAIDs play a major role in the early management of rheumatoid disease. These drugs have an important role as central analgesics, but also reduce inflammation peripherally by affecting the enzyme systems responsible for the synthesis of eicosanoids, which are major components of the inflammatory response. NSAIDs alone, however, will not modify the course of rheumatoid disease, and therefore form only the first level of treatment.

The use of NSAIDs is particularly important during the early stages of evolution of rheumatoid arthritis. The course of this disease is notoriously unpredictable and, in community studies, some patients who fulfill the ARA criteria for rheumatoid arthritis will undergo a spontaneous remission. Such remissions are more usually seen in the early phases of the disease, and it is clearly inadvisable to proceed to the more dangerous second-line drugs until it is reasonably certain that the rheumatoid disease has entered a stage of progression. It is still not clear whether cases that show an early remission should be regarded as a mild form of rheumatoid arthritis, or whether they represent a misclassification. It is, for instance, recognized that a number of viruses, including parvovirus and the rubella virus, may produce a self-limiting form of arthritis that may sometimes last for several years.

The selection of an appropriate NSAID will be based on factors such as cost and patient tolerance. All of the drugs in this category are associated with significant adverse effects (see Chapter 9), and since some of these, including especially gastrointestinal side effects, may represent a significant hazard, it may be appropriate to consider prophylactic therapy with one of the cytoprotective agents (such as misoprostol) in high-risk cases.

Second-Line Drugs

A number of agents have been established, in careful clinical studies, to modify the progress of rheumatoid disease, and in some cases to actually slow the onset of radiological bone erosions. These agents were once called "remittive" drugs, but this term has become less popular, since it has become evident that a true remission in rheumatoid disease is relatively uncommon. They appear to modify the course of the disease and are sometimes referred to as disease-modifying antirheumatic drugs (DMARDs). Most of them also have in common the fact that the onset of their therapeutic effect is slow, and also are referred to as slow-acting antirheumatic drugs (SAARDs). Since many of these agents have a high toxicity profile, their use should be restricted to patients whose disease appears to be progressing relentlessly. However, since there is little or no hope of reversing joint damage once it has occurred in rheumatoid disease, their use should not be delayed beyond the point at which joint damage begins to appear.

Antimalarial Drugs The first choice of second-line agent will often be one of the antimalarial drugs, hydroxychloroquine (400 mg/day) or chloroquine (250 mg/day). These agents have been shown to be effective in comparison with placebo in the treatment of patients with early rheumatoid disease. They have a significant profile of adverse effects (see Chapter 9).

The most serious complication, however, is the presence of retinal and corneal lesions, which in extreme cases may lead to total loss of vision. The probability of visual impairment is very significantly reduced if an ophthalmological examination is performed before the antimalarial therapy begins and if repeated tests are carried out at intervals of 6 months. The patient also may be encouraged to use an Amsler grid, a simple printed sheet, supplied free on request by the manufacturers of the antimalarial drugs. This consists of a grid of dots and a fixation point, and may enable the patient to identify small defects in the visual field in between visits to the ophthalmologist. If any visual impairment is suspected, the patient should be encouraged to consult their physician immediately.

While 70% of patients may be expected to show a response to antimalarials during the early stages of rheumatoid disease, 50% will relapse in the first 2 years and 90% after the first 5 years. At this stage, it will be appropriate to consider one of the other second-line drugs.

Gold Salts Intramuscular injections of sodium aurothiomalate will lead to a diminution of disease activity in 60–70% of patients with rheumatoid disease. The usual regimen consists of an intramuscular injection of 10 mg test dose followed by 25 mg 1 week later, and then 50 mg each week. In 30% of patients, significant adverse effects to gold treatment will be seen, such as skin rashes, and more seriously, hematological effects (see Table 9-9).

If patients with rheumatoid disease show a significant therapeutic response to gold, the frequency of injections may be reduced to 50 mg every 2 weeks and subsequently to 50 mg every 3, 4, or 6 weeks. When the rheumatoid disease is in remission, treatment with gold may be discontinued, but it is not clear how often this will be followed by a relapse. If rheumatoid disease shows no response to gold after the administration of a total dose of 1–1.5 g, there is little point in continuing with this treatment. Eighty percent of patients responding to gold will show a reactivation of their disease within 5 years. When this occurs, it will be necessary to consider one of the other therapeutic agents.

Methotrexate Methotrexate, in an initial dose of 7.5 mg/week given orally, is effective in reducing disease activity in 70–80% of patients with RA. Some of the toxic effects of methotrexate (see Table 9-12) may be reduced by the simultaneous administration of folic acid in a dose of 1 mg/day. The dose of methotrexate may be gradually increased, up to a maximum of 30 mg/week, if a therapeutic effect is not achieved at a lower dose.

Methotrexate may cause bone marrow depression and acute pneumonitis, which can occasionally be fatal. Large doses may lead to the development of fibrosis of the liver and eventually to irreversible cirrhosis. Therefore, it is usually recommended that treatment with methotrexate be given only to individuals who agree to abstain completely from the consumption of alcohol. Liver function tests are needed at intervals of 1–3 months and, if abnormal, a liver biopsy will be required.

Sulfasalazine Enteric-coated sulfasalazine, given in a gradually increasing dose up to a total of 1–2 g twice daily, will result in reduced disease activity in 80% of patients with RA. There is a high incidence of adverse effects in the early stages of treatment, but 20% of patients can be expected to show a continuing therapeutic effect with this drug 5 years after starting treatment.

Penicillamine Penicillamine has been shown in controlled studies to reduce the activity of RA when used up to a maximum dose of 750 mg/day. Proteinuria and thrombocytopenia are common side effects, and like other second-line drugs, only 10–20% of patients will still show a useful therapeutic effect after 5 years.

Azathioprine Given in a dose up to 150 mg/day, azathioprine also may be an effective second-line agent in some patients with rheumatoid arthritis. Significant toxicity includes bone marrow depression and hepatitis.

Cyclophosphamide Cyclophosphamide is one drug shown to delay the rate of development of bony erosions on joint radiographs in patients with RA.[9] However, there is a significant increase in the incidence of lymphoreticular neoplasms after long-term treatment of cyclophosphamide. While this drug may sometimes be used to treat RA, it should not be considered unless the patient is fully aware of, and prepared to accept, the long-term risks.

Cyclosporin A Cyclosporin A has been shown to be highly effective in reducing transplant rejection, and also to modify the activity of rheumatoid disease.[10] It has, however, a high profile of toxicity, including the development of hypertension and interstitial nephritis.

Use of Combination Therapy Some rheumatologists now recommend the use of several second-line agents together in the treatment of intractable rheumatoid disease.[10] While this may sometimes be helpful in individual cases, the high level of toxicity associated with each of these drugs limits the use of combination therapy for RA. It is critical for patients being treated with several of these drugs simultaneously to be monitored with great care for the development of serious side effects.

Systemic Corticosteroids Early observations in patients with RA at the Mayo Clinic showed that oral cortisone had a dramatic effect in reducing the pain and stiffness of active RA. In subsequent studies, however, it became clear that the long-term use of systemic corticosteroids was accompanied by severe adverse effects (see Chapter 9). These included osteoporosis, sometimes leading to multiple vertebral collapse, diabetes, thinning of the skin, and lowered resistance to infection. The use of oral corticosteroids became much less popular, but there is now a consensus that small doses of oral prednisone (10–20 mg/day) may be very helpful in severe RA during the period before long-acting drugs have taken effect, or to help in the control of a severe flare of disease activity. A higher dose (40–60 mg/day) may be required to control some of the systemic manifestations of rheumatoid disease, such as vasculitis. Emphasis should be placed on reducing the dose to the lowest acceptable level, to minimize complications.[11]

Intra-articular Corticosteroids Injections of sustained action corticosteroids (see Chapter 9) may be valuable for the short-term control of inflammation in individual joints.[12] While not effective in the long-term control of rheumatoid inflammation, they are of great value during the early stages of the use of long-acting drugs, and their effect may last for several months. Large joints, such as the knee or shoulder, may remain inflamed after smaller joints begin to respond to antimalarial drugs or gold therapy, and in these circumstances, local steroid injections may provide effective control of symptoms. It is usually felt that injections of any individual joint should be limited in frequency, perhaps to once in 6 months, and that any individual joint should probably not be injected more than five times.

Other Intra-articular Agents In patients with resistant inflammatory synovitis of isolated joints that fails to respond to generalized medical treatment, radioactive phosphorus and radioactive yttrium have been used and will sometimes control the local inflammation.

Rheumatoid disease should be regarded as a systemic disorder, in which the joints often are the primary target organs.

Surgical Management

Despite early diagnosis and appropriate management by a therapeutic team, including the use of medications, some patients with RA will prove to be extremely resistant to treatment and may proceed through increasing levels of disability and handicap. When it is impossible to control joint inflammation by physical and medical means, joints may be progressively destroyed. At this stage, surgical intervention and joint replacement would be appropriate. The replacement of the hip joint is now a standard procedure and is often extremely successful when pain and limitation of ambulation are severe enough to prevent the patient from carrying out activities of daily living and impact adversely on the patient's quality of life.

Total replacement of the knee also has become a practicable operation, and will often be required in individuals with serious secondary degeneration of the joint. Following hip or knee replacement, intensive physical therapy (PT) will be required to ensure that the patient regains a full range of movement (ROM) postoperatively. It also is of great importance that patients be educated in the necessity of continuing with ROM exercises in order to maintain mobility after they return to their home environment.

Prosthetic shoulder joints now are becoming available, and while they do not always increase the range of movement to the damaged shoulder, they will frequently reduce pain to a significant extent. Other prosthetic joints, such as the elbow and the wrist, are in an early stage of development and are not, in general, widely used. For serious disease of the ankle and midfoot, surgical fusion is usually recommended. For deformities of the fingers, it is sometimes possible to offer corrective surgery. For deformities of the toes, resection of the heads of the metatarsals and of the base of the proximal phalanges often will result in great reduction in pain and enable the patient to return to normal ambulation.

Some surgeons recommend early synovectomy for the management of inflammatory disease of the small joints of the hand, wrist, and occasionally the knee. Synovectomy of the knee now can be carried out satisfactorily through an arthroscope. Arthroscopic synovectomy may have a role in retarding the progress of a joint when medical measures and intra-articular corticosteroids have failed. For further detail on surgical management, see Chapter 6.

Seronegative Spondylarthropathy

The term **seronegative spondylarthropathy** refers to inflammatory arthritic conditions that have their primary effect on the axial skeleton. They are referred to as "seronegative" because the serological test for **rheumatoid factor**, which is often helpful in diagnosing RA, is characteristically negative in this group of conditions. The primary disorder of this group is **ankylosing spondylitis (AS)**. However, a group of other conditions including Reiter's syndrome, psoriatic arthritis, and enteropathic spondylitis may show significant evidence of inflammatory arthritis of the spine. Juvenile ankylosing spondylitis also is recognized as a distinct clinical entity. Seronegative spondylarthritis often begins by affecting the sacroiliac joints and, later, the apophyseal joints of the spine. The site of insertion of ligaments into bone (enthesis) also may be involved in and around peripheral joints (**enthesitis** or **enthesopathy**). All the diseases in this group show a tendency to occur in families.

Ankylosing Spondylitis

AS is characterized by the gradual development of inflammation and stiffness in the spine. The prevalence of AS varies in different ethnic groups. It is extremely rare in Japanese, in Australian aborigines, and in Black Africans. The prevalence in Caucasians may be 1 per 1,000, while in adult male Haida Indians it may be as high as 4.2 per 1,000. The prevalence is higher in males than in females, by a ratio of about 3:1.[1]

Association with HLA-B27

AS and the related members of the group of seronegative spondylarthropathies tend to occur with increased incidence in families containing an affected member.[13] In 1973, a very significant relation between AS and the histocompatibility antigen HLA-B27 was demonstrated.[14,15] In most studies, up to 90% of Caucasian patients with AS are positive for HLA-B27. A quantitative expression, relating the frequency of AS and B27 is the relative risk. This indicates the probability of developing AS in a population positive for the antigen HLA-B27. In a number of series, the relative risk is found to be between 90 and 100.

Criteria for Diagnosis

Diagnostic criteria for AS were developed in Rome in 1961 and have since been modified (New York 1966, 1984) (see Table 2-2).[1]

Pathology

AS begins as inflammation in the sacroiliac and lower spinal joints. It is said to involve the sacroiliac joints in all patients. In many patients, the process spreads slowly up the spine. The inflammation involves the synovium of the spinal diarthrodial joints but more characteristically targets joint ligaments at insertion points into bone (**enthesitis**).

The enthesitis affects ligaments of the intervertebral disk joints, the apophyseal or facet joints, as well as the paraspinal ligaments. Lymphocytes dominate the inflammatory response. Typically, the inflammation waxes and wanes over many years and eventually subsides. Active inflammation is associated with bone resorption (erosion) at the enthesis. Inflammation is followed by a "healing phase," where fibrous ligaments are transformed to bone beginning at the insertion point. The end point is bony fusion, or ankylosis (hence the name **ankylosing** spondylitis). Ossification of the annulus fibrosus (Fig. 4-11) and spinal ligaments is the pathological basis for the radiographic "bamboo spine" seen in advanced disease (Fig. 4-12). Bony fusion of spinal joints (Fig. 4-13) produces the marked limitation of spinal movement in late disease.

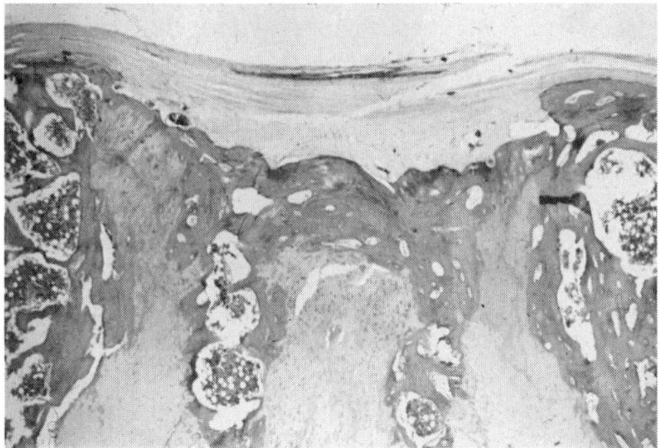

Figure 4-11. A low-power histologic view of bridging ossification in the outer fibers of the annulus fibrosis in ankylosing spondylitis (a syndesmophyte).

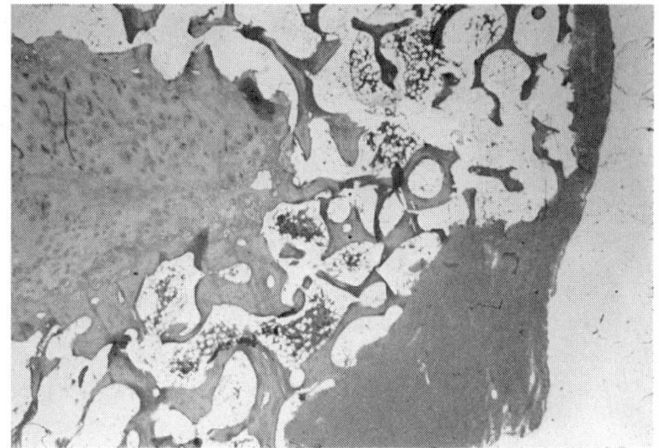

Figure 4-13. A low-power histologic view of the periphery of a facet (apophyseal) joint in advanced ankylosing spondylitis. This demonstrates peripheral ossification. The location of the ossification is compatible with bony transformation of the joint capsule—a late outcome of enthesitis involving the joint capsule ligament.

Peripheral synovial joints are sometimes involved, exhibiting a rheumatoid-like synovitis. Peripheral diarthrodial joint involvement is much more likely to develop into bony ankylosis in AS than in RA. This is likely due to enthesitis-associated joint capsule ossification, which resembles the process that occurs in the capsular ligaments of the spinal apophyseal joints.

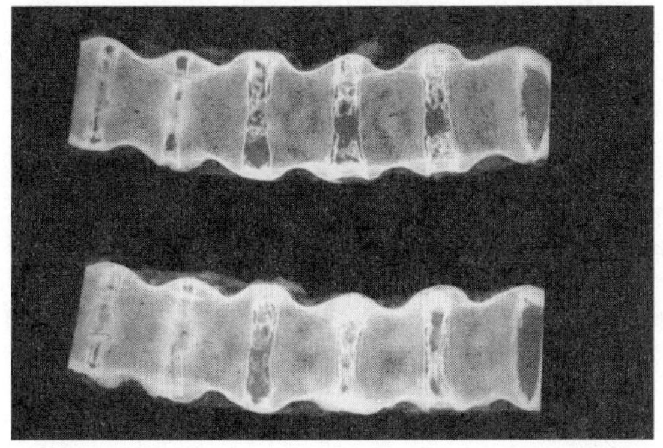

Figure 4-12. A radiograph of a coronal plane slab of the spine in ankylosing spondylitis (AS) that shows the characteristic changes of syndesmophyte formation or bambooing. Ossification is present deep to the lateral collateral ligaments, follows the contour of the intervertebral disk spaces, and involves the outer layers of the intervertebral disk (annulus fibrosus). In contrast, degenerative spurs will extend almost at right angles to the vertebral bodies rather than snugly following the contour of the disk as seen in AS.

Inflammation of peripheral entheses also is characteristic. An example is inflammation at the insertion of the Achilles tendon into the posterior aspect of the calcaneum, and at the insertion of the plantar fascia into the plantar surface of the calcaneum. Such involvement may lead to the formation of a painful bony spur.

Clinical Presentation

The onset of AS is usually insidious, and is most frequently seen in males under the age of 40.[16] The symptoms are initially in the lumbosacral region, with pain and stiffness in the lower back. In common with other forms of inflammatory arthritis, these symptoms are usually worse after a period of immobility, and are frequently most severe on rising in the morning. As in RA, the early-morning stiffness may be relieved by exercise and is frequently alleviated by a hot bath or shower. Initially, the stiffness may be due to muscle spasm associated with underlying joint inflammation, though in the later stages the apophyseal joints may develop fibrous or bony ankylosis. In the final stages of this disease, bony fusion between vertebrae may restrict all movement of the spinal column to a few degrees of flexion and extension in the upper cervical spine (Fig. 4-14).

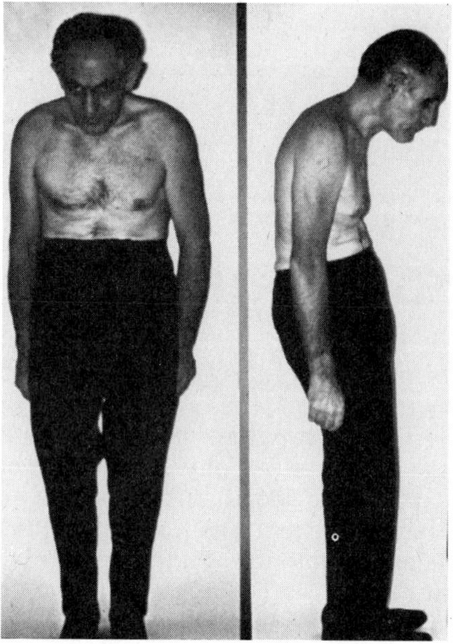

Figure 4-14. On the left a frontal view of a patient with ankylosing spondylitis (Marie-Strümpell disease) demonstrates the characteristic upward gaze of the eyes when looking straight ahead, necessitated by the flexion deformity of the neck. These postural changes are typical of the more advanced forms of this disease. The lateral view of the same patient demonstrates forward protrusion of the head, flattening of the anterior chest wall, thoracic kyphosis, protrusion of the abdomen, and flattening of the lumbar lordotic curvature. Slight flexion of the hips is also present due to hip involvement. The partially fixed thoracic cage is primarily responsible for the muscular atrophy seen in the chest muscles. (Reprinted from the Clinical slide collection on the Rheumatic Diseases, copyright 1991, used by permission from the American College of Rheumatology.)

Physical Examination

In the early stages, patients with AS may show loss of lumbar lordosis due to muscle spasm. There will be limitation of forward flexion of the lumbar spine that can be demonstrated by the Schöber test. In the later stages, the sacroiliac joints may become fused, and the "tide" of inflammation may spread slowly upwards through the lumbar, thoracic, and cervical spine. As the disease progresses, there will be increasing loss of mobility of successive segments of the spine.

Peripheral Joint Involvement

Thirty percent of patients with AS may develop enthesopathy or peripheral joint involvement. Enthesopathy will frequently affect the insertion of the Achilles tendon into the posterior surface of the calcaneum, or the origin of the long plantar ligament from the undersurface of the calcaneum. The patellar tendon also may be involved at its insertion into the tibia. Peripheral involvement is frequently seen in the lower limb, where inflammation may be asymmetric, frequently involving the ankle or knee.

While synovitis in the affected joint may be persistent, with significant effusion and limitation of movement, it is less common to develop severe deformity and erosions in the peripheral joints. Ankylosis, however, is sometimes seen in the lower limbs, particularly in the smaller joints of the feet. While involvement of the hip joint is less common, it can occasionally be severe and progressive, leading to disability and requiring total joint replacement. See Chapter 8 for description of spinal assessment techniques.

Radiological Changes

The earliest radiological change in the sacroiliac joints may consist of blurring of the joint margin, with erosive changes and sclerosis of the underlying bone (Fig. 4-15). As sacroiliitis progresses, the sclerosis becomes more marked and the joint is narrowed as cartilage is lost. In the final stages, the sacroiliac joints are completely obliterated, and the sacrum and ilium are joined by bony fusion (Fig. 4-16).

As the disease progresses, early changes may be seen in the lumbar spine with squaring of the vertebral bodies and the development of erosions at the anterior margin of the vertebral body, known as Romanus lesions. The outer fibers of the annulus fibrosus become calcified and then ossified, and vertebral bodies become linked by syndesmophytes. The final stage is the development of bony fusion of the entire spinal column, producing the radiological appearances known as "bamboo spine" (see Fig. 4-12). This ossification may extend to the posterior longitudinal ligament and the interspinous ligament. In some cases, the only movement is in the superior cervical spine.

Laboratory Findings

In the early stages, the ESR may be raised. The rheumatoid factor test is characteristically nega-

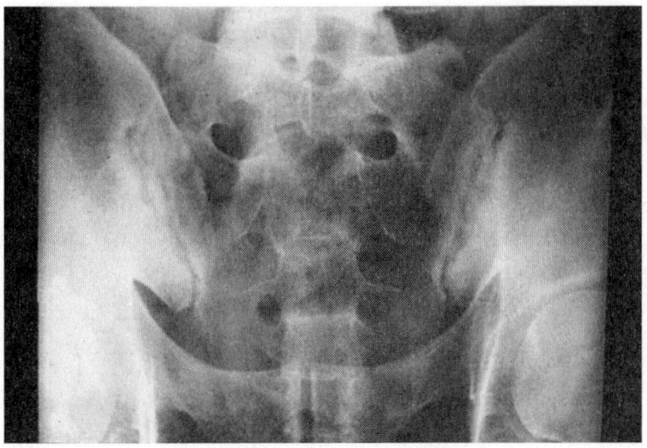

Figure 4-15. The sacroiliac joints are shown in Ferguson projection with the patient supine and the tube angled caudocephalad approximately 30 degrees. This allows the entire length of the sacroiliac joints to be viewed symmetrically. Sacroiliac joints should not be studied in the anteroposterior projection of the pelvis only; supplementary oblique views should be obtained for accurate evaluation. In this instance subchondral bone resorption and irregularity of the sacroiliac joint spaces give rise to the so-called rosary bead effect and apparent pseudowidening. Increased sclerosis is present around the sacroiliac joints. These are relatively early changes. (Reprinted from Berens DL: Roentgen features of ankylosing spondylitis. Clin Orthop 1971; 74:23. With permission.)

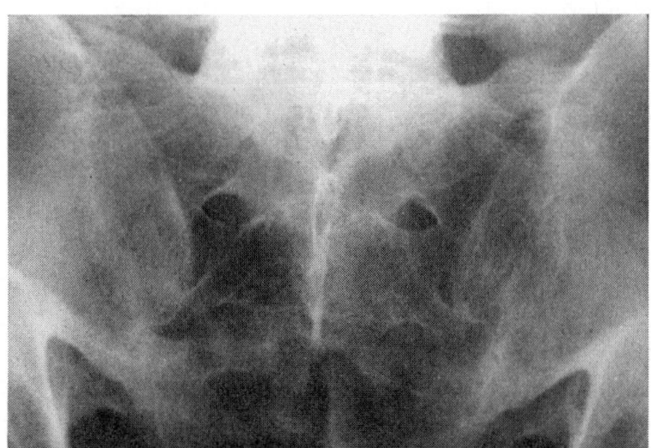

Figure 4-16. There is almost complete obliteration of the sacroiliac joints. Bony trabeculae are noted crossing the residual sacroiliac joint space. There is no gross sclerosis at this time. A moderate degree of osteopenia is present. (Reprinted from Berens DL: Roentgen features of ankylosing spondylitis. Clin Orthop 1971; 74:23. With permission.)

tive. Testing for the HLA-B27 antigen is not usually necessary, since the diagnosis may be established on clinical and radiological grounds.

Seronegative inflammatory arthritic conditions have a primary effect on the axial skeleton, and the serological test for rheumatoid factor is characteristically negative.

Nonarticular Manifestations

Constitutional Symptoms In the early stages, patients may note features of a systemic illness, including fever, weight loss, and fatigue. A mild anemia may develop.

Iritis An inflammatory response in the anterior compartment of the eye (the uveal tract) may be seen in up to 20% of patients with AS. This may eventually lead to scarring of the uveal tract, with secondary glaucoma. Early diagnosis and treatment of eye involvement is essential to prevent serious visual impairment. Patients positive for the HLA-B27 antigen have an increased frequency for anterior uveitis even in the absence of a diagnosis of AS.

Aortic Insufficiency Cardiac involvement, particularly leading to aortic incompetence, may develop late in the course of AS, and has been reported in up to 10% of patients followed for 30 years. In about 1% of patients, cardiac enlargement may be found, and atrioventricular conduction block has been described as a rare complication.

Pulmonary Fibrosis Chronic fibrotic changes may develop in the upper lobes of the lungs, late in the course of AS, in 2–5% of patients. Inflammatory changes and fusion may involve the costovertebral joints, leading to impaired chest expansion and a depression in pulmonary ventilation.

Management

The management of AS requires a deliberate effort of collaboration between physician and physiotherapist. The major long-term disability associated with this disease is the development of severe and permanent deformity of the spine, associated with a lordotic posture. If this is allowed to progress, the patient will have great difficulty in walking because of limitation of the field of forward vision, and will have increasing impairment of respiratory capacity because of ankylosis of the costovertebral joints. It is essential, therefore, that health professionals be involved from the beginning in a sustained educational program to teach the importance of postural back exercises (especially involving extension) to maintain spinal alignment as near to normal as possible. For detail of physical therapy management, see Chapter 15. NSAIDs may be required to control the pain and stiffness (see Chapter 9), and features such as uveitis may require treatment with topical steroids.

Reiter's Syndrome

Hans Reiter described in 1916 a patient who, following an episode of abdominal pain and diarrhea, developed symptoms of arthritis, urethritis, and conjunctivitis. This combination of symptoms is now described as Reiter's syndrome.[17] The syndrome is characteristically precipitated by an infectious episode, which may be either genitourinary or gastrointestinal. The genitourinary infection may be caused by *Chlamydia* species. Gonococcal infections do not cause Reiter's syndrome. A preceding gastroenterstinal infection with *Shigella*, *Salmonella*, *Campylobacter*, or *Yersinia* may provoke Reiter's syndrome, including urethritis. In this case, the arthritis is often described as "reactive," since the infected organisms are not found in the joint. The term "reactive arthritis" is often used as a synonym for Reiter's syndrome.

Pathogenesis

HLA-B27 is found in 80–90% of patients with Reiter's syndrome. The relative risk is estimated at about 10–15 higher in those with HLA-B27.

Clinical Manifestations

Joint involvement usually occurs after a delay, following urethritis or diarrhea, and conjunctivitis. Weight-bearing joints are most commonly affected, and the distribution may be asymmetrical. There is often swelling, redness, and pain of affected joints, but the arthritis may vary from mild to severe. While the joint involvements are usually transient, 20–30% may develop a chronic relapsing arthritis, and a small percentage may even progress to AS. As in AS, patients with Reiter's syndrome frequently develop enthesopathy. Periostitis may develop in the fingers, giving a generalized diffuse swelling of a finger or toe that is sometimes referred to as a "sausage" digit.

Skin Lesions

Painless ulcers on the tip of the penis and around the urethral meatus are common (**balanitis circinata**). Lesions may develop on the soles of the feet or the palms of the hands, presenting initially as papules and later developing into hyperkeratotic lesions (**keratoderma blennorrhagica**). Dystrophic lesions in the nails of the fingers and toes also may be seen.

Radiologic Changes

Sacroiliitis may be found in early Reiter's syndrome and is often asymmetrical. Erosions may occur at the site of insertion of tendons and ligaments into bones.

Management

NSAIDs are used for treating the arthritis. In severe or recurrent cases, methotrexate, azathioprine, or sulfasalazine may be considered.

Enteropathic Arthritis

Ulcerative colitis and Crohn's disease (inflammatory bowel disease) may be associated with a peripheral arthritis and spondylitis resembling those seen in Reiter's syndrome.[18] The clinical course may be influenced by the course of the inflammatory bowel disease, and treatment of the joint symptoms will resemble that for Reiter's syndrome. NSAIDs, however, may provoke severe gastrointestinal hemorrhage in patients with inflammatory bowel disease, and should be avoided. In severe cases, corticosteroids may be required.

Psoriatic Arthritis

Psoriasis is a relatively common skin condition, found in about 1.2% of the general population.[19] Almost 7% of patients with psoriasis may have arthritis. A number of HLA antigens are associated with psoriasis. When psoriatic patients carry the antigen HLA-B27, there is a higher risk for the development of psoriatic spondylitis. When they are positive for the antigen HLA-DR4, they are more liable to develop an arthritis similar to that found in patients with rheumatoid disease.

Pathology

Different patterns of arthritis are seen in patients with psoriasis. One form, affecting the sacroiliac joints and the joints of the lower spine, has pathology similar to that seen in AS, and enthesitis is prominent. With chronicity and "healing," there is a tendency to bony spur formation and bony ankylosis. Spinal arthritis in patients with psoriasis is often associated with HLA-B27 and is frequently described as "spotty" or asymmetric. Extensive bony ankylosis is not common.

Arthritis of hand joints also is common. The DIP joints are prominently involved in one form that is usually associated with severe psoriatic nail involvement. Psoriatic arthritis of the small joints of the hands appears to start as a synovitis. The process leads to progressive destruction of the articular surface. Sometimes, the joint inflammation leads to prominent bone destruction (resorption) adjacent to the joint. The destroyed bone is replaced by granulation tissue (reparative fibrous tissue).

Patterns of Presentation

The commonest age for the occurrence of psoriatic arthritis is between the ages of 30 and 55. Males and females are affected in about equal proportion and the pattern of joint disease is very variable.

Group 1—Classic Psoriatic Arthritis In this form, there is a predominant involvement of the DIP (Fig. 4-17), often associated with nail lesions (Fig. 4-18).

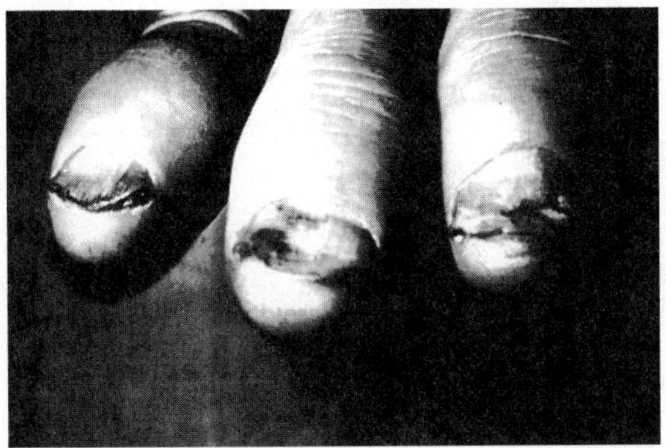

Figure 4-17. Swelling and deformity of the distal interphalangeal joints and uplifting of the distal portion of the nails (onycholysis) are typical of psoriasis. Fragmentation and brown discoloration of the nails are present; total nail destruction may occur. (Reprinted from the Clinical slide collection on the Rheumatic Diseases, copyright 1991, used by permission from the American College of Rheumatology.)

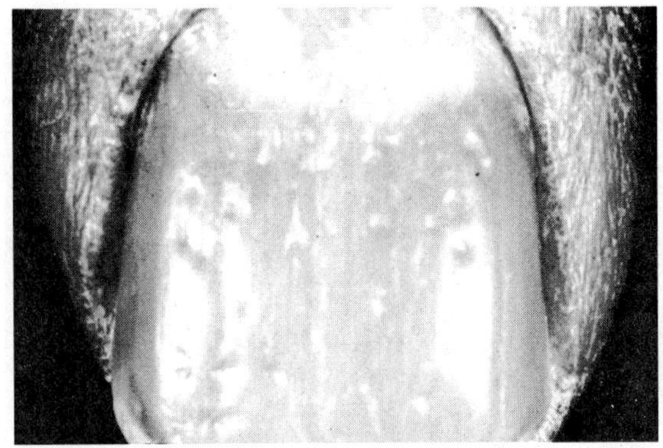

Figure 4-18. Pitting of the nail is a characteristic finding in many patients with psoriasis and is often associated with arthritis of the distal interphalangeal joints. (Reprinted from the Clinical slide collection on the Rheumatic Diseases, copyright 1991, used by permission from the American College of Rheumatology.)

Group 2—Arthritis Mutilans This is associated with severe, destructive lesions of the fingers, often associated with radiological changes known as the "pencil-and-cup" deformity.

Group 3—Symmetric Polyarthritis This form resembles rheumatoid arthritis, and often involves the joints of the fingers symmetrically. In contradistinction to rheumatoid arthritis, the DIP joints are frequently involved. Bony ankylosis frequently develops in psoriatic arthritis of the digits.

Group 4—Oligoarticular Arthritis In this form of the disease there is an asymmetric involvement of individual digits, frequently involving the MCP or MTP, PIP, and DIP joints of a single finger, giving marked swelling of the whole digit with the appearances of a "sausage" finger or toe (Fig. 4-19).

Group 5—Psoriatic Spondylitis This is found particularly in patients positive for the HLA-B27 antigen. Sacroiliitis can occur frequently in an asymmetrical pattern, and stiffening and ossification of the spine can occur, sometimes in an unpredictable pattern.

Management

NSAIDs may be used in the early stages of the disease. Intra-articular corticosteroids may be of

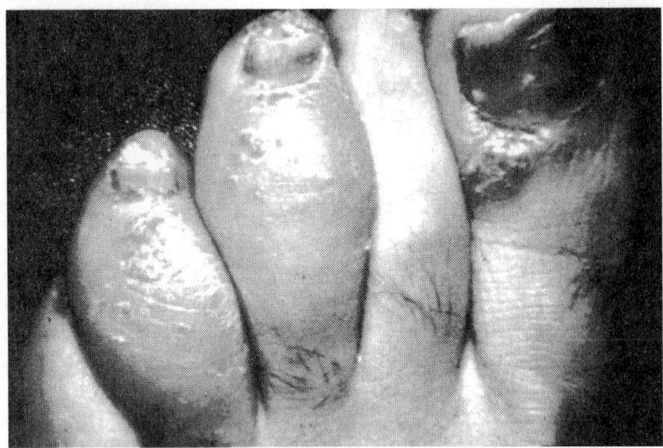

Figure 4-19. Psoriasis can be seen involving the first, third, and fourth toes. This is accompanied by psoriatic arthritis of interphalangeal joints of the third and fourth toes. The sausage shape of these toes is caused by soft tissue swelling more marked than that usually seen in rheumatoid arthritis. (Reprinted from the Clinical slide collection on the Rheumatic Diseases, copyright 1991, used by permission from the American College of Rheumatology.)

benefit when a small number of joints are involved. If the disease becomes chronic, gold or methotrexate may be used. Aggressive treatment for the psoriasis, such as the use of extended exposure to ultraviolet light, may sometimes help to control the associated arthritis. The presence of extensive skin lesions will often limit the physiotherapist in the choice of treatment modalities, since such patients will usually not be suitable for hydrotherapy.

Osteoarthritis

Osteoarthritis (OA) (**degenerative joint disease, osteoarthrosis**) is characterized by thinning and destruction of the hyaline cartilage of joints, followed by remodeling of the underlying bony surfaces. Over the years there has been a debate over which term to use to designate OA. *Osteoarthritis*, with "-itis," suggests an inflammatory reponse, while *osteoarthrosis* is preferred by British writers in recognition that, in comparison to rheumatoid arthritis, OA is essentially noninflammatory. In this text, the term osteoarthritis is used. Workers today recognize OA of totally unknown cause to be *primary OA* and within that category recognize primary generalized and primary inflammatory forms of OA. *Secondary OA* is a form with clearly defined and underlying causative factor(s); for example, joint hypermobility, and hypo- and hyperthyroidism.

In a British radiological survey it was found that 80% of the population above the age of 55 have a significant amount of OA.[20] The prevalence of the disease increases steadily with age. Men outnumber women before the age of 45, and above the age of 45, women show a higher prevalence than men.

Repeated heavy stress on joints as a result of occupation may increase the prevalence of OA. OA of the fingers, knees, and elbows has been found with higher frequency in dockworkers when compared with civil servants. The dominant right hand is frequently more severely involved than the left hand. There is, however, little evidence that marathon running is associated with an increased incidence of OA in the knees or hips. Genetic factors may be involved in some forms of OA, especially with symmetrical nodular involvement of the DIP and PIP joints of the hand. This form of OA is found more commonly in women and appears to have a strong familial association. Recently, one form of familial OA has been associated with a genetic defect in collagen synthesis.[21]

Biochemical Changes in Early Osteoarthritis

Animal models of OA make it possible to study the earliest changes in osteoarthritic cartilage using biochemical methods. In dogs, in whom OA can be produced by surgical division of the anterior cruciate ligament, the earliest biochemical change is an increase in the water content of cartilage. The proteoglycans of cartilage are held in position and restrained by arcades of collagen fibers, tethered to the subchondral bone, and looping upwards to the articular surface. It is thought that early failure of the collagen fibers may enable the proteoglycans to attract more water molecules, and to swell. In the next stage of degeneration, the proteoglycans of cartilage contain a lower concentration of keratan sulfate than normal, while the concentration of chondroitin sulfate increases. In subsequent changes, proteoglycan concentration in the cartilage falls. At this stage the cartilage loses its elasticity, becomes less resistant to repeated mechanical stresses, and the process of disintegration begins.[22]

Pathology

The essence of OA is a noninflammatory degeneration of articular cartilage. Early events include increased water content and increased turnover of the chondroid matrix. Peripendicularly oriented fissures appear in the superficial zone of the cartilage and gradually extend deeper (Fig. 4-20). These fissures promote detachment of small articular cartilage fragments into the joint space, where they are eventually degraded. Progressive thinning of the articular cartilage occurs and the end stage is full-thickness loss of articular cartilage. At this point, the articular surface is composed of a bony articular plate polished from the grinding interaction of bone articulating with bone (Fig. 4-21).

Concurrent with the loss of articular cartilage is a profound remodeling of the juxta-articular bone, which gradually leads to thickened (sclerotic) bone. The shape of the end of the bone often changes with this remodeling. A characteristic component is the formation of new bone at the joint margin (osteophyte or a bony spur). The thickened bony articular plate that forms the articular surface in advanced OA often develops microfractures. These microfractures are important in the pathogenesis of small spherical defects (geodes) in the subarticular bone that are a frequent finding in advanced OA. Microfractures also may result in bone debris being dislodged into the joint space (Figs. 4-22 and 4-23). Such debris can induce a secondary synovitis that is usually mild. This kind of secondary synovial response is often referred to as a "detritus synovitis" (see Fig. 4-20).

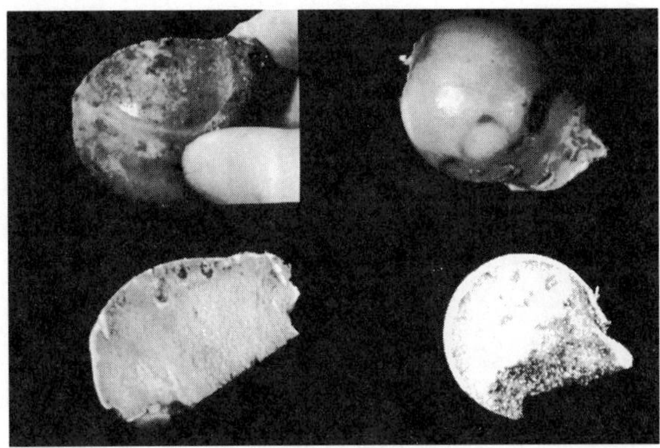

Figure 4-21. A composite gross photograph demonstrating an external and cut surface view of two femoral heads. The left-sided specimen illustrates typical changes of "end-stage" osteoarthritis including extensive loss of articular cartilage, an articular surface composed of polished bony articular plate, and a remodeled bone end with osteophyte formation. The right-sided specimen is a normal femoral head (from a subcapital fracture) for contrast.

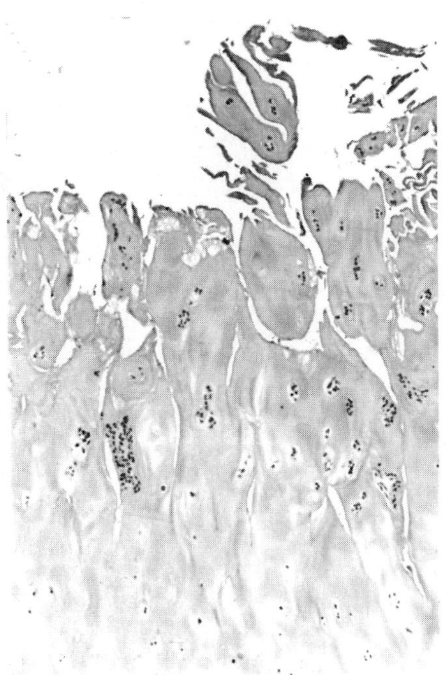

Figure 4-20. A medium-power histological view of the superficial zone of articular cartilage demonstrating characteristic osteoarthritic degeneration including dislodgement of small cartilaginous fragments.

Clinical Features

Joints affected early in the course of OA will tend to be painful after sustained use.[23] Resting will frequently relieve the pain. However, sometimes an inflammatory component can be significant in OA, and many patients will also complain of pain and stiffness on rising in the morning, and after periods of immobility. As the degeneration progresses, any active or passive movement may be painful, and later, pain may occur at rest. In the later stages of OA, where hyaline cartilage has been damaged, patients may complain of a sensation of crunching or crackling on joint movement; this may be detected on palpation or auscultation as crepitus. Degenerative changes of the weight-bearing joints (particularly the hips and knees) tend to occur more frequently in obese individuals.

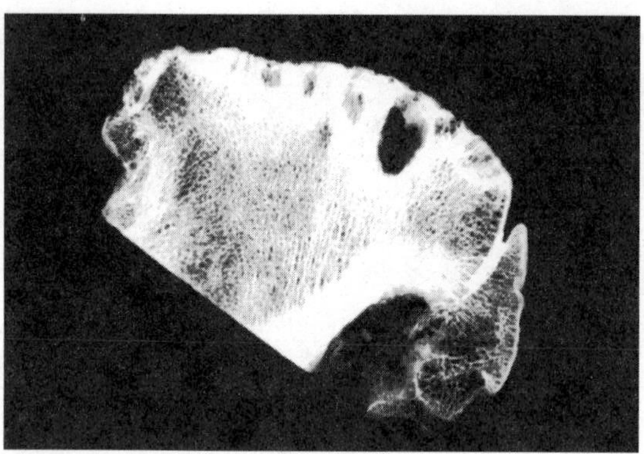

Figure 4-22. A photograph of a radiograph of a coronal slice of a femoral head with "end-stage" osteoarthritis. It illustrates flattening of articular surface contour, osteophyte formation, thickening of the bony articular plate, and subarticular cysts (spherical defects in the bone associated with microfractures).

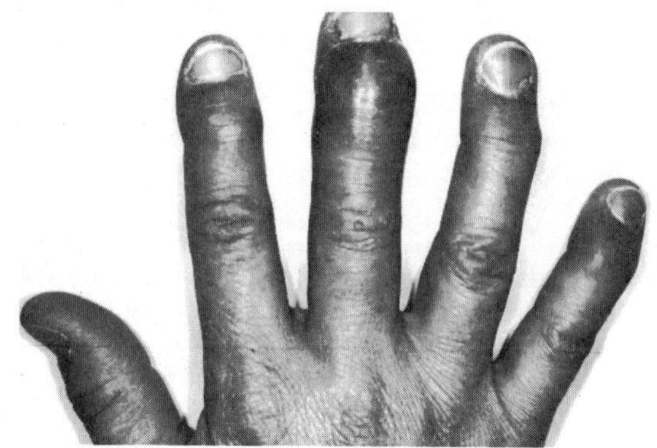

Figure 4-24. Heberden's nodes are present on all the distal interphalangeal joints. The distal joint of the middle finger is red and inflamed. Inflammatory changes consisting of tenderness and soft tissue swelling may occur in early stages of Heberden's node formation, but this reaction usually subsides in the more chronic stages. (Reprinted from the Clinical slide collection on the Rheumatic Diseases, copyright 1991, used by permission from the American College of Rheumatology.)

Hands The DIP and PIP joints of the fingers are commonly affected by OA. Osteophytes formed on the DIP joints are Heberden's nodes (Fig. 4-24). Osteophytes on the PIP joints are Bouchard's nodes (Fig. 4-25). The soft tissues overlying osteophytes may become inflamed, and cyst-like swellings may appear on the digit. As degeneration proceeds in the finger joints, the distal segments of the finger may develop radial or ulnar deviation. The MCP

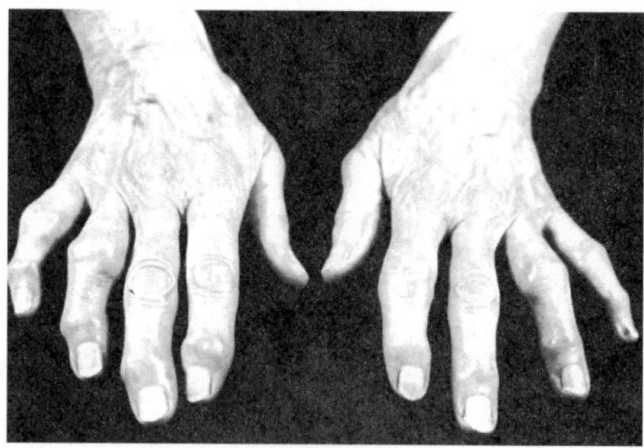

Figure 4-25. Bony enlargement can be seen in distal and proximal interphalangeal joints. The changes in proximal interphalangeal joints (Bouchard's nodes) and distal interphalangeal joints (Heberden's nodes) are common findings in degenerative joint disease of the hands. These changes are more frequently found in women after menopause and often show a genetic predisposition. (Reprinted from the Clinical slide collection on the Rheumatic Diseases, copyright 1991, used by permission from the American College of Rheumatology.)

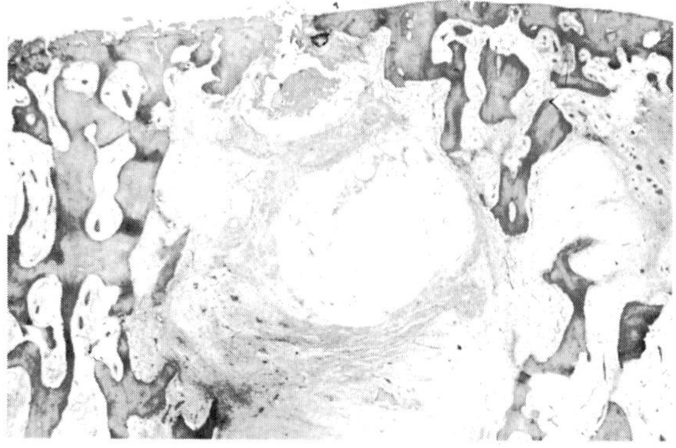

Figure 4-23. A medium-power histological view in "end-stage" osteoarthritis showing a microfracture of the articular plate and an evolving subarticular defect (geode).

joints are usually spared in OA of the hand, although the carpometacarpal joint of the thumb is frequently involved.

In the majority of patients, the deformities of OA in the hands develop slowly and frequently do not lead to major disability. The early stages, particularly associated with the formation of inflamed cysts, are frequently painful. As the disease progresses and deformity develops, the pain is frequently less. The joints of the wrist are usually not severely involved in OA, though degenerative changes may occur at the trapezioscaphoid joint.

Feet The first MTP joint of the foot is often involved in OA. This is frequently associated with the gradual development of a hallux valgus deformity with swelling and pain over the medial aspect of the first MTP joint. Bony osteophytes may project onto the medial aspect of the foot, producing the characteristic bunion deformity.

Knees The medial compartment of the knee joint transmits a higher proportion of body weight than the lateral compartment. As the cartilage begins to degenerate, the stress of weight bearing frequently leads to narrowing of the medial compartment of the knee before the lateral compartment. This will be associated with the development of a varus deformity (**genu varum**). The patellofemoral joint also undergoes a major compressive force when the body is raised from a kneeling or squatting position, and on climbing stairs and hills. Patellofemoral OA may precede other manifestations in the knee joint. Pain associated with OA of the knee often will be worse on activities involving climbing or prolonged standing, and may be relieved at rest. In the early stages there may be synovitis with a joint effusion. Crepitus may be detected by palpating over the patella and asking the patient to extend the knee against gravity. Active and passive movements may be limited by pain, and in advanced cases, as cartilage is lost, the joint may demonstrate anteroposterior and lateral instability.

Hip OA of the hip is common in older individuals. Cartilage loss will occur initially in the upper and outer aspects of the hip joint, and osteophyte formation will occur at the margins of the joint. As cartilage destruction proceeds, cyst-like erosions may develop in the femoral head and in the acetabulum (Fig. 4-26). Patients will complain of pain on walking and standing. On examination, flexion, abduction, and lateral rotation of the hip will frequently reproduce the pain. When walking, patients frequently demonstrate an antalgic gait or limp that develops in an attempt to relieve pressure in the affected joint. On standing on the affected hip the contralateral hip may drop (Trendelenburg's sign). Eventually, a flexion contracture may develop, with a positive Thomas' test.

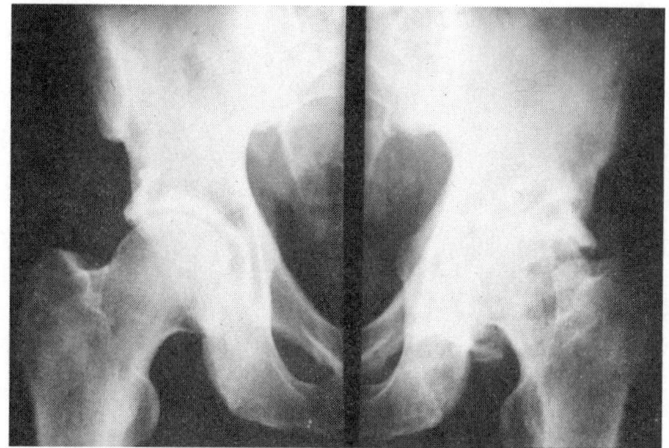

Figure 4-26. An anteroposterior view reveals almost complete loss of joint space in the hip on the right associated with sclerosis, osteophyte formation, and extensive cyst formation of adjacent margins of the head and acetabulum. The hip on the left shows only mild sclerosis and early osteophyte formation. (Reprinted from the Clinical slide collection on the Rheumatic Diseases, copyright 1991, used by permission from the American College of Rheumatology.)

Axial Skeleton Degenerative disease of the spine is closely associated with aging. By the age of 70, 90% of the population will show evidence of degeneration of the axial skeleton not necessarily symptomatic. The areas first affected are those where the spine shows the greatest angulation and the most pronounced angular movement. These are the lower cervical and upper thoracic region, and the lower segments of the lumbar spine. The initial change appears to be a loss of elasticity of the fibers of the **annulus fibrosus**. This enables the jelly-like **nucleus pulposus** to bulge either anteriorly or posteriorly, with consequent reduction of the height of the intervertebral disk. Since the **facet**, or **apophyseal**, joints are aligned obliquely, the change in intervertebral disk height will cause these joints to become malaligned. The normally apposed cartilaginous surfaces slip apart, and bone now articulates with bone. The consequences are similar to those found in OA of peripheral joints, with the development of osteophytes from bony surfaces that lose their hyaline cartilage (Fig. 4-27). When the osteophytes project anteriorly, they may be asymptomatic. When they project posteriorly they may impinge on nerve roots, where they emerge through the intervertebral foramina, causing sensory or motor loss, whose location will depend on the site of the compression. Massive osteophytes may cause compression of the underlying spinal cord, with circulatory impairment (**spinal stenosis**).

The symptoms of spinal OA will often consist of postural pain and stiffness either in the lower cervical or lower lumbar regions. In contrast to the symptoms of inflammatory disease of the spine, which are usually worse after immobility and relieved by exercise, the symptoms of degenerative disease are usually directly related to exertion.

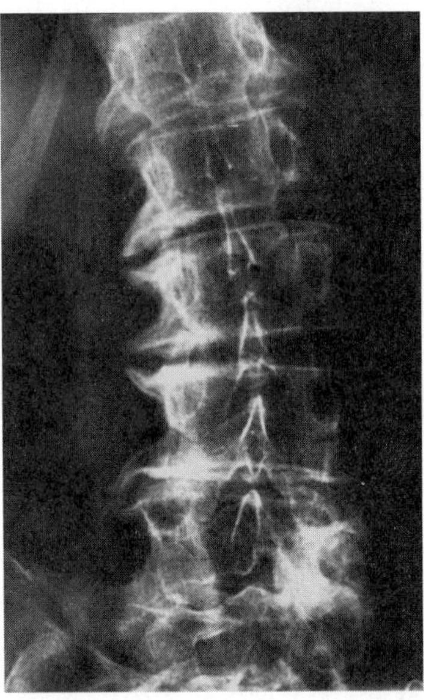

Figure 4-27. This anteroposterior projection of the lumbar spine shows scoliosis and narrowing of the intervertebral spaces on the concave side where extensive osteophyte formation is present. The osteophytes are thick and project laterally in contrast to the thin vertical syndesmophytes of ankylosing spondylitis. Adjacent bony margins are sclerosed. The zygapophyseal articulations are not well demonstrated, but show narrowing and sclerosis, particularly on the concave aspect of the spine. (Reprinted from the Clinical slide collection on the Rheumatic Diseases, copyright 1991, used by permission from the American College of Rheumatology.)

Laboratory Findings

In contrast to rheumatoid arthritis, a systemic inflammatory disorder associated with laboratory changes, such as an increased ESR, anemia, and a positive rheumatoid factor, OA is, in general, limited to the joints and no characteristic abnormalities are found in the blood. In patients treated over a long period with NSAIDs, the blood tests may show evidence of anemia, or of secondary abnormalities caused by NSAIDs, leading to liver or renal damage.

Radiological Findings

Radiographs of affected joints will show loss of joint cartilage in the early stages, with the later development of osteophytes, and malalignment of the affected joint. The subchondral bone underlying damaged cartilage becomes increasingly dense (subchondral sclerosis) and marginal osteophytes develop. As cartilage deteriorates, cyst-like lesions may develop in the underlying bones.

Symptoms of inflammatory disease of the spine are usually worse after immobility and improved by exercise. In contrast, symptoms of degenerative disease are usually directly related to exertion.

General Management

Patient education plays a primary role in the management of OA. For patients with hand involvement, it is important to recognize that this condition, while progressive, rarely leads to severe disability and handicap. The use of assistive devices may reduce forces on damaged joints. Weight loss is important in reducing the pain in weight-bearing joints, and may slow the rate of progress of OA of the hip and knee. When obesity contributes to the problem, referral to a dietician may be an important aspect of management.

Medical Management

Analgesic drugs such as acetaminophen have an important role in the management of pain. Since there is frequently an inflammatory component, particularly in the early stages of OA, there is a rationale for the use of anti-inflammatory medications such as aspirin and other NSAIDs. Their prolonged use in OA, however, is controversial, and there is recent evidence that some of these anti-inflammatory agents may depress the synthesis of essential proteoglycans in cartilage. Since OA occurs with increasing frequency in older individuals, and since this is the group with the highest incidence of adverse affects from NSAIDs, many physicians are now reluctant to prescribe NSAIDs in OA. There appears to be no role for the slow-acting antirheumatic drugs, such as the antimalarials, gold, and cytotoxic drugs.

Intra-articular injections of corticosteroids may relieve the symptoms in individual joints for a brief period, and may be useful in the early stages of the disease. However, it is suspected that the repeated use of corticosteroids may accelerate joint deterioration. Surgical treatment with total joint replacement is the ultimate choice for individuals with OA of the hip and knee.

Weight loss is important in reducing pain in weight-bearing joints; a referral to a dietician is part of management.

Crystal-Induced Arthritis (Gout)

Crystal-induced arthritis (CIA) includes gout and calcium pyrophosphate dihydrate (CPPD) crystal deposition disease. Gout is a term used to describe a group of disorders characterized by an increase of urate concentrations in the plasma, recurrent attacks of acute arthritis, associated with monosodium urate crystals in synovial fluid.[24] In the chronic stages, sodium urate crystals may collect outside joints and in soft tissues producing tophi. The prevalence of gout appears to be about 2.6 per 1,000. After puberty, levels of serum urate are higher in males than in females. Following the menopause, urate concentrations rise in females and the level is equivalent to that found in males.

In the early stages of the disease an acute gouty attack may settle spontaneously within a week. A symptom-free period lasting several months, or several years, may separate the early attacks of gouty arthritis. As the disease progresses, if the condition is untreated, attacks may become more frequent and more severe and will spread to involve other peripheral joints. The spine is rarely involved.

Investigations include radiographs, which in the later stages may show bony erosions around the margins of affected joints and laboratory tests that are positive for negatively birefringent needle-shaped crystals within cells in the joint fluid[25] (Fig. 4-28) and serum uric acid levels. The latter are usually elevated before and after attacks of acute gouty arthritis.

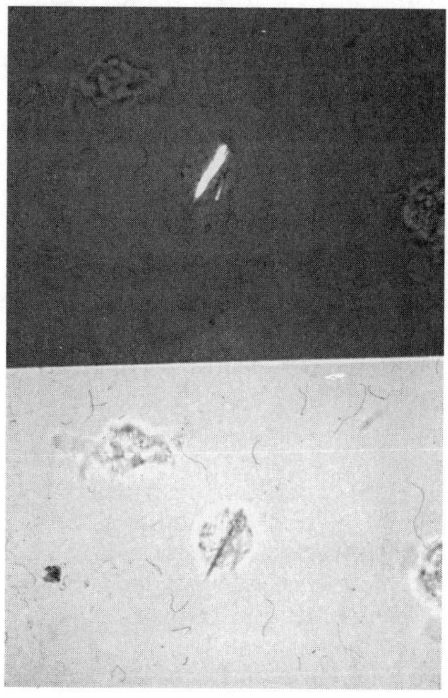

Figure 4-28. This photograph shows monosodium urate crystals that have been phagocytosed by a polymorphonuclear leukocyte in the joint fluid during an acute attack of gout. In the top section, compensated polarized light clearly demonstrates two longer crystals (~13 μm) and one shorter crystal (~9 μm). The bottom section shows the same field under ordinary light. Here only one of the longer crystals is identifiable. This demonstrates the superiority of compensated polarized light over ordinary light microscopy when evaluating joint fluid for crystals. The top section is diagnostic, the bottom section is not. (Reprinted from the Clinical slide collection on the Rheumatic Diseases, copyright 1991, used by permission from the American College of Rheumatology.)

Commonly used drugs in gout are colchicine, allopurinol, uricosurics, and NSAIDs. Aspirin should not be used in an acute attack of gout, since in low doses it tends to inhibit renal excretion of urate. Since gout is now medically a well-controlled condition, it is rarely seen in physical therapy practice. For further detail of crystal-induced arthritis, consult appropriate textbooks.

Rheumatic Diseases in Childhood

Juvenile rheumatoid arthritis (**JRA**) has an incidence in population studies of approximately 14 per 100,000 per year. Although considerably less common than arthritis in adults, JRA is a major cause of childhood disability and, in particular, may be associated with severe eye disease. Girls are more often affected than boys; however, sex and age ratios vary in the different subtypes of JRA. JRA may develop at any age during childhood.[26]

Clinical Manifestations

Pauciarticular Juvenile Arthritis

In about half of children affected, the incidence is pauciarticular. In this type of arthritis where, by definition, four or fewer joints are involved, inflammation often begins in a single joint. The knee is commonly affected, but any other joint may be involved at the time of presentation. The long-term outcome for pauciarticular disease is usually good, with complete functional recovery, though joint inflammation may persist for many months. The early introduction of physiotherapy and occupational therapy is particularly important in this group. The major complication of pauciarticular JRA is a severe inflammatory condition of the anterior chamber of the eye (**anterior uveitis**). This may occur in up to 20% of patients with pauciarticular disease, and is particularly common in females who are positive for antinuclear antibody. Untreated, this may lead to blindness. Careful surveillance by an experienced ophthalmologist is therefore of great importance, since early treatment with local corticosteroids may prevent the development of visual impairment.

Polyarticular Juvenile Arthritis

Thirty to 40% of patients have a presentation involving more than four joints. The onset is common between 1 and 3 years and between 8 and 10 years of age. The pattern of joint involvement may spread, and frequently the small joints of the hands and feet may be involved. Bony erosions may develop as in adult RA. The temporomandibular joint may be affected, producing an underslung jaw (**micrognathia**) that may require supervision by an orthodontist. In severe cases, subcutaneous nodules may develop. In children where the rheumatoid factor tests are consistently positive, the prognosis is worse.

Systemic-Onset Juvenile Arthritis (Still's Disease)

Clinical Manifestations

About 10% of children have a systemic onset. This may begin at any age. The clinical features include a high spiking fever, which returns to baseline each day (quotidian), a salmon-pink rash over the upper trunk with lesions that have a "target" appearance, with a pale center, surrounded by pink, and a white outer circle. Lymphadenopathy and hepatosplenomegaly are frequently found, and there may be effusions in the pericardium and pleura. A high white cell count and anemia may be found. Rheumatoid factor and antinuclear antibodies are usually negative. A polyarticular chronic arthritis may develop within weeks or months of the clinical presentation.

Management

A multidisciplinary team approach involving pediatric rheumatologist, social worker, physical therapist, occupational therapist, nurse and, if necessary, a specialized orthopedic surgeon is important from the very onset of JRA. Education of the child and of the family plays an important role. The simplest and most conservative measures will be the first applied. Aspirin and other NSAIDs are used initially, together with physical measures to control pain and restore motion and function in the musculoskeletal system.

If the disease does not respond to this type of treatment, second-line drugs of the categories used in adult RA may be tried. As in the management of RA, local injections of corticosteroids may be indicated when individual joints fail to respond to systemic treatment.

After 15 years of follow-up, 50% of children are likely to experience complete remission of their symptoms. For the remainder, joint inflammation may persist into adult life, resulting in considerable handicap. For this group, it is important to consider the development of transition clinics, staffed by experts in the care of both children and adults, to facilitate the passage from a pediatric setting to an adult rheumatology clinic.

Systemic Lupus Erythematosus

Systemic lupus erythematosus (SLE) is an inflammatory disease affecting many organs of the body and associated with the presence of autoantibodies in the serum.[27] The etiology of SLE is unknown, although it is known that genetic factors play an important role. Diseases resembling lupus have been found in experimental animals (in particular, in the NZB/NZW mouse). SLE occurs more frequently in females, with a female-to-male ratio of 9:1. The prevalence is about 1 per 2,000. Recent studies suggest that the prognosis of SLE has improved steadily over the last 30 years. In the earlier studies, 50% of patients died within 6 months of diagnosis. In more recent series, 95% are functioning normally 10 years after diagnosis. It is not certain whether this is related to improvements in treatment or to the early diagnosis of milder cases of the disease.

Pathology

The pathological findings in SLE are many, correlating with the wide range of clinical manifestations. The histologic abnormalities are a reflection of the immunologic attack that is the essence of the disease process. Some of the common changes are briefly described.

Active skin involvement is characterized by damage in the interface zone between epidermis and dermis. Liquefactive or vacuolar necrosis of the basal layer of the epidermis occurs, and is associated with deposits of immune complexes. These deposits can be demonstrated using immunohistological techniques. Other cutaneous changes include epidermal atrophy, hyperkeratosis, perifollicular and perivascular dermal inflammation, dermal edema, and fibrosis and loss of skin appendages.

Kidney pathology is present in most patients. Glomerular changes dominate and are related to the trapping and formation of immune complexes in glomeruli. Different patterns of glomerular disease are seen that have different prognostic significance. One pattern is diffuse thickening of the glomerular basement membrane.

Electron dense immune complexes (Fig. 4-29) are seen on electron microscopy intimately associated with this basement membrane thickening.

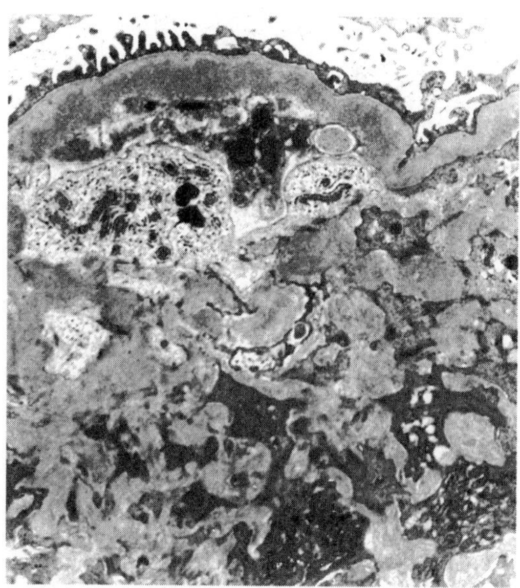

Figure 4-29. This is an electron micrograph of an abnormal glomerulus in lupus erythematosus. It shows diffuse thickening of the capillary basement membrane by electron dense deposits. These electron dense deposits represent immune complex deposits. Glomerular involvement is a common manifestation of systemic lupus erythematosus.

Other patterns of glomerular involvement are characterized by fibrin deposition and proliferation of cells. An uncommon expression of lupus involvement of the kidney is vasculitis in large vessels. Advanced kidney disease is characterized by small, atrophic, and scarred kidneys.

Fibrinous inflammation of pleura and pericardium is a common finding. The heart commonly shows small fibrinous vegetations on valve leaflets near lines of closure. Such vegetations are known as Libman-Sacks endocarditis. They are not related to infection and are usually not important clinically.

Lung involvement is sometimes a dramatic manifestation. It is characterized by a diffuse capillaritis that typically presents with a syndrome of acute lung hemorrhage.

Clinical Presentation

Many organ systems are involved in SLE and the presentation will vary depending on which system is involved first.

Skin

The skin rash of SLE is frequently found after exposure to sunlight. A classical presentation is the **butterfly blush** (Fig. 4-30), which is seen on both cheeks and across the bridge of the nose. In some cases, the rash may extend onto a sun-exposed area on the upper chest (often in a V-shaped distribution) and to sun-exposed areas on the arms and forearms. Frequently, maculopapular lesions of a more chronic nature are found distributed over the same area in SLE. Three other types of SLE with skin lesions are **subacute cutaneous LE, discoid LE, and livedo reticularis.**

Musculoskeletal System

Patients with SLE frequently complain of arthralgia, and the joints may be swollen, tender, and inflamed. This joint involvement is frequently fleeting, and in most cases responds well to anti-inflammatory drugs, usually resolving completely without leaving any deformity. Occasionally, when the joint involvement has been chronic and persistent, deformities may occur, particularly over the fingers, producing a pattern known as **Jaccoud's arthropathy**. In this condition, deformities similar to those found in RA, including swan-neck and boutonnière deformities, ulnar deviation, and volar subluxation of the MCP joints, may occur. In contrast to the deformities found in RA, those seen in SLE are usually completely reducible, and are associated with laxity of periarticular tendons and ligaments.

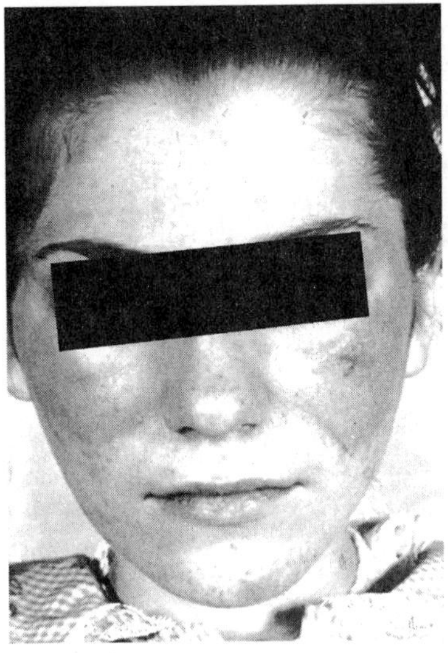

Figure 4-30. This slide reveals a facial eruption in a patient with systemic lupus erythematosus. The rash consists primarily of erythema on the malar and chin areas. Telangiectasia are also present. This type of lesion is suggestive but not diagnostic of systemic lupus. (Reprinted from the Clinical slide collection on the Rheumatic Diseases, copyright 1991, used by permission from the American College of Rheumatology.)

Heart and Lungs

About one third of patients with SLE may develop acute pericarditis or pleurisy. These inflammatory changes in the pericardial and pleural membrane produce a sharp chest pain related to breathing, exercise, and position. In more severe cases, lupus can be associated with myocarditis and endocarditis. In the lungs, acute pneumonitis is occasionally found, associated sometimes with pulmonary hemorrhage. Pulmonary embolism may occur as a complication of thrombosis of a peripheral vein.

Vasculitis

Inflammation in the blood vessels may develop in SLE as a result of the deposition of immune complexes and complement in the walls of small arteries and capillaries. This may lead to a variety of skin lesions, including purpura when small vessels are involved, and papular lesions when larger vessels are involved. Occasionally, major arterial thrombosis may occur, jeopardizing the circulation to a limb.

Gastrointestinal Complications

Ulcers may occur on the mucous membrane of the mouth and throat in SLE. Sterile peritonitis is occasionally seen and pancreatitis may occur as a serious complication. If vasculitis affects vessels leading to the bowel, segments of small or large intestine may become ulcerated, and may finally infarct. This complication will require immediate surgical intervention.

Kidney Involvement

One of the most important long-term complications of SLE is inflammatory disease of the kidney (**glomerulonephritis**). This is found in almost half of patients with SLE, and may vary between mild inflammation, producing almost no clinical problems, to rapidly progressive glomerulonephritis, which may lead to renal failure. Renal involvement will be suggested by abnormalities in the urine, and may eventually lead to a rising urea and creatine in the blood. A renal biopsy may be required to determine the exact pattern of renal involvement in SLE.

Central Nervous System Involvement

Ten to 15% of patients with SLE may develop neuropsychiatric involvement. This may vary between periods of depression, ischemic episodes involving the brain, peripheral neuropathy, and coma or seizures.

Hematological Involvement

Patients with SLE may develop a hemolytic anemia, due to the development of antibodies directed against red blood cells. A low white count (**leukopenia**) is often seen in active lupus, and a low platelet count (**thrombocytopenia**) may occur. This may predispose to hemorrhagic skin lesions (**purpura**) and to hemorrhage at mucosal surfaces.

Laboratory Findings

The characteristic laboratory finding in patients with SLE is the presence of antinuclear antibodies and antibodies to DNA. The pattern of antibodies, and their level in the serum, may give some indication of the disease severity. Many of the inflammatory lesions in blood vessels, which characterize SLE, are due to the combination of antibodies with antigens in the circulation to form **immune complexes**. These may deposit in the wall of capillaries and arterioles, after fixing complement. The deposited immune complexes will attract polymorphonuclear cells, and may lead to tissue destruction by inflammation. The presence of high levels of immune complexes will lead to reduced levels of serum complement.

Antiphospholipid Antibody Syndrome

About 30% of patients with SLE show antibodies to cardiolipin, a form of phospholipid. These antibodies are sometimes associated with the **lupus anticoagulant**. They are associated with a high risk of venous and arterial thrombosis.

Management

Patient education has an important role in the management of SLE. The patient should recognize that the disease frequently has a fluctuating course and may require shorter or longer periods of treatment continued over many years. The disease will, however, often enter periods of remission, sometimes lasting for several years, during which patients with SLE may be free of all symptoms.

The drug treatment required for SLE will depend on the degree of disease activity and on the organs involved. In milder forms of lupus, where the major symptoms are in the joints, the use of NSAIDs may be adequate to control the symptoms. At this stage, physiotherapy, to increase strength and range of movement, and occupational therapy, to splint affected joints and minimize the risk of longstanding deformity, will be of particular importance. Antimalarial drugs may be used for both musculoskeletal and cutaneous manifestations of SLE. If the disease involves other organs such as the heart, lungs, or kidneys, or fails to respond to NSAIDs, it will be necessary to use corticosteroids. Oral prednisone is the most frequently used corticosteroid, and may be used in a dose of 0.5 mg/kg for mild disease or 1 mg/kg for more serious disease. Occasionally, very severe or acute SLE patients may require an intravenous bolus of 1 g of methylprednisone. This may be repeated on three consecutive days. The clinical symptoms of SLE often respond rapidly to corticosteroids, and once the symptoms are controlled, the dose will be slowly reduced. An increase in the dose of corticosteroid will be required if the disease flares.

Azathioprine in a dose of 75–150 mg/day may be given with prednisone, if prednisone alone is not effective, or in an attempt to reduce the prednisone dose, if the dose required is high enough to produce serious side effects. Cyclophosphamide, given orally or by intravenous bolus, may be used for treating the most severe forms of lupus, particularly those with active kidney disease.

Scleroderma

Scleroderma (**systemic sclerosis**) is a generalized disorder of collagen, characterized by gradually spreading fibrosis in the skin, synovium, muscles, and gastrointestinal tract.[28] It occurs with a frequency of between 5 and 10 cases per 1 million annually in all populations studied. The female-to-male ratio is about 3:1.

Clinical Features

The onset of scleroderma is usually gradual. The first complaint may be Raynaud's phenomenon, which is characterized by sudden episodes of pallor of the distal portion of the fingers on exposure to cold (Fig. 4-31). On rewarming, the fingers often become red or purple.

Skin Involvement

Involvement of the skin is characterized by gradual development of thickening and induration, often beginning with the terminal phalanges of the fingers, and slowly spreading centrally. The toes also may be involved. At the onset, the digit may be swollen and stiff, and an early complaint is difficulty in flexion of the finger. As the thickening progresses, the fingers may become increasingly rigid and, finally, are often fixed in partial flexion, with no possibility of flexion or extension (Fig. 4-32). In some cases of scleroderma, the thickening in the skin will gradually resolve, while in others, particularly where the induration has extended above the elbow, it may progress steadily to involve the whole of the upper trunk. The skin of the face may be involved, producing puckering around the lips and difficulty in opening the mouth (Fig. 4-33).

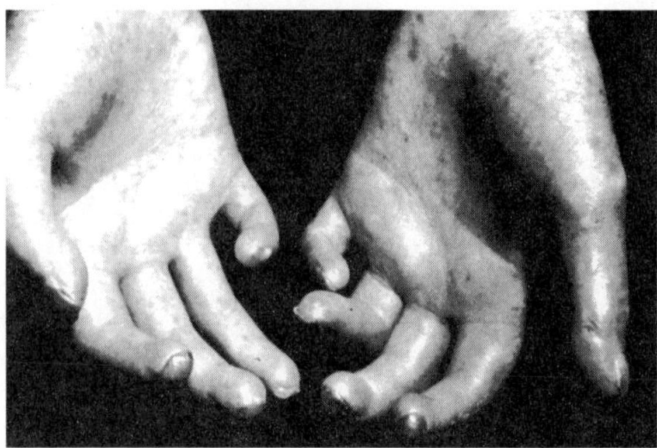

Figure 4-32. The terminal phalanges of both the second and third fingers are shortened and the nails are deformed as a result of bony resorption of the distal phalanges. Flexion contractures and a tightened indurated skin (sclerodactyly) are also shown. (Reprinted from the Clinical slide collection on the Rheumatic Diseases, copyright 1991, used by permission from the American College of Rheumatology.)

CREST Syndrome

The CREST syndrome is associated with *c*alcinosis (calcium deposits around joints on the hand), *R*aynaud's phenomenon, *e*sophageal dysmotility, *s*clerodactyly (thickening of the skin of the finger), and *t*elangiectases. This tends to have a rather more benign course.

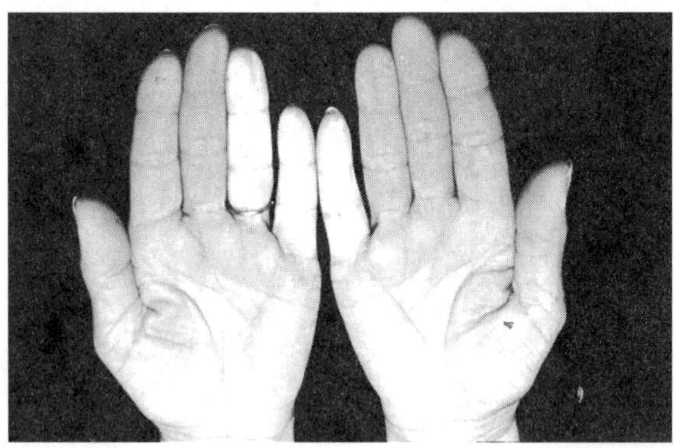

Figure 4-31. The marked pallor of the fourth and fifth digits of the left hand and of the fifth digit of the right hand is characteristic of Raynaud's phenomenon. Vasospastic changes are common in systemic sclerosis, but may also occur in rheumatoid arthritis, systemic lupus erythematosus, and idiopathic Raynaud's disease. (Reprinted from the Clinical slide collection on the Rheumatic Diseases, copyright 1991, used by permission from the American College of Rheumatology.)

Musculoskeletal System

Collagen deposits in the synovial lining tissues are associated with joint pain in the initial stages and subsequently with increasing stiffness and flexion contractures. The tendon sheaths also may be involved. Muscle weakness, particularly affecting the muscles of the hip and shoulder girdles, is frequently seen in scleroderma. This is associated with a progressive myositis or inflammatory change in the muscles.

Gastrointestinal Tract

Ninety percent of patients with scleroderma develop difficulty in swallowing, due to impaired contraction of the muscles of the lower esophagus. In severe cases, the remainder of the bowel may be involved, sometimes producing wide-mouthed diverticula of the large bowel, and constipation. Rarely, the small intestine also is involved.

Lung and Heart Involvement

Lung involvement may occur, with pulmonary infiltrates associated with increasing breathlessness. Less commonly, the heart may be involved.

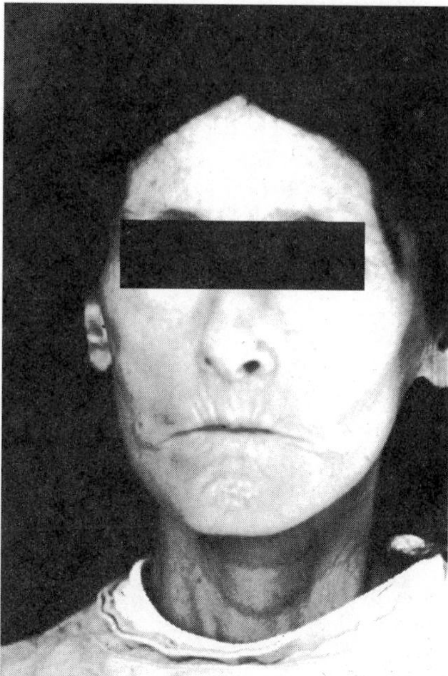

Figure 4-33. The face of this young woman demonstrates many features of systemic scleroderma including drawn pursed lips; shiny skin over the cheeks and forehead; and atrophy of muscles of the temple, face, and neck. These changes in the face are known as *Mauskopf* (mousehead). (Reprinted from the Clinical slide collection on the Rheumatic Diseases, copyright 1991, used by permission from the American College of Rheumatology.)

Renal Involvement

In severe scleroderma the arterioles of the kidney may develop intimal hyperplasia, leading to severe hypertension, with retinopathy and seizures.

While in many cases of scleroderma the course is slow, and may show a spontaneous remission, occasional cases may have a rapid progressive course, leading to death from renal failure, cardiac involvement, or gastrointestinal infiltration.

Management

In the early stages of mild scleroderma, active and passive exercises of the fingers and any other affected joints will be important to maintain range of motion. In patients with Raynaud's phenomenon, education will be important to help the patient to protect themselves from cold exposure. If Raynaud's phenomenon is severe, calcium channel blocking agents such as nifedipine may be used to promote vasodilatation. There is some evidence that the progression of scleroderma may be slowed by treatment with penicillamine. Topical agents have not been shown to have any value in the treatment of sclerodema or Raynaud's phenomenon.

Polymyositis and Dermatomyositis

Polymyositis and dermatomyositis are idiopathic inflammatory diseases of skeletal muscle.[29] The prevalence is about 8 cases per 100,000.

Clinical Features

Polymyositis is characterized by symmetrical weakness of the proximal muscles affecting particularly the shoulder and pelvic girdles, and in severe cases, spreading peripherally. The onset is usually gradual, but in severe cases may progress to a level where patients are barely able to rise from a lying position. In dermatomyositis, a similar distribution of muscle weakness is found, in association with a rash on the face, which characteristically has a deep red color, and may be associated with Gottron's papules (small flat-topped papules on the dorsal surface of the interphalangeal joints of the hands). Cardiac involvement and pulmonary disease may be found. In older patients, polymyositis and dermatomyositis may be associated with cancer. In occasional cases, resection of the cancer may be followed by remission of the myositis.

Laboratory Findings

Enzymes associated with muscle, including transaminases, creatine kinase, and lactate dehydrogenase, are elevated during the acute phase of the illness. Electromyography may show characteristic findings of inflammatory myopathy.

Pathology

A skeletal muscle biopsy is often helpful in confirming the diagnosis of polymyositis or dermatomyositis. Active disease shows an inflammatory infiltrate in the interstitium encasing muscle fibers. It is composed of lymphocytes, histiocytes, and sometimes plasma cells, and is associated with muscle fiber degeneration and necrosis (Fig. 4-34). Older foci show fibrosis, muscle fiber atrophy, and

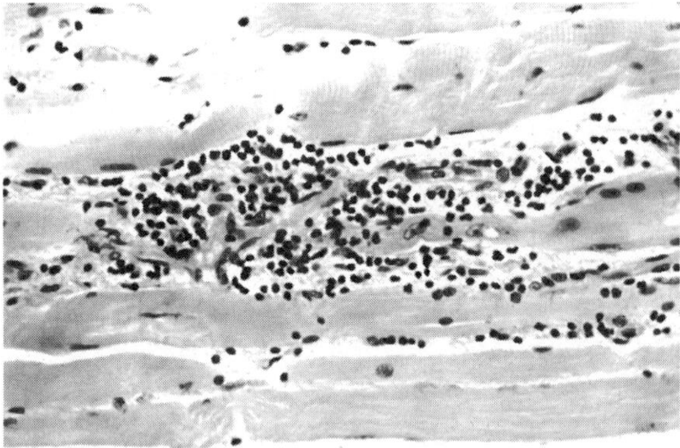

Figure 4-34. A medium-power photomicrograph shows a focus of reactive lymphocytic infiltration in skeletal muscle. A muscle fiber near the center shows inflammatory destruction. This pattern is typical of the muscle inflammation seen in polymyositis and dermatomyositis.

evidence of muscle fiber regeneration. Some biopsies are negative. This likely reflects a sampling error, since the pathology of polymyositis is focal in nature and could be missed.

A skin biopsy in dermatomyositis may show dermal edema, lymphohistiocytic inflammatory cells around superficial blood vessels, dermal calcification, and epidermal atrophy. Changes in acute disease can be indistinguishable from those in acute lupus erythematosus.

Medical Management

Oral corticosteroids are used initially and frequently produce a rapid recovery of muscle strength. If steroids are ineffective, azathioprine or methotrexate may be added.

Polymyalgia Rheumatica and Temporal (Giant Cell) Arteritis

Polymyalgia Rheumatica

Polymyalgia rheumatica is a fairly common syndrome characterized by the gradual development of aching and stiffness in the muscles of the shoulders, neck, and pelvic girdle that persists for 1 month.[30] The stiffness is frequently worse on rising in the morning. The disease usually occurs above the age of 50 and is more common in women than in men, with a ratio in several patient series of 3:1. The prevalence may be about 500 per 100,000. Physical examination will reveal great difficulty in abduction of the shoulders and in lateral rotation. The muscles may be tender, and sometimes joint swelling may be found in the joints of the upper and lower extremities.

Laboratory Findings

The characteristic finding in polymyalgia rheumatica is an elevation of the ESR. A moderate anemia is sometimes found.

Medical Management

Prednisone in a dose of 15–20 mg/day will usually produce a rapid relief of symptoms, often within 24 hours. The steroid dose will be continued for many months, followed by an attempt at gradual reduction. Frequently, the disease will recur as the steroid dose is reduced; in this case, prednisone will be resumed in a higher dose.

Temporal (Giant Cell) Arteritis

Ten percent of patients with polymyalgia may develop temporal arteritis. Found in older subjects, it is more common in women than in men.[30] Chronic inflammatory change is found in the arteries arising from the external carotid circulation. A characteristic clinical finding is a throbbing temporal headache, associated with thickness and tenderness of the temporal artery.

The most dangerous complication of temporal arteritis is sudden loss of vision due to inflammatory narrowing of the ophthalmic arteries. The consequent loss of vision is irreversible. Visual loss will be prevented by adequate early treatment. Pain on chewing may occur (**jaw claudication**).

The disease may be diagnosed by temporal artery biopsy that shows an arteritis. The inflammation involves all layers of the arterial wall. Multinucleated histiocytic giant cells are frequently a prominent feature (**giant cell arteritis**) but are not always seen (Fig. 4-35). The segmental and frequently multifocal process usually results in significant luminal narrowing. Healed or inactive lesions show replacement of normal vessel wall by fibrosis (scar tissue). About 50% of patients with giant cell arteritis may have symptoms of polymyalgia rheumatica.

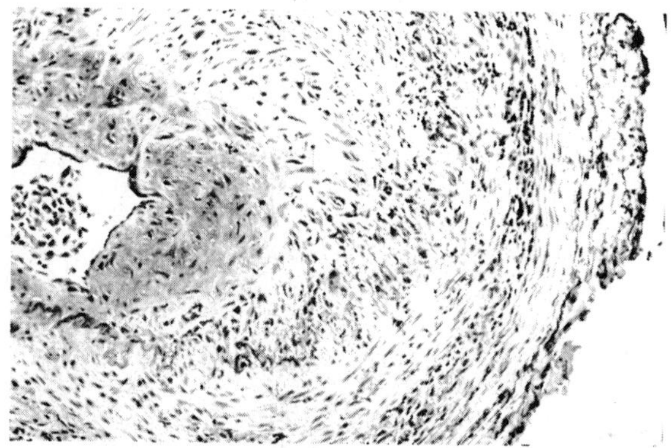

Figure 4-35. This medium-power photomicrograph (orcein-Giemsa stain) of a temporal artery biopsy shows inflammation affecting all layers (i.e., a panarteritis). Giant cells, that more precisely are referred to as multinucleated histiocytes, are a frequent feature of the reaction and have led to the alternative term of giant cell arteritis. The "giant cells" appear to be reacting to altered elastic fibers.

Medical Management

Prednisone should be given as soon as the diagnosis is made. If there is evidence of visual impairment, intravenous steroids may be used initially. Prednisone will be given by mouth in doses of 60–80 mg/day, followed by a gradual reduction, as in polymyalgia rheumatica.

References

1. Felson DT: Epidemiology of the rheumatic diseases. In McCarty DJ, Koopman WJ (eds): Arthritis and Allied Conditions, 12th edition, vol 1, pp 17–47. Philadelphia, Lea & Febiger, 1993.
2. Wilder RL: Rheumatoid arthritis. A. Epidemiology, pathology, and pathogenesis. In Schumacher HR Jr (ed): The Primer on the Rheumatic Diseases, 10th edition, p 86. Atlanta, Arthritis Foundation, 1993.
3. Arnett FC, Edworthy S, Bloch DA, et al: The 1987 revised ARA criteria for rheumatoid arthritis. Arthritis Rheum 1987; 30:S17.
4. Steinbrocher O, Traeger CH, Batterman RC: Therapeutic criteria in rheumatoid arthritis. JAMA 1949; 140:659–662.
5. Baum J, Zwillich SH, Ziff M: Laboratory findings in rheumatoid arthritis. In McCarty DJ, Koopman WJ (eds): Arthritis and Allied Conditions, 12th edition, vol 1, pp 841–860. Philadelphia, Lea & Febiger, 1993.
6. Schrohenloher RE, Koopman WJ: Rheumatoid factor. In McCarty DJ, Koopman WJ (eds): Arthritis and Allied Conditions, 12th edition, vol 1, pp 861–876. Philadelphia, Lea & Febiger, 1993.
7. McCarty DJ: Clinical picture of rheumatoid arthritis. In McCarty DJ, Koopman WJ (eds): Arthritis and Allied Conditions, 12th edition, vol 1, pp 781–810. Philadelphia, Lea & Febiger, 1993.
8. Williams HJ: Rheumatoid arthritis. C. Treatment. In Schumacher HR Jr (ed): The Primer on the Rheumatic Diseases, 10th edition, p 96. Atlanta, Arthritis Foundation, 1993.
9. Fosdick WM, Parsons JL, Hill DF: Long-term cyclophosphamide therapy in rheumatoid arthritis. Arthritis Rheum 1968; 11:151–161.
10. Fauci AS, Young KR Jr: Immunoregulatory agents. In Kelley WN, Harris ED Jr, Ruddy S, Sledge CB (eds): Textbook of Rheumatology, 4th edition, vol I, pp 797–821. Philadelphia, WB Saunders Co, 1993.
11. Axelrod L: Glucocorticoids. In Kelley WN, Harris ED Jr, Ruddy S, Sledge CB (eds): Textbook of Rheumatology, 4th edition, vol I, pp 779–796. Philadelphia, WB Saunders Co, 1993.
12. Gatter RA: Arthrocentesis technique and intrasynovial therapy. In McCarty DJ, Koopman WJ (eds): Arthritis and Allied Conditions, 12th edition, vol 1, pp 711–720. Philadelphia, Lea & Febiger, 1993.
13. Moll JMH, Haslock I, Macrae I, et al: Associations between ankylosing spondylitis, psoriatic arthritis, Reiter's disease, the intestinal arthropathies and Behçet's syndrome. Medicine 1974; 53:343.
14. Brewerton DA, Caffrey M, Hart FD, et al: Ankylosing spondylitis and HL-A 27. Lancet 1973; 1:904–907.
15. Schlosstein L, Terasaki PI, Bluestone R, et al: High association of an HL-A antigen, W27, with ankylosing spondylitis. N Engl J Med 1973; 288:704–706.
16. Khan MA: C. Seronegative spondylarthropathies. B. Ankylosing spondylitis. In Schumacher HR Jr (ed): The Primer on the Rheumatic Diseases, 10th edition, p 155. Atlanta, Arthritis Foundation, 1993.
17. Fan PT, Yu DTY: Seronegative spondylarthropathies. C. Reiter's syndrome. In Schumacher HR Jr (ed): The Primer on the Rheumatic Diseases, 10th edition, p 158. Atlanta, Arthritis Foundation, 1993.
18. Mielants H, Veys EM: Seronegative spondylarthropathies. E. Enteropathic arthritis. In Schumacher HR Jr (ed): The Primer on the Rheumatic Diseases, 10th edition, pp 163–166. Atlanta, Arthritis Foundation, 1993.
19. Vasey FB: Seronegative spondylarthropathies. D. Psoriatic arthritis. In Schumacher HR Jr (ed): The Primer on the Rheumatic Diseases, 10th edition, pp 161–163. Atlanta, Arthritis Foundation, 1993.
20. Kellgren JH, Lawrence JS: The Epidemiology of Chronic Rheumatism. Vol 2. Atlas of Standard Radiographs of Arthritis. Oxford, England, Blackwell Scientific Publications, 1963.
21. Kellgren JH, Lawrence JS, Bier F: Genetic factors in generalized osteoarthrosis. Ann Rheum Dis 1963; 22:237–255.

22. Howell DS, Pelletier J-P: Etiopathogenesis of osteoarthritis. In McCarty DJ, Koopman WJ (eds): Arthritis and Allied Conditions, 12th edition, vol 2, pp 1723–1734. Philadelphia, Lea & Febiger, 1993.
23. Moskowitz RW, Goldberg VM: Osteoarthritis. B. Clinical features and treatment. In Schumacher HR Jr (ed): The Primer on the Rheumatic Diseases, 10th edition, pp 188–190. Atlanta, Arthritis Foundation, 1993.
24. Terkeltaub R: Gout. A. Epidemiology, pathology, and pathogenesis. In Schumacher HR Jr (ed): The Primer on the Rheumatic Diseases, 10th edition, pp 209–213. Atlanta, Arthritis Foundation, 1993.
25. McCarty DJ: Calcium pyrophosphate dihydrate crystal deposition disease. In Schumacher HR Jr (ed): The Primer on the Rheumatic Diseases, 10th edition, pp 219–222. Atlanta, Arthritis Foundation, 1993.
26. Singsen BH: Pediatric rheumatic diseases. A. Nonarticular rheumatism, juvenile rheumatoid arthritis, juvenile spondylarthropathies. In Schumacher HR Jr (ed): The Primer on the Rheumatic Diseases, 10th edition, pp 171–175. Atlanta, Arthritis Foundation, 1993.
27. Pisetsky DS: Systemic lupus erythematosus. A. Epidemiology, pathology, and pathogenesis. In Schumacher HR Jr (ed): The Primer on the Rheumatic Diseases, 10th edition, pp 100–105. Atlanta, Arthritis Foundation, 1993.
28. LeRoy EC, Silver RM: Systemic sclerosis and related syndromes. A. Epidemiology, pathology, and pathogenesis. In Schumacher HR Jr (ed): The Primer on the Rheumatic Diseases, 10th edition, pp 118–120. Atlanta, Arthritis Foundation, 1993.
29. Plotz PH, Leff RL, Miller FW: Inflammatory and metabolic myopathies. In Schumacher HR Jr (ed): The Primer on the Rheumatic Diseases, 10th edition, pp 127–131. Atlanta, Arthritis Foundation, 1993.
30. Healey LA: Polymyalgia rheumatica. In Schumacher HR Jr (ed): The Primer on the Rheumatic Diseases, 10th edition, pp 148–149. Atlanta, Arthritis Foundation, 1993.

Plate 1

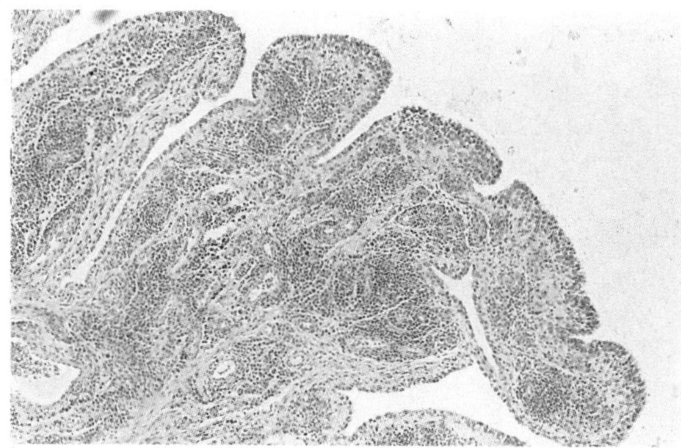

Figure 4-1. See page 48.

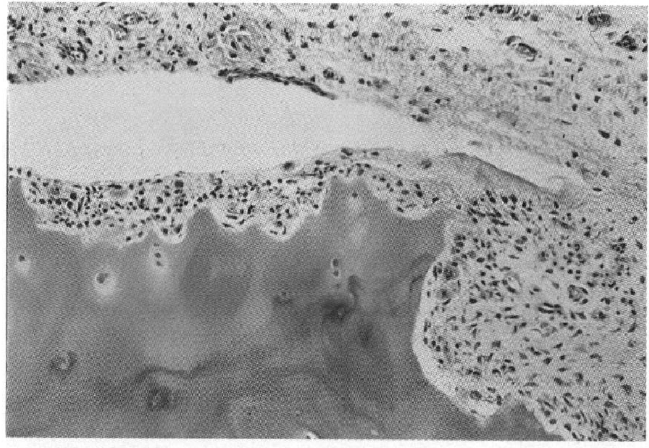

Figure 4-4. See page 49.

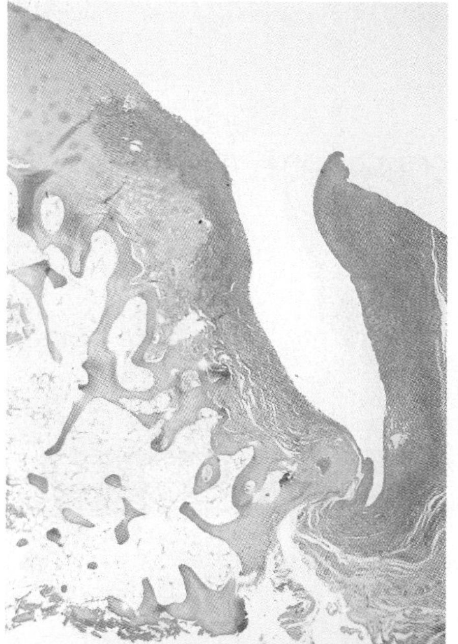

Figure 4-2. See page 49.

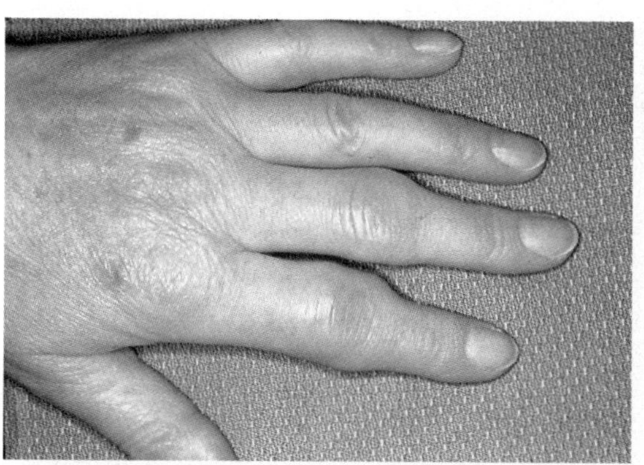

Figure 4-5. See page 50.

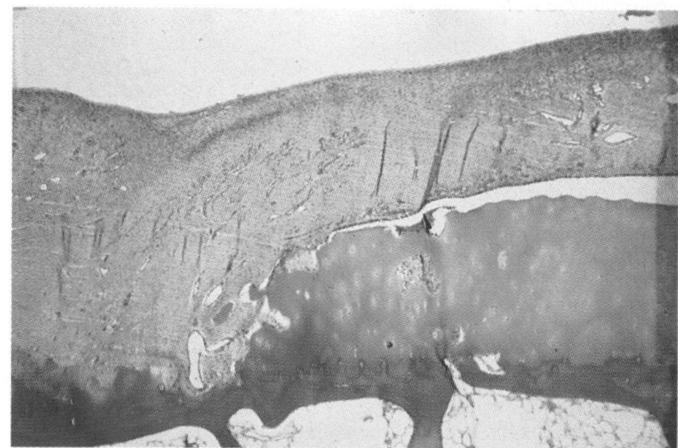

Figure 4-3. See page 49.

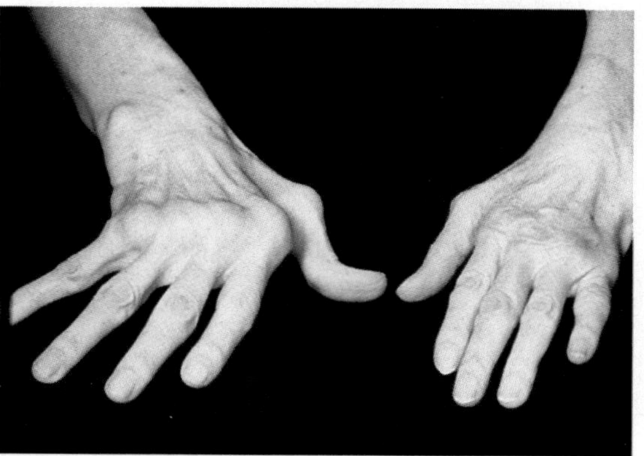

Figure 4-6. See page 52.

Plate 2

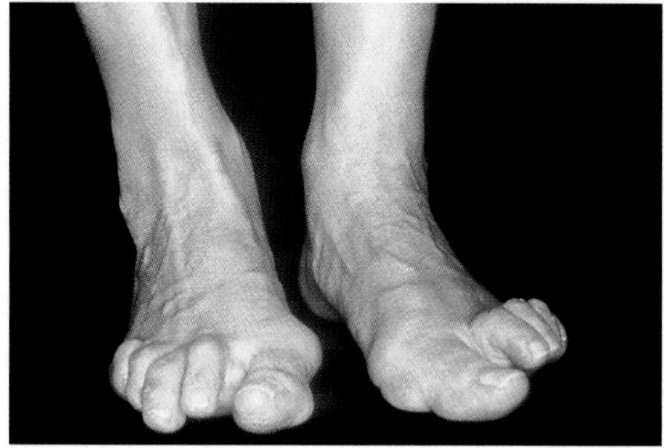

Figure 4-7. See page 53.

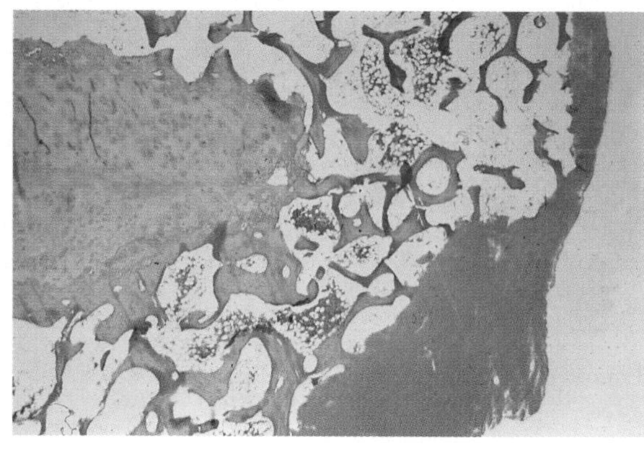

Figure 4-13. See page 61.

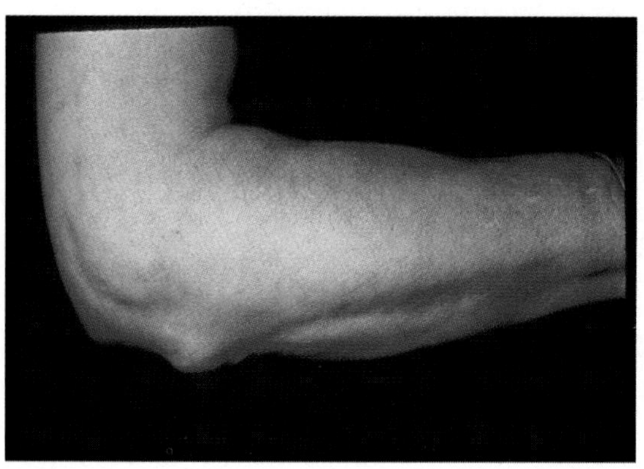

Figure 4-9. See page 54.

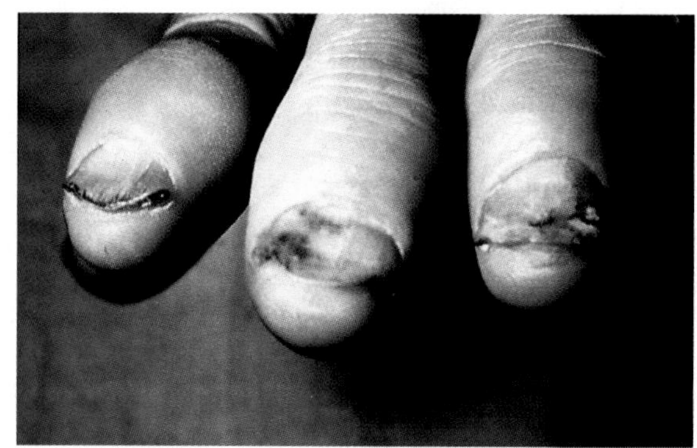

Figure 4-17. See page 65.

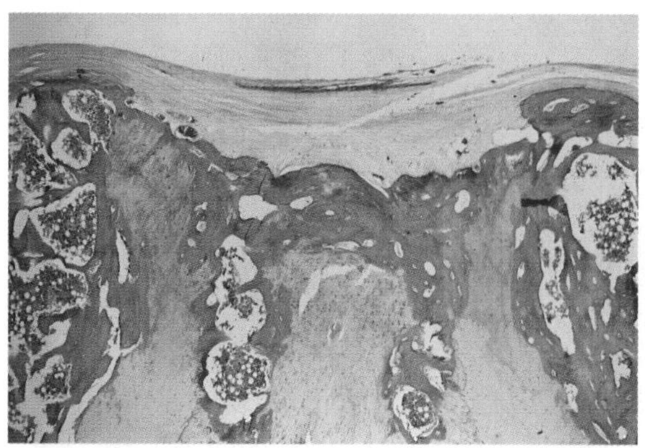

Figure 4-11. See page 61.

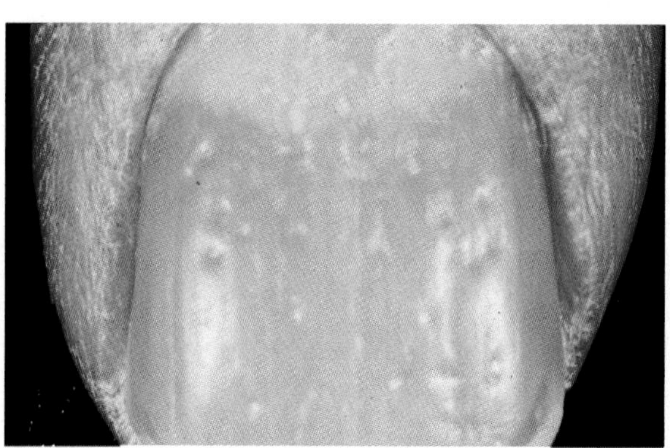

Figure 4-18. See page 65.

Plate 3

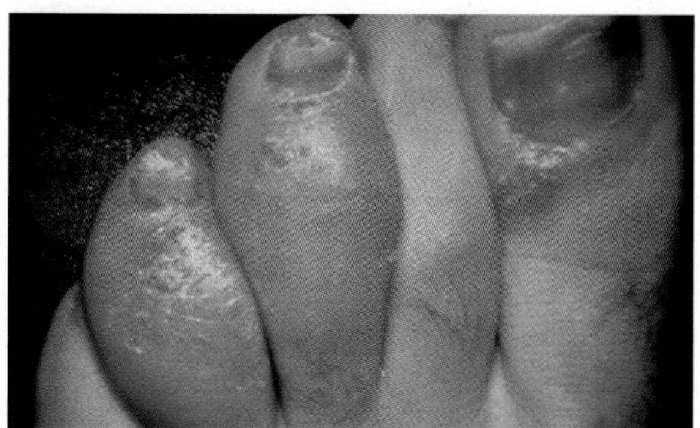

Figure 4-19. See page 66.

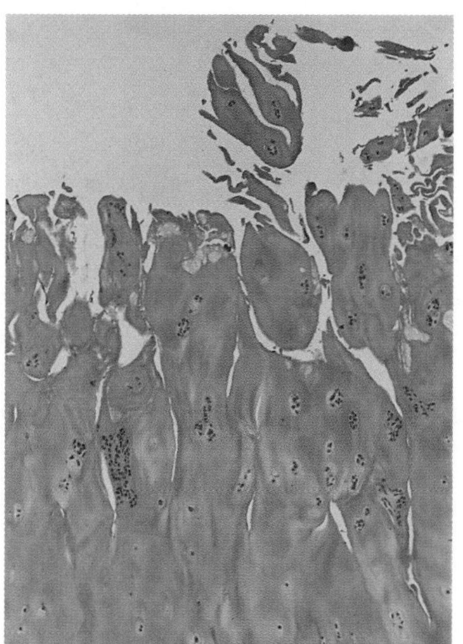

Figure 4-20. See page 67.

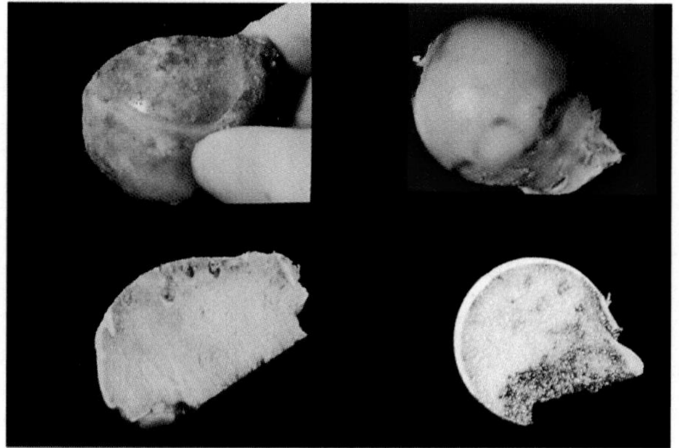

Figure 4-21. See page 67.

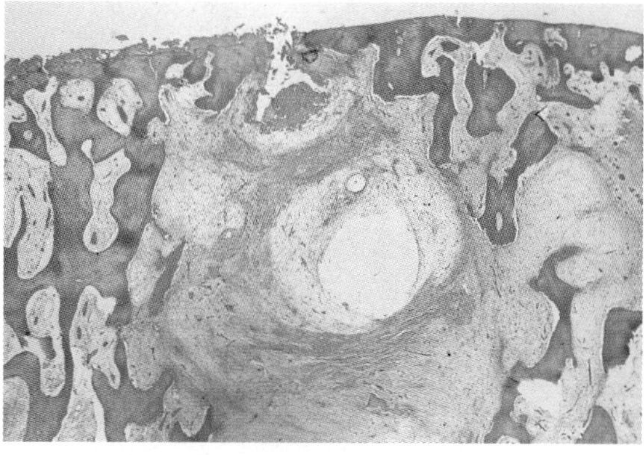

Figure 4-23. See page 68.

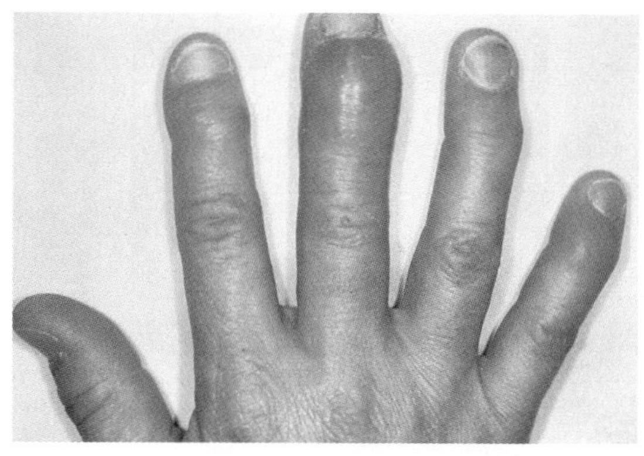

Figure 4-24. See page 68.

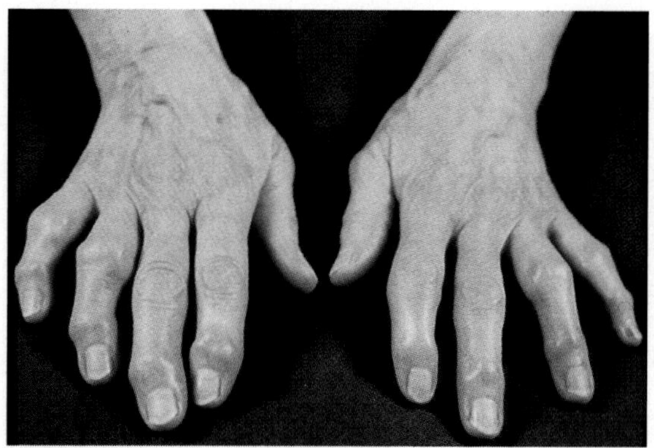

Figure 4-25. See page 68.

Plate 4

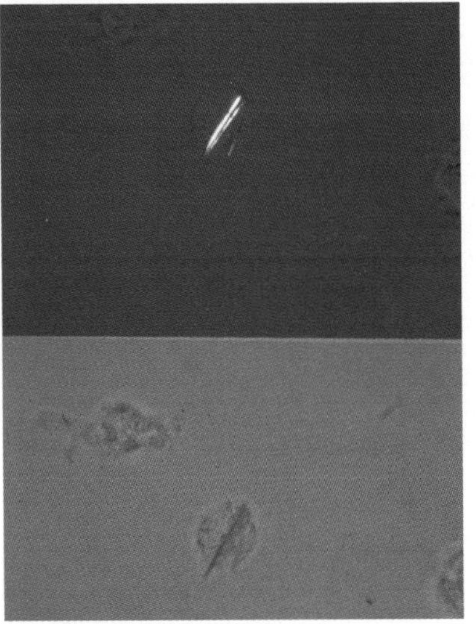

Figure 4-28. See page 71.

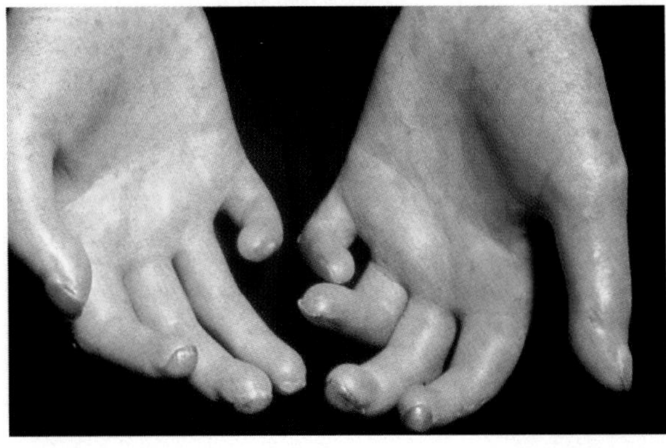

Figure 4-32. See page 76.

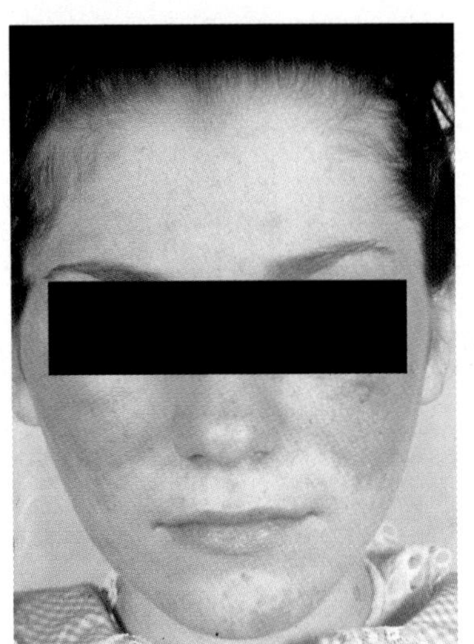

Figure 4-30. See page 74.

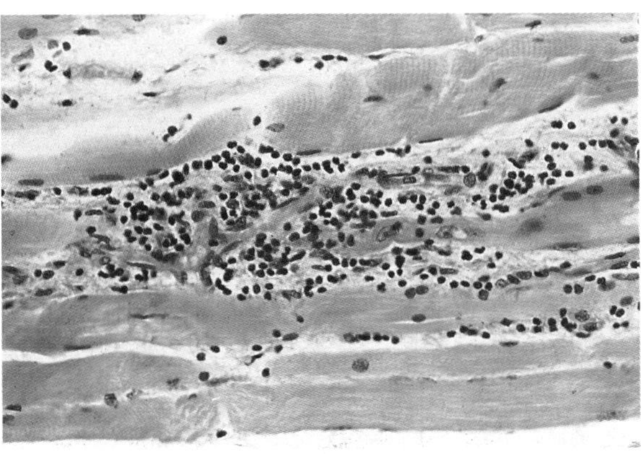

Figure 4-34. See page 78.

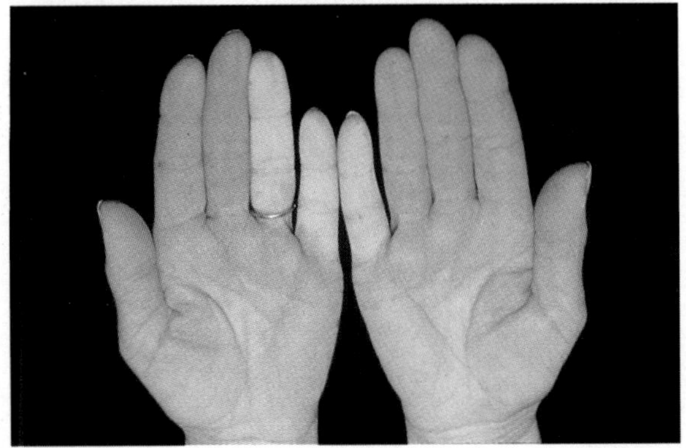

Figure 4-31. See page 76.

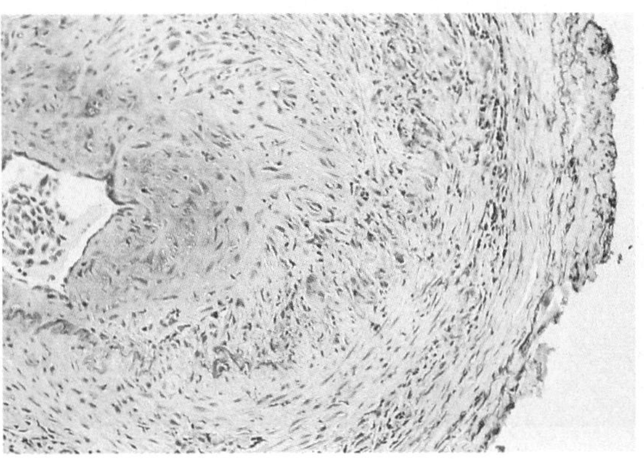

Figure 4-35. See page 79.

CHAPTER 5

Pain and Tender Points: Fibrositis/Fibromyalgia and Related Syndromes

Hugh A. Smythe, MD, FRCP[C]

PHYSICAL THERAPY IN ARTHRITIS, Joan M. Walker, PhD, PT, and Antoine Helewa, MSc(Clin Epid), PT, W.B. Saunders Company © 1996.

Chronic Pain Syndromes, Overview

Chronic pain syndromes remain a major source of concern and controversy. Many of these patients remain without proper diagnosis, problem definition, and effective treatment. Many health professionals have no defined approach to patients presenting with pain and fatigue, but who have normal findings on routine physical examination. Laboratory investigations and imaging strategies are not helpful. All of us concerned with cost-efficient care are aware of the major increases in costs relating to these problems and the need to deliver appropriate help while avoiding inappropriate medical and insurance costs.

The commonest and best studied of these syndromes is now termed fibromyalgia (FM), formerly "fibrositis." From studies over two decades, new, internationally recognized criteria for the diagnosis of FM have emerged.[1] The combination of *widespread pain and tenderness at 11 or more of 18 defined sites* yielded sensitivity of 88% (88% of patients preselected with this diagnosis met these criteria) and specificity of 81% (meaning that 19% of patients with other pain syndromes met these criteria). This happy simplicity was as unexpected as it is welcome. The addition of any other criteria reduced sensitivity or specificity. Accompanying symptoms of fatigue, headache, and sensitivity to a variety of stimuli in the external and internal environment were equally common in all subgroups; so "at the diagnostic or classification level, the distinction between primary . . . and secondary-concomitant fibromyalgia . . . is abandoned." The statistical power of the criteria came from the addition of the disciplined tender point count (Fig. 5-1).

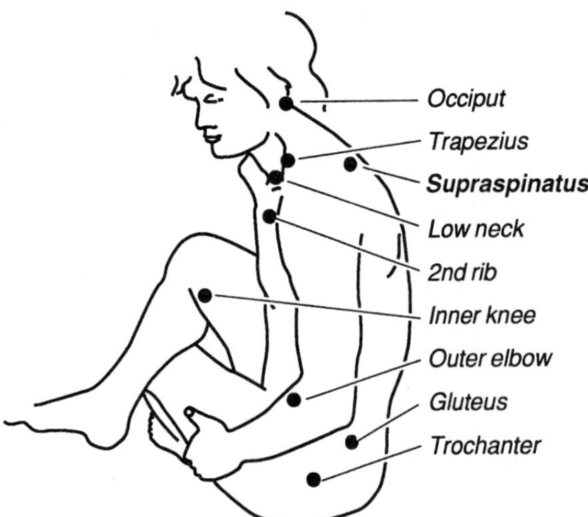

Figure 5-1. The tender points in the ACR criteria set.

Think of it; "fibromyalgia" translates as widespread pain, and "fibrositis" as points of tenderness.

The **pathogenesis** of these features also can be summarized simply. The location of the pain and the different locations of the tender points are determined by the patterns of referred pain associated with mechanical problems in the lower neck and back. The severity of the pain and the presence of the accompanying symptoms are further influenced by amplifying factors, such as sleep disturbance and physical deconditioning. Vicious cycles develop. Stresses during sleep aggravate neck pain, so that sleep is nonrestorative. Morning pain stiffness and fatigue inhibit activity, with rapid physical deconditioning.

It follows that diagnosis depends on the understanding that nonarticular pain may often be due to referred pain mechanisms. Assessment of such patients requires a systematic examination for characteristic patterns of unexpected tenderness and nontenderness, and a knowledgeable search for the source of such referred pain.

It follows also that treatment requires *two phases*: in the first, correction of ongoing mechanical problems in the *neck and back*; and in the second, long-term efforts to *develop a high level of general fitness*. The second phase is often harder, because fitness activities demand energy, which is in short supply and which may increase pain.

Prevalence

Epidemiological studies have shown that over 10% of adults, when questioned, have widespread pain. Applying the American College of Rheumatology (ACR) criteria for fibromyalgia, there was a prevalence of 3.8% in adult females and 0.5% in males, increasing with age.[2] There are many with regional problems, similar in nature to those underlying fibromyalgia, but with fewer tender points. Patients with other forms of arthritis are at increased risk, and the coexistence of arthritis with fibromyalgia may lead to inappropriate and even dangerous treatment.[3]

Phenomena Associated with Pain

Deep Pain Differs From Surface Pain

Injury to a finger (which is richly represented in our cerebral cortex and consciousness) is felt in a fraction of a second, located precisely, with accurate information about the injurious agent; sharp, burning, cold, or crushing. This effect is so strong that you can still feel a hand, even if it is amputated—it exists in the brain, as well as at the end of your arm.

None of this is true of deep structures. The joints of the spine, for example, are not represented in our conscious brain, and cannot be pictured in our imagination. Pain from a deep structure *must* be referred; that is, misrepresented as arising in some other region.

Referred Pain and Referred Tenderness

A deep spinal origin is obvious when there is a continuous band of pain spreading from the spine to the hand or foot; but this situation is uncommon. The pain is often discontinuous and variable in quality, and, most difficult of all, the central site of origin may be without any symptoms at all! Pain arising deep in the neck is never perceived to arise in structures about the 5–6 and 6–7 disks. It is commonly felt as pain in the (nontender) back of the neck (massage gives comfort), but also may be felt as headache; or chest wall, shoulder, or elbow pain, or as numbness in the hand.[4] This makes diagnosis and treatment very difficult for patients and health professionals alike.

In response to the pain, protective effects occur, including spasm and weakness of muscle, increased blood flow, and enhanced tenderness. When the pain is deep in origin, these responses also are misplaced to regions remote from the site of injury, just as the pain is referred. There is one key difference. The location of referred pain and allied sensations is quite variable from patient to patient, but the sites of referred tenderness are precisely predictable in location. These sites are themselves deep, and usually are not central to the areas of referred pain, so are generally unknown to the patient.

Exactly the same points are tender in regional as in general pain syndromes, and understanding of pathogenesis and treatment of widespread pain syndromes requires a clear grasp of the nature and treatment of regional pain.

Pain Equivalents

When pain is referred to the leg, or to the forearm or hand, it often changes character. The distress that is felt as an *aching* or *pressure* centrally, may feel like *burning* elsewhere, or not like pain at all, but *swelling*. When pain from the neck is referred to the forearm or hand, it often changes to a feeling of *numbness* or *tingling*, and loss of nerve function (carpal tunnel syndrome) may be suspected. This can be checked by a simple test. When the sensation of numbness is present, rub the fingers over a piece of clothing. If the patient can tell the difference between cloth and paper, major nerve damage is extremely unlikely.

Headache behind and above the eyes is similarly common,[5] and mislabeled "tension headache." This is simply referred pain from the neck, and relates to the complex neural links between eyes and fingers that gives us our human hand skills. Similarly, dizziness, an *unsteadiness* rather than a spinning feeling, is common in patients with neck problems.

Tender-Point Assessment as an Objective Pain Measure

Pain can be exaggerated or suppressed, but it is a personal experience, not objectively accessible for independent evaluation. In contrast, the *tenderness* is unknown to the patient, and can be measured objectively, as the force required to produce pain at the characteristic "active" sites. Equally characteristic "control" points have been identified, which remain nontender despite being located in regions to which pain is often referred. The naiveté of the patient about the tender and control points is almost total, and the pattern is not subject to psychological bias. These patterns will be described in more detail later.

The precisely predictable tenderness in areas without symptoms, contrasted with unexpected lack of tenderness at control sites, permit objective assessment of subjective pain.

Cervical Syndromes

Frequency and Location of Neck Problems

Low neck problems are as common as low back problems. Symptoms and tenderness long predate radiographic changes. By the age of 30, 30% of one population studied had neck/shoulder/arm pain, but in 90% of these, the radiographs showed minimal or no changes.[6] By the age of 50, 50% showed radiographic changes. At 65, 90% showed damage. These changes are concentrated in the lower neck, exactly where we find the tenderness; but the tenderness appears decades earlier.

The pain is referred to a wide variety of possible sites determined by the problems in the low neck, and so is the quite different location of the tender points. The multiplicity and pattern of tenderness is important. If only one point is found, a diagnosis such as "tennis elbow," "bursitis," or "tendonitis" is reasonable. It is important that the alternative diagnosis, of a referred pain syndrome, be carefully considered. When examination reveals many tender points in a characteristic pattern, the local injury hypothesis becomes untenable. When pain is confined to a local region, it is helpful to know of characteristic points additional to those defined in the 1990 criteria (see Fig. 5-1). With neck support, the 5–6 cervical level and related referred sites may lose their tenderness. However, the 6–7 cervical interspace, inadequately supported during sleep, may remain very tender, and with changes in the pattern of referred tenderness (Fig. 5-2). The "tennis elbow" sites will be much less tender than the medial epicondyle. The trapezius no longer will be tender, but the origin and insertion of pectoralis minor will be tender, behind the outer breast and at the tip of the coracoid. The pain may be lower, between the scapulae, or about or below the breasts. These associations are all characteristic of the **syndrome of the 6–7 cervical segments.**[4]

The Biomechanics of Cervical Strain

It has been observed that degenerative changes in humans occur at sites that are anatomically unique. What is special about the human neck? It is not our neck that is different; it is our shoulders. We can swing our arms through 360 degrees; dogs and horses cannot. We can climb, swim, and throw. Humans have broad shoulders that permit great versatility of upper limb function. So we can do all sorts of things through the day that other animals cannot. But there is one drawback; we cannot *sleep* on our side without stressing our neck. The chest part of the spine is supported by our ribs and shoulders, but the lower neck is unsupported, and sags, and locks, with tight ligaments and crushed bone (Fig. 5-3).

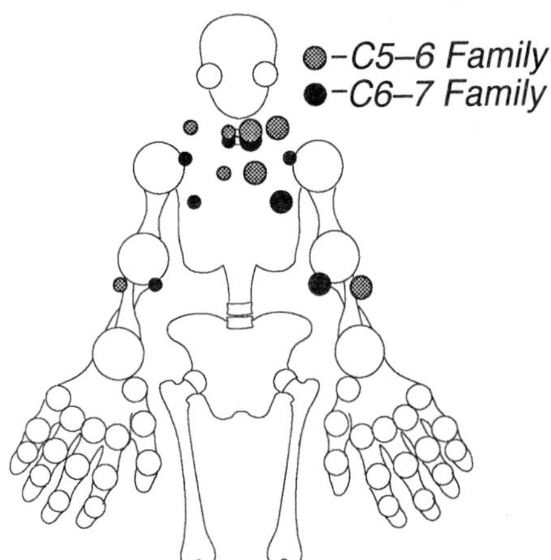

Figure 5-2. Distribution of tender points associated with chronic neck strain. The location and quality of the pain are variable, but the location of the tenderness is different, constant, and predictable, with a different pattern of points related to the C6–7 level from those defined in the ACR criteria.

Treatment of Neck Problems

The solution is to deliver precisely focused support to the key site, the lower neck, throughout sleep (Fig. 5-4). This can be a difficult learning process, because the patient is unaware of the very tender site deep in the front of the lower neck, just above the medial end of the clavicle. The thoracic spine is curved to accommodate the heart and lungs, and has limited flexibility in its upper half. During sleep, the forward curve of the upper thoracic spine should be continued into the neck. An erect posture of the head and neck requires extension of the lower neck, tightening the tender structures in the front of the lower vertebrae.

Further, there is a problem with the lower shoulder. It tends to rise to the level of the chin, displacing support away from the lowest levels in the neck where it is needed. Look carefully at the

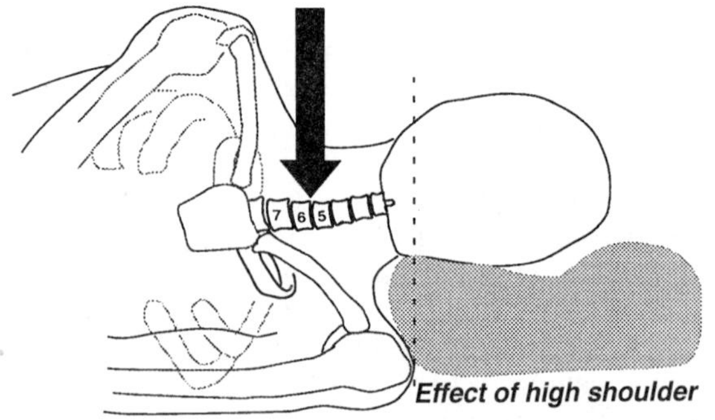

Figure 5-3. Problems in the lower neck during sleep. The ribs and shoulders support the chest. The lower neck is unsupported and the vertebrae sag until ligaments tighten, then lock and twist.

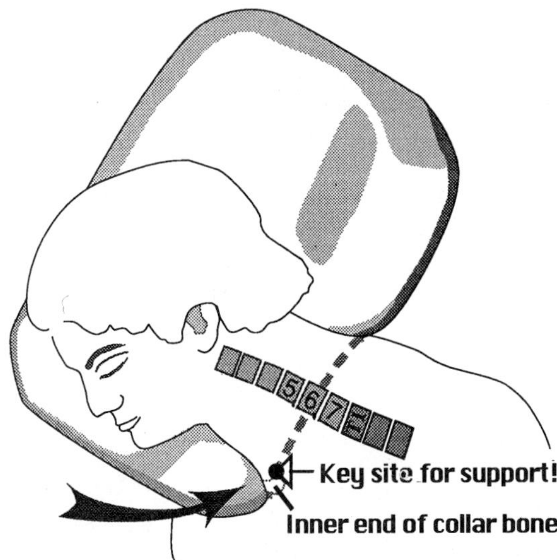

Figure 5-4. The neck is forward, continuing the curve of the spine in the upper chest. This relaxes ligaments in the front of the low neck and opens space for support to the lower cervical vertebrae.

dotted line in Figure 5-4, the 5–6 level is supported, the 6–7 level is not.

A solution is to roll the upper shoulder and neck forward, to open space between chin and shoulder, allowing access to the lower neck by the neck support. This will only be comfortable if a large pillow is placed under the chest and waist, raising the trunk so that the neck is not twisted, and relieving pressure on arm and shoulder.

Significance of the C6–7 Syndrome

When neck support has caused disappearance of tenderness at the 5–6 level in the neck, this is often associated with disappearance of tenderness at the trapezius, second rib, and outer elbow sites. This strongly argues that the earlier tenderness at these sites was determined segmentally, and by mechanical factors in the spine. It also points to revised treatment strategies, which seem to be effective.[4]

By extension, it also argues that other syndromes featured by the association of pain and characteristic tender sites may be determined segmentally by referred pain mechanisms, and especially with pain due to mechanical factors in the spine. If so, it would predict that treatment programs that ignore these factors and depend solely on centrally acting medication or behavioral modification (or alternatively, on treatments primarily directed at the peripheral sites of referred tenderness) will be equally disappointing. The common automatic association of tricyclic medications with "fibromyalgia," or stretch-and-spray or "trigger point" injections with "myofascial pain syndromes," indicates the distortions that may arise simply from the terminology used.

Suspect a referred pain syndrome when patients present with regional "myofascial" pain.

Back Problems

Ten to 30% of adults have back pain at any time. Pain sufficient to impair ability to work affects 3–12% of the population. No group is immune. Young and fit athletes are at risk, just as are sedentary workers. Generally, the prognosis is benign; 90% of those forced to lose time return to work within 2 months. About 5% remain disabled after 1 year, and most of the social and financial costs relate to this chronic pain group.

Developmental Changes in the Human Spine

Damage is concentrated in the two lower lumbar segments. Other animals show neither this prevalence nor distribution. At birth, the lumbar spine and sacrum are straight in humans, as in all other mammals (Fig. 5-5). At about 1 year of age we begin to walk, at a time when abdominal muscle strength is not yet developed, so that the tummy sags, the rump is prominent, and the characteristically sharp human lumbosacral angle appears. The upright posture allowed humans to develop the special skills of our arms and hands. This freedom was obtained at the cost of locking our low back, hips, and knees at the limit of the range of travel. Locked joints are subject to much greater crushing forces than those that are free to move. The strong position for the back is the "ready" position of an athlete, with knees, hips, and back gently flexed.

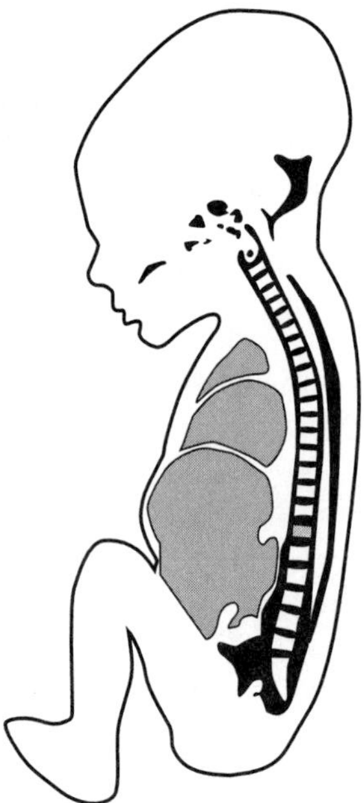

Figure 5-5. Infant spine; no lumbar curve.

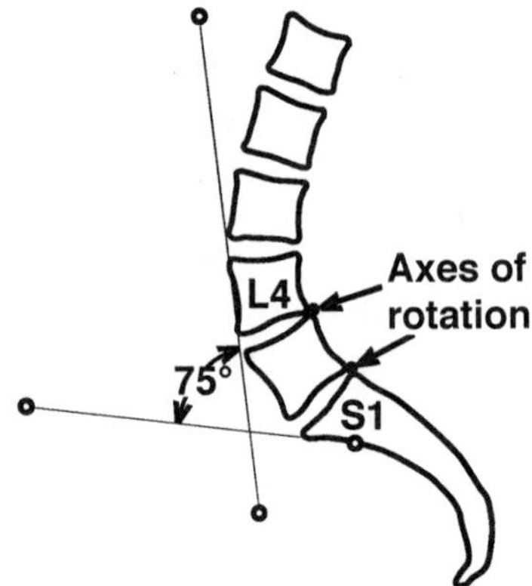

Figure 5-6. Locked low back in humans. At the limit of extension, crushing forces are greatest at the axes of rotation.

Figure 5-6 shows the angles in the low back when we stand erect. The problem is not just that we have a curve in the low back, but that the two lower levels may be *locked* at the limit of their range of travel. The force through a locked joint rises dramatically.[7]

The Mechanics of a Locked Joint

In explaining this problem, body language may be more convincing than words. Hold the subject's middle finger firmly. If the finger is slightly bent forward, at the metacarpophalangeal joint, you can load the base of the finger with all your force and produce no pain. Move the finger back until ligaments tighten, and the joint is locked. It begins to hurt *even if the pressure is directed away from the joint!* The pain is due to the interaction between tight ligaments and crushed bone. This is the nature of pain of mechanical origin, in the low back or low neck.

Patterns of Referred Tenderness in Back Syndromes

Quantitative tender-point assessment permits objective assessment of the relative severity of pain for scientific or legal purposes. The naiveté of the patient about tender and control points is so valuable that I am almost reluctant to divulge my trade secrets!

Consider, for example, the region of the knee. Most often the pain is felt posteriorly or laterally, but these regions remain nontender and offer excellent control points. The inner knee is usually not symptomatic, but marked tenderness is found there, with a complex inner anatomy. There is tenderness in the fat pad posterior to vastus medialis, 7 cm above the joint line, and 7 cm below the joint line there is less tenderness at the level of the joint itself, and much less on the outer side, where the pain may be felt (Fig. 5-7). Another very characteristic and useful point lies in the instep, in the origin of the short flexor muscle to the great toe. This again will be unknown to the patient, and is sharply localized; tissues 1 cm away can tolerate 20 times as much pressure. These points indicate a spinal origin of obscure knee or foot complaints.

Importance of the Abdominal Muscles

The two lower disks are the site of most problems in the low back, and locked extension is the reason for this special vulnerability. Why do some recover less well than others? There are a number of factors, but the most common and reversible is abdominal muscle weakness. In one study, abdominal muscle strength in males with back pain was 40% less than in asymptomatic subjects at the same work site.[8] No examination of a patient with back or leg pain is complete without an assessment of abdominal muscle strength. A simple clinical method is shown in Figure 5-8. Studies have shown this method to be statistically as efficient as more complex measures. If abdominal muscles remain weak, the lower spine is doomed to sag into locked lumbar hyperextension. Other causes of lumbar hyperextension must be identified, such as flexed hips, due either to joint disease or to tight surrounding ligaments. A pelvic tilt, due to unequal leg length or spinal problems, may be a correctable factor.

The Fibrositis/Fibromyalgia Syndrome

The ACR criteria[1] for the classification of fibromyalgia are designed to identify groups of patients for study. They are not more than a guide to the evaluation of an individual patient, and a second definition deals more specifically with cause and treatment. The **location** of pain, and the different locations of the points of referred tenderness, are determined by the patterns of referred pain associated with mechanical problems in the lower neck and back. The **severity** of the pain, and the presence of the accompanying symptoms, are further influenced by **amplifying factors**, such as sleep disturbance and physical deconditioning. In brief, fibromyalgia is about necks, backs, sleep, and fitness.

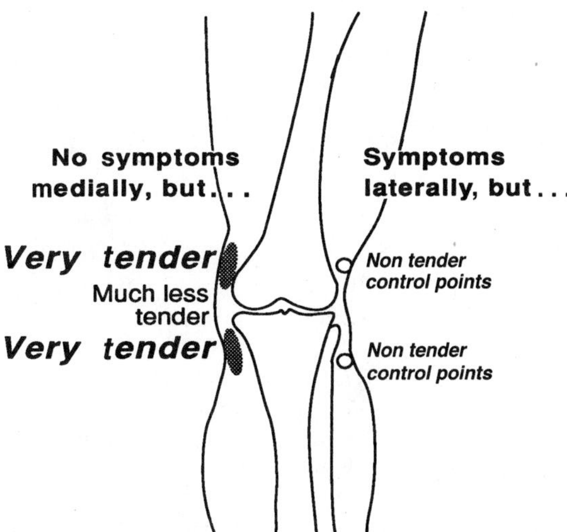

Figure 5-7. Tender and control sites near the left knee with referred pain from the back.

The outstanding symptoms of the fibrositis/fibromyalgia syndrome are pain, stiffness, and fatigue. In addition, there are a cluster of other symptoms, describable as an excess sensitivity to unpleasant stimuli other than pain. These include cold; weather change; and other irritants in the external environment such as noise, bright lights, and cigarette smoke. Their eyes may feel dry or sensitive, but tear formation is normal. In addition, they are sensitive to unpleasant internal stimuli and may have an irritable stomach, irritable bowel, irritable bladder, or persistent nonproductive cough. Exercise may cause marked increase in muscle soreness. An amplification of pain is related to poor sleep and physical deconditioning, and the modulation of other unpleasant stimuli is similarly affected. Let us review some data (Table 5-1).

The "neurological" symptoms often are not recognized to be part of chronic pain syndromes, even by health professionals. Two common misdiagnoses are carpal tunnel syndrome because of the sensation of numbness, and the chronic fatigue syndrome because of abrupt onset, headache, impaired thinking, and profound sense of weakness.

Nonrestorative Sleep and Physical Unfitness

In early studies, fibromyalgic patients described a morning increase in pain and stiffness, associated with profound exhaustion; they were worsened rather than refreshed by their sleep. When measured, dreaming sleep was essentially normal in "fibrositic" patients. What emerged unexpectedly was a profound disturbance in deep nondreaming sleep,[9] with intrusion of alpha rhythms into deep non–rapid eye movement (REM) sleep. This was studied further.[10]

> Two groups of young, healthy, nonathletic volunteers were subjected to selective sleep stage deprivation. Six subjects were deprived of stage 4 sleep and seven subjects of REM sleep. The stage 4 deprived group reported more musculoskeletal symptoms during the deprivation than the REM deprived group. The stage 4 deprived group also showed a significant increase in muscle tenderness, between the baseline and deprivation conditions and an altered pattern of overnight change in muscle tenderness in re-

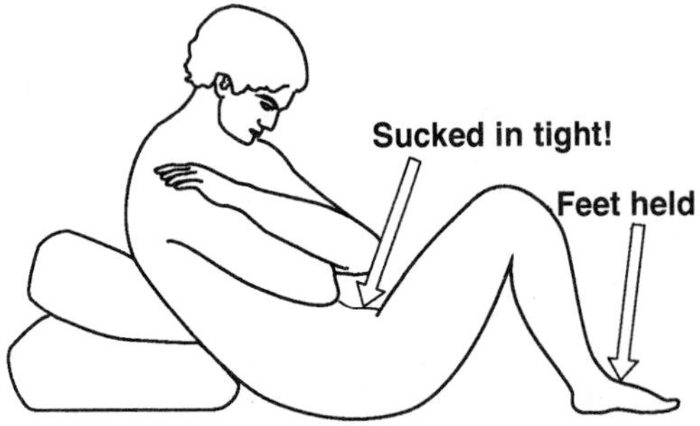

Figure 5-8. Safe, tough situp. This is graded on a 0–6 scale: grade 1 when a situp can be done only with a two- or three-pillow head start; grade 2 when lying flat with arms extended over thighs; and 3–6 when hands are at opposite elbows, shoulders, behind the neck, or behind the head to the opposite ears.

sponse to deprivation. The REM deprived group did not show either of these changes.

However, the stage 4 sleep deprivation condition alone is not responsible for the emergence of musculoskeletal symptoms. Physical fitness may be an important variable. All our subjects did not exercise regularly and tended to lead sedentary lives. Furthermore, in a pilot study, three subjects who were quite physically fit and accustomed to running 2–7 miles per day did not develop pain symptoms or changes in dolorimeter scores while undergoing the stage 4 deprivation experiment. [They did show alpha intrusion when a buzzer was used to disturb their sleep.]

Sleep apnea[11] and sleep-related myoclonus[12] have both been associated with fibromyalgia in some but not all subjects. These sleep anomalies are not in themselves sufficient or specific causes of fibromyalgia; there must be other factors. In pain-tolerant subjects, or in those with resolved regional pain, sleep disturbance can lead to chronic fatigue, daytime drowsiness, or to no symptoms at all.

Measurement of Tenderness

Tenderness has been measured as a simple count of tender points, as scored tenderness, or by dolorimetry, determining the force needed to reach pain threshold. Palpation is statistically as effective as dolorimetry, though the latter may be useful for medicolegal or research purposes. Females, steroid-treated, lupus, and rheumatoid patients were more tender, after controlling for the other effects. The tender points of subjects with both rheumatoid arthritis and concomitant fibromyalgia were

Table 5-1. Fibromyalgia Criteria Study (n = 558)*†

Symptom	Sensitivity	Specificity	Accuracy
Symptoms of Pain			
Neck pain	85.3%	49.6%	67.5%
Low back pain	78.8%	54.4%	66.6%
Widespread pain	97.6%	30.9%	65.9%
Headache	52.8%	72.6%	62.3%
Symptoms of Excess Sensitivity			
Irritable bowel	29.6%	87.5%	57.1%
Irritable eyes	35.8%	77.0%	55.4%
Irritable bladder	26.3%	84.5%	54.2%
Dysmenorrhea	40.6%	68.3%	53.4%

*Adapted from Wolfe F, Smythe HA, Yunus MB. The American College of Rheumatology 1990 criteria for the classification of fibromyalgia; report of the multicenter criteria committee. Arthritis Rheum 1990; 33:160–172. With permission.

†Sensitivity was the proportion of fibromyalgia patients with the complaint or symptom, specificity the proportion of controls without the manifestation, and accuracy the mean of the two.

considerably more tender than actively inflamed rheumatoid joints, even in the same subjects.[3,13]

The Muscles in Fibromyalgia

Reduced oxygen uptake, fiber atrophy, and other noninflammatory changes have been demonstrated in the muscles of patients with fibromyalgia. These are present throughout the muscles, at nontender as well as tender sites, occur in a variety of other conditions, and likely represent the effects of deconditioning defined.[14]

Memory and Concentration

A prominent and disturbing symptom for many patients is forgetfulness and impaired concentration. These symptoms have perhaps not been adequately documented in classic studies and review of fibromyalgia, and are given greater prominence in accounts of the chronic fatigue syndrome, and in whiplash injuries.[5]

The Treatment Program

As summarized in the introduction, the treatment program usually has two separate phases. In the first, we concentrate on strategies to **correct mechanical problems in the neck and low back**. With a safe back and neck, the second, harder stage is begun: long-term efforts to **develop a high level of general fitness**. In controlled studies, aerobic exercise has improved maximum oxygen uptake and symptom tolerance in patients with FM. Postexercise myalgia was a problem and we learned not to try to achieve "too much too soon."[15,16]

Without a safe neck and back, fitness activities may cause flares; without fitness, the return of energy, restorative sleep, and tolerance to pain can be only partially successful, and dependent on the use of imperfect medications.

Pain Relief

A variety of physical measures may give some relief, and generally without side effects. These include heat, cold, massage, liniments, and electrical stimulation. All release the body's own internal morphine-like pain relievers. All work similarly, so choose that which is readily available, not that which is trendy and expensive.

Medicines are only modestly helpful and not ideal for long-term use. The most effective agents—the tricyclics—are given in small doses to help correct the nonrestorative sleep problem. Studies of their effectiveness have shown modest benefit, particularly in the first few months, but with evidence of loss of effect with time.[17] Withdrawal may precipitate symptom increase. Formulations currently available persist in the body, with half remaining in about 30 hours. Doses adequate to help sleep are often followed by daytime fogginess, making return to high levels of mental or physical activity more difficult. Short-acting hypnotics are less effective in correcting the specific sleep disturbance, but may be prescribed for short periods to control stress and anxiety.

Strategies: Cope or Control, Passive or Active

Some programs have emphasized coping strategies such as relaxation and stretching exercises, as well as the use of heat, massage, and electrical stimulation. These measures may give temporary comfort and a feeling of greater control, but are ineffective in relieving pain and restoring energy, drive, and function.[14,18] The responsibility for improvement is focused on the health professional, with the patient a passive recipient. Effective therapies described are neither obvious nor easy and are certainly more demanding. The program described here restores responsibility to the patient, is available 7 days a week, and provides a sound path to recovery. The emphasis is on hope, not cope.

Setbacks: Avoiding, Active Recovery

Active programs may be punctuated with a temporary increase in symptoms if some of the built-in safety techniques fail for one reason or another. The details of a safe sit-up, of neck support, and of exercise strategies are very important. Because deep structures are involved, accurate and timely feedback may not be consciously registered in time to prevent flares. Some patients have had such disappointments, so many blows to their confidence and self-esteem, and so much pain and exhaustion, that it is difficult for them to believe that *they* can improve, and that the discipline and effort will pay off. The good news is that they *can* be much better; the bad news is that *only they* can make it happen. The therapist points the way and checks the details, but it is the patient's job to improve.

With the active treatment program described, about half of subjects studied have achieved major or complete relief in 6 months, and about 75% in 18 months.[4] This may seem too slow, but it is better to set realistic goals and adhere to a consistent strategy.

Evaluation of the Patient with Chronic Pain

Assessment for the purpose of diagnosis can be simple, as most of the information about tenderness is contained in a subset of eight of the ACR points (four right and four left; see Fig. 5-9).[19] Often, as part of the treatment strategy, the assessment must include an educational component. The patient needs to learn the relevance of neck support, situp exercises and aerobic fitness, and the interview becomes more complex and time-consuming. Evaluation of relative severity is even more demanding, especially if there are insurance or medicolegal issues. Evidence of exaggerated pain behavior should be recorded but interpreted with caution. Opinion about prognosis may be requested. In this review, we will concentrate on an efficient basic examination, with indications of the elements of more extensive approaches.

Examination for Tenderness

How hard should you press? About 4 kg. This is a learned skill. Observer variation can be halved with training, and it is helpful to have a dolorimeter or even a bathroom scale. The pressure is delivered by the bone in the end of your terminal phalanx. Learn not only the feel of 4 kg, but also observe the associated degree of blanching in and beside the nail bed.

Measuring Tenderness

Tender points can be counted as present or absent, scored as to severity, or measured by dolorimetry, in terms of the kilograms of force required to reach pain threshold. With a limited number of points,

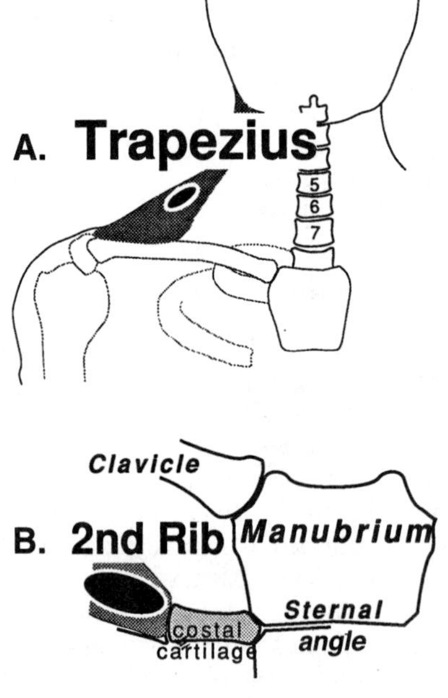

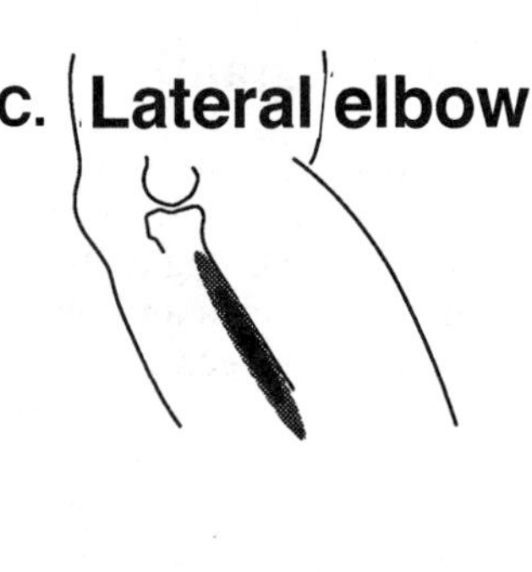

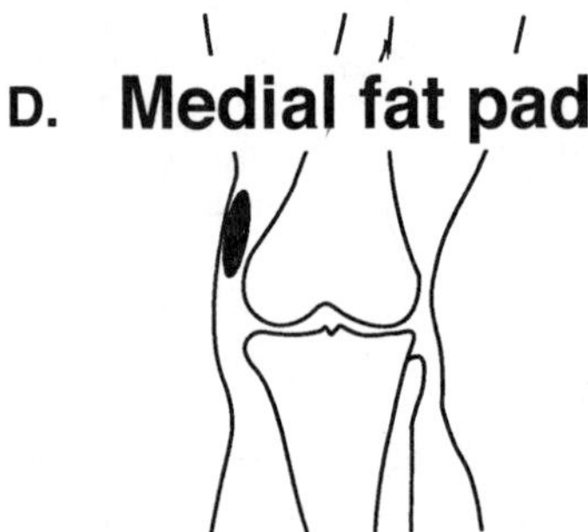

Figure 5-9. Sites for screening exam. *A*, Trapezius, the tender point is in the muscle at the midpoint of the upper border. *B*, Second rib, the tender point is in the origin of the pectoralis major muscle, near the costochondral junction. *C*, Lateral elbow, the tender point is about 3–6 cm from the epicondyle, in the extensor muscle of the middle finger, rotating with the radius. *D*, Medial fat pad located 3–6 cm above the knee joint line, just posterior to the vastus medialis.

a tenderness score can function well statistically and is easily translated into counts. Variation among examiners can be a problem with any of these techniques, and formal testing of interobserver variation can identify difficulties and provide the feedback that ensures uniformity of technique. The following scoring system has been used extensively.

0 = None
1 = Mild; expressed, but no withdrawal
2 = Moderate; expressed plus withdrawal
3 = Severe; immediate exaggerated withdrawal
4 = Patient untouchable; withdraws without palpation

Results are recorded on the form shown in Table 5-2. For the ACR point count, if tender circle on Figures 5-1 or 5-2: occiput R, L; supraspinatus origin R, L; neck R, L; gluteus R, L; trochanter R, L.

Accessory Points

For regional pain syndromes, other points are helpful, and points relevant to the neck and low back were discussed and illustrated earlier.

Possible Neck Problems

With the patient lying, examine for tenderness at the upper body sites defined in the ACR criteria study (see Fig. 5-1), at the **key site** in the low anterior neck just above the inner end of the clavicle; and at the C6–7 sites, coracoid tip, lateral pectoral, and medial epicondyle (see Fig. 5-2).

Possible Low Back Problems

Check for abdominal muscle weakness (Fig. 5-7), locked lumbar hyperextension, and accessory sites of referred tenderness (Fig. 5-6 and text). Check for limited forward flexion in terms of finger-floor distance, limited straight leg raising, pain on dorsiflexion of the foot, popliteal nerve tenderness, muscle weakness, and reflex loss.

Table 5-2. Four-Site Screening Examination Form (For scoring, see text.)

Sites	Palpation, Score 0–4 Right	Left
Trapezius		
Second rib		
Lateral elbow		
Medial knee		

Control Sites

Examination of "control" sites may be very helpful. In most patients, these remain nontender to palpation, even though these lie in regions to which pain is commonly referred. The ACR criteria for FM did not require this characteristic, but other criteria sets do. The sites used in the ACR study were: the dorsal aspect of the distal third of the forearm, the thumbnail, and the midpoint of the third metatarsal dorsally. Other useful sites include the vastus lateralis above the outer knee, and the origin of tibialis anterior, to contrast with tenderness in the fat pads medially proximal and distal to the knee joint line. By dolorimetry, these sites are more tender in some patients with chronic pain syndromes, but this is not often detectable on palpation. In the absence of steroid therapy or autoimmune disease, widespread control point tenderness may reinforce other evidence of exaggerated pain behavior.

Pain Behavior

Many signs of exaggerated pain behavior have been described, with the implication that these are markers of malingering. This is of course a very important issue, but none of these signs have been validated by published experimental studies to separate cultural or individual responses to real pain from deliberate faking or abnormal pain behavior. Control site tenderness certainly suggests exaggerated responses, but can be seen in severe physical deconditioning, or in subjects with autoimmune diseases, or on steroid therapy. In a group of subjects, some normal and some with pain syndromes of varying severity, examined when responding normally and when exaggerating, the following markers[20] were found to be helpful in distinguishing normal from exaggerated responses: (1) grimacing, (2) bracing, (3) sighing, (4) rubbing, (5) guarding, (6) leap, (7) alert and passive anticipation, (8) inconsistency, (9) groans, (10) histrionic behavior, and (11) tremor. One study has reported that individuals with FM and such markers are just as responsive to therapy as more stoical subjects.[21]

Relative Severity

The current level of symptoms may be recorded using

A pain scale
A pain diagram, or standard questionnaire
Level of function, by informal or formal questionnaire, or task performance

These subjective evaluations should be supported by objective measurements of tenderness, by quantitative point counts, scored tenderness, or dolorimetry, in each case checking for inappropriate control site tenderness or other evidence of exaggerated pain behavior.

For legal purposes, use objective, qualitative tender point assessment.

Disability Assessment

For most purposes, the task is simple. The patient can describe the severity of their pain, stiffness, and fatigue on a 0 to 10 scale. They can further describe endurance, variation with time of day, and specific tasks that give trouble. Examination of the characteristic tender sites can be very helpful, because the patient is unaware of their existence, and the severity of the unexpected tenderness, contrasted with lack of tenderness at control sites, gives an independent measure of the severity of their pain syndrome. The examiner can record evidences (or lack) of exaggeration or inconsistency, which may be verbal, in reactions during examination, or during performance tasks such as grip strength or situps. But well-motivated patients can be theatrical, or apprehensive.

"The problem . . . is face validity. Patients with FM don't look ill. Clinically, they are not weak. They would appear to be able to do most tasks and ADL activities in ways that would appear to belie their HAQ scores."[22, p 71,74] "The type of information needed to support or oppose a claim usually is not present in ordinary medical records."[22, p 81] Expert opinion is unusually important in leading to a fair evaluation. However, the physician's responsibility to serve the best interests of the patient may appear to be in conflict with the duty to society, and the physician may seem to "substitute compassion and intelligence for medical truth in these circumstances."[22, p 82] Carefully gathered and presented data are to be preferred to an opinion possibly biased on either side.

Cathey et al compared FM and rheumatoid arthritis (RA) patients to normal controls, using a computerized work simulator. The FM patients initially did well, but decreased their rate of performance or discontinued because of pain. For both the RA and FM patients, there were strong correlations (*r* values between .50 and .77) between work performance and other measures, such as disability index (HAQ scores), grip strength, patient assessments of global severity, and pain scores.[23] These observations seem to validate these measures of disability; however, it should be recognized that other interpretations are possible. Statements of functional limitation(s) should be verifiable on testing. There may be advantages in the consistent use of well-designed questionnaires or structured assessments, but all in common use are as vulnerable as a visual analogue scale to biased perceptions by patient, observer, or both.

If doubt remains, follow-up assessments may give new insights. At the first visit, they have all performed a situp; perhaps with a three-pillow head start, but painlessly. I will have made much of this, because the load through their lower back during a situp is quite large, but by avoiding hyperextension they have had two victories; first the situp effort, and second, freedom from pain when the back is in a safe position. At the next visit, they are to have continued this exercise. If they have not, it is made very clear that they are not trying hard enough to get better. More often, one is rewarded to find that this initially frightened patient has in fact worked hard, and has been rewarded by decreased lower body pain and tenderness.

Relation to Specific Precipitating Events

Are the patient's undoubted symptoms and disability attributable to a specific reported injury? A history of previous vigorous good health, changed by a significant trauma to unrelenting pain, is often offered, but previous medical records may reveal that related symptoms have occurred in the recent past. When compensation is claimed, it may be very important to check all medical documentation, particularly that available for the period before the event. It is therefore in the patient's best interest to respond honestly to questions about past health, as misleading statements will destroy credibility.

There is a sequence common to many injuries of deep spinal structures, with features that may be misunderstood. As stated earlier, a finger is richly represented in our cerebral cortex; an injury is felt at once, localized accurately, and identified as sharp, burning, or crushing. Injury to a deep spinal structure may not be perceived for hours or days, can never be accurately localized, and the referred distress may have the quality of numbness, tingling, or swelling in distal sites, and aching, tension, or burning more centrally. The same injury may produce all of these diverse qualities simultaneously! At first the symptoms are confined to a single region but with time may become widespread. This is particularly true of neck injuries. Aggravation by stresses during sleep results in increased morning pain, stiffness, and fatigue. Physical deconditioning follows, which may particularly affect abdominal muscle strength, leading to back and lower limb pain. Poor sleep and deconditioning lead to sensitivity to a variety of external and internal irritants, from weather to irritable bowel or bladder. This sequence is sufficiently familiar to be known as "metastasizing fibromyalgia." Many consultants cannot understand the mechanisms involved, and dismiss the whole chain of events as incredible.

Prognosis

Patient Factors

The patient who has always kept fit and been free of chronic pain symptoms can reasonably expect to return to that high level of function. Previous headache, abdominal or musculoskeletal pain, and multiple surgical procedures all warn of slower progress. In the young, hypermobility is a risk factor for neck and back complaints. Later, obesity is a daunting problem. Is the patient actively accepting responsibility for improvement, or are passive coping strategies favored? Are there firmly held, alternative belief structures about the cause and remedy of their symptoms?

The social setting also is important. If a job change is needed, does the patient have the educational and other resources to adapt, and support structures at home, at work, and in society to enable that change? Or is their life such that their best survival strategy is to remain disabled?

Health Care System Factors

Ideally, there should be no need for consultants, but an informed and responsive primary care team, sensitive to the symptom language of referred pain syndromes, and to the need for early active and appropriate therapy. Ideally, much of the "work hardening" should be available at the work site. Ideally, the primary care providers would be competent and professional and keep records adequate to determine if neck problems have been identified and treated; abdominal muscle weakness identified and treated; fitness problems identified and treated. A multidisciplinary and coherent program should be available, including an educational program with support material for the patient.

Summary

The diagnosis in patients with chronic pain syndromes presents problems. Because the quality of pain may differ from region to region, and because of accompanying symptoms such as numbness, weakness, dizziness, fatigue, or impaired concentration, the same patient may be perceived, investigated, and advised very differently by different health professionals. The possibility of early, serious neurological diseases, such as multiple sclerosis or amyotrophic lateral sclerosis, may lead to deep anxiety and extensive, fruitless investigations. In this presentation I have dealt perhaps too briefly with these varying but common symptom patterns.

The name attached to the syndrome may dictate treatment responses and prognosis. The label "fibromyalgia" may lead to tricyclic medications as a primary treatment response, to gloomy predictions, and to emphasis on coping strategies. The same patient, assessed elsewhere, may be given a variety of diagnostic labels, including migraines, various myofascial pain syndromes, carpal tunnel syndromes, and various forms of "-itis"—tendinitis, bursitis, epicondylitis, neuritis, costochondritis (what bad luck to have all these separate entities at once!). Treatment routines are prescribed with more optimism, more costs, but no more benefit.

For brevity, these complexities have been described in a condensed, perhaps simplistic account. In particular, the treatment program has been presented only in outline; but the devil is in the details. What do you do on the second visit, when the patient reports that he/she cannot do the prescribed situps, disliked the neck support, has had no improvement, and has forgotten all of the explanations and techniques demonstrated in such detail at the first visit? Furthermore, they have had contradictory advice from other health professionals. Who are they to believe? An effective response requires patience, empathy, and above all, time—that which is always in short supply. Stern authority is not appropriate; the patient must share the evidence that underlies the details of the long-term strategy.

References

1. Wolfe F, Smythe HA, Yunus MB: The American College of Rheumatology 1990 criteria for the classification of fibromyalgia; report of the multicenter criteria committee. Arthritis Rheum 1990; 33:160–172.
2. Wolfe F, Ross K, Anderson J, et al: The prevalence and characteristics of fibromyalgia in the general population (abstr 57). Arthritis Rheum 1993; 36(Suppl):S48.
3. Buskila D, Langevitz P, Gladman DD, et al: Patients with rheumatoid arthritis are more tender than those with psoriatic arthritis. J Rheumatol 1992; 19:1115–1119.
4. Smythe HA: The C6–7 syndrome—clinical features and treatment response. J Rheumatol 1994; 21: 1520–1526.
5. Radanov BP, Sturzenegger M, De Stefano G, et al: Relationship between early somatic radiological, cognitive and psychological findings and outcome during a one-year followup in 117 patients suffering from common whiplash. Br J Rheumatol 1994; 33: 442–448.
6. Lawrence JS: Disc degeneration: its frequency and relation to symptoms. Ann Rheum Dis 1969; 28: 121–138.
7. Smythe HA: The mechanical pathogenesis of generalized osteoarthritis. J Rheumatol 1983; 9(Suppl): 11–12.
8. Nachemson A, Lindh M: Measurement of abdominal and back muscle strength with and without low back pain. Scand J Rehabil Med 1969; 1:60–65.
9. Moldofsky H, Scarisbrick P, England R, et al: Musculoskeletal symptoms and non-REM sleep disturbance in patients with "fibrositis syndrome" and healthy subjects. Psychosom Med 1975; 37:341–351.
10. Moldofsky H, Scarisbrick P: Induction of neurasthenic musculoskeletal pain syndrome by selective sleep stage deprivation. Psychosom Med 1976; 38: 35–44.
11. Molony RR, MacPeek DM, Schiffman PL, et al: Sleep, sleep apnea and the fibromyalgia syndrome. J Rheumatol 1986; 13:797–800.
12. Moldofsky H, Tullis C, Lue FA: Sleep related myoclonus in rheumatic pain modulation disorder (fibrositis syndrome). J Rheumatol 1986; 13:614–617.
13. Smythe H, Lee D, Rush P, et al: Tender shins and steroid therapy. J Rheumatol 1991; 18:1568–1572.
14. Kalyan-Raman UP, Kalyan-Raman K, Yunus MB, et al: Muscle pathology in primary fibromyalgia syndrome: a light microscopic, histochemical and ultrastructural study. J Rheumatol 1984; 11:808–813.
15. Klug GA, McAuley E, Clark S: Factors influencing the development and maintenance of aerobic fitness: lessons applicable to the fibrositis syndrome. J Rheumatol 1989; (Suppl 19)16:30–39.
16. McCain GA, Bell DA, Mai FM, et al: A controlled study of the effects of a supervised cardiovascular fitness training program on the manifestations of primary fibromyalgia. Arthritis Rheum 1988; 31: 1135–1141.
17. Carette S, Bell M, Reynolds J, et al: Comparison of amitryptiline, cyclobenzaprine, and placebo in the treatment of fibromyalgia. Arthritis Rheum 1994; 37: 32–40.
18. Deyo RA, Walsh NE, Martin DC, et al: A controlled trial of transcutaneous electrical nerve stimulation (TENS) and exercise for chronic low back pain. N Engl J Med 1990; 322:1627–1634.
19. Smythe HA, Buskila D, Gladman DD: Performance of scored palpation, a point count, and dolorimetry in assessing unsuspected nonarticular tenderness. J Rheumatol 1993; 20:352–357.
20. Waddell G: Understanding the patient with back pain. In Jayson M (ed): The Lumbar Spine and Back Pain, 4th edition, pp 469–485. New York, Churchill Livingstone, 1992.
21. Clark S, Burckhardt C, Campbell S, et al: Pain behavior and treatment outcomes in fibromyalgia patients (abstr PO391). Arthritis Rheum 1992; 35(Suppl):S350.
22. Wolfe F: Disability and the dimensions of distress in fibromyalgia. J Musculoskeletal Pain 1993; 1(2):65–87.
23. Cathey MA, Wolfe F, Kleinheksel SM, et al: Functional ability and work status in patients with fibromyalgia. Arthritis Care Res 1988; 1:85–98.

CHAPTER 6

Surgical Interventions

Ira Richterman, MD
Mary Ann Keenan, MD

General Considerations

While the majority of patients with arthritis will be successfully managed with nonsurgical approaches, surgical intervention plays an important role in the management of both inflammatory and degenerative forms of arthritis. A team approach and consultative management is critical in patient treatment, particularly for the patient with inflammatory arthritis. Unlike osteoarthrosis (degenerative arthritis), in which surgery may be needed for one or two joints, the patient with inflammatory arthritis may require surgery for several joints. Also, in inflammatory arthritis, the disease process will continue following surgery.

Rheumatoid arthritis (RA) affects all synovial joints, bone, muscle, fascia, ligaments, and tendons. Because it is a systemic disease it also can affect internal organs.[1] Immune mechanisms are involved as evidenced by the presence of large numbers of lymphocytes in the synovial tissue and by the presence of rheumatoid factor (IgM antibodies) in the serum and synovial fluid of 80% of the patients. These antigen-antibody reactions activate the complement system and attract neutrophils to the joint fluid. The immune complexes then are phagocytized and lysosomal enzymes are released into the synovial fluid. These enzymes and the inflammatory synovial pannus are, in part, re-

PHYSICAL THERAPY IN ARTHRITIS, Joan M. Walker, PhD, PT, and Antoine Helewa, MSc(Clin Epid), PT, W.B. Saunders Company © 1996.

sponsible for the destruction of articular cartilage and periarticular structures. Tendons also are directly invaded by the inflammatory synovium and may attenuate and rupture. Ligaments and joint capsules become weakened by the chronic inflammatory process and may become stretched by repeated joint effusions.

The erosion of articular cartilage is greatly enhanced by the superimposition of mechanical derangements on a joint weakened by chronic inflammation and enzymatic deterioration. Osteoporosis results from the hyperemia of inflammation. Disuse of limbs secondary to pain, weakened muscle action, and mechanical derangements enhance the osteoporosis.[2]

Optimum management requires an interdisciplinary team approach involving many specialists. The orthopedic surgeon should be involved early in the course of the patient's disease and not merely be called upon when medical management has failed to be effective. A knowledge of biomechanics, gait dynamics, and energy requirements can be useful in preserving function for the patient. Because the disease is an ongoing and progressive process, the goal of management is to prevent deformities and maintain function for the patient over a lifetime.

Factors in the Decision Process

Many factors must be considered in the decision of whether to intervene surgically in the management of the patient with arthritis. Each patient is unique, an individual, with differing sets of perceptions, expectations, socioeconomic needs, and reactions to disability. The risk/benefit balance must be carefully considered and the patient fully involved in the decision process. Questions that the orthopedist must ask are:

- Will surgery alleviate the symptoms related to weakness, instability, and pain?
- Will surgery make the patient more independent, more self-sufficient?
- Will surgery stabilize the patient's condition, prevent further loss of function?
- Will surgery enable the patient to continue or return to employment?
- Will surgery facilitate care giving?

In selected situations early surgical intervention may prevent excessive deterioration of joint structure and function. Synovectomy has been shown to be effective in preventing tendon rupture in the hand.[3,4] Arthroscopic synovectomy and débridement of cartilage lesions of the knee and shoulder show promise for slowing joint destruction.[5,6] Fusion of an unstable cervical spine can prevent the disastrous effect of a spinal cord injury.[7,8]

The majority of surgical intervention is reconstructive. Since relief of pain is the most consistent result of reconstructive surgery, pain is the primary indication for surgery. Restoration of motion and function and the correction of deformity are additional indications for surgical intervention.[9] Preoperative assessment is a meticulous process. The surgeon must attempt to elicit sufficient information from the patient, family, and therapists, in addition to clinical examination and radiographic evaluations, in order to ascertain which deformities are causing the greatest functional losses. The patient can only tolerate a finite number of surgical procedures, and these must be carefully staged in order to obtain the maximal result.

Joint scoring systems (Tables 6-1 and 6-2) are available and used in assessment of the patient's suitability for surgery. The Einstein-Moss scoring system is a recent modification of the well-known Harris scoring system for total joints.[10] It was developed by a team of orthopedic surgeons and physical therapists in order to incorporate objective values of functional tasks into the scoring system. However, the indication for surgery is not based on a single, cumulative total preoperative score. All scoring systems should include consideration of the following factors:

Pain

Is the patient's pain associated with movement or weight bearing? Does the pain require control with narcotic drugs? Pain that is not easily controlled is a strong indicator for surgery.

Function and Activities of Daily Living (ADL)

The patient should be assessed or questioned on their ability to perform required ADL, and to participate in recreational activities. Quantitative tests appropriate to the involved joint(s) should be used whenever possible. These include such measures as distance walked; gait velocity; number of stairs ascended/descended; ability to get in and out of a car, to manipulate objects, and to dress. Function in ADL impacts significantly on the patient's quality of life. Quantitative tests allow for assessment of the surgical intervention that may follow.

Ability to Work

Is the patient employed? Has the patient had to restrict or cease employment?

Table 6-1. The Einstein-Moss Hip Score

Pain		
None/ignores		44
Slight, occasional, no complaints in activity		40
Mild, no effect on ordinary act; pain after unusual act		40
Moderate, tolerable, makes concessions, occasional codeine		30
Marked, serious limitations		10
Totally disabled		0
Function		
Gait (Condition After Walking Maximum Distance)		
Limp		
None		11
Slight		8
Moderate		5
Severe		0
Unable to Walk		0
Support		
None		11
Cane, long walks		7
Cane, full time		5
Crutch		4
Two canes		2
Two crutches		0
Unable to walk		0
Distance walked		
Unlimited		11
Six blocks		8
Two to three blocks		5
Indoors only		2
Bed and chair		0
Functional Activities		
Stairs		
Normally		4
Normally with banister		2
Any method		1
Not able		0
Sox/tie shoes		
With ease		4
With difficulty		2
Unable		0
Sitting		
Any chair, 1 hour		5
High chair, 1/2 hour		3
Unable to sit, any chair 1/2 hour		0
Deformity		
Fixed Add.	10 degrees	
Fixed M.R.	10 degrees	
Perm. flex contracture	30 degrees	
Leg length discrepancy	3 cm	
None of the above deformities		4
Any of the above deformities		0

Table continued on following page

Table 6-1. Continued

Range of Motion				
Flexion to	________	degrees	211–260	6
Abduction to	________	degrees	161–210	5
Adduction to	________	degrees	101–160	4
L.R. in extension to	________	degrees	61–100	3
M.R. in extension to	________	degrees	31–60	2
			0–30	1
TOTAL MOTION	________	degrees		
TOTAL HIP FUNCTION SCORE ________ (Max 100 points)				

Table 6-2. The Einstein-Moss Knee Score

Pain (Max 30 pts)	
Pain with walking	
No pain	15
Mild pain	10
Moderate pain	5
Severe pain	0
Pain at rest	
No pain	15
Mild pain	10
Moderate pain	5
Severe pain	0
Function (Max 22 pts)	
Walking	
Walking and standing unlimited	12
Walking five to ten blocks and standing ability 1/2 hour	10
Walking one to five blocks and standing ability up to 1/2 hour	8
Walking less than one block	4
Cannot walk	0
Stairs	
Climbing stairs	5
Climbing stairs with support	2
Transfer	
Transfer activity	5
Transfer activity with support	2
Range of Motion (Max 18 pts)	
1 point for each 8 degrees of arc of motion	
Total degrees of knee motion ________ / 8 = ________	________
Muscle Strength (Max 10 pts)	
Excellent: cannot break quadriceps power	10
Good: can break quadriceps power	8
Fair: moves through the arc of motion	4
Poor: cannot move through the arc of motion	0

Table continued on opposite page

Table 6-2. Continued

Flexion Deformity (Max 10 pts)	
No deformity	10
Less than 5 degrees	8
5–10 degrees	4
More than 10 degrees	0
Instability (Max 10 pts)	
None	10
Mild: 0–5 degrees	8
Moderate: 5–15 degrees	5
Severe: more than 15 degrees	0
Aids/Lag/Deformity (Subtract from total)	
One cane	−1
One crutch	−2
Two crutches	−3
Extension lag of 5 degrees	−2
Extension lag of 10 degrees	−3
Extension lag of 15 degrees	−5
Each 5 degrees of varus	−1
Each 5 degrees of valgus	−1
TOTAL KNEE FUNCTION RATING ______________ (Max 100 points)	

Joint Condition

Assessment of a joint encompasses range of motion (ROM), stability, and the presence and degree of deformity or malalignment. The status of contiguous joints also must be assessed, as their condition may significantly impact surgical success. For example, when knee surgery is contemplated, the surgeon needs to assess whether the foot can be placed plantigrade. Can the contralateral limb support the operative leg during postoperative rehabilitation, and can the upper limbs manage ambulatory aids?

Age

Physiologic age is more important than the patient's chronological age. Age is a critical factor in the potential life of the planned procedure and in the patient's expectations of surgery.

Weight

Particularly in osteoarthrosis (OA) with a limited number of joints being affected, obesity negatively impacts success of surgical interventions of lower limb joints. Morbid obesity is a relative contraindication to hip or knee arthroplasty.

Ability of the Patient to Cooperate

Ultimately, a positive outcome from surgical interventions depends on the patient's ability to actively cooperate with postoperative rehabilitation. In some cases, however, when surgical intervention may facilitate care, surgery may be undertaken despite the perception that the patient will not be cooperative.

Since relief of pain is the most consistent result of reconstructive surgery, pain is the primary indication for surgery.

Patient Perceptions and Expectations

It is important to establish clearly what the patient perceives surgery may accomplish, and what their expectations of outcome may be. Some patients may see surgery as curative, allowing full resumption of former life and recreational activities. Others may perceive surgery as cosmetic, to

Table 6-3. Factors that Compromise Surgical Intervention

1. Morbid obesity
2. Active infection
3. Overwhelming poor general health
4. Inadequate motor control (paresis or paralysis)
5. Inadequate bone stock
6. Emotional instability

correct deformity; however, this may be a minor factor in the decision process if adequate function exists despite the presence of deformity. Other patients' main expectation may be improvement in function. It should be established clearly whether these expectations are realistic. Expectations must be viewed in the light of comorbidities.

General Health

The presence of coexisting medical conditions will impact the patient's ability to participate in postoperative rehabilitation. Cardiovascular and respiratory conditions may present concerns regarding the choice of anesthetic technique. An unstable or rigid cervical spine may necessitate flexible fiberoptic intubation.

Factors that compromise a positive outcome from surgical intervention are given in Table 6-3. The presence of an active infection, obesity, or emotional instability may necessitate a delay in scheduling surgery until an improvement or resolution has been achieved. Other factors, such as inadequate bone stock, may completely negate surgical intervention.

Types of Surgical Procedures

Table 6-4 lists the various surgical procedures and their goals that may be employed in patients with arthritis. Pain relief with improvement or restoration of function are desired outcomes of all pro-

Table 6-4. Surgical Procedures and their Main Purpose

Procedure	Purpose
Débridement	Removal of damaged cartilage fragments, loose bodies, and inflamed synovium. Smooth irregular surfaces.
Osteotomy	Improve joint or limb alignment to redistribute forces.
Arthrodesis	Provide stability, prevent further malalignment and/or compression of neural elements.
Arthroplasty	Improve or restore function. Decrease disability. Eliminate severe pain.
Synovectomy	Remove inflamed synovium to protect articular cartilage or tendons from enzymatic damage.
Bursectomy	Removal of inflamed bursa (i.e., olecranon).
Tendon transfer	Correct malalignment, restore function, arrest deterioration of tendons.
Nerve decompression	Relieve nerve compression (i.e., ulnar nerve transposition at the elbow).
Nodule resection	Cosmesis, pain relief.

cedures. Procedures may be combined, such as débridement with ligament release, or elbow joint synovectomy with radial head excision. The more commonly employed procedures are osteotomy, débridement, arthrodesis (fusion), and arthroplasty (joint replacement surgery).

In patients with inflammatory arthritis who have uncontrolled synovitis and good articular cartilage, a synovectomy is a palliative approach.[3,4] Removal of synovium retards cartilage destruction due to release of cartilage degradative enzymes by the synovium. Synovium, however, tends to regenerate. An osteotomy may delay the need for a total joint replacement and is often employed in young, active individuals with degenerative arthritis, where extensive destruction of articular cartilage is present.[11-13]

Synovectomy can be a palliative approach; however, synovial tissues tend to regenerate.

Arthrodesis is a primary procedure where there is spinal instability associated with intractable pain and/or neural compression. In both the cervical and lumbar regions, arthrodesis is combined with neural decompression, of either the spinal cord or the nerve roots. Arthrodesis may be the only reasonable alternative to arthroplasty, or the end result with failure of an arthroplasty. Local intercarpal fusions serve to provide stability while maintaining some wrist ROM and function. Contiguous joints should be mobile and functional when considering arthrodesis. When planned for the hip or knee joint, it is imperative for function that the other large joint has adequate, pain-free motion and motor control. Arthrodesis also is a primary procedure when there is inadequate bone stock for an arthroplasty.

Arthroplasties have been performed on most joints; however, they are mainly used for hip, knee, and shoulder joints. This procedure requires adequate bone stock and motor control and is particularly indicated in the presence of severe pain and disability. A partial joint hemiarthroplasty (i.e., only one surface, such as at the hip only the femoral surface, or at the knee unicompartmental) or a total joint arthroplasty may be performed.[13-16] A variety of metal alloys, high-density polymers, and ceramic materials are used to resurface joints. Problems exist in loosening of implants and the creation of wear particles that produce an inflammatory response at the bone-impact interface with eventual bone erosion.[17,18]

Surgical Considerations in Inflammatory Arthritis

Surgery in inflammatory arthritis usually is not an isolated event as it may be in osteoarthrosis. RA is a systemic disease and will continue to progress after surgery. In RA, multiple joint involvement is an important factor. Benefit of surgery to one joint may be negated by the extent of involvement of a contiguous joint. For example, hand surgery is affected by the condition of the elbow and shoulder, and when these joints are severely involved the patient may not be able to use any improved hand function. In such cases priority of operations becomes important.

Priority of Operations

In the patient with multiple joint involvement, cervical instability with myelopathy takes priority. Generally operations are performed on the lower limb joints before upper limb joints (Table 6-5). If upper limb function is so poor, however, that the patient could not tolerate ambulatory aids, then upper limb surgery will take priority over lower limb procedures. Correction of malalignment and contractures may be essential to the outcome of other procedures. For example, malalignment of the ankle/foot complex can affect knee replacement outcome.[19]

Table 6-5. Priority of Surgical Procedures

Lower limb:	Foot ⇒ hip ⇒ knee ⇒ ankle
Upper limb:	Wrist ⇒ hand ⇒ elbow ⇒ shoulder
	Nondominant before dominant side

Limb dominance must be considered in multiple surgeries, not only for scheduling but also in type of procedure. A wrist arthrodesis may be more appropriate to the "helping hand" (nondominant) and joint replacements to the dominant hand to provide motion. A stable, pain-free wrist is needed for successful hand surgery, and functional motion in the elbow and shoulder is needed for hand and wrist procedures.

Surgeries and Medications

Collaboration and consultation between the orthopedic surgeon and the rheumatologist is essential throughout planned surgeries. A patient should achieve maximum benefit from medication prior to surgery, and the disease should be controlled for a good surgical outcome. Consideration must be given to the patient's medications.[1] There is a need to continue to ensure that other joints remain quiescent so the postoperative rehabilitation can be achieved. Nonsteroidal anti-inflammatory drugs (NSAIDs) will need to be stopped 5 days preoperatively to decrease postoperative bleeding. In the postoperative period, deep vein thrombosis is a complication that can be fatal, and its prophylaxis cannot be overlooked. Thus, the NSAIDs need to be balanced with deep vein thrombosis prophylaxis to avoid bleeding complications and minimize the risks of thrombosis. With lower limb procedures, medication dosage may need to be changed so that the patient can properly use ambulatory aids in a relatively pain-free manner.

Surgical Procedures for Specific Anatomic Locations

Spine

Surgery in the spine has the goals of providing stabilization, relief, or prevention of pain and neurologic complications. Surgery is indicated in the presence of one or more of the following:

- intractable pain
- excessive instability
- neurologic deficit

Involvement of the cervical spine in rheumatoid arthritis is classically divided into three categories.[7,8,20] The most common form of involvement is atlantoaxial instability resulting from erosion of the transverse and alar ligaments. These ligaments normally maintain the odontoid process of the axis within the anterior one third of the ring of the atlas where the two bones articulate with one another. Disruption of the ligaments results in excessive motion between C1 and C2. Forward flexion of the head causes anterior subluxation of the atlas on the axis and possible impingement of the spinal cord or occlusion of the vertebral arteries.

The second common form of arthritic spine disease is the category of subaxial instability. This can be manifested by subluxation occurring between two or more cervical vertebrae below the level of C2. When the degree of subluxation is severe or its appearance sudden, pressure can be exerted on the spinal cord. This pressure may be sufficient to cause permanent and complete quadriparesis. Commonly, the subluxation occurs slowly and the spine adapts to a severe degree of deformity before clinical symptoms appear.

The least common pattern of cervical spine deformity is superior migration of the odontoid process of C2 resulting from severe bone erosion. As the dens migrates proximally, radiographic detail is lost secondary to the overlapping of bony structures. Computed tomography (CT) is most useful in elucidating the exact nature of the deformities.

Orthotic supports are useful in controlling the patient's symptomatology. Posterior cervical fusion is indicated when the spinal cord is at risk of damage. The common level of fusion is C1–C2, supplemented by wire fixation. When the subluxation is irreducible or severe osteoporosis is present, fusion to the occiput may be necessary. Occasionally, it is useful to supplement the bone graft with polymethyl methacrylate (PMMA) fixation.[7]

Cervical spine disease in patients with erosive polyarticular arthritis often presents difficulties in endotracheal intubation at the time of surgery. The stability of the cervical spine should be assessed prior to any surgical procedure on a patient with RA. Lateral flexion-extension radiographs taken within 1 year of surgery are sufficient to detect any significant instability. Use of the flexible fiberoptic bronchoscope for such problems is helpful. The indications for fiberoptic intubation in the patient with arthritis are:

1. An unstable cervical spine on flexion and extension
2. Limited mobility of the cervical spine
3. Impaired motion of the temporomandibular joints with or without associated micrognathia

In patients with severe erosive disease of the cervical spine and proximal migration of the odontoid process, a rotational deviation of the larynx occurs, which mandates using a flexible fiberoptic scope.[20,21]

In OA with spinal stenosis, decompression is often accomplished using a posterior approach with decompressive laminectomy and foraminotomy. If multiple levels are decompressed or if facet joints are resected, then fusion is required, because spinal instability has been created. In addition, fusion is indicated when treating degenerative spondylolisthesis that has not responded to the conservative therapy of rest, NSAIDs, and physical rehabilitation.

Upper Extremity

Shoulder

The shoulder is a common site of arthritic involvement.[22] Normally, the glenohumeral joint has more motion than any other joint. This motion is rotation and the glenoid is very shallow in shape to allow greater freedom of motion. In RA, shoulder involvement is generally insidious in onset, with episodic increases in pain. The pain is not constant early in the course of the disease and therefore shoulder disease is often not appreciated until a significant amount of destruction is present. It is important to examine the shoulder on a regular basis to detect early loss of motion and function.

The rotator cuff muscles are central to the normal functioning of the shoulder. They provide stability to the humeral head and also provide rotation. In RA, attenuation and rupture of the rotator cuff is common. Trauma or degenerative arthritis also causes rotator cuff tears. When the rotator cuff has ruptured, the humeral head migrates proximally and is subjected to abnormal muscle forces. This results in the rapid deterioration of the glenohumeral joint.

Arthroscopy provides a new and useful tool in examining the shoulder. The integrity of the rotator cuff, biceps tendon, and glenoid labrum can be assessed. In the patient with RA, synovectomy can be performed arthroscopically using motorized shavers or the holmium:yttrium-aluminum-garnet (Ho:YAG) laser with minimal morbidity. Impingement of a chronically inflamed rotator cuff against the undersurface of the acromium also can be treated by arthroscopic acromioplasty.

When the rotator cuff ruptures, repair should be performed. If the rupture is detected early, excessive damage to the glenohumeral joint can be avoided. If extensive joint damage is already present, then repair or reconstruction is done at the time of prosthetic arthroplasty. The extensively damaged glenohumeral joint can be successfully reconstructed by prosthetic arthroplasty.[16,23–27] Preoperative radiographic evaluation should include anteroposterior, lateral, and axillary radiographs to assess the alignment of the glenoid. The glenoid is often eroded asymmetrically and the prosthetic glenoid component must be accurately aligned for optimum functional result and to minimize the abnormal forces that might lead to prosthetic loosening. If the glenoid is normal in shape and articular surface, then only a hemiarthroplasty is performed (i.e., replacing only the proximal humerus). Pain is effectively alleviated by total shoulder replacement. The functional result is dependent on the integrity of the soft tissues and muscle function. A careful postoperative therapy program is essential to maximize function.

The anterior portion of the deltoid muscle provides forward elevation of the humerus. This is the position of function and the common arc of motion for activities using the upper extremity. It is therefore important to preserve these muscle fibers and their attachments when performing any surgery of the shoulder. Without a functioning anterior deltoid, shoulder arthroplasty is contraindicated.

The tendon of the long head of the biceps muscle stabilizes the humeral head against riding upward. It also reduces subacromial impingement. The intra-articular portion of the tendon should be preserved whenever possible.

Post-traumatic osteoarthrosis is another major etiology of glenohumeral joint dysfunction. Degeneration of the joint may occur following multiple dislocations, multidirectional instability, and fracture of the proximal humerus. Pain with motion often is the main symptom for which patients seek medical attention.

Elbow

The elbow joint consists of three separate articulations: the radiocapitellar, ulnotrochlear, and radioulnar. These articulations allow the hand to rotate 180 degrees around the longitudinal axis of the forearm. Hand function is dependent on being placed correctly in space as required for use. The elbow is the most important joint for positioning the hand. Unlike the shoulder or wrist, if the elbow is fused the functional loss is great. The goal of treatment is to maintain a painless arc of motion.

Subcutaneous rheumatoid nodules are common along the extensor surface of the ulna. These often cause problems with pressure when resting the arm on any surface. They may interfere with the use of forearm troughs on walking aids. If bothersome, they should be surgically excised, but the patient must be advised that they can recur.

Radiocapitellar arthritis often is the predominant feature of elbow involvement following radial head fractures and can cause marked pain and a decreased range of motion. The pain is most pronounced with pronation and supination of the forearm. Radial head excision and synovectomy is effective in relieving the pain and often results in an improved arc of motion.

Ulnohumeral arthritis does not always require surgical intervention. When the joint destruction is severe but ligamentous stability remains, prosthetic arthroplasty can be done.[28] Several designs of elbow prostheses are available. They can be classified into semiconstrained and unconstrained designs. An unconstrained design is preferable, as the mechanical forces leading to loosening are not directly transferred to the bone. The shoulder should be evaluated carefully prior to prosthetic elbow arthroplasty. A patient with limited shoulder motion will exert greater forces on the elbow in an effort to compensate for the decrease in shoulder function.

Wrist and Hand

Reconstructive hand surgery can be considered for the patient with inflammatory or degenerative arthritis. Evaluating a patient with hand deformities and developing a rational plan for treatment can be a complex task. Many joints, tendons, and ligaments are involved in a linked system of structure and function.

Synovitis Dorsal tenosynovitis is common in RA. It is significant because it often results in rupture of the extensor tendons.

Extensor tendon ruptures occur as the result of attenuation of the tendon from chronic inflammation, ischemia secondary to interference with the normal circulation to the tendon, attenuation of the tendon from rubbing against abnormal bony surfaces that are prominent secondary to ligamentous laxity, and from direct invasion of the tendon by synovium. Tenosynovectomy should be performed in patients who have persistent synovitis for a 4- to 6-month interval that has not been responsive to medical treatment. Recurrence of the synovitis is rare following synovectomy and the procedure has been shown to prevent extensor tendon rupture.[3,4]

The common tendons to rupture in order of frequency are the extensors of the fifth finger, the ring finger, and the extensor pollicis longus (EPL) tendon. The results of surgical repair by tendon transfer are inversely proportional to the number of tendons involved. Prompt diagnosis and treatment are essential for a successful outcome. For a single tendon rupture in the fifth and ring fingers, a side-to-side repair using the adjacent extensor tendon is advised. The extensor indicis tendon also may be transferred for repair of the EPL tendon or for rupture of two finger extensors. For more complex ruptures, the wrist extensors or flexor digitorum superficialis tendons (FDS) may be transferred dorsally to restore function.

Synovitis in the flexor tendon sheaths is manifested by crepitation palpable in the palm with finger flexion and extension. Triggering of the fingers may result from the inflamed synovial tissue catching on the flexor pulleys with motion. Carpal tunnel syndrome also may occur secondary to the swelling within the carpal canal, causing pressure on the median nerve. Early treatment consists of local steroid injection to reduce the inflammation, splinting, and medical management of the underlying synovitis. Persistent synovitis may require carpal tunnel release and synovectomy. Rupture of the flexor tendons is rare.

Wrist The wrist joint is a frequent site of synovitis. The wrist begins to deviate in a radial direction and sublux volarly. The radioulnar joint is commonly inflamed and painful. Radial deviation of the carpus can be rebalanced by transfer of the extensor carpi radialis longus tendon to the extensor carpi ulnaris.

> **RA is a systemic disease and will continue to progress after surgery.**

When the wrist becomes unstable, several choices of surgical treatment are available. If the deformity is mild, bone stock can be preserved and motion maintained by a limited carpal fusion. The lunate and scaphoid are fused to the distal radius to prevent further displacement of the carpus. The distal ulna can be fused to the distal radius to provide a platform to support the wrist. A segment of the ulna is removed just proximal to the fusion to allow for pronation and supination of the forearm. If the intercarpal joints are severely involved by the arthritis, the base of the capitate can be removed and a spacer inserted to preserve motion at the intercarpal row.

Another option is to perform a prosthetic arthroplasty of the wrist. More bone stock is removed with these procedures, but revision is still possible in the event of fracture of the prosthesis. Several designs of total joint prosthesis have been developed for the wrist.

Fusion of the wrist joint provides a stable and pain-free joint and remains a reasonable surgical choice for selected individuals. Fusion may interfere with personal hygiene tasks and so it is advisable to avoid fusing both wrist joints. Several conditions requiring limited fusions include chronic instability patterns of the wrist, fixed flexion contractures, and congenital deformations.

Wrist and finger deformities commonly occur together in a collapsing zig-zag pattern. The wrist deviates in a radial direction and the fingers then drift ulnarward at the metacarpophalangeal (MCP) joint level. When both deformities are present, it is important to realign the wrist prior to correcting the finger deformities or the ulnar deviation of the fingers will recur.

MCP Joints Ulnar deviation and volar subluxation of the fingers at the MCP joint level is common (Fig. 6-1*A*). In RA with ulnar deviation, the extensor tendons sublux into the valleys between the metacarpal heads. This can be confused with extensor tendon rupture. When the joint surfaces are preserved, a synovectomy, soft-tissue release of the volar capsule, and realignment of the extensor tendons will improve function. If the joint surfaces are destroyed, then a Silastic interposition arthroplasty is indicated (Figs. 6-1*B* and 6-2). If the joints are unstable secondary to ligament loss, it may be necessary to reconstruct the radial collateral ligament using a portion of the volar plate to provide a stable pinch. Tightness of the intrinsic tendons occurs in conjunction with the subluxation of the MCP joints. When this occurs, a release of the intrinsic tendons is performed along with

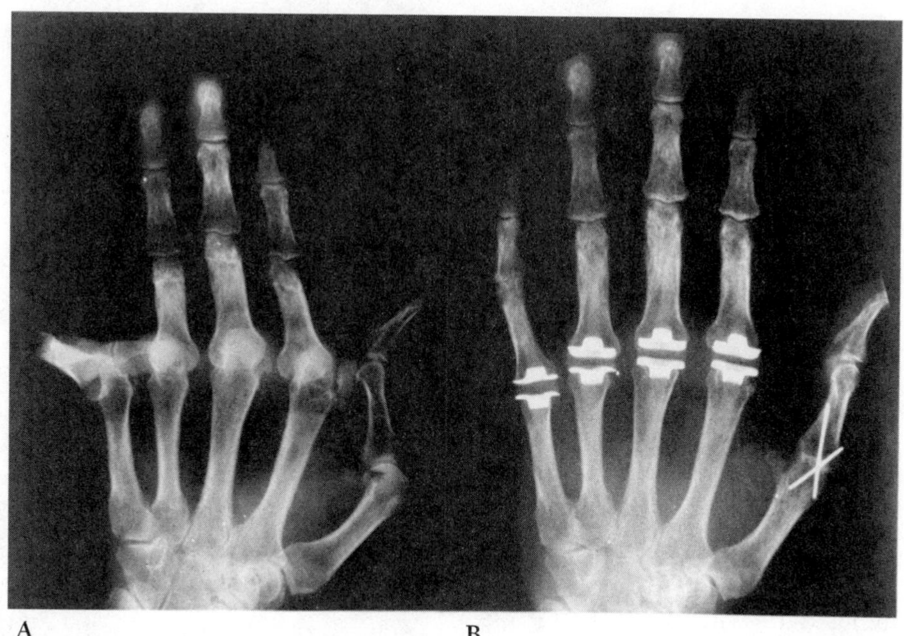

Figure 6-1. *A*, Preoperative radiograph of a patient with RA that shows a boutonnière deformity of the thumb. The metacarpophalangeal (MCP) joints of the fingers are dislocated volarly and the fingers are ulnarly deviated. *B*, Postoperative radiograph showing reconstruction of the hand using Silastic interposition arthroplasties of the MCP joints and fusion of the MCP joint of the thumb. (Courtesy Wright Medical Technology, Inc, Arlington, TN 38002.)

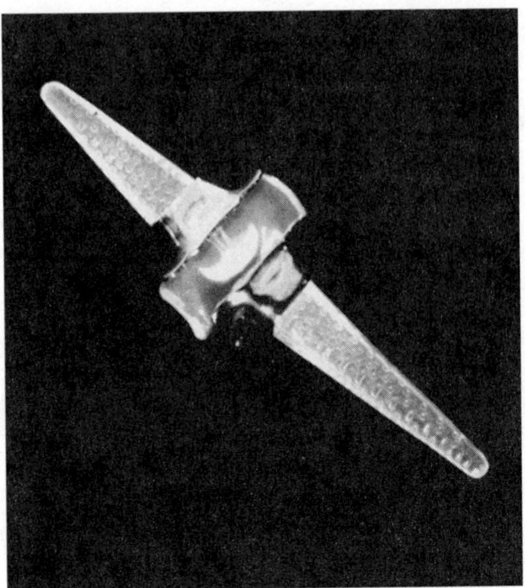

Figure 6-2. A Silastic prosthesis used for interposition arthroplasties of the MCP joints. The metal grommets help to prevent erosion of the bone ends. (Courtesy Wright Medical Technology, Inc, Arlington, TN 38002.)

the arthroplasty. Dynamic splinting of the fingers to maintain alignment while allowing motion is used continuously for 6 weeks following surgery and then for an additional 6 weeks at night.

Proximal Interphalangeal (PIP) Joints Continued synovitis causes gradual attenuation of the capsular and ligamentous structures, with resulting tendon imbalance. The fingers can develop either a flexion or an extension type of deformity.

A flexion deformity results from rupture or attenuation of the central slip of the extensor mechanism with gradual volar displacement of the lateral bands. As the lateral bands sublux volarly, a hyperextension deformity of the distal IP joint results. This flexion malalignment also is called a boutonnière deformity (see Fig. 3-8*A*). A boutonnière deformity interferes with grasping large objects but does not usually impede pinch function used for picking up small items.

Interposition arthroplasty using a Silastic spacer has given unpredictable results. Fusion of the IP joints gives dependable results when the boutonnière deformity is fixed (see Fig. 6-1*B*). In the index and long fingers, stability for pinch is required for good function rather than a large arc of motion. Motion is more important in the ring and small fingers to provide a functional grasp. When arthroplasty is considered, the ring and fifth fingers are usually selected.

Hyperextension (swan-neck) deformities can be either primary or secondary (see Fig. 3-8*B*). Primary deformities are due to stretching of the volar plate from synovitis or rupture of the FDS tendon. A flexion deformity of the MCP joints with tightness of the intrinsic muscles proximally combined with a mallet deformity distally results in a secondary swan-neck deformity. Swan-neck deformities interfere with picking up small objects but do not cause much difficulty with grasping larger objects. If the deformity is treated early and is secondary to intrinsic tightness, a release of the in-

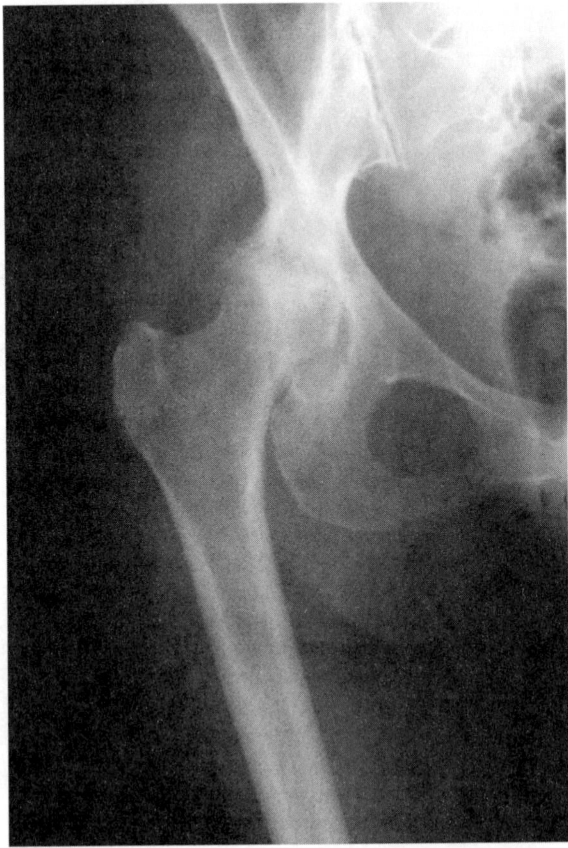

Figure 6-3. Preoperative radiograph of the hip showing extensive osteoarthrosis. (Courtesy Wright Medical Technology, Inc, Arlington, TN 38002.)

trinsic tendons will correct the imbalance. When the deformity is seen late and is rigid, the choices of surgical treatment are fusion or arthroplasty.

Derangements of the distal IP joints are either mallet deformities secondary to rupture of the extensor tendon or lateral deformities from loss of capsular and ligamentous support. When the deformities interfere with function, fusion of the joint is indicated.

Thumb Flexion of the thumb MCP joint with extension of the IP joint is the equivalent of a boutonnière deformity (see Fig. 6-1*B*). The reverse deformity can also be seen with extension of the MCP joint and flexion of the IP joint. An adduction deformity of the metacarpal places increased stress on the MCP joint, producing lateral instability and hyperextension. Adduction of the thumb occurs when the carpometacarpal joint has subluxed radially.

Arthritic derangements of the first carpometacarpal joint is a common disorder with a higher incidence in women. The clinical symptoms include pain and weak grasp. This condition can be treated with fusion, but arthroplasty is desirable to maintain motion. Interpositional arthroplasty can be performed by excising the trapezium and inserting soft tissue in its place.

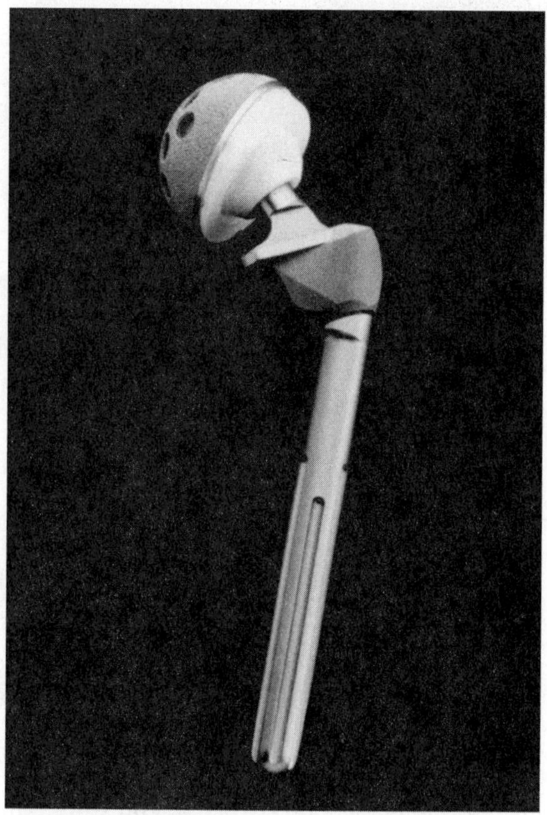

Figure 6-4. A total hip prosthesis that has porous surfaces on the femoral and acetabular components allowing for fixation by bony ingrowth. (Courtesy Wright Medical Technology, Inc, Arlington, TN 38002.)

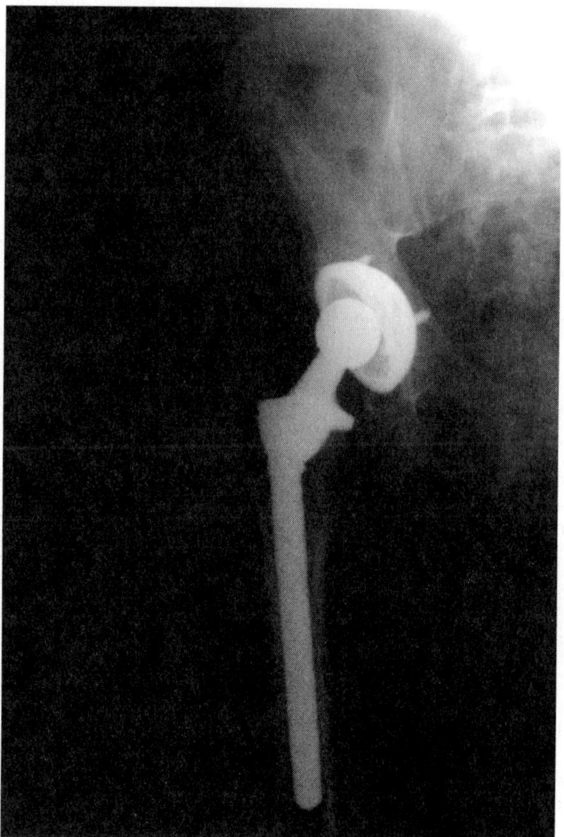

Figure 6-5. Postoperative radiograph taken 2 years after total hip arthroplasty. There is excellent apposition of the bone surfaces against the prosthetic components. (Courtesy Wright Medical Technology, Inc., Arlington, TN 38002.)

Careful postoperative therapy programs are essential to maximize function gained from surgical procedures.

Lower Extremity

Hip

Total joint replacement has vastly improved the quality of life for the patient with arthritis. Special problems exist in the patient with RA when considering total hip arthroplasty. Osteoporosis is very pronounced and fracture can occur easily during the surgery. Protrusio acetabulae also is common and may require bone grafting. Delayed wound healing can occur, especially if the patient has been taking systemic steroids. The risk of infection also is increased in this population. In the patient with juvenile rheumatoid arthritis, excess femoral anteversion may be present, distorting the anatomy. Also, the small size of the bone may require a special prosthesis. Despite these problems, total joint arthroplasty remains the treatment of choice for the arthritic hip. Total joint arthroplasty provides a stable joint with excellent functional potential. Fixation of the prosthetic components may be obtained using PMMA or by bony ingrowth into a porous surface.[29–31] The following case study illustrates a typical case.

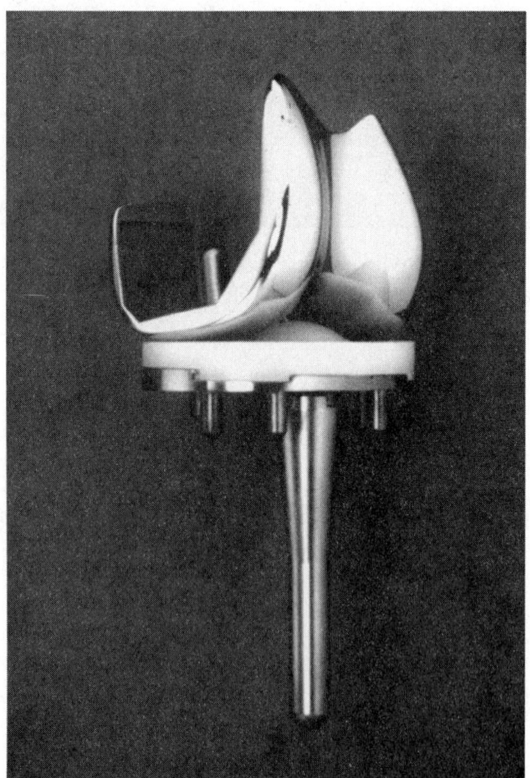

Figure 6-6. A modular total knee prosthesis that can be inserted using polymethyl methacrylate (PMMA) cement fixation or as a porous ingrowth device. (Courtesy Wright Medical Technology, Inc, Arlington, TN 38002.)

Case History JF is a 60-year-old male without any significant medical conditions. He complained of severe pain in his left hip. He could ambulate, with the aid of a cane, a maximum of one city block. His symptoms worsened with activity, and there had not been any symptomatic relief from conservative treatment, which consisted of NSAIDs, therapy, and exercise. Radiography of his left hip revealed the classic radiographic findings of OA: joint space narrowing, subchondral sclerosis, and osteophyte formation (Fig. 6-3).

Preoperatively, his Einstein-Moss hip score was 40. After meeting with an orthopedic surgeon, a clinical nurse coordinator, and a therapist, he elected to have a total joint replacement for his left hip (Fig. 6-4).

His postoperative rehabilitation began on day 2 with gentle, limited ROM and gait training. Once he achieved independence (average time is about 2 weeks), which included self-dressing and stair climbing, he was discharged home, with therapy continued as an outpatient. Over the next several months, he worked on increasing his ROM and strength.

At 1 year postoperative time, he was very satisfied with his functional outcome as an unlimited, unassisted, pain-free walker, with a total hip function score of 96 (Fig. 6-5).

Knee

Valgus deformity is commonly seen in the patient with RA. This is the result of a valgus deformity of the hindfoot which then places excessive stress on the knee proximally.[19] Mild medial knee pain can be relieved with the use of an ankle-foot orthosis that corrects hindfoot valgus. Knee flexion deformity also is common. In the presence of a joint effusion, the intra-articular pressure and therefore the pain are minimized by placing the knee in 30 degrees of flexion. This encourages the formation of flexion contractures.

When evaluating a patient with OA of the knee, the physician must determine which joint spaces are involved. There are three potential compartments: the medial joint compartment, the lateral joint, and the patellofemoral joint. Often a patient has involvement only of the medial or lateral joint space. If the patient is less than 55 years old, has no systemic disease, is active and has no varus or valgus thrust while walking, has at least 90 degrees of knee flexion and less than a 15-degree flexion contracture, then a high tibial osteotomy is indicated.[11–13] This procedure will change the mechanical axis of the leg such that during weight bearing, the mechanical axis will pass through the unaffected compartment. This procedure often will delay the need for total knee arthroplasty for up to 10 years.

Recently, arthroscopic evaluation of the knee has demonstrated the importance of the meniscus in the degeneration of the knee. In the patient with RA, the synovium directly invades the body of the meniscus, which causes tears. The mechanical derangement resulting from the torn meniscus then causes rapid deterioration of the articular surfaces, which have been rendered abnormal by the action of enzymes. Synovectomy of the joint line and partial meniscectomy is easily accomplished under arthroscopic control and may have a role in preventing articular damage in the rheumatoid knee.[5,6] In the mildly osteoarthritic knee, arthroscopic débridement is very successful in alleviating painful symptoms. With the advent of the Ho:YAG laser, rough, fraying articular cartilage can be smoothed, and loose bodies can be removed. Finally, the degradative enzymes of the inflammatory process can be washed from the joint.

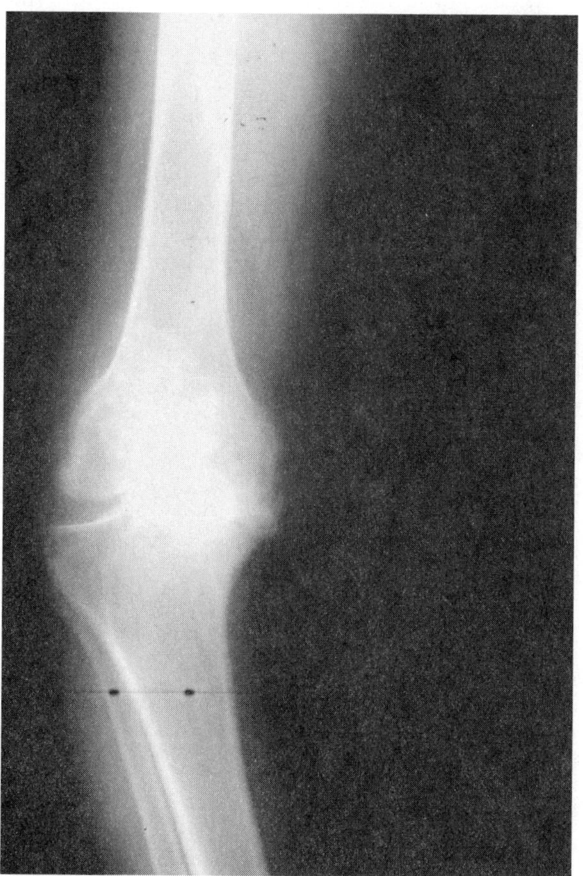

A

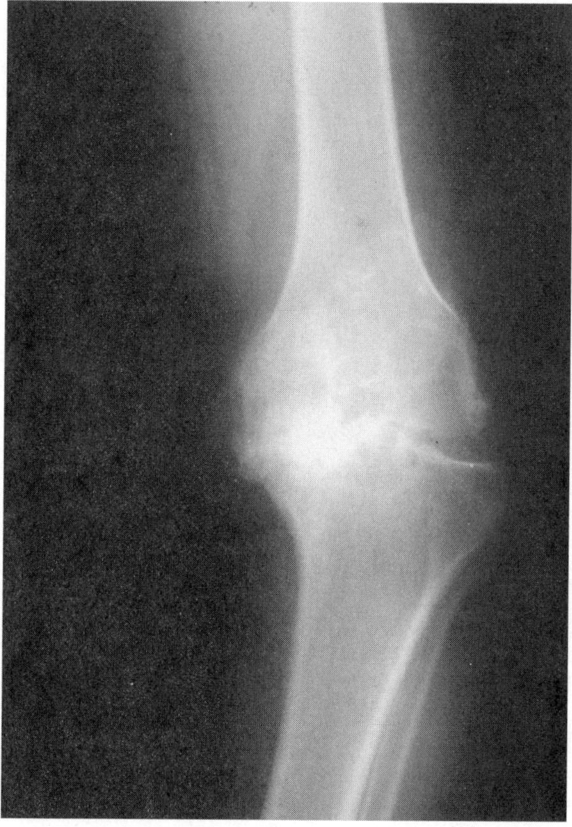

B

Figure 6-7. Preoperative radiograph of both knees showing extensive osteoarthrosis and significant varus malalignment.

Total knee arthroplasty has been proven to be an effective procedure to restore knee alignment and motion and to relieve pain (Figs. 6-6 through 6-8).[14,15,18,32–35] When a valgus deformity is present, serial soft tissue releases should be done to realign the limb prior to cutting the bone for insertion of the prosthetic components. The lateral retinaculum, popliteus tendon, proximal iliotibial band, posterolateral capsule, and lateral collateral ligament can be released in this sequence to provide soft tissue balance. A flexion deformity is corrected at the time of arthroplasty by release of the posterior capsule from the femur or by removing additional bone from the distal femur in severe cases. The following case study illustrates a typical case.

Case History LG is a 59-year-old male who was very athletically active as a young man. He presented with severe bilateral knee pain and bowing deformity of his legs. Although his walking potential was unlimited, he chose to have bilateral total knee replacement to alleviate his severe pain, which did not allow him to sleep at night (Fig. 6-6). His preoperative radiographs demonstrate severe OA and varus malalignment (Fig. 6-7). His initial Einstein-Moss total knee score was 62.

His postoperative rehabilitation began on day 2 with gait training and ROM exercises. He was discharged home 2 weeks later after achieving 90 degrees of flexion and independent ambulation. At 1 year following operation, his total knee score improved to 75, but significant pain in his nonoperated knee led him to have his second knee replacement. His postoperative therapy was identical to his previous course. One year later his knee score improved

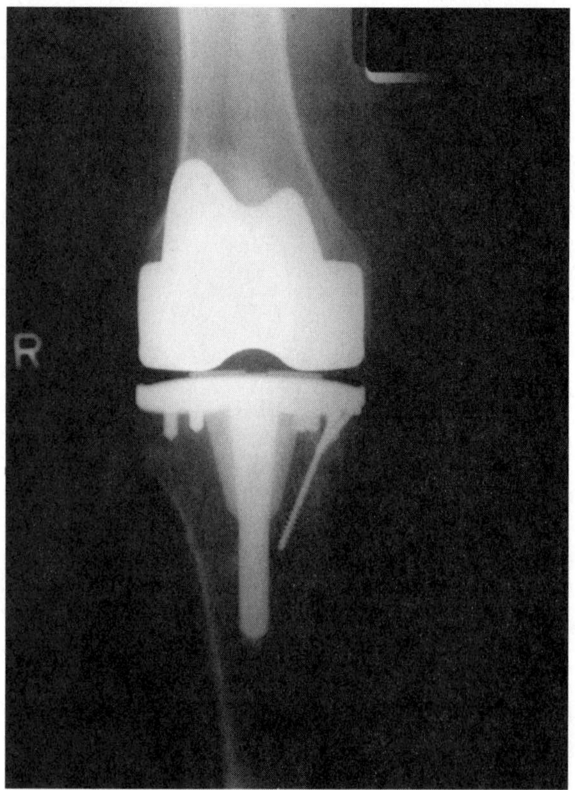

A

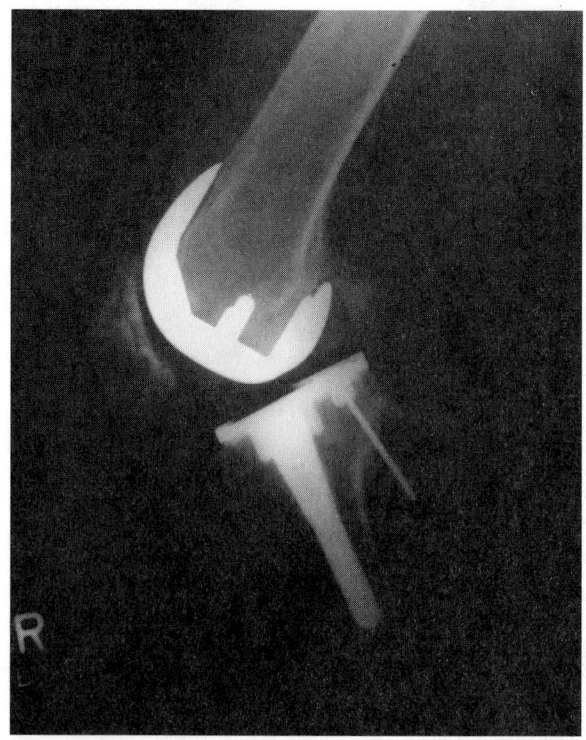

B

Figure 6-8. *A,* Anteroposterior radiograph of knees showing bilateral total knee arthroplasty. The normal valgus alignment has been restored by the surgery. *B,* Lateral radiograph of a total knee arthroplasty. (Courtesy Wright Medical Technology, Inc, Arlington, TN 38002.)

to 91, with excellent correction of his malalignment (Fig. 6-8).

Foot

Forefoot involvement is common in RA. Claw toe deformities with plantar subluxation of the metatarsal heads result in painful callosities on the plantar surface of the forefoot. This is usually accompanied by a hallux valgus deformity. Skin ulcerations may form over bony prominences. Forefoot pain prevents the patient from transferring body weight over the foot during terminal stance and results in a shortened step-length. Extra-depth shoes with wide toe boxes and moulded pressure-relieving inserts may be sufficient to relieve pain and improve gait (see Chapter 10). When the deformities are marked, resection of the metatarsal heads in conjunction with fusion of the metatarsophalangeal joint of the great toe is indicated.

Hindfoot involvement also is common and results in a planovalgus or pronation deformity.[19] A longitudinal arch support or similar shoe insert is not sufficient to hold the hindfoot in alignment. When the deformity is supple, an ankle-foot orthosis with a well-moulded arch support will control the position of the heel and subtalar joint during gait. This also will reduce the valgus thrust on the knee joint. If the deformity is fixed, a triple arthrodesis will align the hindfoot.

Summary

Arthritis is a disease that can be extremely debilitating. When conservative medical therapy has failed, however, surgical intervention can significantly alleviate the symptoms of arthritis, and either stabilize or improve function. When indicated, surgical intervention is an effective and powerful tool used for the treatment of arthritis.

References

1. Katz WA: Modern management of rheumatoid arthritis. Am J Med 1985; 79(Suppl 4C):24–31.
2. Akeson WH, Amiel D, Abel MF, et al: Effects of immobilization on joints. Clin Orthop 1987; 219:28–37.
3. Janet W, Zukerman J, Sledge C: Synovectomy: its use in the treatment of rheumatoid arthritis. Res Staff Physician 1984; 32(10):34.
4. Wynn Parry CB, Stanley JK: Synovectomy of the hand. Br J Rheumatol 1993; 32:1089–1095.
5. Cohen S, Jones R: An evaluation of the efficacy of arthroscopic synovectomy of the knee in rheumatoid arthritis: 12–24 month results. J Rheumatol 1987; 14(3):452–455.
6. Highgenboten CL: Arthroscopic synovectomy. Orthop Clin North Am 1982; 13:399–405.
7. Conaty JP, Mongan ES: Cervical fusion in rheumatoid arthritis. J Bone Joint Surg 1981; 63A:1218–1227.
8. Pellicci P, Ranawat CS, Tsairis P, et al: A prospective study of the progression of rheumatoid arthritis of the cervical spine. J Bone Joint Surg 1981; 63A:342–350.
9. Charter RA, Nehemkis AM, Keenan MA, et al: The nature of arthritis pain. Br J Rheumatol 1985; 24:53–60.
10. Harris WH: Traumatic arthritis of the hip after dislocation and acetabular fractures: treatment by mold arthroplasty. An end-result study using a new method of result evaluation. J Bone Joint Surg 1969; 51A:737–755.
11. Coventry MB, Ilstrup DM, Wallrichs SL: Proximal tibial osteotomy. A critical long-term study of eighty-seven cases. J Bone Joint Surg 1993; 75A:196–201.
12. Rudan JF, Simurda MA: High tibial osteotomy. A prospective clinical and roentgenographic review. Clin Orthop 1990; 255:251–256.
13. Weale AE, Newman JH: Unicompartmental arthroplasty and high tibial osteotomy for osteoarthrosis of the knee. A comparative study with a 12- to 17-year follow-up period. Clin Orthop 1994; 302:134–137.
14. Jackson RW, Burdick W: Unicompartmental knee arthroplasty. Clin Orthop 1984; 190:182–185.
15. Klemme WR, Galvin EG, Petersen SA: Unicompartmental knee arthroplasty. Sequential radiographic and scintigraphic imaging with an average five-year follow-up. Clin Orthop 1994; 301:233–238.
16. Lee DH, Niemann KMW: Bipolar shoulder arthroplasty. Clin Orthop 1994; 304:97–107.
17. Buechel FF, Drucker D, Jasty M, et al: Osteolysis around uncemented acetabular components of cobalt-chrome surface replacement hip arthroplasty. Clin Orthop 1994; 298:202–211.
18. Wasielewski RC, Galante JO, Leighty RM, et al: Wear patterns on retrieved polyethylene tibial inserts and their relationship to technical considerations during total knee arthroplasty. Clin Orthop 1994; 299:31–43.
19. Keenan MA, Peabody TD, Gronley JK, et al: Valgus deformities of the feet and characteristics of gait in patients who have rheumatoid arthritis. J Bone Joint Surg 1991; 73A:237–247.
20. Keenan MA, Stiles CM, Kaufman RL: Acquired laryngeal deviation associated with cervical spine disease in erosive polyarticular arthritis. Anesthesiology 1983; 58:441–449.
21. Stiles CM, Patel M, Keenan MAE: Anesthesia for rehabilitation surgery. In Nickel VL, Botte MJ (eds):

Orthopaedic Rehabilitation, 2nd edition, pp 105–115. New York, Churchill Livingstone, 1992.
22. Lawrence R, Hochberg MC, Kelsey JL, et al: Estimates of the prevalence of selected arthritis and musculoskeletal diseases in the United States. J Rheumatol 1989; 16:427–441.
23. Barrett WP, Franklin JL, Jackins SE, et al: Total shoulder arthroplasty. J Bone Joint Surg 1987; 69A: 865–872.
24. Bromstrom LA, Wallensten R, Olsson E, et al: The Kessel prosthesis in total shoulder arthroplasty. A five-year experience. Clin Orthop 1992; 277:155–160.
25. Cofield RH: Total shoulder arthroplasty with the Neer prosthesis. J Bone Joint Surg 1984; 66A:899–906.
26. Freidman RJ, Thornhill TS, Thomas WH, et al: Nonconstrained total shoulder replacement in patients who have rheumatoid arthritis and class IV function. J Bone Joint Surg 1989; 71A:494–498.
27. Thomas BJ, Amstutz HC, Cracchiolo A: Shoulder arthroplasty for rheumatoid arthritis. Clin Orthop 1991; 265:125–128.
28. Ewald FC, Simmons ED, Sullivan JA, et al: Capitellocondylar total elbow replacement in rheumatoid arthritis. Long-term results. J Bone Joint Surg 1993; 75A:498–507.
29. Eftekhar NS: Long-term results of cemented total hip arthroplasty. Clin Orthop 1987; 225:207–217.
30. Phillips FM, Pottenger LA, Finn HA, et al: Cementless total hip arthroplasty in patients with steroid-induced avascular necrosis of the hip. A 62-month follow-up study. Clin Orthop 1994; 303:147–154.
31. Shih CH, Du YK, Lin YH, et al: Muscular recovery around the hip joint after total hip arthroplasty. Clin Orthop 1994; 302:115–120.
32. Healy WL, Seidman J, Pfeifer BA, et al: Cold compressive dressing after total knee arthroplasty. Clin Orthop 1994; 299:143–146.
33. Hosick WB, Lotke PA, Baldwin A: Total knee arthroplasty in patients 80 years of age and older. Clin Orthop 1994; 299:77–80.
34. Laskin RS: Total condylar knee replacement in patients who have rheumatoid arthritis. A ten year follow-up study. J Bone Joint Surg 1990; 72A:529–535.
35. Levy AS, Marmar E: The role of cold compression dressings in the postoperative treatment of total knee arthroplasty. Clin Orthop 1993; 297:174–178.

CHAPTER 7

Psychological Distress and Clinical Outcomes

Donna J. Hawley, RN, MN, EdD

Clinical Outcomes

The impact of any chronic disease is evaluated by examining the short- and long-term effects of the disease on the general health status of the individual. Fries and Spitz[1] describe a hierarchical framework with five categories or dimensions of health status. These categories include disability, discomfort, financial costs, iatrogenic effects (e.g., drug side effects), and mortality (see Fig. 7-1). The discomfort category includes both pain and psychological distress. These five areas obviously are interrelated, with one area affecting and overlapping the other. For example, the financial costs of arthritis and significant drug side effects interact with the pain and the psychological distress. Pain management cannot be isolated from managing depression. Adapting to functional loss is inherently connected to pain and emotional distress. The relationships between disability, chronic pain, and psychological distress are complex and difficult to separate. Nonetheless, current research indicates that the psychological dimension of arthritis is independent of, although related to, other outcomes of chronic disease. In this chapter, the psychological aspects of arthritis are explored. These factors are examined both as independent components of disease and as they relate to other disease outcomes, particularly pain and disability.

Although there are over 100 different types of arthritis and related rheumatic disorders, the majority of the research on psychological aspects has been centered on rheumatoid arthritis (RA). Research recently has been increasing in areas of os-

PHYSICAL THERAPY IN ARTHRITIS, Joan M. Walker, PhD, PT, and Antoine Helewa, MSc(Clin Epid), PT, W.B. Saunders Company © 1996.

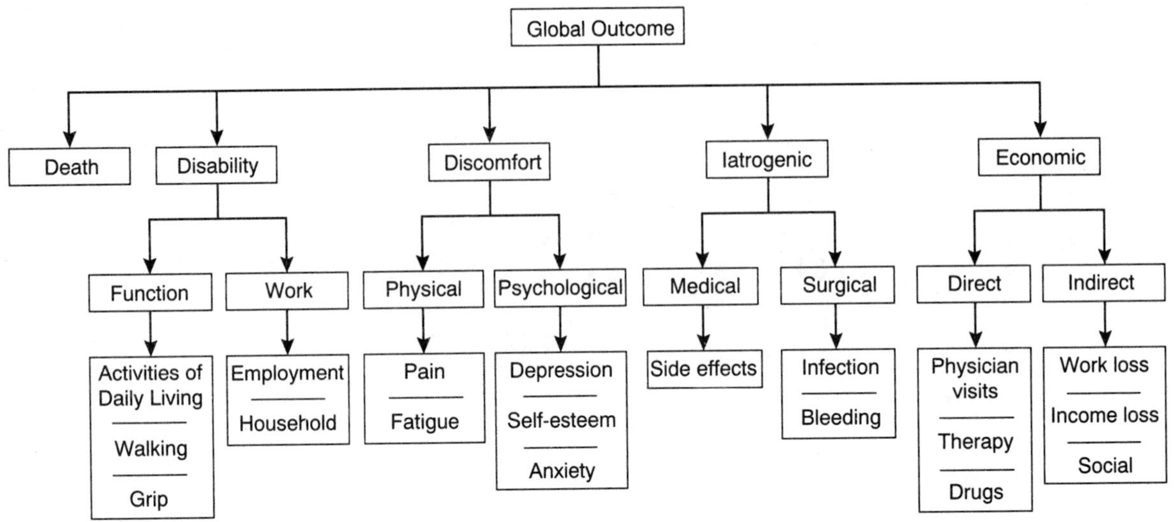

Figure 7-1. The outcomes of rheumatic disorders are shown as a hierarchy with global outcome at the top and becoming more specific under each of the subcategories. (Adapted from Fries JF, Spitz PW: In Spilker B [ed]: Quality of Life: Assessments in Clinical Trials, pp 25–35. New York, Raven Press Ltd, 1990. With permission.)

teoarthritis (OA),[2–5] fibromyalgia,[6–8] and systemic lupus erythematosus (SLE).[9,10] Nonetheless, RA, as the most prevalent of the systemic rheumatic disorders, remains the most commonly studied form of arthritis. Information from rheumatoid arthritis may be used as a model for looking at other types of arthritis.

Early Studies of Psychological Distress

Early studies of the psychological characteristics of people with RA found evidence of a "rheumatoid personality" and suggested that certain psychological traits were present prior to disease onset or were even etiological.[11] People with rheumatoid arthritis were reported to be "over-reacting to their disease, self-sacrificing, masochistic, rigid, moralistic, conforming, self-conscious, shy, inhibited, and perfectionistic."[12] Most of the studies that led to these conclusions were flawed. Properly controlled studies failed to support the notion of psychological underpinnings to rheumatoid arthritis. The idea of a rheumatoid personality is no longer considered valid or useful in explaining disease onset or outcome.[13,14]

The early studies often lacked control or comparison groups, provided limited demographic and diagnostic information about study subjects, and used methods and instruments with questionable validity and interrater reliability.[12,15] During the last 15–20 years, validated psychological instruments have largely replaced unstructured interviews. Statistically sophisticated studies have considered the multivariate relationships of social factors, demographic characteristics, and disease severity to observed psychological abnormalities. In recent years, investigators have examined abnormalities of emotional or mental status in arthritis, both cross-sectionally and longitudinally, using depression or depressive symptoms as the psychological factor studied. Depression or depressive symptoms may be considered surrogates for a general state of emotional health. Creed indicates that "anxiety neurosis and depressive illness overlap" and suggests use of the term depression for a state of emotional distress that he describes as a mixture of anxiety and depression.[16] This convention will be used throughout this chapter. The term depression will be used in this broad context and not as a specific psychiatric diagnosis.

Clinicians should recognize that the idea of a rheumatoid personality is not considered valid or useful in explaining disease onset or outcome.

Prevalence of Depression

Prevalence Studies

Depression has long been accepted as a major problem for people with rheumatoid arthritis.[14] Early studies reported prevalence rates as high as 80%,[17] but consensus from recent investigations of depression estimate a prevalence near 20%.[8,16,18] Depression in RA is similar to that in other chronic diseases, such as pulmonary disease, diabetes, cancer, chronic cardiovascular disease, and hypertension,[19] and somewhat less than depression in patients with chronic pain.[20] The prevalence of depression for people with RA is two to three times that of the general population.[21–23] Estimates of the prevalence of current depression in the general population have been reported between 5 and 13%. Percentages vary with gender, race, education, and income, as well as varying with the methodologies and definitions used in different studies.[21,22]

Hawley and Wolfe compared depressive symptoms among the various rheumatic disorders[8] (Table 7-1). People with RA report similar levels of depressive symptoms compared to those with OA of the knee, hip, or axial skeleton; low back pain; neck pain; and other chronic musculoskeletal problems commonly seen in a rheumatology referral practice. Only patients with OA of the hand had consistently lower depression scores than patients with RA. Fibromyalgia patients had consistently higher depressive levels, with almost 30% reporting serious depressive symptoms. The finding that fibromyalgia patients have high depression scores is consistent with other studies.[24–27]

Recently, Katz and Yelin[18] reported data from a large panel study of patients with RA in northern California. Patients were interviewed yearly from 1986 through 1990. The sample ranged from 648 patients in 1986 to 486 in 1990. About 4% of the patients were depressed each year of the four years; yet over 29% experienced depressive symptoms in one or more years. Individuals reporting depressive symptoms in one year were much more likely to report depression in subsequent years.[18]

Table 7-1. Percentage of Rheumatic Disease Patients who are at Risk for Serious Depressive Symptoms*

Diagnostic Category	N	Percentage of Patients with Probable Depression
Rheumatoid arthritis	1,152	20.4
Fibromyalgia	543	29.3
Osteoarthritis: knee or hip	463	16.8
Osteoarthritis: hand	379	14.2
Neck pain	160	23.1
Low back pain	547	22.7
OA/Axial overlap†	464	19.6
Other diagnoses†	2,445	18.4

*From Hawley DJ, Wolfe F: Depression is not more common in rheumatoid arthritis: a 10 year longitudinal study of 6,608 rheumatic disease patients. J Rheumatol 1993; 20:2025–2031. With permission.

†OA/Axial pain overlap group included patients with more than one diagnosis of osteoarthritis, neck pain, or low back pain. The last clinic group, "other diagnoses," included patients with all other rheumatic disease diagnoses.[8]

In summary, 70–80% of people with RA do not have serious depressive symptoms and seem to be managing their lives and their disease. They adapt and develop strategies that enable them to cope with the pain and disability of rheumatoid arthritis. However, a very significant minority is experiencing depressive symptoms and many with arthritis have periods in their disease course in which depressive symptoms are problematic.

Most people with rheumatoid arthritis do not present with serious depressive symptoms and cope with their disease. Clinicians, however, should note that depression is a problem in some patients with RA.

The challenge for physical therapists and for all health professionals is to assist those individuals who are experiencing psychological distress. To meet this challenge, an understanding of relationships between psychological distress and arthritis is necessary. Three areas are essential to such an understanding: (1) depressive symptoms and psychological distress demonstrated by people with arthritis, (2) the relationships between disease severity and depressive symptoms, and (3) appropriate interventions and strategies that may improve depression. These three areas are discussed in the remainder of this chapter.

Recognition of Depression and Psychological Distress: Assessment

Characteristics of Depression and Depressive Symptoms

The diagnosis of psychological disturbance or depression requires the use of comprehensive clinical interviews using standard diagnostic classification systems.[28] Such diagnosis is beyond the purview of this chapter and is done only by specially prepared health care professionals. However, recognition of psychological distress and depressive symptoms is a part of routine, daily rheumatological practice. Every health care professional working with an individual with arthritis can learn to recognize signs and symptoms of depression and psychological distress and intervene as needed.

Determining depression in clients requires alertness to symptoms of depression. Typical symptoms of depression are feelings of sadness, loss of interest in surroundings and in the family, difficulty concentrating, and sluggish thinking. People may withdraw from family and friends, lose interest in work or daily activities, and have feelings of guilt or loss of self-esteem. Certain somatic complaints also are part of depression. Changes in appetite, most frequently but not always a decrease in appetite, increased fatigue or lethargy, and problems with sleep including either excessive somnolence, insomnia, or early morning awakening are common symptoms. Many of the somatic symptoms typical of depression are an inherent part of a systemic inflammatory process. Sleep disturbances, loss of appetite, and fatigue may be part of the disease and may not necessarily be indicative of depression[29,30] (Table 7-2). Separating, for example, the fatigue caused by the disease and fatigue as a symptom of depression can be challenging for the health care professional. Evaluating these common symptoms and complaints of psychological distress (e.g., sadness, sluggish thinking, anorexia, lethargy), in combination with the physical measures common to inflammatory rheumatic disease (e.g., erythrocyte sedimentation rate [ESR] and swollen joint count), is necessary for the identification of psychological distress in this group of patients/clients.

Self-Report Measures for Depressive Symptoms

In addition to being cognizant of depressive symptoms, self-report scales are available and may be used as part of professional practice. The Center for Epidemiological Studies–Depression Scale (CES-D),[31] the Beck Depression Inventory,[32] and the depression subscale of the Arthritis Impact Measurement Scales (AIMS)[33] have been used extensively in studies of patients with arthritis. The AIMS depression scale is short (i.e., six items) and can be easily administered in a busy clinic setting. The six items relate to mood (e.g., enjoyment of activities, low spirits) during the past month. Somatic items such as fatigue, appetite, or weight loss or gain are not part of the scale. The AIMS depression scale is strongly correlated with the CES-D scale ($r = .81$).[35] The Beck Depression Inventory and the CES-D are both longer than the AIMS depression scale with 21 and 20 items, respectively; however, the length is certainly not prohibitive for use in practice and research settings.

Table 7-2. Common Characteristics of Depression*

General Characteristics	Somatic Complaints	Common Signs and Symptoms in Systematic Rheumatic Disorders†
Feelings of sadness; feeling "blue"	Fatigue	Fatigue
Inability to "shake off" feelings of sadness; cannot be "cheered up" by others	Appetite change Anorexia Overeating	Anorexia
Cognitive problems: sluggish thinking; inability to concentrate; memory problems	Sleep problems Hypersomnia Insomnia Early awakening Waking up fatigued	Sleep problems resulting in fatigue
Discouraged about the future Frequent crying	Weight loss or gain Psychomotor agitation or retardation	Weight loss
Loneliness Feelings of being disliked Finding little enjoyment in life Loss of interest in surroundings Suicide		

*Data from Center for Epidemiological Studies Depression Scale,[31] Beck Depression Inventory,[32] the depression subscale of the Arthritis Impact Measurement Scales,[33] and Short Geriatric Depression Scale.[34]

†Data from Pincus et al: Arthritis Rheum 1986; 29:1456–66[29]; Callahan et al: Arthritis Care Res 1991; 4:1–11[30]; and Blalock et al: Arthritis Rheum 1989; 32:991–997.[35]

Recognition and Referral

Regardless of the assessment methods used, clinicians need to recognize depressive symptoms and other types of psychological distress in their patients. Interventions as described in the rest of this chapter may be useful for a majority of patients; however, referrals to other health care professionals should be considered and are appropriate in cases of serious depression. Of course, *patients expressing suicidal thoughts require an immediate referral.*

Relationship between Clinical Factors and Psychosocial Factors

The relationship between disease severity and psychological distress is not direct. Anecdotally, every clinician knows that certain people with severe disability and pain are not depressed and seem to manage despite their disease. Likewise, some people with apparent mild disease complain of considerable pain, are depressed, and complain of distress that appears to be excessive based solely on the disease process. Specifically, chronic long-term pain that is characteristic of arthritis may lead to a depression, or chronic pain as stated by Magni et al may be the expression of "an underlying depressive disturbance which is made manifest through the symptom of pain."[21] Similarly, frustrations with inability to perform usual activities of daily living or inability to complete required work may deepen depressed moods. The corollary, that general psychological health may exacerbate pain and disability, also is true. Researchers have attempted to sort out these apparent incongruities using correlational or cross-sectional studies and recently in longitudinal studies.

Cross-Sectional Studies

People with depressive symptoms also report higher levels of pain than do those who are not depressed,[36–38] although the relationship may be only moderate. However, the picture is more complicated as other factors are examined. Bishop et al[39] determined that the number of painful joints, grip strength, and number of medications taken by hospitalized patients with rheumatoid arthritis were not correlated with depression. Frank et al,[38] using structured interviews, found that depression was not related to common disease severity indicators including grip strength, ESR, total joint count, or walking time. Similarly, Murphy et al also reported that depression was not related to disease severity measures, such as ESR, joint scores, rheumatoid factor, morning stiffness, as well as duration of disease.[40] They did find significant relationships between depression and the Stanford Health Assessment questionnaire, a self-report instrument that asks patients about their ability to do various activities of daily living.[40] In a sophisticated analysis of 158 individuals with rheumatoid arthritis, Newman et al ascertained that certain disease severity measures were important contributors to depression scores.[41] They reported that demographic variables (especially being female but also education, marital status, age, and social class), functional ability, social isolation, and "economic deprivation" contributed significantly in explaining depression scores. Disease duration, ESR and, unexpectedly, pain were not important predictors of depression in that study.[41]

Longitudinal Studies

Longitudinal studies have provided additional clues concerning the relationship between disease characteristics, pain, depression, and various social factors. Hawley and Wolfe,[36] in a 4-year study of 400 patients with RA, showed that worsening depression was associated with increasing age, lower education level, being unmarried, lower family income, but was not associated with any clinical variable such as pain, disability, or joint count. McFarlane and Brooks[37] reported similar results in their 3-year study of 30 patients. They did not find significant relationships between psychological variables and various disease severity measures or disease duration. In a study of 75 patients with early rheumatoid arthritis that were followed for 2 years, Raspe reported that pain intensity and functional capacity decreased slightly and work disability increased among participants, as did the number of erosive changes seen on radiography, but "mental suffering" was stable for the group as a whole, and for individuals.[42]

A recent study by Wolfe and Hawley[43] examined changes in self-report depression scores between routine clinic visits to a referral rheumatology practice. They found that changes in depression scores were related to the clinical variables of self-report functional disability scores and pain scores, as well as to education level, grip strength, disease duration, and length of morning stiffness. These findings suggest that over short periods of time (i.e., time between routine outpatient clinic visits), depressive symptoms may fluctuate with disease severity measures such as pain, functional disability, and grip strength. However, over longer periods of time and over the course of a chronic disease, depressive symptoms remain essentially stable.[43]

Emerging from these cross-sectional and longitudinal studies are two important points. First, although there are relationships between depression, pain, functional ability, and some severity measures, the relationships are moderate.[44] Functional disability, pain, and psychological status are separate concepts and operate to a considerable degree independently of disease severity, disease duration, and even long-term outcome. Second, the characteristics and causes of depression and psychological distress among people with RA are multifactorial and are related more to individual personality, family, and social circumstances than to disease severity. Social factors such as age, education, sex, marital status, economics, social isolation, and social support are important to our understanding of psychological distress in arthritis. In the next section, we will look at some of these social factors and at interventions addressing these factors.

Social Support

Social support in its broadest interpretation is important to the successful management of any chronic disease. Lanza and Revenson define social support as the "process by which interpersonal relationships promote well-being and protect people from health declines, particularly when they are facing stressful life circumstances."[45] Using this broad definition, social support includes family and friends, health care professionals, community groups such as church organizations or clubs, self-help educational programs, and formal support groups.

Individuals with RA reporting support from family (particularly spouses) and friends have an advantage over those reporting less support in areas such as self-esteem and psychological well-being,[46] adjustment of illness,[46,47] and depression.[48–50] Support from family and friends may buffer the coping skills of individuals.[45] Brown et al studied the possible buffering effects of social support in the management of arthritis pain. They reported that individuals with higher satisfaction for emotional support (from a variety of sources) were less depressed at all levels of pain severity.[51]

In examining the support from family and friends, Revenson et al warn that support can be both helpful and nonhelpful or a "double-edged sword."[49] In their study of 101 newly diagnosed individuals with rheumatoid arthritis (82% women), these authors found that positive or helpful support was related to lower depression scores and problematic or nonhelpful support was related to higher scores.[52] Affleck et al[47] asked people with arthritis to describe helpful and unhelpful types of support. In order of frequency mentioned by study participants, opportunities to express feelings and concerns, encouragement of hope and optimism, and being offered useful information were most helpful. Unhelpful approaches included minimizing the severity of an illness, expressions of pity, pessimistic statements about the future, and unnecessarily solicitous behavior.[47]

In the context of social support, studies most frequently have concentrated on the support from family, friends, and various social and self-help groups. The importance of support from health professionals is an additional component of social support and is an area where additional research could be helpful. In two separate studies reported by Revenson et al in a single publication, health care professionals have been rated as the "source of most helpful support" by 33–45% of patients.[52] Concrete professional activities related to solving disease-related problems (e.g., prescribing treatments or medications) were listed significantly more often than less tangible areas of support, such as providing information or emotional support.[52]

Strategies and Interventions

In addition to support from family, friends, and professionals that are provided on a one-to-one basis, specific strategies have been tested and have been shown to improve depression and psychological well-being for patients with arthritis. These strategies included various coping mechanisms, exercise, cognitive behavioral interventions, and psychoeducational interventions. Each of these strategies except exercise will be discussed. The beneficial effects of exercise are described in Chapters 11, 13, and 14.

Coping Strategies

Coping strategies used by people with arthritis may be positive or negative as well as helpful or nonhelpful. Coping strategies may attenuate the effects of stresses such as pain or may even exacerbate problems. Furthermore, the effectiveness of coping strategies may be independent of pain severity or the degree of disability.[53,54] Brown et al[54] demonstrated that passive coping behaviors such as depending on others; limiting social activities; and suppressing anger, depression, or frustration are positively related to depression. On the other hand, active coping behaviors such as staying busy, ignoring pain, or using activities to distract one from pain are negatively related to depression. In fact, they found that passive coping behaviors may actually intensify the relationship between pain and depression.[54] Similar descriptive evidence when studying a variety of chronic diseases including RA has been reported.[55] A positive affect is related to two major active coping strategies; that is, cognitive restructuring and information seeking while negative affect was related to emotional expressions, fantasy, and self-blame. These findings support clinical observations and make intuitive sense.

Table 7-3 lists various coping strategies used by individuals with chronic disease and chronic pain. The strategies are divided into groups labeled as passive and active coping strategies. While the studies described above indicate that active coping strategies are more effective in the self-management of chronic disease, the effectiveness of any coping strategy depends on the situation.[55] For example, after initial diagnosis, denial may be a very logical and useful defense mechanism or coping strategy. When a person hears a diagnosis that has a very uncertain and potentially serious outcome, denial is both protective and useful for a short period of time. However, continuing to deny a diagnosis for an extended period of time is not useful. Although seeking help from others is listed as passive coping activity, under some circumstances it is an active approach. Seeking help from others when such help is necessitated by physical limitations is essential, appropriate, and an active strategy. It is only when one depends unnecessarily on others that this strategy becomes a passive activity and ineffective.

Table 7-3. Commonly Used Coping Strategies*: A Comparison of Passive and Active Strategies

Passive Coping Strategies	Active Coping Strategies
Denial	
Focusing on the pain or problem	Distraction
	Selectively ignoring the pain
	Activity
	Imagery
	Avoidance
Isolation from family, friends, social activities	Participation in activities
	Being physically active
	Leisure activities
Seeking comfort from others	Seeking information from knowledgeable others
Telling others about the pain	Professionals
Praying	Read materials about the disease
	Attend self-management classes
Fantasizing/wishing for better medications from the physician	Cognitive restructuring: reappraise situation
	Find positive aspects to life
Dreaming the problem will disappear	Make illness less important in one's life
Daydreaming	Adapt new approaches to managing disease
Blaming others or self	
Dependence on others	Independence
Calling for professional help	Get appropriate help for major tasks
	Maintain as much independence as possible

*Data from the work of Brown et al: J Consult Clin Psychol 1989; 57:652–657,[54] Felton et al: Soc Sci Med 1984; 18:889–898,[55] and Brown and Nicassio: Pain 1987; 31:53–64.[56]

Generally speaking, active coping strategies are more effective than passive approaches, but the effectiveness of any strategy depends on the situation and the individual at a given point in time.

Interventions

The goal for the clinician is determining how to use this information about effective and noneffective coping strategies in practice. Assisting people to adapt strategies such as distraction or information seeking rather than ineffective strategies such as fantasizing or blaming oneself is well recognized as a vital component of clinical practice. The challenge then for the physical therapist and for all health care professionals is how to achieve this goal.

Descriptive studies as summarized above have provided very useful information concerning the characteristics of psychological distress and the effectiveness of coping strategies and of social support. While useful diagnostically for the clinician, the next logical step is to move from cross-sectional and longitudinal descriptive studies of social support and coping strategies to studies that test interventions for patients experiencing psychological distress. Findings from descriptive studies have been used as the basis for psychological intervention studies. The typical psychological interventions used in studies of people with RA have been collectively labeled as cognitive-behavioral therapies or self-management therapies.[57] These types of treatments feature activities such as relaxation techniques, imagery, coping strategies, problem-solving techniques, pain management techniques (e.g., diversion, biofeedback), and communication. Specifics differ from study to study, but generally interventions focus on teaching patients techniques that will enable them to manage their own disease. The overall goal is to increase confidence that pain and other symptoms are under the individual's control. This confidence or belief that one can master or control a situation is called "self-efficacy."

Cognitive Behavioral Therapies

Preliminary studies using relaxation training and biofeedback[58] and cognitive strategies such as deep muscle relaxation and visual imagery[59] show beneficial effects on pain. Parker et al, studying primarily elderly men with rheumatoid arthritis, found that participants in the cognitive-behavioral group demonstrated greater use of coping strategies and increased confidence for pain management than control groups.[60] Reduced pain behavior, disease activity, and trait anxiety were demonstrated following a cognitive-behavioral treatment program.[57]

In a comprehensive controlled clinical trial, Radojevic et al[61] examined the effectiveness of both cognitive-behavioral therapy and family support. A total of 59 people with RA was randomly assigned to one of three intervention groups, to a control or a no-treatment group. The three interventions included (1) a cognitive-behavioral therapy group with family support, (2) a cognitive-behavioral therapy group without family support, and (3) education with family support. All groups improved over the study; however, the two behavioral therapy groups showed decreases in disease severity measures compared to the control and the education groups. Immediately following the intervention, the behavioral therapy group with family support demonstrated more improvement in health status than any of the other study groups. Family support may be an important factor to consider when designing and implementing treatment programs.[61]

Psychoeducational Interventions

An additional area within the broad rubric of cognitive-behavioral therapy is the psychoeducational interventions. Education of the patient is an important component of practice for health professionals from all disciplines. Historically, the effectiveness of educational interventions has been evaluated by determining if there was an increase in a participant's knowledge about his/her disease. During the last 20 years emphasis has changed. Behavioral outcomes rather than knowledge have become the key measure of success. Since the major outcome variables for individuals with RA and OA are disability, pain, and depression, these are logical variables for evaluating the efficacy of psychoeducational interventions.[62] A meta-analysis of psychoeducational intervention studies found that participants in these types of interventions had improvements of 16% in pain, 22% in depression, and about 8% in disability compared to untreated groups.[62] While these results are considered only "modest,"[62] such improvement in a chronic painful disorder must be considered clinically important. As Deyo[63] and Fitzpatrick et al[64] have pointed out, improvement and beneficial effects of therapy in rheumatoid arthritis are often "quite subtle."[64]

The Arthritis Self-Management Course (ASMC), developed by Kate Lorig et al, exemplifies the effectiveness of psychoeducational interventions.[65] The program has been evaluated extensively for behavioral, health status, and cost outcomes with over 2,500 people during an 11-year period. Since 1982, the ASMC has been sponsored by the Arthritis Foundation and is offered by the local chapters of the Arthritis Foundation throughout the United States. The program is now offered in Canada, Australia, New Zealand, and several other countries throughout the world.

The important variables studied during the first 5 years of controlled clinical trials examining the ASMC were pain, depression, and disability.[66] In addition, the number of times the participant exercised, used relaxation techniques per month, and the number of physician visits in a 4-month period were used as indicators of increased self-care activities. Knowledge of arthritis also was included.[66]

During these early randomized, controlled clinical trials, subjects completing the ASMC had increased knowledge, as expected, but more importantly they had less pain and participated in more self-management activities such as exercise than did controls. This improvement in clinical outcome for the group participating in the course continued for up to 20 months with only minor reductions.[66] Depression scores improved for participants but not for controls. Although the improvements were statistically significant in some trials,[67] they were not in other studies.[68] Disability scores did not improve significantly in any study, but they did not worsen either.[66–68] In many forms of arthritis, disability is progressive; thus, stability over time is an excellent clinical outcome, regardless of the statistical finding. Such variability in results confirms the importance of ongoing evaluation of the clinical outcomes of this particular course and for other psychoeducational interventions.

Despite the favorable results of the ASMC, Lorig et al determined that the relationship between the changes in behavior that occurred following the educational program (e.g., increased relaxation, exercise) and the improvements in health status measures (pain, depression, functional disability) was weak.[68] Correlations ranged from −0.01 for knowledge and disability to −0.14 for exercise frequency and pain. On the basis of these findings, Lorig et al did extensive follow-up discussions with participants from the self-management courses. From these discussions, the researchers learned that a participant's belief in his/her capacity to manage the disease improved during the course even though the disease itself did not change.[67] In other words, the course improved people's belief in their own ability or increased their perceived power over the disease. People believed they could manage their arthritis better and such a belief influenced the clinical outcome. Indeed, they learned to manage their disease better. This belief is similar to the psychological concept of self-efficacy. In response to this finding, Lorig began in the mid 1980s to study the relationship of self-efficacy and arthritis self-management.

Self-efficacy is a belief that one can accomplish certain activities. Self-efficacy is behavior specific rather than a characteristic or trait. An individual can believe or have high self-efficacy in one area such as the ability to exercise regularly but at the same time believe that he or she cannot control the pain or the fatigue of arthritis. Since this belief is dynamic, perceived self-efficacy can be modified through a variety of mechanisms including education. For example, Parker et al have shown that learning and using coping strategies for pain management also will increase confidence that pain is manageable.[60] Consistent with self-efficacy theory, Lorig et al have demonstrated that perceived self-efficacy is related to both present and future health status for participants in the Arthritis Self-Management Course.[67]

Nontraditional Treatments

Nontraditional treatments, unconventional treatments, complementary medicine, alternative medicine, and unorthodox therapies are terms frequently used to describe those treatments or therapies that are not in the mainstream of standard, Western health care. Boisset and Fitzcharles define such therapies as interventions not "widely taught in North American medical schools or generally available in North American hospitals."[69]

These treatments range from harmless folk treatments (e.g., copper bracelets) to a few expensive and potentially harmful therapies. Recent reports describe usage among arthritis patients between 34%[69] and 84%.[70] A recent study in the United States estimated use by the general population at 34% and costs estimated at almost $14 billion for 1990.[71]

Individuals with arthritis use nontraditional or unorthodox treatments for two reasons. First, the current treatments for arthritis are not curative. Despite advances in treatments, many of the inflammatory rheumatic diseases are progressive, painful, and disabling. Second, the course of the rheumatic diseases is variable. There may be periods of remission that last a few days to, in rare cases, years. These positive changes occur in response to therapy or may occur spontaneously. Individuals may mistakenly associate improvement with the visit to the uranium mine, to the change in diet, to the medication, or to physical therapy, all of which were completed recently. Thus the two factors of inadequate treatment and variable disease course coupled with a large market (36 million people in the United States alone have arthritis) provide a fertile environment for the advent of unconventional treatments.[72]

Examples of nontraditional treatments include acupuncture, massage, reflexology, homeopathic medications, herbs, vitamins, minerals, special diets of various kinds, fish oil, DMSO, WD-40, urine injections, folk remedies (copper bracelets, vinegar and honey), venom from various animals, and even sitting in uranium mines. While usage of these treatments is high among persons with arthritis, two recent reports, one in Canada[69] and one in the United States,[70] indicate that the problem may not be as serious as previous reports indicated.[73,74] While usage of these types of therapies is common, both of these recent studies indicate that the use of costly or dangerous treatments is not. Boisset and Fitzcharles in their study in Canada estimate cost at about $100 per year per individual.[69] Similarly, Cronan et al in the United States reported that most people use "inexpensive, harmless remedies, such as exercise, prayer, and relaxation."[70]

Physical therapists and other health care professionals need to be aware of the types of unconventional therapies, their costs, and their potential for harm.

Establishing an environment that encourages the patient to share information about the various types of nontraditional treatments that he/she is using is essential.

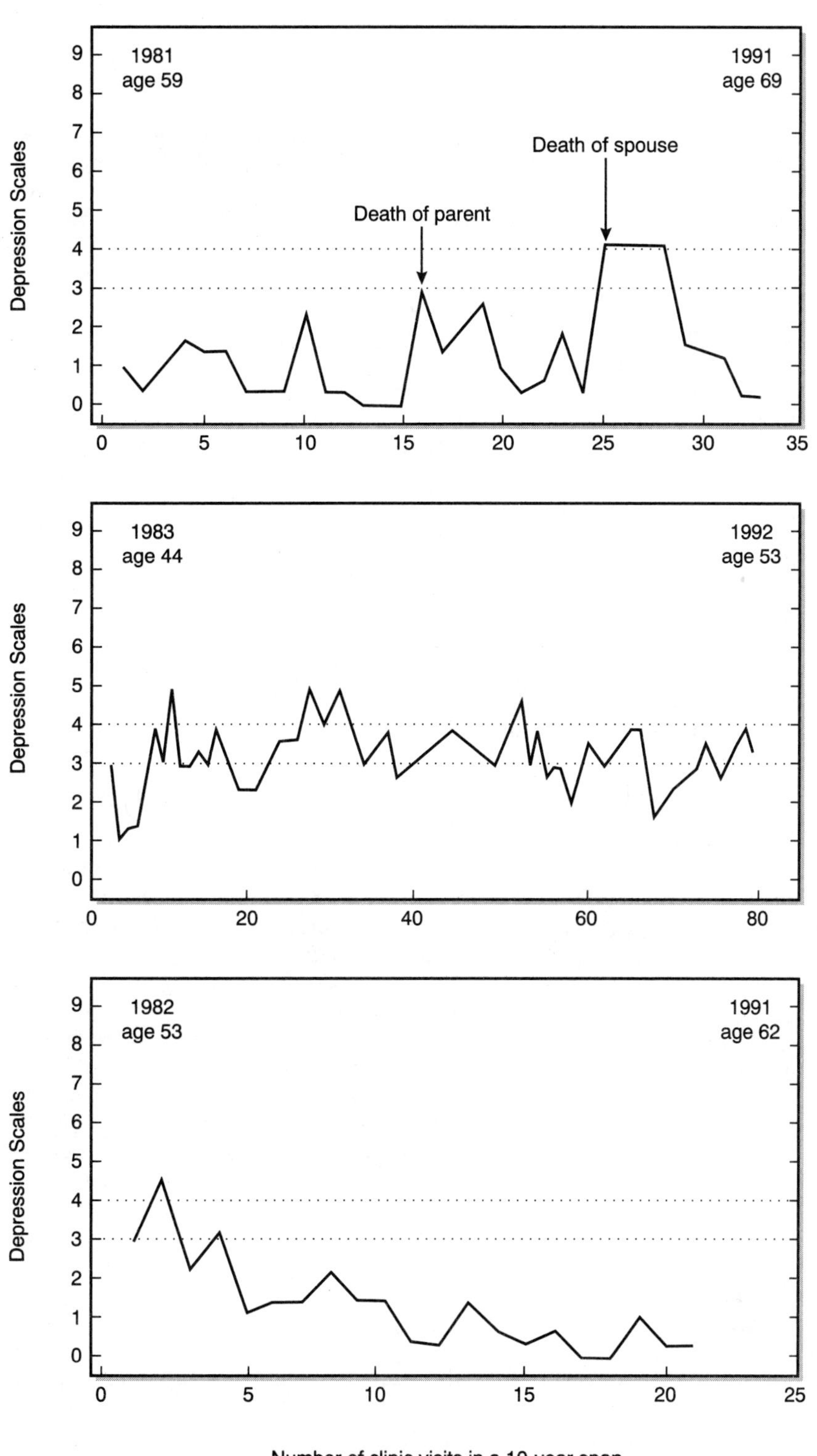

Figure 7-2. Three patterns for the changes in depressive symptoms over time are illustrated. The Y or vertical axis represents the scores on the AIMS depression scale with scores ranging from 0 to 10. The X or horizontal axis represents visits to a specialty rheumatological clinic over about a 10-year period. The horizontal lines at 3 and 4 on the Y-axis are the levels at which depressive symptoms are possibly and probably, respectively, indicative of depression on this particular depression scale. (From Hawley DJ, Wolfe F: J Rheumatol 1993; 20:2025–2031. With permission.)

Providing information that allows patients to make informed decisions about what treatments to use and not use is an important aspect of the role for all health care providers.

Summary

While the majority of people with arthritis manage their disease reasonably well, depressive symptoms and psychological distress are common. Relationships between disease characteristics and psychological distress are complex. Strategies for managing the symptoms, the long-term outcomes, and the psychological distress of chronic rheumatic diseases are issues important for health care providers, patients, and their families.

Case Studies

Three case studies of patients with rheumatoid arthritis illustrate only how depression scores change over time and may offer clues for understanding individual differences among people who happen to have a chronic disabling disease. These cases are described below. They illustrate three characteristic patterns of psychological distress as seen in people with RA over the course of the disease. Similar patterns can probably be found when examining the clinical course of other chronic disorders. Three graphs, shown in Figure 7-2, depict these three courses for depressive symptoms over time. All three women have RA that does not remit for any extended period of time. They each experience progressive disease with gradually increasing disability. AIMS depression scores are shown for each visit to a specialty clinic over about a 10-year period. AIMS depression scores range from 0 to 9.9, with scores above 3.00 indicating the presence of possible depressive symptoms, and scores above 4.00 probable depression.

Case History

Case 1. This case is a woman first seen in the clinic at age 59 years. She exhibited little depression at the time of her diagnosis and her depression scores remain stable and low during the entire 10-year period. Two peaks in her depression scores can be noted at the time her parent and her spouse died. Except during times of stress or family crisis unrelated to her disease, this lady is managing her disease quite effectively from, at least, a psychological point of view.

Case 2. This case illustrates a second pattern. This patient is a woman first diagnosed at age 44. Her depression scores are high at the time of diagnosis and remain high throughout the disease course. She struggled with depression throughout the 10-year period for a variety of reasons. Her scores are relatively stable but are consistently high. Her depressive symptoms probably are not related to any great extent to her disease.

Case 3. This case illustrates a pattern of high depression early in the disease with a decline soon after diagnosis. As an individual adapts to the disease, he learns to cope or adapts to the situation. Depressive symptoms then are reduced to "normal" or a state of essentially non-depression with such adaptation. This woman experienced high depression scores at the time of her diagnosis. The diagnosis caused her distress, as reflected in her initial depression score. Her scores decreased quickly after diagnosis and remained low during the remaining time that she was followed. She has adapted with time to her disease and has learned to cope with her disorder.

These cases illustrate that the interaction between psychosocial factors and disease are complex and include much more than the severity or the characteristics of the disease. They also demonstrate that many people do manage their disease using various coping strategies. Patients gain support from family, friends, and health care professionals. They attend formal support groups and participate in educational programs, such as the Arthritis Self-Management program. Many people manage very well, while others do not. The role for all health professionals is to provide assistance to those who are having difficulties managing their disease and to support the independence of those who are managing.

References

1. Fries JF, Spitz PW: The hierarchy of patient outcomes. In Spilker B (ed): Quality of Life: Assessments in Clinical Trials, pp 25–35. New York, Raven Press, 1990.

2. Salaffi F, Cavalieri F, Nolli M, et al: Analysis of disability in knee osteoarthritis—relationship with age and psychological variables but not with radiographic score. J Rheumatol 1991; 18:1581–1586.
3. Weinberger M, Tierney WM, Booher P, et al: Social support, stress and functional status in patients with osteoarthritis. Soc Sci Med 1990; 30:503–508.
4. Rene J, Weinberger M, Mazzuca SA, et al: Reduction of joint pain in patients with knee osteoarthritis who have received monthly telephone calls from lay personnel and whose medical treatment regimens have remained stable. Arthritis Rheum 1992; 35:511–515.
5. Dexter P, Brandt K: Distribution and predictors of depressive symptoms in osteoarthritis. J Rheumatol 1994; 21:279–286.
6. Goldenberg DL: Psychiatric and psychologic aspects of fibromyalgia syndrome. Rheum Dis Clin North Am 1989; 15:105–114.
7. Uveges JM, Parker JC, Smarr KL, et al: Psychological symptoms in primary fibromyalgia syndrome: relationship to pain, life stress, and sleep disturbance. Arthritis Rheum 1990; 33:1279–1283.
8. Hawley DJ, Wolfe F: Depression is not more common in rheumatoid arthritis: a 10 year longitudinal study of 6,608 rheumatic disease patients. J Rheumatol 1993; 20:2025–2031.
9. Liang MH, Rogers M, Larson M, et al: The psychosocial impact of systemic lupus erythematosus and rheumatoid arthritis. Arthritis Rheum 1984; 27:13–19.
10. Cornwell CJ, Schmitt MH: Perceived health status, self-esteem and body image in women with rheumatoid arthritis or systemic lupus erythematosus. Res Nurs Health 1990; 13:99–107.
11. Hoffman AL: Psychological factors associated with rheumatoid arthritis. Nurs Res 1974; 23:218–234.
12. Moos RH: Personality factors associated with rheumatoid arthritis: a review. J Chronic Dis 1964; 17: 41–55.
13. Spergel P, Ehrlich GE, Glass D: The rheumatoid arthritic personality: a psychodiagnostic myth. Psychosomatics 1978; 19:79–86.
14. Anderson KA, Bradley LA, Young LD, et al: Rheumatoid arthritis: review of psychological factors related to etiology, effects, and treatment. Psychol Bull 1985; 98:358–387.
15. Baum J: A review of the psychological aspects of rheumatic diseases. Semin Arthritis Rheum 1982; 11:352–361.
16. Creed F: Psychological disorders in rheumatoid arthritis: a growing consensus? Ann Rheum Dis 1990; 49:808–812.
17. Rimon R: Depression in rheumatoid arthritis. Ann Clin Res 1974; 6:171–175.
18. Katz PP, Yelin EH: Prevalence and correlates of depressive symptoms among persons with rheumatoid arthritis. J Rheumatol 1993; 20:790–796.
19. Mason JH, Weener JL, Gertman PM, et al: Health status in chronic disease: a comparative study of rheumatoid arthritis. J Rheumatol 1983; 10:763–768.
20. Magni G: On the relationship between chronic pain and depression when there is no organic lesion. Pain 1987; 31:1–21.
21. Magni G, Calidieron C, Rigati-Luchini S, et al: Chronic musculoskeletal pain and depressive symptoms in the general population. An analysis of the 1st National Health and Nutrition Examination Survey data. Pain 1990; 43:299–307.
22. Weissman MM, Myers JK: Affective disorders in a US urban community: the use of research diagnostic criteria in an epidemiological survey. Arch Gen Psychiatry 1978; 35:1304–1311.
23. Crook J, Rideout E, Browne G: The prevalence of pain complaints in a general population. Pain 1984; 18:299–314.
24. Ahles TA, Yunus MB, Masi AT: Is chronic pain a variant of depressive disease? The case of primary fibromyalgia syndrome. Pain 1987; 29:105–111.
25. Alfici S, Sigal M, Landau M: Primary fibromyalgia syndrome—a variant of depressive disorder? Psychother Psychosom 1989; 51:156–161.
26. Yunus MB, Ahles TA, Aldag JC, et al: Relationship of clinical features with psychological status in primary fibromyalgia. Arthritis Rheum 1991; 34:15–21.
27. Gaston-Johansson F, Gustafsson M, Felldin R, et al: A comparative study of feelings, attitudes and behaviours of patients with fibromyalgia and rheumatoid arthritis. Soc Sci Med 1990; 31:941–947.
28. American Psychiatric Association: Diagnostic and Statistical Manual of Mental Disorders (DSM-III-R), 567 pp. Washington, DC, American Psychiatric Association, 1987.
29. Pincus T, Callahan LF, Bradley LA, et al: Elevated MMPI scores for hypochondriasis, depression and hysteria in patients with rheumatoid arthritis reflect disease rather than psychological status. Arthritis Rheum 1986; 29:1456–1466.
30. Callahan LF, Kaplan MR, Pincus T: The Beck Depression Inventory, Center for Epidemiological Studies-Depression Scale (CES-D), and General Well-Being Schedule Depression Subscale in rheumatoid arthritis: criterion contamination of responses. Arthritis Care Res 1991; 4:1–11.
31. Radloff L: The CES-D scale: a self-report depression scale for research in the general population. Appl Psychol Measurement 1977; 1:385–401.
32. Beck AT, Steer RA, Gabin MG: Psychometric properties of the Beck Depression Inventory: twenty-five years of evaluation. Clin Psychol Rev 1988; 8:77–100.
33. Meenan RF, Gertman PM, Mason JH: Measuring health status in arthritis: the arthritis impact measurement scales. Arthritis Rheum 1980; 23:146–152.
34. Sheikh JI, Yesavage JA: Geriatric depression scale (GDS). Recent evidence and development of a shorter version. Clin Gerontol 1986; 51:165–173.

35. Blalock SJ, deVellis RF, Brown GK, et al: Validity of the Center for Epidemiological Studies depression scale in arthritis populations. Arthritis Rheum 1989; 32:991–997.
36. Hawley DJ, Wolfe F: Anxiety and depression in patients with RA: a prospective study of 400 patients. J Rheumatol 1988; 15:932–941.
37. McFarlane AC, Brooks PM: An analysis of the relationship between psychological morbidity and disease activity in rheumatoid arthritis. J Rheumatol 1988; 15:926–931.
38. Frank RG, Beck NC, Parker JC, et al: Depression in rheumatoid arthritis. J Rheumatol 1988; 15:920–925.
39. Bishop D, Green A, Cantor S, et al: Depression, anxiety and rheumatoid arthritis activity. Clin Exp Rheumatol 1987; 5:147–150.
40. Murphy S, Creed F, Jayson MIV: Psychiatric disorder and illness behaviour in rheumatoid arthritis. Br J Rheumatol 1988; 27:357–363.
41. Newman SP, Fitzpatrick R, Lamb R, et al: The origins of depressed mood in rheumatoid arthritis. J Rheumatol 1989; 16:740–744.
42. Raspe HH: Social and emotional problems in early rheumatoid arthritis. 75 patients followed up for two years. Clin Rheumatol 1987; 6:20–25.
43. Wolfe F, Hawley DJ: The relationship between clinical activity and depression on rheumatoid arthritis. J Rheumatol 1993; 20:2032–2037.
44. Peck JR, Smith TW, Ward JR, et al: Disability and depression in rheumatoid arthritis: a multi-trait, multi-method investigation. Arthritis Rheum 1989; 32:1100–1106.
45. Lanza AF, Revenson TA: Social support interventions for rheumatoid arthritis patients: the cart before the horse? Health Educ Q 1993; 20:97–117.
46. Fitzpatrick R, Newman S, Lamb R, et al: Social relationships and psychological well-being in rheumatoid arthritis. Soc Sci Med 1988; 27:399–403.
47. Affleck G, Pfeiffer C, Tennen H, et al: Social support and psychological well-being in rheumatoid arthritis. Arthritis Care Res 1988; 1:71–77.
48. Fitzpatrick R, Newman S, Archer R, et al: Social support, disability, and depression: a longitudinal study of rheumatoid arthritis. Soc Sci Med 1991; 33:605–611.
49. Revenson TA, Schiaffino KM, Majerovitz SD, et al: Social support as a double-edged sword: the relation of positive and problematic support to depression among rheumatoid arthritis patients. Soc Sci Med 1991; 33:807–813.
50. Goodenow C, Reisine ST, Grady KE: Quality of social support and associated social and psychological functioning in women with rheumatoid arthritis. Health Psychol 1990; 9:266–284.
51. Brown GK, Wallston KA, Nicassio PM: Social support and depression in rheumatoid arthritis: a one year prospective study. J Appl Soc Psychol 1989; 19: 1164–1181.
52. Revenson TA, Cameron AE, Lanza AF: Perceived helpfulness of patient-provider support transactions: findings from two studies (abstr). Arthritis Care Res 1991; 4:S19.
53. Felton BJ, Revenson TA: Coping with chronic illness: a study of illness controllability and the influence of coping strategies on psychological adjustment. J Consult Clin Psychol 1984; 52:343–353.
54. Brown GK, Nicassio PM, Wallston KA: Pain coping strategies and depression in rheumatoid arthritis. J Consult Clin Psychol 1989; 57:652–657.
55. Felton BJ, Revenson TA, Hinrichsen GA: Stress and coping in the explanation of psychological adjustment among chronically ill adults. Soc Sci Med 1984; 18:889–898.
56. Brown GK, Nicassio PM: Development of a questionnaire for the assessment of active and passive coping strategies in chronic pain patients. Pain 1987; 31:53–64.
57. Bradley LA, Young LD, Anderson KO, et al: Effects of psychological therapy on pain behaviour of rheumatoid arthritis patients. Treatment outcome and six-month follow up. Arthritis Rheum 1987; 30: 1105–1114.
58. Denver DR, Laveault D, Girard F: Behavioral medicine: biobehavioral effects of short-term thermal biofeedback and relaxation in rheumatoid arthritis patients (abstr). Biofeedback Self Regul 1979; 4: 245–246.
59. Randich SR: Evaluation of a pain management program for rheumatoid arthritis patients (abstr). Arthritis Rheum 1982; 25(Suppl):S11.
60. Parker JC, Frank RG, Beck NC, et al: Pain management in rheumatoid arthritis patients. A cognitive-behavioral approach. Arthritis Rheum 1988; 31:593–601.
61. Radojevic V, Nicassio PM, Weisman MH: Behavioral intervention with and without family support for rheumatoid arthritis. Behav Ther 1992; 23:13–30.
62. Mullen PD, Laville EA, Biddle AK, et al: Efficacy of psychoeducational interventions on pain, depression, and disability in people with arthritis: a meta-analysis. J Rheumatol 1987; 14:33–39.
63. Deyo RA: Measuring the quality of life of patients with rheumatoid arthritis. In Walker SR, Rosser SR (eds): Quality of Life: Assessment and Application, pp 205–222. Lancaster, MTP Press Limited, 1988.
64. Fitzpatrick R, Ziebland S, Jenkinson C, et al: A comparison of the sensitivity to change of several health status instruments in rheumatoid arthritis. J Rheumatol 1993; 20:429–436.
65. Lorig K: Arthritis Self-help Course: Leader's Manual and Reference Materials. Atlanta, Arthritis Foundation, 1990.
66. Lorig K, Lubeck D, Kraines RG, et al: Outcomes of self-help education for patients with arthritis. Arthritis Rheum 1985; 28:680–685.
67. Lorig K, Chastain RL, Ung E, et al: Development and

evaluation of a scale to measure perceived self-efficacy in people with arthritis. Arthritis Rheum 1989; 32:37–44.
68. Lorig K, Seleznick M, Lubeck D, et al: The beneficial outcomes of the arthritis self-management course are not adequately explained by behaviour change. Arthritis Rheum 1989; 32:91–95.
69. Boisset M, Fitzcharles MA: Alternative medicine use by rheumatology patients in a universal health care setting. J Rheumatol 1994; 21:148–152.
70. Cronan TA, Kaplan RM, Posner L, et al: Prevalence of the use of unconventional remedies for arthritis in a metropolitan community. Arthritis Rheum 1989; 32:1604–1607.
71. Eisenberg DM, Kessler RC, Foster C, et al: Unconventional medicine in the United States. N Engl J Med 1993; 328:246–252.
72. Hawley DJ: Nontraditional treatments of arthritis. Nurs Clin North Am 1984; 19:663–672.
73. Arthritis Foundation: Basic Facts: Answers to Your Questions. Atlanta, Arthritis Foundation, 1983.
74. Price JH, Hillman KS, Toral ME, et al: The public's perceptions and misperceptions of arthritis. Arthritis Rheum 1983; 26:1023–1028.

CHAPTER 8

Assessment of Joint Disease

Hugh A. Smythe, MD, FRCP[C]
Antoine Helewa, MSc(Clin Epid), PT

This chapter emphasizes a general approach to musculoskeletal diagnosis, and specific clinical skills that are not described in standard texts. In other systems, the physical examination is organized as inspection, palpation, percussion, and auscultation. In the musculoskeletal system, we assess **inflammation, damage**, and **function**. We define a screening examination, for those with few complaints, as well as a thorough exploration of more challenging problems. At the end of each section is a format that is quickly completed when there are few findings, comprehensive when there are many.

The section on peripheral joint problems details the techniques needed to assess inflammation separately from damage, because anti-inflammatory and reconstructive therapies are so different. Damage is discussed in a general approach rather than a joint-by-joint description of the many possible patterns. Function is reviewed separately, as restoration of function is an important part of the treatment plan (see Chapter 4 for laboratory and radiographic features).

The section "Pain Amplification Syndromes" is important, not only because the entities are com-

PHYSICAL THERAPY IN ARTHRITIS, Joan M. Walker, PhD, PT, and Antoine Helewa, MSc(Clin Epid), PT, W.B. Saunders Company © 1996.

Table 8-1. Musculoskeletal Disorders

Inflammatory joint diseases
Traumatic, mechanical, and **degenerative** disorders
Metabolic disorders with skeletal manifestations
Nonarticular rheumatic syndromes
Miscellaneous disorders

mon but also because they may coexist with other diseases and, if unrecognized, present difficulties in assessment and the risk of inappropriate treatment.

In the section "Assessment of Spinal Disease" the phenomena associated with referred pain are described, as are the skills needed to localize the site of origin of spinal pain or restriction of movement. Different disease entities affect different parts of the spine. Therapy of the mechanical problems requires a recognition of the pathogenetic forces acting at vulnerable levels.

The diagnostic classification of Schumacher[1] in the Primer on the Rheumatic Diseases is difficult to memorize and a simplified grouping is offered in Table 8-1, which gives a basic division into inflammatory, degenerative, metabolic, and nonarticular syndromes, and Table 8-2, which gives a subclassification of the inflammatory types. The group of seronegative forms of chronic polyarthritis associated with the antigen HLA-B27 and the common but neglected "benign polyarthritis" group are separated from the seropositive diseases because the genetic and immunologic features are so different.

Problem Identification and Quantitative Assessment: Peripheral Joints

The classic medical history led to a provisional diagnosis, and the prognosis and plan of management was implicit in this label. The shortcomings of this approach are very apparent in the chronic musculoskeletal disorders. A diagnosis of rheumatoid arthritis (RA) is consistent with any prognosis from the most benign to the most horrible, and the variety of treatment programs that may be appropriate is very wide.

For all health professionals, a more useful objective is the definition of the **problems** challenging the patient, with a quantitative assessment of severity. In persons with rheumatoid arthritis, the commonest are:

1. Uncontrolled polyarthritis
2. Structural damage and deformity

Table 8-2. Subclassification of Inflammatory Joint Diseases

Group	Examples
1. Seropositive chronic polyarthritis (rheumatoid arthritis and variants)	Rheumatoid arthritis Sjögren's syndrome
2. Diffuse connective tissue disorders ("collagen") diseases	Systemic lupus erythematosus
3. Seronegative chronic polyarthritis	
B27-associated diseases	Ankylosing spondylitis Reiter's syndrome
Other	Arthritis with psoriasis
4. Juvenile chronic polyarthritis group	Systemic form Oligarticular form
5. Benign polyarthritis group (due to immune mechanisms)	Rheumatic fever Serum sickness
6. Due to infectious agents	Gonococcal arthritis
7. Associated with systemic disease	Sarcoidosis Hypertrophic osteoarthropathy
8. Crystal-induced synovitis	Gout Pseudogout

3. Functional loss
4. Pain amplification syndromes
5. Inappropriate drug therapy and non-compliance
6. Focus on coping or passive therapies, rather than on control or cure
7. Drug side effects
8. Extra-articular involvement
9. Incorrect or incomplete diagnosis
10. Exaggerated pain behavior

While assessing patients, avoid leading questions.

While performing the assessment, the observer is constantly making choices, influenced by the interaction of preliminary hypotheses as to the nature of the patient's problems, and the evidence emerging from history and examination. As each patient is unique, so the assessment process will be unique. It is easy to assess the severity of inflammation, unless the patient has important non-articular pain. This issue must not be ignored, but may be set aside in a few moments if unsupported by the clinical evidence; or it may dominate the assessment process. The **objective of the assessment is to produce a plan of management.** Past treatment efforts are of great importance. Often it emerges that appropriate therapy was discontinued after inadequate trials, or for "side effects" not characteristic of that therapy, with decisions made without adequate evidence or advice. In rheumatic diseases the outcome of a treatment strategy becomes clear after many months or years. It follows that the chosen strategies must be followed consistently over time, with ongoing quantitative monitoring of markers of success, failure, or toxicity, with an information system understood and available to all members of the treatment team, especially including the patient. Compliance is so important, that the patient should be given both full information and a high level of responsibility.

Each treatment plan is a miniature therapeutic trial, presenting difficulties comparable to those arising in controlled studies of new drugs. From these we learn the need to define in advance the duration and objectives of the trial period, and to choose numerical measures of treatment effect. These permit subsequent decisions to be made on the basis of a quantitative evaluation of progress.

Measures of Inflammatory Activity

A study by the Cooperating Clinics Committee of the American Rheumatism Association (ARA) identified four measures of special value in measuring activity of rheumatoid arthritis,[2] and their scheme has been used in a large number of published studies.

- duration of morning stiffness, minutes ____
- grip strength, mm Hg R____/20
  L____/20
- number of active joints ____
- sedimentation rate, mm/hr ____

An important additional measure used in recent studies asks the patient to score their symptoms as a mark on a line, 10 cm long, anchored at the ends as "none" or "worst possible"—the Visual Analogue Scale (VAS). Measuring marks on a line with a millimeter rule can be tedious, and comparable results can be obtained by asking patients to put a number to their symptoms, on a 0–10 scale, with 10 being the worst possible.

Other measures have been proposed, some of which may become standard.[3] These include disability and quality of life questionnaires, such as the Health Assessment Questionnaire (HAQ),[4] the Arthritis Impact Scale, second version (AIMS2)[5] (see Appendix III), and patient's and observer's global assessments. There are also ongoing studies about the strategies for combining multiple individual measures into a single summary measure of severity or treatment outcome.[6]

Specific Clinical Techniques

Pain, Stiffness, and Duration of Morning Stiffness

To avoid leading questions, ask "How do you feel when you first get up—is that a good time or a bad time?" "Was this morning typical of the last week?" (If this morning was very unusual, settle for typical or average experience in the past week.) "What time did you get out of bed?" "Five minutes later, what were your symptoms?" Avoid leading questions if possible; but if necessary, specifically ask about pain, stiffness, and fatigue, and score on a 0–10 scale. For duration of morning stiffness, ask "At what time did the stiffness ease?"

Grip Strength

Roll your blood pressure cuff loosely (so that your index finger can fit inside) into a cylinder about 6 cm (2.5 inches) in diameter, and secure with two broad rubber bands, 7 × 1 cm. Inflate the system to 100 mm Hg, then deflate to 20 mm Hg (Fig. 8-1*A*). Encourage the patient to squeeze, . . . *hard!*, and record the highest level reached and maintained for 3 seconds. (For greater sensitivity and reproducibility, the bladder is removed from the cuff and sewn permanently into a special bag 14 × 9 cm, Fig. 8-1*B*). The modified blood pressure cuff also is an excellent device for measuring strength of any muscle (see later under "Functional Assessment"). A 20-mm Hg rise in pressure is about equal to 2 kg of force on the bag; about 5 lb.

The absolute level of grip strength may be affected by time of day, fitness, deformity, or pain of any origin, so that a single measure of grip strength is not a specific measure of inflammation. *Change* in grip strength, however, is quite sensitive to treatment effects.

Actively Inflamed Joints

Active joint inflammation is deemed to be present if *any* of the following three signs are present:

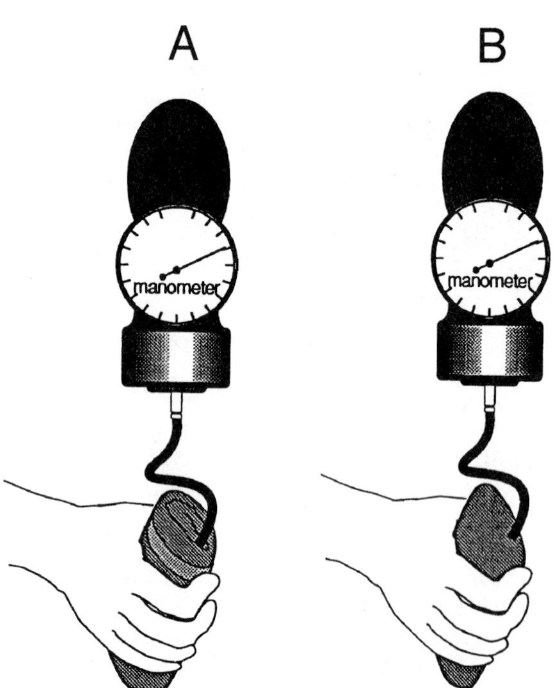

Figure 8-1. *A*, Grip strength using a rolled cuff. *B*, Grip strength using a sewn bag. (Copyright H. Smythe, MD, FRCP[C].)

effusion, tenderness, or **stress pain**. It is often helpful to diagram the distribution of active joints as in Figure 8-2, and to count the total number. Rubber stamps or printed formats are available for the more elegant drawing, but the stick figure gives equal information. In reviewing charts over time, the visual display gives more key information than long written accounts.

In other schemes, joints are given scores weighted according to their size or the severity of the inflammation, but the gain in sensitivity in weighted joint counts is offset by greater interobserver variation. Just as important is the ability to communicate information. A statement that there are 15 actively inflamed joints is easily understood, but few can decipher the meaning of a "Lansbury index[7] of 56." The presence of excess joint fluid is so central to the recognition of inflammatory disease, that effusions are often counted separately.

Synovial Effusions

The most reliable general sign is the demonstration of *fluctuation*, an increase of fluid pressure produced by force in one direction that is transmitted equally in all directions (the hydraulic effect). Fluid moves. If you wish to palpate the back of a joint, passively move it into extension, tightening the anterior capsule and forcing the fluid into the area to be examined (or punctured). Fig-

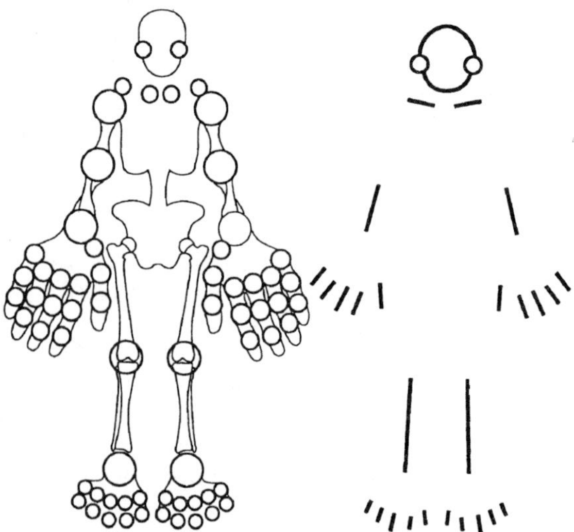

Figure 8-2. Distribution of active joints. Provides a visual format for recording data on active joints. (Copyright H. Smythe, MD, FRCP[C].)

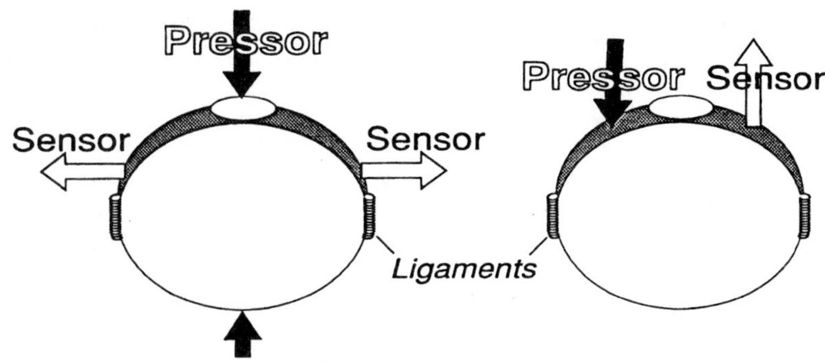

Figure 8-3. Two ways of detecting joint effusions. (Copyright H. Smythe, MD, FRCP[C].)

ure 8-3, left, illustrates the **four-finger technique** to detect fluid in an interphalangeal joint. It is relatively easy to learn, but applicable only when the joint can be surrounded. The placement of the examiner's "sensor" fingers is critical. The collateral ligaments are outside the synovium, and prevent the fluid from bulging. The "sensors" must be dorsal to the ligaments and proximal to the base of the middle phalanx (Fig. 8-4).

For most joints, the examiner must use the **two-finger technique** (Fig. 8-3, right), one pressing downward, the other feeling the upward lift. These techniques can be practiced on a fresh but well-massaged grape. The push of the pressor finger should be directed slightly away from the sensor finger, to prevent a shift of periarticular fat giving a false impression of a fluid lift. Score as normal unless there is thoroughly convincing evidence of fluid. Expressions such as "boggy" swelling, or "soft tissue" swelling, indicate only uncertainty, provided perhaps by a lack of skill and an excess of fat. When fat is deposited about joints, its distribution may mimic an effusion; being fluid at body temperature, fat may fluctuate. If subcutaneous, it can be pinched up to establish that it is superficial to deep fascia. Muscle bellies also will fluctuate across the long axis of the fibers, but not parallel with them.

The **bulge** sign is a sensitive and dramatic indication of a small effusion. In the knee joint, the pouch of synovium medial to the patella is emptied of fluid by a gentle upward stroke, and refilled by an upward or downward stroke on the lateral side. A similar sudden bulge can be seen over the radial head when the elbow is gently moved from midflexion to full extension.

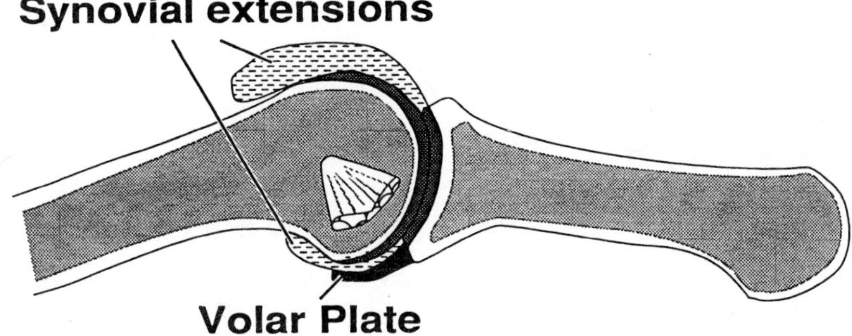

Figure 8-4. Anatomy of MCP or MTP joint. Only the origin of the collateral ligament is indicated, the insertion is into the volar plate and the phalanx. (Copyright H. Smythe, MD, FRCP[C].)

The most reliable general sign of synovial effusion is the demonstration of *fluctuation*.

Specific Joint Tenderness

When studying articular or nonarticular tenderness, it is extremely important to work at "threshold" levels. Unlike the bulge of fluid, tenderness is usually **most marked under the collateral ligaments**. Patients with pain syndromes also may report tenderness of their joints elsewhere; so be sure to control for this. There must be distinctly more tenderness on direct pressure over the joint line, and less tenderness with firmer pressure on bone adjacent to the joints. These techniques are especially useful in the wrist, finger, and toe joints.

Stress Pain

Stress pain is produced when a joint at the limit of its range of movement is nudged a little further. This is especially useful in the shoulder (limit of medial and lateral rotation), wrists, metacarpophalangeal (MCP) joints, and joints in the ankle region. (NOTE: Pain *during* the arc of movement may be due to bare bone rubbing on bare bone [due to loss of articular cartilage]; it is not a reliable sign of inflammation.)

How hard should you press to test for tenderness or stress pain? Determine the patient's general level of tenderness by squeezing the triceps and the lower calf muscles, and by pressing over the manubrium, metacarpals, and proximal phalanges. The pressure used on joints should be about 20% less than that reaching pain threshold elsewhere. When in doubt, record as inactive. The risks of overcounting are greater than undercounting, as error may lead to overdiagnosis, overtreatment, and unnecessary complications.

The ARA joint count includes a brilliant simplification that permits essential information to be gathered in a few minutes. The wrists and ankles include many separate synovial spaces, but are treated as one. The neck and hips are not indicated at all, because it requires skill and time to determine if pain in these regions is truly inflammatory in origin. Simpler schemes with even fewer joints have been used.

Relative Severity

In the ARA Cooperating Clinics Committee study,[2] four measures of inflammatory activity were assessed in 499 patients with peripheral rheumatoid arthritis. For each measure, the findings were divided in ten grades of relative severity as shown in Table 8-3. A typical patient had about 90 minutes of morning stiffness, a grip strength of about 120 mm Hg, 15 active joints, and an erythrocyte sedimentation rate (ESR) of about 45 mm/hr. Patients with mild disease had values in the first few col-

Table 8-3. ARA Cooperating Clinics Committee Study of Inflammatory Measures*

	Percentile Grade Limits								
Measures of Inflammation†	**10**	**20**	**30**	**40**	**50**	**60**	**70**	**80**	**90**
Morning stiffness, minutes	5	30	60	75	90	120	160	220	300
Grip strength, mm Hg									
Males	250	190	160	140	125	105	90	75	55
Females	190	150	130	110	100	85	75	60	50
Number of active joints	4	6	9	12	15	20	25	30	36
Sedimentation rate	10	20	28	35	40	50	60	70	90

*Data from The Cooperating Clinics Committee of the American Rheumatism Association: A seven-day variability study of 499 patients with peripheral rheumatoid arthritis. Arthritis Rheum 1965; 8:302–335.

†A typical RA patient would fall in the 50th percentile and would have morning stiffness of 90 minutes, grip strength of 125 if male or 100 if female, 15 active joints, and a sedimentation rate of 40. Similarly, a severely involved patient would fall in the 80th percentile with morning stiffness of 220, grip strength of 75 if male and 60 if female, 30 active joints, and a sedimentation rate of 70.

umns, and those with very active arthritis would fit in the right side of the table.

The observations were repeated on the same patients one week later, without treatment change. While variation of a measure into adjacent grades was common (~30%), change of more than two grades or more occurred uncommonly (~5% of cases). Thus, if major changes are observed, these likely reflect real changes in the patient's condition and not chance variation.

Composite Indices

The relative severity indicated by any one measure rarely agrees exactly with others (or else, only one would be needed). In older patients, for example, the ESR tends to be high, and may be insensitive to a changing clinical state. Grip strength is one of the most repeatable and sensitive measures, but may be affected markedly by age and established deformities. Schemes have been evolved to combine separate observations into a single numerical index. Lansbury described an Articular Index,[7] which gave extra weight to large or more severely involved joints, and an Activity Index[7] combining this with grip strength, morning stiffness, sedimentation rate, duration to fatigue, and acetylsalicylic need. Goldsmith and others have described a Pooled Index,[8] in which the various measures were standardized to a common scale of standard deviation units. The Pooled Index (and other indices of inflammation) is commonly used in clinical trials, and has been shown to be responsive to treatment effects.[8]

Destruction and Deformity in Inflammatory Joint Disease

Patterns of Damage

Stiffening may be the outstanding feature of damage. Stiffening results from intra-articular adhesions in the synovial extensions (see Fig. 8-4) and deep to the collateral ligaments, or from adhesion of surrounding tendons and ligaments to a thickened capsule. Ultimately, this stiffening may progress to a bland, painless bony fusion. The first sign will be loss of range of motion, which urgently *must* be treated aggressively. This may seem more characteristic of aging, but it is a severe threat in juvenile-onset arthritis. Damage also may result in instability or **loosening**. Destruction of supporting structures may allow displacement of controlling tendons, and joint structures. Finally, loss of articular cartilage will leave bare bone, with characteristic **bone-on-bone crepitus**, which must be distinguished from crepitus due to synovial villi or loose fragments, or the benign clicks produced by ligaments or bones (such as the patella) when these slip over the mismatched curves of underlying joint surfaces.

The **mechanisms of damage** vary, affected by the anatomy and function unique to each joint. To produce **angular deformities**, there must be a *deforming force*, and *damage to a supporting structure*. For ulnar deviation at the MCP joints to occur, radial collateral ligaments must be attenuated or destroyed by the inflammatory process, which is most aggressive between collateral ligaments and bone. The pull of flexor tendons is the deforming force, and the angular deformity progresses more rapidly if the flexor or extensor tendons are themselves displaced by damage to *their* supporting ligaments.

In the MCP joints of the hands, the structures attached to the volar plate determine the patterns of deformity. The volar plate is a fibrocartilaginous extension of the articular surface of the base of the proximal phalanx (see Fig. 8-4), to which it is firmly attached. The flexor tendon is held close to the volar plate by the tendon sheath, thickened here to form a pulley or sling ligament. With flexion grip, the palmar pull of the flexor tendon is transmitted through the volar plate to the collateral ligaments. When these stretch, the base of the proximal phalanx is displaced in a palmar direction. The angle of pull of the second tendon means that this deforming force falls most on the radial collateral ligament. If the sling ligament stretches, the tendon is pulled to the ulnar side of the joint. Superficial to the collateral ligaments are the transverse fibers of the extensor hood, also anchored to the volar plate. These keep the extensor tendon centered over the center of the dorsal aspect of the joint and, if damaged, also allow ulnar subluxation of the extensor tendons. The displaced flexor and extensor tendons now are powerful ulnar deviators.[9] In the fifth finger, the ulnar pull of the short flexors in the hypothenar eminence overpower the weak radial pull of the long flexor.

In the metatarsophalangeal (MTP) joints of the feet, displacement of the flexor tendons from under the metatarsal heads permits the unopposed extensors to pull the proximal phalanx into hyperextension. The unsupported metatarsal heads prolapse, cutting through the protective fatty-fibrous pad and, eventually, the skin. Calluses form to prevent skin penetration, and *should not be pared.* Orthoses at this stage will not correct the tendon displacement; the ideal time for carefully fitted metatarsal mounds was much earlier.

In addition to inflammation, **shear instability** in joints produces rapid loss of articular cartilage. Severe crushing forces develop in joints that are **locked**, because of capsular adhesions, or because they are loaded at the limit of their normal range of travel.

Quantifying Damage

Joint destruction may be assessed clinically or radiologically. In evaluating rheumatoid damage, osteoarthritic changes in the terminal interphalangeal (IP) joints, fifth proximal interphalangeal (PIP), first carpometacarpal (CMC), and first MTP joints are ignored. No simple method of describing these often complicated changes has yet achieved international acceptance. For clinical use, we recommend a simple count of damaged joints, applying to this problem the same technique we have used for quantifying inflamed joints. On a skeleton diagram (see Fig. 8-2), record signs of damage such as loss of range, lax collaterals, bone or tendon subluxation, malalignment, metatarsal prolapse, hammer toes, or bone-on-bone crepitus. Such crepitus must be distinguished from the snapping sensations that occur when some normal joints move under load, as the contours of the bony components rarely match, and from the localized fine painless crepitus of deteriorating cartilage, or the villous crepitus of hypertrophied synovium. Bony crepitus is hard, may cause sudden pain, and may be felt well away from the joint line.

Damage-Duration Index

The number of "damaged" joints is related to the duration of the disease and its aggressiveness. The count of "damaged" joints is divided by the disease duration in years, giving an index of the rate of destruction. Obviously, a patient with ten damaged joints after only 2 years of disease (damaged-duration index = 5) is much more threatened than a patient with ten damaged joints after 40 years of disease (damage-duration index = 0.25). These two examples illustrate the extreme values seen in clinical studies. A median value for the index is about 0.75.

The number of "damaged" joints is related to the duration of the disease and its aggressiveness.

Use of These Measures in Prognosis and as a Guide to Treatment

The disease may run a benign, malignant, or intermediate course, requiring different approaches to treatment and follow-up. Guides to prognosis are needed that can be determined early in the course of the disease. Age and sex have relatively little predictive value. An abrupt, severe onset, forcing the patient to bed within weeks of the onset, paradoxically suggests a rather favorable course. The following factors are of some value and may indicate a more unfavorable outlook:

- rapid accumulation of damage to date, assessed clinically or radiologically
- presence of extra-articular features, such as nodules or nailfold infarcts
- a psychologically adverse passive reaction to disease, particularly when symptoms are used to manipulate family or health care workers
- high levels of rheumatoid factor

Extra-articular Features

Each family of arthropathies has its own pattern of extra-articular features. In rheumatoid disease, look for tendon sheath involvement, tendon nodules, subluxation, or rupture. As well, look for other nodular sites, Raynaud's phenomenon, nailfold infarcts (appearing like dark slivers about the base of the nails), peripheral neuropathy, palmar erythema, leg ulcers, all indicative of vasculopathy. Dry or inflamed eyes, pleural pain, or lung fibrosis can occur. Check for anemia clinically (compare pallor of the palm with your own, check the nailbed and look inside the eyelid), or by reviewing the hemoglobin levels in relevant reports.

In ankylosing spondylitis or Reiter's syndrome, inquire about urethritis, colitis, and examine for conjunctivitis, iritis, skin and mucosal lesions, and enthesitis (tender spurs) at the heel or elsewhere. Figure 8-5 provides a polyarthritis assessment form for clinical use.

POLYARTHRITIS ASSESSMENT

Patient's Name________________________ Age______ Assessment Date __________

Inflammatory Activity

Duration of morning stiffness, hours ________
Grip strength, mm. of Hg. Right ________/20
Left ________/20
Number of active joints ________
Sedimentation Rate ________

Joint Pain Now (Circle number):

No Pain: 0 — 1 — 2 — 3 — 4 — 5 — 6 — 7 — 8 — 9 — 10 : *Worst possible*

Damaged Joints: Include lax collaterals, subluxation, bone on bone crepitus, malalignment, loss of more than 20 % of normal passive range of motion. Exclude Heberden's nodes.

Extra-Articular Features

Nodules
Eye
Vasculitis
Other (Specify) ______________________________
____

Active Joints

Number active ______

Damaged Joints

Number damaged ______

"FIBROMYALGIC" POINT COUNT

Point Count

	Right	Left
Occiput		
Trapezius		
Supraspinatus		
Low neck		
2nd rib		
Inner knee		
Outer elbow		
Gluteus		
Trochanter		

Total (of 18) ________

Problem List ______________________________
____
____
____

Functional Class

Extend to one decimal place. Best possible score is 1.0, worst is 4.9. Class:__________

1. COMPLETE ability to carry on all usual duties without handicaps.
2. ADEQUATE FOR NORMAL ACTIVITIES despite handicap of discomfort or limited motion.
3. LIMITED only to little or none of duties of usual occupation or self-care.
4. INCAPACITATED. Bedridden or confined to a wheelchair; little or no self-care.

Observer: ______________________________

Figure 8-5. Polyarthritis Assessment Form. (Copyright H. Smythe, MD, FRCP[C].)

Functional Assessments

Joint Range

Gently assess full passive range of movement (ROM) with the patient fully relaxed, and usually supine, to remove restrictions due to action of antigravity muscles. Be sensitive to hypermobility as well as stiffness. Record range in degrees, using the anatomical position, palms forward, as the starting point. A fully extended knee is at 0 degrees, not 180 degrees. Avoid ambiguous minus signs; is a knee at −15 degrees hyperextended, or demonstrating a loss of full extension? Use 15 degrees E or F instead. **Active range** can be used in a 1-minute assessment of a well patient with no skeletal symptoms.

Muscle Strength

Measure with the modified blood pressure cuff (Fig. 8-6). The 0–5 scale of muscle strength is of no use in musculoskeletal disease. Virtually all patients can move against gravity, but are somewhat weak. So all would be scored 4, with no way of measuring change. The manometer method is safe, cheap, portable, and can be quickly adapted to any muscle group, independent of gravity.[10–12] The cuff is placed distally as far as possible, without crossing a (possibly painful) joint. Pressure is applied with a flat hand, not gripping the cuff. The examiner increases pressure over a period of about 5 seconds, and records the highest force the patient can sustain.

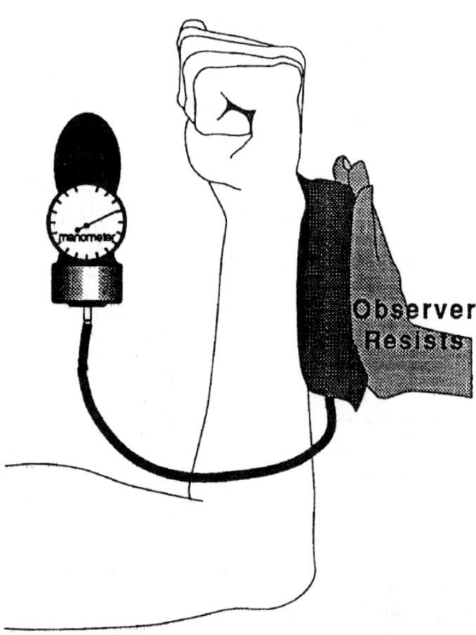

Figure 8-6. Use of modified blood pressure cuff to measure isometric triceps strength. (Copyright H. Smythe, MD, FRCP[C].)

Activities of Daily Living (ADL)

Dimensions of Function

- mobility
- self care—eating, dressing, washing, grooming, use of toilet
- hand functions—door handles, keys, coins, jar tops, carrying, pen, scissors
- work/play activities—work outside home, light and heavy work in house, hobbies, sports

Questionnaire measures of the total impact of disease, such as the HAQ[4] and AIMS[5] have become accepted as standard outcome measures, sensitive to meaningful change, and relevant to the patient's concerns. They are of particular use when the information is gathered for entry into a computer-based study, as in a therapeutic trial or an epidemiological study. More information can be gathered more quickly about the needs of an individual patient by thoughtful, less rigidly structured inquiry.

ARA Functional Class

1. Normal function without or despite symptoms
2. Some disability, but function is adequate for normal activity without special devices or assistance
3. Restricted activities, and special devices or personal assistance are required
4. Totally dependent

This scheme has too few grades to be of use in therapeutic trials or in assessing progress, and works better if a decimal place is used to indicate variation within the classes. Thus a "good 2" might be scored as 2.2, and a "bad 2" as 2.9.

Narrative Description

Narrative description emphasizes recent changes in ability to perform specific functions. Define reasons for loss of function (i.e., pain, stiffness, weakness, instability, fatigability) or any of these increasing with duration of activity.

Exaggerated Pain Behavior and Disability Assessment

Health professionals are increasingly asked by third parties to make judgments about disability that can be difficult if the complaints seem to be out of proportion to evidence of disease, or if there are words or actions that seem inappropriately dramatic. Given the rise in costs associated with disability awards over the past decade, it is evident that these assessments are an important responsibility, and that we do not do them well. Signs of "exaggerated" pain behavior have been described,[13] but not validated, not informed by knowledge of referred pain patterns, and not sensitive to cultural effects that may affect the observer and the client. An early well-designed study on pain behavior[14] did not assume that pain behavior is necessarily abnormal. In a study of patients with fibromyalgia, markers of pain behavior did not predict treatment outcome.[15] We have found (unpublished data) that quantitative scoring of a list of adjectives describing the patient's reactions to examination to be a valuable assistance to blinded observers asked to judge whether volunteer patients were giving honest responses, or exaggerating their tenderness in a modest way. These adjectives are included in the format for recording findings on the assessment of spinal disease at the end of this chapter.

Pain Amplification Syndromes

There is increasing interest in the specific neural mechanisms that modulate the response to painful stimuli. Endorphins ease pain and substance P is involved in pain mediation, but there remains inadequate knowledge of the neurobiochemical mechanisms by which pain is increased. Many pain amplification syndromes can be recognized. Though not inflammatory in nature, all can occur in patients with RA, enormously complicating assessment and treatment. These include:

- referred pain syndromes
- the "fibromyalgia" syndrome
- reflex dystrophy syndromes
- the painful shins of steroid therapy
- narcotic withdrawal pain

The "Fibromyalgia" Syndrome

The commonest and best studied of these syndromes is now termed fibromyalgia (FM), formerly "fibrositis." Arising from major studies over two decades, new, internationally recognized criteria for the diagnosis of fibromyalgia have emerged.[16] The combination of **widespread pain** and **tenderness at 11 or more of 18 defined *bilateral* sites** (Fig. 8-7) yielded sensitivity of 88% (88% of patients preselected with this diagnosis met these criteria) and specificity of 81% (meaning that 19% of patients with other pain syndromes met these criteria). The statistical power of the criteria came from the addition of the disciplined tender point count. Think of it: "fibromyalgia" translates as widespread pain, and "fibrositis" as points of tenderness.

The primary purpose of these criteria was to define groups of patients for research studies. They are only a guide to diagnosis and assessment of severity. Symptoms of fatigue, headache, and sensitivity to a variety of stimuli in the external and internal environment were common, and are important in the clinical assessment.

The **pathogenesis** of these features also can be summarized simply. The *location* of the pain and the different locations of the tender points are determined by the patterns of referred pain associated with mechanical problems in the spine. **Upper body tender points relate to mechanical problems**

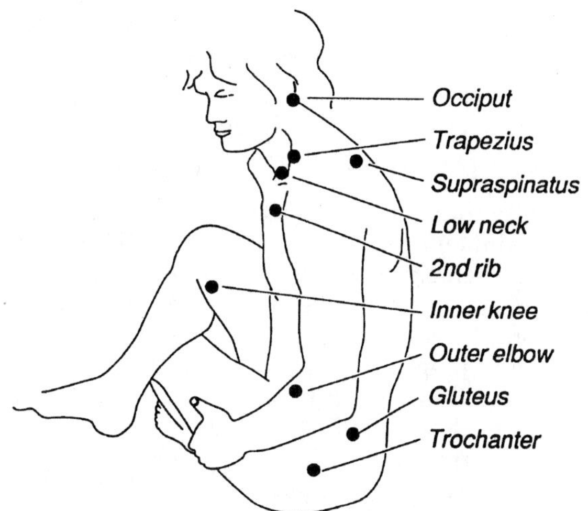

Figure 8-7. The tender points in the ACR criteria set; possible total of 18 points bilaterally.

in the neck, and lower body points to problems in the low back. The *severity* of the pain and the presence of the accompanying symptoms are further influenced by **amplifying factors**, such as sleep disturbance and physical deconditioning.

It follows that diagnosis depends on the understanding that nonarticular pain, "numbness," or "swelling" may often be due to **referred pain mechanisms**. Assessment of such patients requires a systematic examination for characteristic patterns of unexpected tenderness and nontenderness, and a knowledgeable search for the sources of referred pain. The most commonly overlooked relevant findings are marked tenderness in the low anterior neck, and great difficulty in performing a sit-up due to profound abdominal muscle weakness.

In the patient with RA, concomitant fibromyalgia often leads to serious overestimation of the amount of inflammatory activity. The patient with FM and concomitant RA (or other joint disease) may describe point pain, stiffness, fatigue, and even "swelling." When joint effusions cannot be demonstrated, it must be recognized that these symptoms *may* reflect the FM rather than uncontrolled inflammation and require totally different treatment strategies (see Chapter 5).

Assessment of Spinal Disease

Health professionals continue to manage spinal disorders poorly. The approach presented here is a supplement to standard approaches. In what structures does the patient's pain originate? What is the nature of the pathology? How much investigation is appropriate for the patient?

Referred Pain: Why is it So Hard to Diagnose?

Diagnosis of the nature and site of origin of deep pain is difficult because the involved structures are not represented in the brain (Fig. 8-8) or in our body image. If a finger is hurt, the pain is felt in a fraction of a second, localized to within millimeters, and the quality of the injury is recognized as sharp, burning, or crushing. None of this is true of pain of deep origin. Deep pain is referred; that is, misinterpreted as arising in tissues other than its site of origin, especially to muscles and bony prominences, usually sharing the same segmental nerve supply. Awareness of the injury may be **delayed** for hours, or days, and the **quality** of the distress may vary from aching, to burning, "swelling," or "numbness," according to the region to which it is referred.

Secondary reflex changes often develop, which may be thought of as protective in intent. Hyperalgesia may develop, often more pronounced in deep structures than in skin, with local points of referred deep tenderness. Circulation may increase. Muscles tend to splint the part, but voluntary muscle action is inhibited. All these signs can lead to an erroneous diagnosis of injury in the area of reference, and the deep, central primary pathology may be overlooked. As a rule, pain is referred distally rather than proximally. A knowledge of the common patterns of pain reference can be quickly gained and the search for the primary site of pathology may be challenging but is usually rewarding.

Regional Tenderness

Exactly the same sites become tender in regional pain syndromes associated with spinal problems, as in the general pain syndrome of fibromyalgia. Lateral elbow pain, aggravated by use, may be called "tennis elbow." Dissatisfaction with simple therapies may lead to closer evaluation. It is found that the tenderness is not at the lateral epicondyle, but about 5 cm distally, in the origin of the extensor muscle to the long finger from the lateral intermuscular septum, close to and rotating with the radius (Fig. 8-9). The marked and sharply localized tenderness still suggests local pathology, but further examination reveals equally marked, unsuspected sites of tenderness at other characteristic sites (Fig. 8-10), much more marked on the symptomatic side, and unassociated with lower body pain or tenderness. The lateral elbow tenderness and nearby pain is part of a referred pain syndrome.

Full examination for referred pain patterns of tenderness is essential for correct diagnosis and effective treatment of "overuse" syndromes.

Overuse Syndromes

The pain may not be restricted to the elbow but extend distally, associated with a sense of numbness or tingling in the hand, strange in that it is often mixed with pain. If the texture of cloth can still be recognized, despite the "numb" feeling,

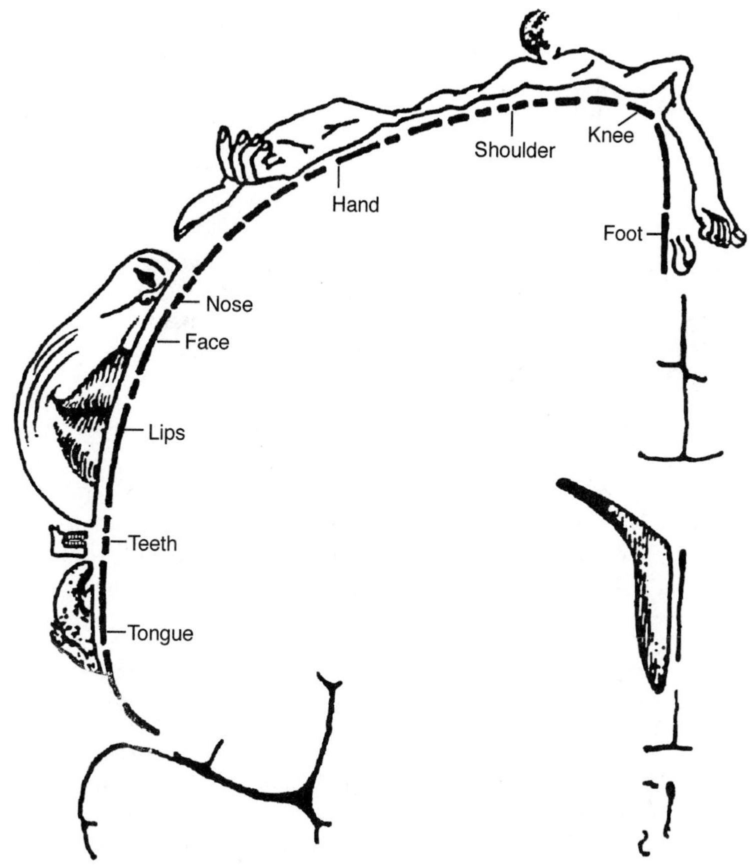

Figure 8-8. The sensory cortex: The hands and feet are represented, but deep structures are not. (Adapted from Penfield W, Rasmussen T: The Cerebral Cortex of Man, p 214. New York, Macmillan, 1955.)

nerve compression is very unlikely. The symptoms disturb sleep, and also are aggravated by use, at work or at play. Two (or more) factors are at work. Loads on the arms are equally loads on the neck. In addition, the pull of a muscle on its very tender origin by the elbow is the mechanical equivalent of the pressure of the examiner's finger—it hurts. Full examination for referred pain patterns of tenderness is essential for correct diagnosis and effective treatment of these syndromes.

Symptom Patterns

Mechanical Lesions

Mechanical lesions include chronic strain, disk disease, apophyseal joint osteoarthritis, spondylolysis, and spondylolisthesis. The commonest problems are mechanical in origin; begin abruptly; and improve quickly with a brief period of rest, analgesic (*not* anti-inflammatory) therapy, and early mobilization. If recovery is delayed or interrupted by recurrences, identification of continuing pathogenetic forces may be the key to therapy. Nearly all of the mechanical problems affect either the lower cervical spine, or the two lowest lumbar spaces, and these two areas will eventually cause symptoms in virtually every member of the population. Why? The lower lumbar spine is locked at the extreme range of hyperextension in virtually everyone with low back pain problems, and close to the extreme range in all of us. The lower neck is vulnerable for a variety of reasons, of which the most important and neglected are compressive and shearing stresses arising during sleep.

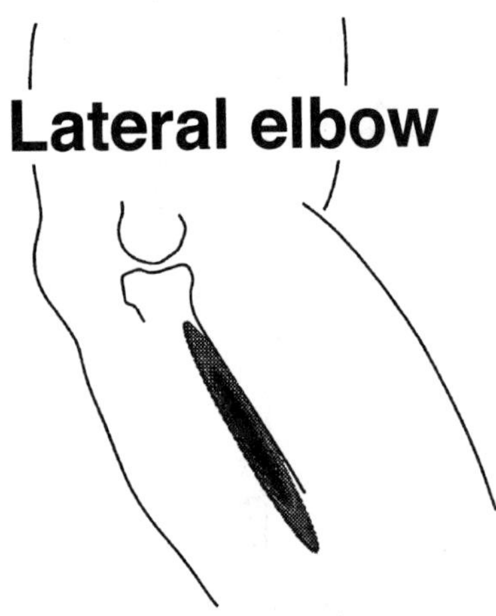

Figure 8-9. The "tennis elbow" site, 3–6 cm from the epicondyle, in the extensor muscle to the middle finger, rotating with the radius. (Copyright H. Smythe, MD, FRCP[C].)

Inflammatory Back Pain

Ankylosing Spondylitis

Ankylosing spondylitis affects just under 1% of all males, and may constitute 2–5% of young men with back pain. Aggressive anti-inflammatory treatment can prevent damage, so early recognition is both difficult and important. Radiologic changes in the sacroiliac joints may be delayed, so that diagnosis may depend on recognition of characteristic symptoms and signs. Involvement of the low lumbar spine is not common in the early stages, so midline lumbosacral pain is uncommon. Buttock pain of insidious onset, with night pain, and morning pain and stiffness eased with exercise are characteristic. Midlumbar paravertebral pain, arising at the thoracolumbar junction and aggravated by turning during sleep, is often the next symptom, and is uncommon in mechanical problems. Precipitation by gastrointestinal or genitourinary infection, heel pain, lower limb arthritis, ocular inflammation, painless mucosal lesions, or a family history may make the diagnosis easy. Physical findings will be discussed later.

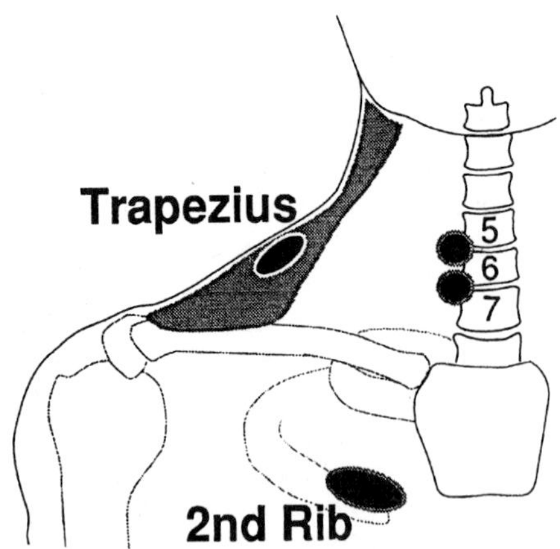

Figure 8-10. Neck and referred points. (Copyright H. Smythe, MD, FRCP[C].)

Spinal Osteomyelitis, Discitis, or Tumor

These are much less common, but difficult though essential to diagnose. Only occasionally is infection linked with clear evidence of systemic sepsis. Often the onset is insidious. As in spondylitis, night pain is common, and the thoracolumbar junction is a favored site, missed in routine spine films, as the lesions may be too low to be seen in the thoracic films, too high for the lumbar films. Pain and tenderness at sites other than low cervical and low lumbar spine lead to appropriate diagnostic investigations.

Polymyalgic Syndromes

Widespread pain, not clearly restricted to swollen or damaged joints, may occur in fibromyalgia, polymyalgia rheumatica, viral or other infection ("influenza"), autoimmune disease, or tumor. The differential diagnosis is as broad as fever of unknown origin.

Important Other Diagnoses

These include osteoporosis and other metabolic bone disease, neurological disorders, and pain referred from viscera. It is, fortunately, unusual for any of these conditions to be primarily located or restricted to the lower cervical spine or lumbosacral angle. Pain and stiffness are often worse during or after rest, and evidence of systemic disease may be present. Pain arising in the midlumbar spine associated with morning stiffness could be due to a mechanical problem, but there is not the overwhelming probability of this diagnosis that would be associated with lumbosacral angle pain, so that the diagnostician must be especially alert. If the anatomical site is wrong, if the pattern of pain does not fit with mechanical aggravation, or if symptoms or signs of other disease are present, beware of missing an important other diagnosis.

Enhanced Pain

Pain amplification syndromes are due to alterations in physiological pain modulation, neurological but not primarily psychological. The most common is the *fibromyalgia syndrome*, readily assessable by the point count. Psychological exaggeration of physical disability for reasons of *secondary gain* also is common and much more difficult to quantify and to separate willful from unconscious components. *Psychogenic regional pain syndromes* include classical hysteria, hallucinatory pain, and others. These are uncommon and typically affect regions with a high emotional significance and a large cortical representation. Under these circumstances, secondary tension and hostility can develop in any normal person.

Red Flags

Most pain syndromes are mechanical in origin and unassociated with nerve root damage or other serious disease. Complex investigations are not warranted and treatment should stress active recovery of function. However, uncommon but serious problems will be seen and must not be missed. Night pain, weight loss, fever sweats, or tenderness in the spine between C7 and L4 are all *red flags*, indicating the need for fuller investigation. Look for:

- evidence of nerve root pressure
- evidence of inflammatory back pain
- evidence of important other diagnoses
- exaggerated pain behavior

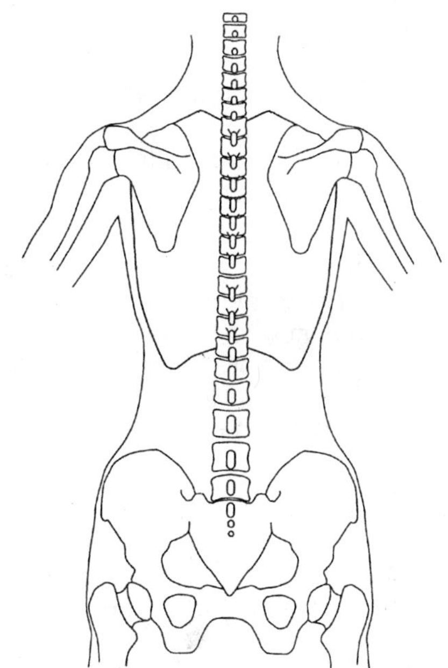

Figure 8-11. Map of the spine to indicate location of spinal pain and tenderness. (Copyright H. Smythe, MD, FRCP[C].)

Techniques of Spinal Examination

Map Pain, Hyperesthesia, Deep Tenderness, and Pain on Movement

Patients should be totally relaxed during this examination. In examination of the spine, a spinal map (Fig. 8-11) may be used to record findings. The position illustrated in Figure 8-12 relaxes tight antigravity muscles and opens lordotic curves to allow better identification of bony landmarks.

Hyperesthesia

Hyperesthesia is more often deep than cutaneous. Begin gently by raising and rolling a skin fold to create traction on the deep fascia. Where this creates pain, deep pressure and movement must be done warily. Reactive reddening of the skin often develops in an area of referred pain and tenderness, and this dermatographia helps document the contribution of reflex factors to a continuing pain syndrome.

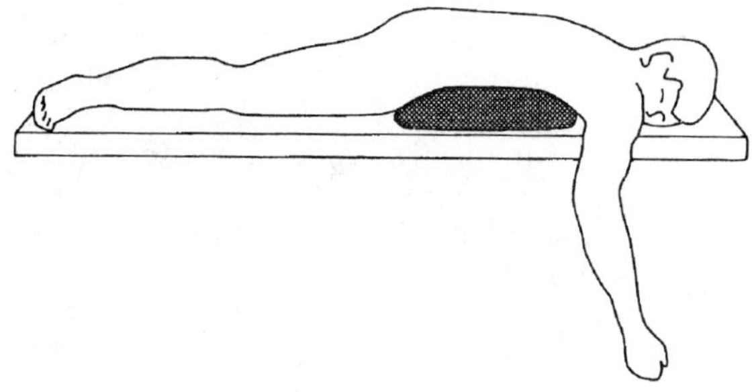

Figure 8-12. Relaxed prone position. A pillow eliminates the lumbar lordosis, and relaxes tight ligaments. (Copyright H. Smythe, MD, FRCP[C].)

Deep Tenderness

Deep tenderness over interspinous ligaments is elicited without moving the deep vertebral structures. It is therefore referred deep tenderness. Once this is appreciated, understanding the nature of other sites of referred deep tenderness is easier.

Pain on Movement

The necessary techniques must be safe, using traction or gliding movements rather than crushing forces. The orientation of the apophyseal joints is different in the cervical, thoracic, and lumbar regions, and determines the direction of movement.

Regional Range of Movement

Measures, such as finger-floor distance, assess overall function of a great number of spinal and extraspinal structures. They are useful in screening, and are sensitive to treatment effects.[17] To identify the anatomical structures involved, the approach must be regional. We wish to determine the maximum range that the condition of the joints permits, and this is achieved with the muscles totally relaxed and the joints not bearing weight. In general, the patient should be lying or otherwise securely supported, and movements carefully assisted by the examiner (i.e., passive range should be recorded). It is not necessary to record every possible movement of every joint. Certain great simplifications can focus and increase rather than sacrifice precision. An assessment of spinal disorder data sheet is attached for recording results, and is largely self-explanatory (Fig. 8-13).

Lateral flexion of the cervical spine cannot occur for anatomical reasons between the skull and C2, so that limited lateral flexion is often the most sensitive indicator of lower cervical pathology. When rotation is restricted, the site of pain or deep tenderness helps indicate whether the pathology is upper or lower cervical. Thoracolumbar rotation is easy to measure badly. The orientation of the apophyseal facets prevents rotation in the lumbar spine, and about half of the total range occurs between T8 and L1. Fix the pelvis by having the patient sit astride the examining table or facing the back of a chair. The shoulder blades get in the way: have the patient place hands on opposite shoulders to move the scapulae laterally, and assist rotation by gentle pressure on the opposite elbow. Don't use the shoulder line as a measure of rotation—movement of the scapulae over the thorax invariably occurs and leads to gross errors. Locate the angles of the ribs at T1, and record range of rotation between T1 and pelvis.

In ankylosing spondylitis, flexion-extension range is first lost at the thoracolumbar junction, and last in the lower lumbar spine. The three 10-cm segment method illustrated later is much more sensitive to the effects of spondylitis than the older Schober techniques.[17]

Stress Pain in Deep Structures

In the lower thoracic spine the most useful technique may be resisted rotation; the examiner's thumb stops rotation at each level in turn while torque is applied to the upper trunk. This technique may be done with the patient prone, or in the sitting position, facing the back of a chair. In this position, long-axis compression may indicate the level of serious bone or disk pathology in the lumbar spine; with the patient prone and totally relaxed, firm quick thrusts on the spinous processes produce anteroposterior movement on each segment in turn and permit very accurate localization.

Tests of Nerve Compression

Limitation of Straight Leg Raising (SLR)

This may occur when excursion of a nerve root is limited as it tightens over a protruding disk, or alternatively because of reflex muscle spasm or apprehension on the part of the patient. The limitations produced by the check-rein effect of root pressure is mechanically consistent; the others will vary under different circumstances.

The *three-phase SLR test* is more informative than the unmodified test. This test, and reflexes, may be hard to assess in the lower limb if the examiner is standing on the contralateral side. If the examination table is hard to move, have the patient switch end for end.

In phase one, gentle elevation of the relaxed, straight limb is continued until stopped by pain; the angle is recorded.

In phase two, the limb is dropped 10–15 degrees until pain is relieved, and only then is the foot sharply dorsiflexed. Discomfort in the calf may be due to stretching of the muscle, but pain in the posterior thigh or back counts as a positive test.

In phase three, this observation is controlled by lowering the limb a further 15 degrees, at which point sharp dorsiflexion of the foot will not cause nerve-root pain, but will still place traction on a

Assessment of Spinal Disorders

Patient's Name______________________________ Age_______ Assessment Date ____________

1. Posture, Spinal Curves and Gait :

Little flexion takes place in the upper thoracic spine, which is curved to accommodate the heart and lungs. The erect posture forces secondary curves in the low cervical and lumbar spine. The neck is resting on T1, which is inclined forward to a greater or lesser degree. Loss of occiput-wall distance often reflects changes in thoracolumbar spine, or even hips.

- cervical
  - — occiput-to-wall distance (neck extended),______ cm.
- thoracic, curve flat or accentuated?
- lumbar
- leg length inequalities
- Gait abnormalities.

1. Spinal Curves

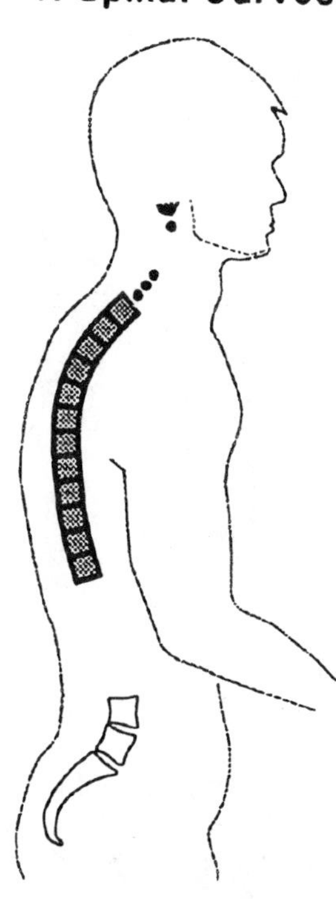

2. Map hyperesthesia, tenderness, pain on motion.

Spinal Pain Now (Circle number):

None: 0 — 1 — 2 — 3 — 4 — 5 — 6 — 7 — 8 — 9 — 10 :*Worst possible*

3. Mobility

			Results	Normal
Cervical	upper	flexion-extension	_______°	90°
	lower	flexion extension	_______°	90°
	(patient	rotation, right	_______°	80°
	supine)	left	_______°	80°
	lateral	right	_______°	> 50°
	flexion	left	_______°	> 50°
Thoracic	chest expansion	infra-mammary	_______	>> 5 cm
	rotation	pelvis to T1	_______°	> 40°

4. Thoracolumbar flexion-extension

In the Schober test, marks are made over the S1 spine and 10 cm higher, with the subject standing. The distance between the 2 marks is remeasured after full flexion, and normally increases by 5 cm.

The 10 cm segment test, has proved more sensitive in measuring losses due to age or disease. Changes of >2.5 cm occur normally in the upper 2 segments, >3 cm in the lowest.

MARK in Flexion

30 cm

20 cm

10 cm

S1 = 0

REMEASURE in Extension

Results:

(mark change, cm)

Upper _________

Mid _________

Lower _________

2. Pain Diagram

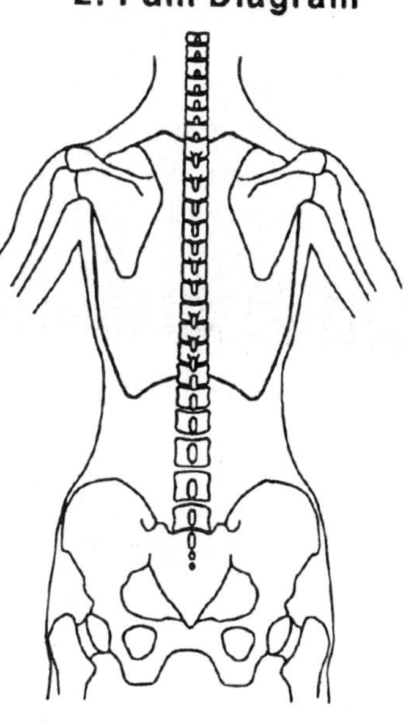

Figure 8-13. Spinal disorders assessment form. (Courtesy of H. Smythe, MD, FRCP[C].) *Illustration continued on following page*

5. Restricted Range

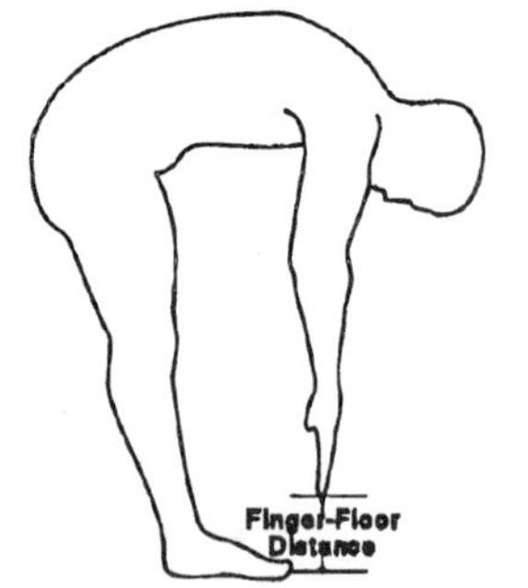

Finger-floor distance, ______cm

7. Three Phase Straight Leg Raising

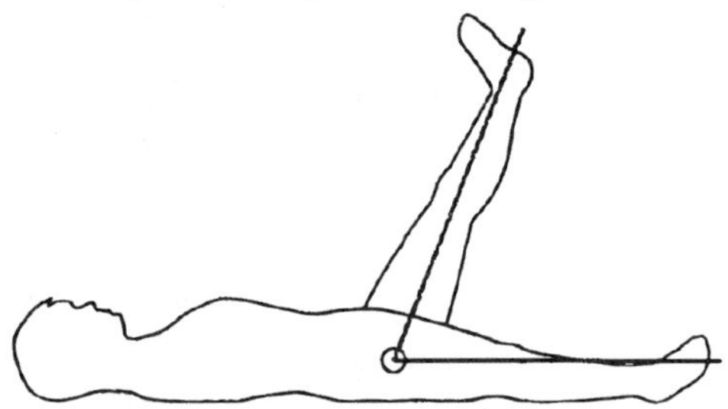

Phase one: Mark location of any pain.
Right _____° Left _____°
Phase two, drop 15° dorsiflex foot.
Pain? Right _____° Left _____°
Phase three; drop another 15°, dorsiflex foot
Pain? Right _____° Left _____°

11. Suck-in Situps

Safety: The exercise must be painless.

The spine must form a smooth, C-shaped curve, with no movement at the belt line. Begin with a strong pelvic tilt, then tilt the head forward until the chin is on the chest. Smoothly bring the elbows to the knees, and lay back pushing the belt line down.

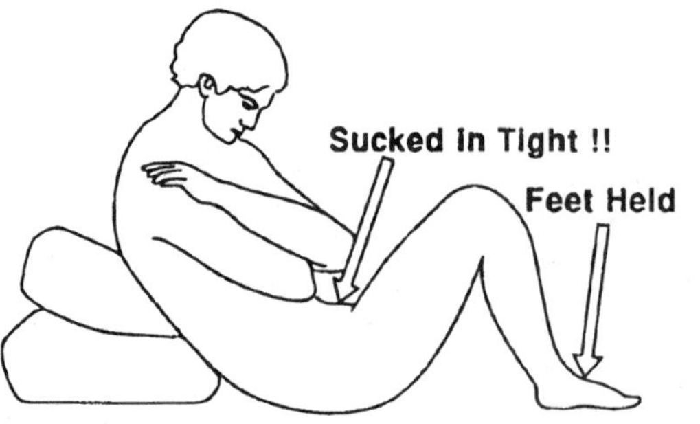

6. Locked Hyperextension

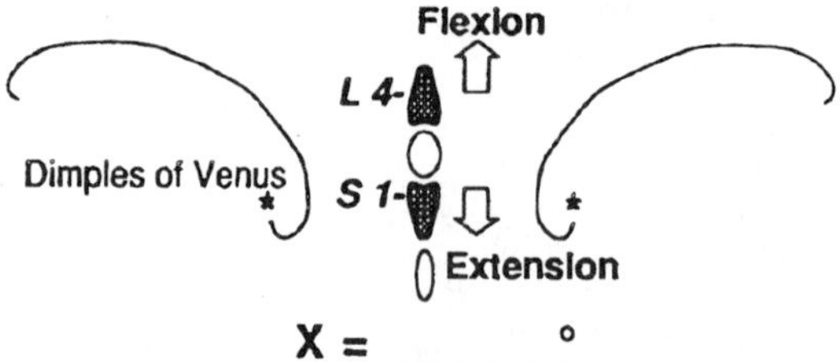

X = ______°

8. Bow-String Sign

Popliteal nerve tenderness

Tender? Right _____ Left _____

9. Reflexes

Score 0 — 4; normal 2.

Site	Right	Left
Knee (L3-4)		
Hamstring (L5)		
Ankle (S1)		

10. Exaggerated Pain Behaviour

(score each 0-4). 1) grimacing __
2) bracing __ 3) sighing __ 4) rubbing __
5) guarding __ 6) leap __ 7) alert, passive, anticipation __ 8) inconsistency __
9) groans __ 10) histrionic __ 11) tremor __
12) Other, score __ and describe.

Situp Scoring Scale:

0. Can't do a sit-up.
1. Needs 2 or more pillows.
2. Flat, arms stretched toward knees.
3. Hands to opposite elbows.
4. Hands to opposite shoulders.
5. Hands behind neck.
6. Arms behind head, fingers touching opposite ears.

Score _______

Observer: ________________________

Figure 8-13. *Continued*

calf tender because of venous thrombosis or rupture of synovial fluid from the knee.

In doubtful cases, mechanical consistency can be further tested by a *three-phase finger-to-floor test*, measured first with the feet together, again with the "involved leg" back, and finally with the "involved leg" forward. In the absence of root pressure, slight improvement usually occurs with each repetition. With root pressure, advancing the "involved leg" (equivalent of SLR) worsens performance. Another modification of SLR can be shared with the patient and used later when there is concern about continuing back pain. The patient sits on the edge of a chair, knees straight, and gently slides the fingertips down the front of the shin. If they can reach within 15 cm of the ankle, continuing nerve root pressure is unlikely.

In the rare instances when only the L3–L4 lumbar roots are involved, SLR will ease rather than aggravate pain, as the femoral nerve trunk passes in front of the hip joint. In the three-phase *femoral stretch* test there is reproduction of pain by passive hyperextension of the hip, relief by slight flexion, and further aggravation by flexion of the knee.

Nerve Trunk Tenderness

Nerve trunk tenderness consistently accompanies nerve root pressure. This is best exemplified by the "bowstring sign," in which the popliteal nerve is found to be sharply more tender than the adjacent hamstring muscles, which are used as a control. In the L3–L4 root syndrome, the femoral nerve will be sharply tender, and in cervical disk disease, the brachial plexus.

Impairment of Nerve Root Function

Impairment of nerve root function must be sought with care. Loss of power must be tested using adequate resistance. Calf power should be tested by having the patient standing on one foot, and asked to rise up on the "toe" ten times. Weakness of dorsiflexion of the foot can be tested with the patient sitting, heels on the ground, when they should be able to support the examiner's full weight, delivered manually. Weakness of dorsiflexion of the big toe may be a more sensitive test of the L5 root damage. Sensory testing is often inconsistent when the patient is apprehensive. The cold edge of a tuning fork may give a more consistent sensory stimulus and thus more consistent results than the most skilfully wielded pin, and the exaggerating patient may report cold while denying heat, equating cold with numbness. Loss of vibration sense is a sensitive test for neuropathy.

Reflex Loss

The most commonly damaged root is L5, so add the medial hamstring reflex to the usual list. If the patient is fully relaxed, reinforcement techniques are rarely necessary. *Record reflexes* on all routine exams, then you can tell if a lost reflex is new or old.

Ongoing Mechanical Factors

The special vulnerability of the lower lumbar spine is due to a posture of extreme hyperextension. Place your index finger and thumb firmly on the L4 and S1 spines with the patient flexed, and feel the movement as the patient rises slowly (Fig. 8-14). At first there is little movement; extension is occurring at the hips. Then the two spines come together until the extreme of hyperextension is reached, after which no further movement in this region occurs. This end point is often reached with the patient's upper trunk still 20 degrees flexed, so record $X = 20$ degrees. Locked lumbar hyperextension is usually due either to postural habit or to weak abdominal muscles, both reversible with some effort. Other less obvious, and less treatable, causes are excessive thoracic curves, and loss of hip extension due to intrinsic hip disease or to tight ligamentous structures anteriorly about the hip, common in obesity, diffuse idiopathic skeletal hyperostosis (DISH), diabetics, or large-boned individuals.

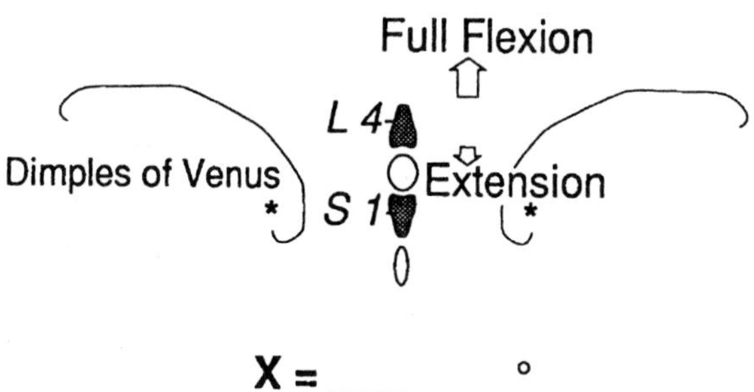

Figure 8-14. Direct assessment of locked lumbar hyperextension. (Copyright H. Smythe, MD, FRCP[C].)

Summary

The quantitative measures of inflammation, damage, and function described in this chapter have been extensively reported in the literature in terms of their validity, reproducibility, and responsiveness. They are an important component of the curricula of graduate medical trainees in rheumatology and of rheumatologically trained physical and occupational therapists, and are part of the undergraduate curricula of these disciplines in certain parts of the United States and Canada. The techniques are intuitive and lend themselves well to communication between specialists and nonspecialists. Since the management of inflammatory arthritis is a team effort, the standardization of these measures of inflammation enhance communication within the treatment team—which always includes the patient—and plays an important role in goal setting and treatment plans.

References

1. Schumacher HR Jr (ed): Primer on the Rheumatic Diseases, 10th edition. Atlanta, Arthritis Foundation, 1993.
2. The Cooperating Clinics Committee of the American Rheumatism Association: A seven-day variability study of 499 patients with peripheral rheumatoid arthritis. Arthritis Rheum 1965; 8:302–335.
3. Felson DT, Anderson JJ, Boers M, et al: The American College of Rheumatology preliminary core set of disease activity measures for rheumatoid arthritis trials. Arthritis Rheum 1993; 36:729–740.
4. Fries JF: Toward an understanding of patient outcome measurement. Arthritis Rheum 1983; 26:697–704.
5. Meenan RF, Mason JH, Anderson JJ, et al: AIMS2: the content and properties of a revised and expanded arthritis impact measurement scales health status questionnaire. Arthritis Rheum 1992; 35:1–10.
6. Conference on outcome measures in rheumatoid arthritis clinical trials. Maastrich, the Netherlands April 29–May 3, 1992. J Rheumatol 1993; 20:525–603.
7. Lansbury J: Methods for evaluating rheumatoid arthritis. In Hollander JL (ed): Arthritis and Allied Conditions, pp 781–845. Philadelphia, Lea & Febiger, 1966.
8. Goldsmith CH, Smythe HA, Helewa A: Interpretation and power of a pooled index. J Rheumatol 1993; 20:575–578.
9. Smith EM, Juvinall RC, Bender LF, et al: Flexor forces and rheumatoid metacarpophalangeal deformity. JAMA 1966; 198:130–134.
10. Helewa A, Goldsmith CH, Smythe HA: The modified sphygmomanometer—an instrument to measure muscle strength: validation study. J Chronic Dis 1981; 34:353–361.
11. Helewa H, Goldsmith CH, Smythe HA: Patient, observer and instrument variation in the measurement of strength of shoulder abductor muscles in patients with rheumatoid arthritis using a modified sphygmomanometer. J Rheumatol 1986; 13:1044–1049.
12. Helewa A, Goldsmith C, Smythe H, et al: An evaluation of four different measures of abdominal muscle strength: patient, order, and instrument variation. J Rheumatol 1990; 17:965–969.
13. Waddell G: Understanding the patient with back pain. In Jayson MIV (ed): The Lumbar Spine and Back Pain, 4th edition, pp 469–485. Edinburgh, Churchill Livingstone, 1992.
14. Richards JS, Nepomuceno C, Riles M, et al: Assessing pain behaviour: the UAB pain behaviour scale. Pain 1982; 14:393–398.
15. Clark S, Burckhardt C, Campbell S, et al: Pain behaviour and treatment outcomes in fibromyalgia patients. Arthritis Rheum 1992; 35:S350.
16. Wolfe F, Smythe HA, Yunus MB, et al: The American College of Rheumatology 1990 criteria for the classification of fibromyalgia; report of the multicentre criteria committee. Arthritis Rheum 1990; 33:160–172.
17. Miller MH, Lee P, Smythe HA, et al: Measurement of spinal mobility in the sagittal plane: new skin contraction technique compared with established methods. J Rheumatol 1984; 11:507–511.

CHAPTER 9

Pharmacology and the Interaction with Physical Therapy

Anne Marie Whelan, BSc(Pharm), PharmD
Joan M. Walker, PhD, PT

Treatment goals and objectives for patients with arthritis may include one or more of the following: (1) reduction of joint pain, (2) reduction of inflammation, (3) preservation of joint function, (4) prevention of disease progression, and (5) maintenance of lifestyle. Goals and objectives will be prioritized depending on the actual disease state and condition of the patient. Pharmacological therapy plays an important role in the achievement of these goals and objectives.

The physical therapist (PT) should be familiar with a client's drug regimen not only because it may influence treatment timing and response but also because the PT can play a role in enhancing compliance with drug therapy. The PT may see the client more frequently than other members of the health care team and can verbally monitor if the client is adhering to the prescribed regimen, as well as monitor for any side effects of drug therapy. As part of physical therapy (PTy), the therapist is in an ideal position to request to see the drugs the client is taking, both by prescription and over-the-counter. The therapist should ensure that drug containers can be easily manipulated by the client with hand involvement.

The physical therapist's role in drug therapy is as follows:

- monitor intake
- monitor adverse reactions
- monitor ability to open containers
- contribute to client's drug education
- consider client's drugs in timing of treatment and effect of modalities

Most arthritis conditions have multifactorial etiology so that therapy is often complex, involv-

PHYSICAL THERAPY IN ARTHRITIS, Joan M. Walker, PhD, PT, and Antoine Helewa, MSc(Clin Epid), PT, W.B. Saunders Company © 1996.

ing several interventions simultaneously. Therapy, especially PTy, in some instances is efficacious; at other times it can be harmful. Careful monitoring of response is essential.

This chapter will focus on the various drugs used in the pharmacological management of arthritis. For further detail, readers are referred to Chapter 4 and individual product monographs.[1,2]

Drugs Used in Treatment

There are many different pharmacologic agents used in the treatment of arthritis. Some provide symptomatic relief, while others are targeted at slowing or arresting the disease process. Acetaminophen, aspirin and its derivatives, and nonsteroidal anti-inflammatory drugs (NSAIDs) provide relief from the pain associated with arthritis. Aspirin, NSAIDs, and steroids provide symptomatic relief from the inflammation. Pharmacologic agents aimed at slowing the disease progression in rheumatoid arthritis (RA) include the antimalarials, gold compounds, penicillamine, sulfasalazine, and cytotoxic agents such as methotrexate and azathioprine. Steroids may play some role in slowing the progression of RA. Some of these drugs also are used in the treatment of other forms of arthritis, such as systemic lupus erythematosus. Agents such as colchicine, allopurinol, and uricosuric agents are used in the treatment of gout and hyperuricemia. Often, combinations of these drugs will be used to provide symptomatic relief while allowing the other agents to slow or arrest the disease process.

This chapter will focus on the common drugs used in the treatment of arthritis. Pharmacology, pharmacokinetics, adverse drug reactions, drug interactions, administration, and availability of the agents will be discussed. The actual approach to treating a particular disorder and role of these drugs in that treatment is discussed in Chapter 4. Special considerations for PTy are included at the end of each drug or drug category.

Acetaminophen

Pharmacology and Pharmacokinetics Acetaminophen is an agent that is effective at reducing pain (analgesic effect) and at reducing fever (antipyretic effect). It is believed to produce its analgesic effect by a mechanism similar to that of acetylsalicylic acid (ASA or aspirin); however, the exact site and mechanism of action is still not clearly understood.[3] Unlike aspirin, acetaminophen possesses no clinically significant anti-inflammatory activity.[4] It differs also from aspirin in that it does not affect uric acid levels and does not inhibit platelet activity.[4]

Acetaminophen is used in the treatment of arthritis for its analgesic activities, and may be used in conjunction with anti-inflammatory therapy. Equivalent doses (650 mg four times daily) of acetaminophen and aspirin produce similar analgesic effects.[5] Acetaminophen is rapidly absorbed from the gastrointestinal (GI) tract following oral administration, with peak plasma concentrations occurring within 30–60 minutes.[6] It has a half-life in the range of 1–3 hours. This may be prolonged in neonates, patients with liver disease, and following ingestion of toxic doses.[6]

Adverse Effects and Drug Interactions Acetaminophen is generally well tolerated. Mild, reversible elevations in liver enzymes may occur, but levels return to normal when the drug is discontinued. At higher doses patients may become excited, disoriented, and/or dizzy.[4] Excessive doses of acetaminophen (10 g) can cause liver toxicity and may be fatal. Early symptoms of toxicity may include nausea, vomiting, diarrhea, and abdominal pain. Acetylcysteine is a specific antidote used to treat acetaminophen toxicity.[4]

Chronic abuse of alcohol may increase the toxicity of large doses or overdoses of acetaminophen. Concurrent administration of barbiturates, carbamazepine, rifampin, phenytoin, or sulfinpyrazone may increase the risk of liver toxicity.[7]

Acetaminophen: Considerations for Physical Therapy

- Acetaminophen will only reduce pain—not inflammation.
- Acetaminophen should provide an analgesic effect within 30–60 minutes following oral administration.
- Acetaminophen rarely causes adverse effects.
- Patients exhibiting symptoms of toxicity should be referred immediately for medical attention.
- Acetaminophen is found in combination with other medicinal ingredients in both nonprescription and prescription drugs, so patients may be taking more acetaminophen than they realize—this may increase the risk of adverse effects.

Salicylic Acid Derivatives

Pharmacology and Pharmacokinetics Acetylsalicylic acid, the prototype of the salicylates, was originally synthesized in 1853 but was not used routinely until 1899, when it was found to be well tolerated and effective in the treatment of arthritis.[4] Aspirin is particularly useful, as it has both analgesic and anti-inflammatory activities. Aspirin also prolongs bleeding time and effectively lowers elevated body temperatures.

Acetylsalicylic acid exerts its anti-inflammatory activity primarily by inhibiting prostaglandin synthesis (Fig. 9-1). Phospholipids are released from cells in response to tissue injury and are converted to arachidonic acid, which is further metabolized via the lipoxygenase and cyclooxygenase pathways. The end products (leukotrienes, prostaglandins, and thromboxane) help to mediate the inflammatory response to tissue injury. Aspirin exerts its anti-inflammatory activity by irreversibly inhibiting the activity of the cyclooxygenase enzyme.[4,8,9] This enzyme also is found in platelets. As platelets cannot resynthesize cyclooxygenase, the effect of aspirin lasts the entire life span (about 7 days) of the platelet and thus interferes with platelet aggregation. This will result clinically in increased risk of bleeding and easy bruisability. The analgesic effect of aspirin is in part mediated by its anti-inflammatory activity. However, it is believed to also suppress pain at the subcortical level.[4]

Many medications may result in an increased risk of bleeding and easy bruisability. This must be considered when handling manually and applying apparatus.

The salicylates are rapidly absorbed from the GI tract following oral administration, with peak plasma levels occurring within 15–120 minutes depending on the specific dosage formulation. Aspirin is partly converted to salicylate during absorption, and both aspirin and salicylate produce anti-inflammatory effects.[6] A dose of 600 mg of aspirin will provide relief from mild to moderate pain. This dose may be repeated every 4 hours. For the treatment of RA and other inflammatory conditions, higher doses, in the range of 3.6–5.4 g/day, are required. This should be divided into several doses through the day. The exact dose is tailored to the specific patient and will be adjusted based on the patient's response, adverse effects, and serum salicylate levels.

The usual serum salicylate level desired for anti-inflammatory effect is 15–30 mg/100 ml. However, there is wide interpatient variability in salicylate kinetics. Therefore, the same dose in different patients may result in very different salicylate levels.[7] Adverse effects are more likely to occur at levels greater than 30 mg/100 ml.[7] Although serum salicylate levels do not always correlate with efficacy, they may be used to monitor for toxicity and compliance. In children with juvenile RA the usual initial dose is 60–90 mg/kg in those under 25 kg in weight, or 2.4–3.6 g/day in children weighing more than 25 kg.[6] The various salicylic acid derivatives available are presented in Table 9-1.

Adverse Effects and Drug Interactions Despite its wide availability, the use of aspirin is limited in many patients because of its high incidence of adverse effects (Table 9-2). At doses used to alleviate inflammation, aspirin's major adverse effect is gastric intolerance, which may manifest as dyspepsia, nausea, indigestion, or heartburn. It also may cause mucosal erosion and ulceration, and fecal blood loss.[10] This is due to direct irritation to the GI mucosa and decreased production of prostaglandins, which protect the gastric mucosa.[10]

The risk of GI toxicity may be increased with advancing age; with concomitant corticosteroid, alcohol, or NSAID use; and in patients with RA or a history of peptic ulcer disease.[10] Gastric irritation may be decreased by taking aspirin with a large glass of water or milk, and by taking it with food.[6] Aspirin also has been buffered and enteric coated to help decrease adverse GI effects. The enteric-coated preparations are most commonly prescribed for the treatment of arthritis, as they cause less GI irritation than the uncoated ASA products.[11] Patients at high risk of mucosal erosion and ulceration may be placed on protective agents such as histamine receptor antagonists (i.e., cimetidine), prostaglandin analogues (i.e., misoprostol), sucralfate, or antacids.[6,10]

At high doses aspirin also can have negative effects on the central nervous system (CNS) by causing tinnitus, altered hearing, dizziness, and vertigo. These are reversible when the dose is reduced. At doses less than 2 g/day, serum uric acid levels may be increased, while levels will decrease at doses greater than 4 g/day.[4] Aspirin may rarely cause liver toxicity. As prostaglandins play a role in maintaining normal kidney function in some instances, use of aspirin may lead to impaired renal function ranging from elevation of serum creatinine levels to acute renal failure.[12,13] Aspirin may cause hypersensitivity reactions (urticaria, angioedema, and bronchospasm) in patients with asthma and nasal polyps. As mentioned previously, ASA irreversibly impairs platelet aggregation and prolongs bleeding time. As new platelets must be released before bleeding time will return to normal and this can take up to 7 days, it is generally recommended that ASA be discontinued about 7 days prior to any surgery.[11]

Tinnitus, dizziness, and vertigo may result from high doses of aspirin and cause balance problems.

As mentioned previously, concomitant administration of ASA with other medications may increase the risk of GI toxicity. Other potential drug interactions are presented in Table 9-3. If patients are on any of these drugs concurrently with ASA, they should be monitored for the potential effects of these interactions.

Availability and Administration Aspirin is available in several dosage forms (tablets, effervescent tablets, suppositories) manufactured by various companies. Most products are available over-the-counter without requiring a physician's prescription. Several analogues of ASA also are available. Choline magnesium trisalicylate, a salicylate salt, is converted to salicylate when ingested.[6] This drug also is used for its analgesic and anti-inflammatory activities (Table 9-4). Choline magnesium trisalicylate, as compared to aspirin, causes less GI irritation, has little effect on platelet function or bleeding time, and is less likely to cause renal problems.[14] Salsalate, the salicylate ester of salicylic acid, is absorbed in the small intestine and also is associated with less GI irritation than ASA.[2] Diflunisal, a difluorophenyl derivative of salicylic acid, does not release salicylate in the blood.[15] Like choline magnesium trisalicylate, it is used for its analgesic and anti-inflammatory properties. Adverse effects occurring with diflunisal are similar to those of aspirin and other NSAIDs.

Salicylic Acid Derivatives: Considerations for Physical Therapy

- Aspirin and its derivatives will reduce pain and inflammation.
- Onset and duration of analgesic activity; avoid aggressive mobilization at peak analgesic activity. Pain decrease may allow excessive motion and further traumatize joint structures.
- Onset and peak anti-inflammatory activity; physical activity can negate drug effects by promoting further release of cartilage destructive enzymes.
- CNS effects (i.e., tinnitus, dizziness) may affect a patient's ability to respond to and participate in physical therapy. Be observant of new balance problems.
- Patients on high doses of aspirin may bruise easily; use care in applying apparatus and in some massage techniques (e.g., deep transverse frictions).
- Patients may experience GI irritation and/or ulceration, which may add to their discomfort.
- Drugs used to offset GI adverse effects may cause CNS adverse effects that may affect a patient's ability to respond to and participate in physical therapy.
- Aspirin is found in combination with other medicinal ingredients in both prescription and nonprescription drugs, so patients may be taking more aspirin than they realize—this may increase the risk of adverse effects. Monitor both prescription and over-the-counter drug intake.

Nonsteroidal Anti-inflammatory Drugs

Pharmacology and Pharmacokinetics NSAIDs were developed in response to the need for aspirin-like drugs without the toxicities of aspirin. There are currently several NSAIDs available in the United States and Canada (see Table 9-1) that are divided into several chemical classes. The anti-inflammatory effect of NSAIDs is mediated through their ability to inhibit the activity of the cyclooxygenase enzyme (see Fig. 9-1). Unlike ASA, this inhibition is reversible; therefore, platelet function returns to normal when the NSAID is cleared from the blood.[11]

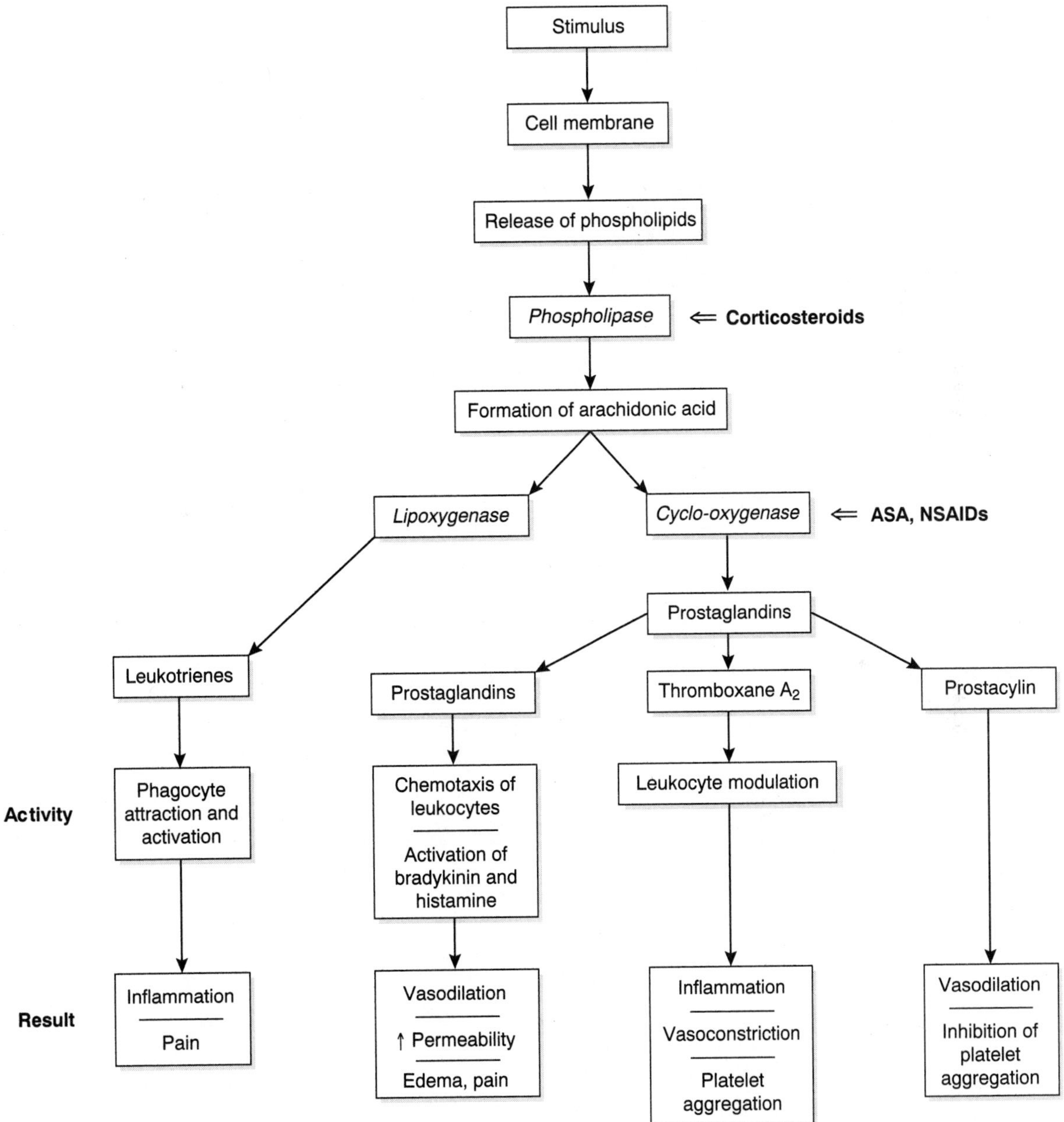

Figure 9-1. Simplified schematic of the inflammatory process. Site of action of corticosteroids, ASA, and NSAIDs. When drugs are effective subsequent effects in the inflammatory process are minimized. (Data from Payan DG, Shearn MA: Nonsteroidal anti-inflammatory drugs; nonopioid analgesics; drugs used in gout. In Katzung BG [ed]: Basic and Clinical Pharmacology, 4th edition, pp 431–450. Norwalk, Appleton & Lange, 1989; and Schuna AA, Coulter L, Lee SS: Rheumatoid arthritis and the seronegative spondyloarthropathies. In DiPiro JT, Talbert RL, Hayes PE, et al [eds]: Pharmacotherapy, A Pathophysiologic Approach, pp 1313–1329. Norwalk, Appleton & Lange, 1993.)

Table 9-1. Nonsteroidal Anti-inflammatory Drugs*

Class	Brand Name[†]	Dose[‡] and Dosing Schedule	Analgesic Effect (hours)		Anti-inflammatory Effect	
			Onset	Duration	Onset (days)	Peak (weeks)
Acetic Acid Derivatives						
Diclofenac	Voltaren® (USA and CAN)	75–100 mg in 3 divided doses	—[§]	—	—	2
Indomethacin	Indocid® (CAN Indocin® (USA)	75–100 mg in 3 divided doses	0.5	4–6	Within 7	1–2
Tolmetin Na	Tolectin® (USA and CAN)	600–1,800 mg in 3–4 divided doses	—	—	Within 7	1–2
Ketorolac	Toradol® (USA and CAN)	100 mg q4–6h (oral) 10–30 mg q4–6h (IM[‖])	IM: 10 min	IM: up to 6	—	—
Etodolac	Lodine® (USA)	800–1,200 mg in divided doses	0.5	4–6	—	—
Nabumetone	Relafen® (USA)	1,000 mg as a single dose	—	—	—	—
Fenamates						
Mefenamic Acid	Ponstel® (USA) Ponstan® (CAN)	250 mg q6h	—	—	—	—
Meclofenamate Na	Meclomen® (USA)	200–400 mg/day in 3 or 4 doses	1	4–6	Few days	2–3
Indole Derivatives						
Sulindac	Clinoril® (USA and CAN)	150 mg twice daily	—	—	Within 7	2–3
Oxicams						
Piroxicam	Feldene® (USA and CAN)	20 mg once daily	1	48–72	7–12	2–3
Tenoxicam	Mobiflex® (CAN)	10–20 mg once daily	—	—	—	—

Propionic Acid Derivatives						
Fenoprofen	Nalfon[R] (USA and CAN)	1.8–2.4 g in 3–4 divided doses	—	—	2	2–3
Flurbiprofen	Ansaid[R] (USA and CAN)	200–300 mg in 3 divided doses	—	—	—	—
Ibuprofen	Motrin[R] (USA and CAN)	800–1,200 mg in 3–4 divided doses	0.5	4–6	Within 7	1–2
Ketoprofen	Orudis[R] (USA and CAN)	150–200 mg in 3–4 divided doses	—	—	—	—
Naproxen	Naprosyn[R] (USA and CAN)	750–1,000 mg in 2 divided doses	1	Up to 7	Within 14	2–4
Naproxen Na	Anaprox[R] (USA and CAN)	275 mg q6–8h	1	Up to 7	Within 14	2–4
Tiaprofenic acid	Surgam[R] (CAN)	600 mg in 2–3 divided doses	—	—	—	—
Pyrazolon Derivatives						
Phenylbutazone	Butazolidin[R] (CAN)		—	—	—	—
Salicylic Acid Derivatives						
ASA	Various	2.6–5.4 g in 3–4 divided doses	—	—	—	—
Choline Magnesium Trisalicylate	Trilisate[R] (USA and CAN)	1–1.5 g twice daily	—	—	—	—
Diflunisal	Dolobid[R] (USA and CAN)	500–1,000 mg in 2 divided doses	1	8–12	—	—
Salsalate	Disalcid[R] (USA)	3,000 mg in divided doses	—	—	—	—
Other						
Floctafenine	Idarac[R] (CAN)	200–400 mg q6–8h	—	—	—	—

*Data from Krogh CME (ed): CPS, 29th edition. Ottawa, Canadian Pharmaceutical Association, 1994.[1] Zurich DB: Physician's Desk Reference. Montvale, Medical Economics Co Inc, 1993.[2] Olin BR (ed): Facts and Comparisons. St Louis, Facts and Comparisons Inc, 1992.[3] McEvoy GK (ed): AHFS Drug Information. Bethesda, American Society of Hospital Pharmacists, Inc, 1993.[6]

†Common brand name in United States (USA) and Canada (CAN).

‡Usual anti-inflammatory dose except for ketorolac, mefenamic acid, etodolac, and idarac. Doses adjusted based on response and occurence of adverse effects.

§Information not available.

‖IM, intramuscular.

Table 9-2. Adverse Effects of ASA*†

Adverse Effects of ASA
Cardiovascular effects
Pulmonary edema
Central nervous system effects
Tinnitus
Altered hearing
Vertigo
Dizziness
Dermatological effects
Skin eruptions and lesions
Gastrointestinal effects
Dyspepsia
Heartburn
Nausea
Vomiting
Diarrhea
Indigestion
Ulceration
Hematological effects
Leukopenia
Thrombocytopenia
Pancytopenia
Purpura
Hepatic effects
Hepatotoxicity
Hypersensitivity effects
Urticaria
Angioedema
Bronchospasm
Renal effects
Renal necrosis
↑ serum creatinine
Acute renal failure

*Data from Krogh CME (ed): CPS, 29th edition. Ottawa, Canadian Pharmaceutical Association, 1994.[1]

†This list is not all-inclusive; it includes effects that are most likely to occur, or if do occur, may be serious.

NSAIDs produce analgesia by their inhibitory effect on the arachidonic acid cascade. For most of the NSAIDs the dose required to reduce inflammation is about double that needed for analgesia.[10] The reason for this is not presently clearly understood. It is known that some of the newer NSAIDs, such as ketoprofen and diclofenac, also inhibit the lipoxygenase enzyme, thereby inhibiting the formation of the leukotriene B_4 (LTB_4), which is known to be a mediator of pain.[10] Ketoprofen and diclofenac are both clinically effective at reducing pain and inflammation. Conversely, one of the most potent inhibitors of cyclooxygenase, indomethacin, is an effective anti-inflammatory agent but has poor analgesic activity.[10]

Adverse Effects and Drug Interactions Adverse effects associated with NSAID use are similar to those seen with the salicylates. Indomethacin, tolmetin sodium, piroxicam, phenylbutazone, and ketorolac tend to cause the most GI irritation. If this becomes a problem, other NSAIDs should be tried or protective agents may be administered (i.e., histamine antagonists, sucralfate, misoprostol).

Most NSAIDs will cause minor adverse effects of the CNS such as headache and dizziness. These effects occur most frequently with indomethacin.[16] Tinnitus occurs most frequently with aspirin as mentioned previously but also can occur with the other NSAIDs, particularly tolmetin sodium, fenoprofen, and naproxen.[10] All NSAIDs have the potential to cause liver toxicities. It is recommended by some that patients should have baseline liver function tests done before starting NSAID therapy and periodically thereafter.[10] Due to the possibility of renal toxicity, NSAIDs should be used cautiously in patients at high risk (i.e., those with congestive heart failure), and renal function should be carefully monitored.[10] As NSAIDs do inhibit platelet function, they should be discontinued approximately 24 hours prior to any surgery to allow bleeding times to return to normal.[10]

Since several drugs may interact with NSAIDs (Table 9-5), patients on concomitant therapy should be monitored carefully. Not all NSAIDs available will interact with concurrently administered drugs to the same degree.

Availability and Administration Table 9-1 lists the NSAIDs currently available along with the most common brand name, usual dose and dosing interval, and onset of analgesic and anti-inflammatory activity. If not effective, another NSAID may be tried. It is not unusual for patients to try several NSAIDs before an effective one is found. As noted in Table 9-1, some NSAIDs are given once daily while others must be given three to four times a day. Frequency of dosing may influence compliance with therapy, as compliance tends to decrease as the number of doses increases. All of the NSAIDs require a prescription, with the exception of the 200-mg strength of ibuprofen, and a 200-mg strength of naproxen sodium which are

Table 9-3. Drug Interactions with ASA*†

Drugs	Effects
Affecting ASA	
Ascorbic acid, ammonium chloride	↓ salicylate excretion
Antacids	↓ salicylate activity
Corticosteroids	↓ salicylate levels
Affected by ASA	
Alcohol	↑ risk of GI toxicities and prolonged bleeding time
Angiotension-converting enzyme inhibitors	↓ antihypertensive effect
Anticoagulants	prolonged bleeding time
β-Blockers	↓ antihypertensive effect
Methotrexate	↑ methotrexate blood levels
NSAIDs	↓ NSAID blood levels and ↑ risk of GI toxicities

*Data from Olin BR (ed): Facts and Comparisons. St Louis, Facts and Comparisons Inc, 1992.[3]

†This list is not all-inclusive; it includes interactions that are likely to occur, or if do occur, may be serious.

available over-the-counter. Approved indications for the various NSAIDs are outlined in Table 9-4.

NSAIDs: Considerations for Physical Therapy

- NSAIDs will reduce pain and inflammation but are not equipotent in their activity.
- Onset and duration of analgesic activity.
- Onset of anti-inflammatory activity; treatment should be progressed slowly over several weeks.
- CNS adverse effects (i.e., dizziness) may affect patient's ability to respond to and participate in PTy.
- Patients may experience GI irritation and ulceration, which may add to their discomfort.
- Drugs used to offset GI adverse effects may cause CNS adverse effects, which may affect patient's ability to respond to and participate in PTy.
- Ibuprofen, 200 mg, and naproxen sodium, 220 mg are available without a prescription, so patients may be taking several NSAIDs or more ibuprofen or naproxen than they realize. This may increase the risk of adverse effects.

Corticosteroids

Corticosteroids are used in the treatment of arthritis because of their anti-inflammatory and immunosuppressive effects. They come in various dosage forms and strengths, and may be administered as short- or long-term therapy. In this section, systemic and intra-articular administration will be discussed separately. It also should be noted that corticosteroids may be given as intravenous (IV) boluses in some forms of arthritis and are often used topically in systemic lupus erythematosus (SLE).

Systemic Therapy

Pharmacology and Pharmacokinetics The adrenal cortex produces and releases various hormones into the circulation. They are divided into three main groups: (1) glucocorticoids (primarily responsible for regulation of fat, carbohydrate, and protein metabolism), (2) mineralocorticoids (primarily responsible for maintaining water and electrolyte balance), and (3) sex hormones (i.e., androgens, testosterone, and estradiol).[17] Natural and synthetic versions of these hormones are used in the treatment of a wide variety of disorders, particularly inflammatory and immunologic diseases.

Corticosteroids exert their anti-inflammatory effect by inhibiting the activity of phospholipase in

Table 9-4. Indications for the NSAIDs*†

Class	Rheumatoid Arthritis	Juvenile RA	Osteoarthritis	Ankylosing Spondylitis	Gout	Pain‡
Acetic Acid Derivatives						
Diclofenac	x✓		x✓	✓		
Indomethacin	x✓		x✓	x✓	x✓	
Tolmetin Na	x✓	x✓	x✓	x		
Ketorolac						x✓
Etodolac			✓			✓
Nabumetone	✓		✓			
Fenamates						
Mefenamic acid						x✓
Meclofenamate	✓		✓			✓
Indole Derivatives						
Sulindac	x✓		x✓	x✓	✓	
Oxicams						
Piroxicam	x✓		x✓	x		
Tenoxicam	x		x	x		x
Propionic Acid Derivatives						
Fenoprofen	x✓		x✓			✓
Flurbiprofen	x✓		x✓	x		x
Ibuprofen	x✓		x✓			x✓
Ketoprofen	x✓		x✓	x		x✓
Naproxen	x✓	x✓	x✓	x✓	✓	✓
Naproxen Na	✓	✓	✓	✓	✓	x
Tiaprofenic acid	x		x			
Pyrazolon Derivatives						
Phenylbutazone				x	x	
Salicylic Acid Derivatives						
ASA	x✓		x	x		x✓
Choline magnesium trisalicylate	x✓		x✓			
Diflunisal	x✓		x✓			x✓
Salsalate	✓		✓			
Other						
Floctafenine						x

*Data from Krogh CME (ed): CPS, 29th edition. Ottawa, Canadian Pharmaceutical Association, 1994.[1] Zurich DB: Physicians' Desk Reference. Montvale, Medical Economics Co Inc, 1993.[2]

†Approved indications as listed in CPS (CAN) product monographs (x) and PDR (USA) product monographs (✓).

‡Mild to moderate pain associated with inflammation.

Table 9-5. Drug Interactions with NSAIDs*†

Drugs	Effects
Affecting NSAIDs	
Cimetidine	↑ or ↓ NSAID blood levels
Probenecid	↑ blood levels of NSAIDs
Salicylates	↓ blood levels of NSAIDs and ↑ risk of GI toxicities
Affected by NSAIDs	
Alcohol	↑ GI toxicities
Anticoagulants	prolonged bleeding time
Angiotension-converting enzyme inhibitors	↓ antihypertensive effect
β-Blockers	↓ antihypertensive effect
Cyclosporine	↑ risk of nephrotoxicity
Phenytoin	↑ phenytoin levels
Lithium	↑ lithium levels
Loop diuretics	↓ effect of diuretic
Methotrexate	↑ risk of toxicity
Penicillamine	↑ bioavailability
Thiazide diuretics	↓ effect of diuretic

*Data from Olin BR (ed): Facts and Comparisons. St Louis, Facts and Comparisons Inc, 1992.[3]

†This list is not all-inclusive; it includes interactions that are likely to occur, or if do occur, may be serious.

the arachidonic acid cascade (see Fig. 9-1). This in turn decreases production of prostaglandins and leukotrienes.[18] Corticosteroids cause an increase in the number of neutrophils, resulting in an overall decrease in the number of cells available at the inflammation site.[19] Corticosteroids also cause a decrease in the number of lymphocytes, monocytes, eosinophils, and basophils, resulting in a decreased ability to respond to antigens.[19] The immunosuppressive activity of corticosteroids is due to a combination of the effects described above.[19]

Corticosteroids have been used in the treatment of RA since the 1940s for their anti-inflammatory and immunosuppressive activities.[9] Studies have shown that corticosteroids reduce both pain and stiffness in patients with RA.[20] Although some initial studies indicated that corticosteroids may inhibit the progression of RA, this has not been proven in long-term, well-designed clinical trials.[21–23]

Adverse Effects and Drug Interactions As the adrenal hormones affect so many functions within the body, administration of exogenous corticosteroids has the potential to cause numerous adverse effects, some of which can be very serious (Table 9-6). With short courses of high doses, patients may experience elevations in serum glucose levels and in white blood cell counts. Corticosteroids cause potassium loss and sodium retention (which may manifest clinically as elevated blood pressure and edema). Psychosis may occur within 5–30 days of onset of therapy; the risk appears to increase with higher doses.[3] Corticosteroids also may cause GI irritation and ulceration.

These same adverse effects also may occur with longer courses of therapy, in addition to other potential complications. As little as 7–10 days of therapy with a corticosteroid may suppress the natural hypothalamic-pituitary-adrenal (HPA) axis. This may result in Cushing's syndrome, with puffiness of the face, redistribution of fat from the extremities to the trunk and face, insomnia, acne, increased hair growth, and increased appetite. With prolonged administration, muscle weakness, thinning of the skin, easy bruisability, and osteoporosis may occur. Healing of wounds is often impaired. Corticosteroid use also may result in visual complications, such as cataract development and glaucoma.

Avascular necrosis (necrosis due to loss of blood supply) has been reported, particularly in

Table 9-6. Adverse Effects of Corticosteroids*†

Cardiovascular effects
Arrhythmias
Hypertension
Atherosclerosis
Central nervous system effects
Convulsions
Vertigo
Headache
Neuritis
Steroid psychosis
Dermatological effects
Impaired wound healing
Thin fragile skin
Petechiae
Ecchymoses
Purpura
Striae
Acneform eruptions
Urticaria
Edema
Focal atrophy
Endocrine effects
Amenorrhea
Cushingoid syndrome
Aggravate/precipitate diabetes mellitus
Secondary adrenocortical and pituitary unresponsiveness
Fluid and electrolyte effects
Sodium retention
Edema
Hypokalemia
Hypertension
Alkalosis
Hypocalcemia
Gastrointestinal effects
Nausea
Vomiting
↑ appetite
Weight gain
Peptic ulcer
Pancreatitis
Musculoskeletal effects
Muscle weakness
Muscle wasting
Osteoporosis
Aseptic necrosis
Delayed skeletal development
Ophthalmic effects
Cataracts
↑ intraocular pressure
Glaucoma
Exophthalmos
Other effects
↑ susceptibility to infection
HPA axis suppression
Agranulocytosis
Coagulation disturbances
Nephrolithiasis
↑ white blood cell counts

*Data from Olin BR (ed): Facts and Comparisons. St Louis, Facts and Comparisons Inc, 1992,[3] and Spruill WJ, Wade WE: In Koda-Kimble MA, Young LY (eds): Applied Therapeutics, The Clinical Use of Drugs, 5th edition, pp 76-1–76-15. Vancouver, Applied Therapeutics Inc, 1992.[24]

†This list is not all-inclusive; it includes effects that are most likely to occur, or if do occur, may be serious.

patients on corticosteroids for the treatment of SLE. These patients may be more at risk because of an associated rheumatoid arteriolar vasculitis occurring in the affected bone. The risk also appears greater with higher doses.[24] Avascular necrosis usually occurs in the head of the femur. Aseptic necrosis (necrosis without infection) of the hip, knee, or shoulder also may occur in patients receiving high doses.

Parenteral administration of corticosteroids may result in scarring, induration, inflammation, paresthesia, and irritation at the site of injection. Hyperpigmentation or hypopigmentation as well as atrophy, sterile abscesses, burning, and tingling also have been reported.[3]

Corticosteroids have the potential to interact with several other medications (Table 9-7). Barbiturates, phenytoin, and rifampin will enhance the clearance of corticosteroids and decrease their pharmacologic effect. Response to vaccinations and toxoids may be decreased, as corticosteroids inhibit the body's antibody response.

Availability and Administration There are several corticosteroids on the market for use in arthritis (Table 9-8). Orally administered corticosteroids are usually intended as temporary therapy

Table 9-7. Drug Interactions with Corticosteroids*†

Drugs	Effect
Affecting Corticosteroids	
Barbiturates	↓ pharmacologic effect of corticosteroid
Cholestyramine, antacids	↓ absorption of corticosteroid
Oral contraceptives	inhibition of corticosteroid metabolism
Phenytoin	↓ corticosteroid effects
Ketoconazole	↑ corticosteroid effects
Erythromycin	↑ corticosteroid effects
Rifampin	↓ corticosteroid effects
Affected by Corticosteroids	
Anticoagulants	dose of anticoagulant may need to be altered
Cyclosporine	↑ levels of both drugs
Digoxin	↑ risk of digoxin toxicity
Isoniazid	↓ isoniazid levels
Diuretics	↑ risk of hypokalemia
Salicylates	↓ salicylate levels
Theophylline	alteration in activity of either drug may occur

*Data from Olin BR (ed): Facts and Comparisons. St Louis, Facts and Comparisons Inc, 1992.[3]

†This list is not all-inclusive; it includes interactions that are likely to occur, or if do occur, may be serious.

until the disease is controlled or therapeutic response from another drug is obtained. They may be used long term, at the lowest dose possible, if patients fail to respond to other treatment. It is usually recommended that the corticosteroid be administered once daily in the morning to mimic the natural release of adrenal hormones and to minimize HPA axis suppression.[25] With higher doses, the total daily dose may be divided and administered twice daily to decrease adverse effects and to provide better symptomatic relief.[26] If patients are on corticosteroids for the long term, the drug should not be stopped abruptly, because symptoms of the disease may reappear or worsen. Symptoms of adrenal insufficiency (i.e., nausea, fatigue, anorexia, hypotension, dizziness) also may occur.[19] In order to minimize the frequency of occurrence of these events, the corticosteroids should be tapered slowly over several months.[19]

Intra-articular Therapy

With intra-articular therapy, the corticosteroid is injected directly into the affected joint. This will reduce pain and inflammation, as well as preserve or restore joint motion.[27] In general, intra-articular therapy is considered adjunctive therapy that is part of a complete management program.

Intra-articular corticosteroid therapy is contraindicated in patients with local infection, generalized infection with bacteremia, and recent serious injury at the injection site. Potentially, the most serious complication of intra-articular administration is the introduction of infection to the joint. Fortunately, this occurs very rarely.[27] Other possible effects of intra-articular therapy include crystal-induced synovitis, cutaneous atrophy, osteonecrosis, steroid arthropathy, and tendon rupture. The risk of systemic effects is low, but they may occur and the risk increases with the frequency of injections.[6] Local adverse reactions, such as postinjection flare, may occur; the pain can be alleviated by local application of ice and oral analgesics. The reaction will usually subside within a few hours.[27]

There are several corticosteroids that may be injected into the affected joint (Table 9-8). The rate of absorption and duration of action are related to the solubility of the compound injected; the least water-soluble compounds (i.e., triamcinolone) have the longest duration of action. The actual agents used and the dose depend on the physician's experience, size of joint, degree of inflammation, and amount of fluid present in the joint. Injection of the corticosteroid directly into the joint results in symptomatic relief for several days to several months.[9]

Table 9-8. Common Corticosteroids Used in Arthritis*

Corticosteroid	Equivalent Dose (mg)	Relative Anti-inflammatory Potency	Relative Mineralocorticord Potency	Examples of Products Available
Short-Acting				
Cortisone	25	0.8	2	Cortone[R] injection (CAN), tablets (CAN and USA)
Hydrocortisone	20	1	2	Solu-Cortef[R] injection (CAN and USA), Cortef[R] tablets (CAN)
Intermediate-Acting				
Prednisone	5	4	1	Deltasone[R] (CAN and USA) tablets
Prednisolone	5	4	1	Various: injection, tablets
Triamcinolone	4	5	0	Kenalog[R] (CAN and USA), Aristospan[R] (CAN and USA) injection
Methylprednisolone	4	5	0	Depo-Medrol[R] (CAN and USA) injection, Medrol[R] (CAN and USA) tablets
Long-Acting				
Dexamethasone	0.75	25–30	0	Decadron[R] injection, tablets (CAN and USA)
Betamethasone	0.6–0.75	25	0	Celestone[R] injection, tablets (CAN and USA)

*Data from Krogh CME (ed): CPS, 29th edition. Ottawa, Canadian Pharmaceutical Association, 1994.[1] Zurich DB: Physicians' Desk Reference. Montvale, Medical Economics Co Inc, 1993.[2] Olin BR (ed): Facts and Comparisons. St Louis, Facts and Comparisons Inc, 1992.[3]

Corticosteroids: Considerations for Physical Therapy

- Corticosteroids will provide symptomatic relief but do not affect the progression of the disease.
- Corticosteroids may cause GI irritation.
- Once-daily morning dose of a corticosteroid is preferred, but patients may be on divided doses spread out evenly over the day to provide symptomatic relief.
- Patients should not stop long-term corticosteroids abruptly, as symptoms of the disease may reappear or worsen, or symptoms of adrenal suppression may occur.
- Corticosteroids may impair vision and cause osteoporosis, weight gain, edema, muscle weakness, dizziness, low blood sugar, and easy bruisability. These and other adverse effects may affect the patient's ability to respond to or participate in PT.
- Caution should be exercised in treatment of patients on long-term corticosteroid therapy (RA, JRA) because of the high potential for fractures with minimal stress.
- Following corticosteroid intra-articular injection of weight-bearing joints, bed rest or nonweight bearing on crutches will be required for a period of 5 days.

Antimalarials

Pharmacology and Pharmacokinetics Hydroxychloroquine and its parent drug chloroquine are two antimalarial drugs that have been used in the treatment of RA. They are considered to be disease-modifying antirheumatic drugs (DMARDs) or slow-acting antirheumatic drugs (SAARDs), although their exact mechanism of action is unknown. It is believed that they have both anti-inflammatory and immunosuppressive activities.[6]

Adverse Effects and Drug Interactions When used as antimalarials, adverse effects with these drugs are usually mild and reversible. However, more serious and sometimes irreversible adverse effects can occur with higher doses used for longer durations, such as seen in the treatment of RA.[6] After oral administration, adverse GI effects such as epigastric discomfort, nausea, vomiting, diarrhea, and cramps may occur. These may be minimized by administering the drugs with food or a glass of milk. Patients may experience pruritus, skin rash, pigmentary changes of the skin, bleaching of the hair, or hair loss.[6] The CNS may be affected with the patient complaining of symptoms such as headache, fatigue, and nervousness. Confusion, personality changes, and depression may also occur. Rarely, peripheral neuritis, neuromyopathy, and adverse hematologic effects may occur.[6]

Patients on antimalarial drugs experiencing new eye problems should be immediately referred to their physician.

A major concern with the antimalarial drugs is their ability to cause visual toxicities, such as keratopathy and retinopathy. Keratopathy, including transient edema or deposits in the cornea, have been reported in 30–70% of patients. It can occur within just a few weeks of beginning therapy and is reversible when the drug is discontinued. It may be asymptomatic in up to 50% of patients; however, other patients may experience visual halos, focusing difficulties, blurred vision, or photophobia.[6]

The risk of retinopathy increases with increasing doses (>250 mg chloroquine; >650 mg hydroxycloroquine).[11] Symptoms of retinopathy include blurred vision, night blindness, light flashes and streaks, and photophobia. Occasionally, retinal changes are reversible if detected early, but they are usually permanent and may result in blindness. The retinal damage may occur even after the drug is stopped. Routine exams are necessary to monitor for these visual toxicities. Hydroxychloroquine is the only antimalarial officially approved for the treatment of RA and SLE in the United States (USA) and Canada (CAN). Long-term therapy with high doses has been associated with fewer adverse effects than similar treatment with chloroquine.[6]

The antimalarial agents should not be used concurrently with phenylbutazone, gold compounds, or penicillamine, due to the increased risk of severe skin reactions. They should be used cautiously with drugs that cause hepatoxicity, as hydroxychloroquine concentrates in the liver and may cause toxicity. Digoxin levels may be increased if used concomitantly with hydroxychloroquine.[3]

Availability and Administration Hydroxychloroquine is available in both the USA and CAN as Plaquenil,[R] 200-mg tablets. Treatment for RA is usually initiated at a dose of 400 mg/day, and when a good response is attained the dose may be reduced by about 50% to 200 mg/day.[1] It may take 6–12 weeks before an effect is seen, and it is usually recommended that the drug be tried for at least 6 months.[28] It is not currently approved for use in juvenile RA, as its safety in children for this indication has not been proven.[1] Hydroxychloroquine also is used in the treatment of SLE. Baseline and periodic eye exams and blood counts should be obtained to monitor for toxicities while patients are being treated with hydroxychloroquine.

Antimalarials: Considerations for Physical Therapy

- Hydroxychloroquine is a SAARD, so it may not provide relief for 6–12 weeks.
- Hydroxychloroquine is generally well tolerated—any GI irritation may be minimized by administering with food or milk.
- Doses used in the treatment of RA may cause serious visual toxicities that may be asymptomatic or cause changes, such as blurred vision, visual halos, difficulty in focusing, photophobia, and fog before the eyes. Permanent damage and blindness may occur. Patients experiencing these effects should be referred to their physician.

Table 9-9. Adverse Effects of Gold Compounds*†

Gastrointestinal effects
Diarrhea
Abdominal cramping and pain
Nausea
Hematological effects
Leukopenia
Thrombocytopenia
Aplastic anemia
Eosinophilia
Agranulocytosis
Pancytopenia
Mucocutaneous effects
Rash
Pruritis
Erythema
Ulceration of oropharynx
Metallic taste
Exfoliative dermatits
Gray to blue pigmentation
Renal effects
Proteinuria
Hematuria
Glomerulonephritis
Nephrotic syndrome
Other effects
↑ liver enzymes
Hepatitis
Headache
Dizziness
Peripheral neuropathy
Nitritoid reaction
Interstitial pneumonitis
Anaphylactic reaction

*Data from McEvoy GK (ed): AHFS Drug Information. Bethesda, American Society of Hospital Pharmacists, Inc, 1993.[6]

†This list is not all-inclusive; it includes effects that are most likely to occur, or if do occur, may be serious.

Gold Compounds

Pharmacology and Pharmacokinetics Gold therapy or chrysotherapy has been used in the treatment of RA for well over 50 years.[29] Gold is available in both intramuscular injection and oral formulations. Intramuscular gold therapy is believed to work by inhibiting the function of mononuclear phagocytes.[30] Data also indicate that this therapy may have an immunoregulatory effect; that is, it causes immunostimulation, as well as immunosuppression.[29,31] Oral gold therapy with auranofin is believed to work in a similar manner and also to have immunoregulatory effects.[32] Chrysotherapy, then, will have anti-inflammatory and immunoregulatory effects with a reduction in pain as a result of the aforementioned effects. Gold therapy will slow the progression of RA but it will not stop or reverse the disease process.[6]

The two injectable formulations, gold sodium thiomalate (water-soluble) and aurothioglucose (oil-soluble), are both intended for intramuscular administration. Gold sodium thiomalate is rapidly absorbed following injection, while aurothioglucose is absorbed slowly and irregularly. Some patients complain of lumps at the site of injection.[11] With administration of oral gold therapy only approximately 25% of the dose is absorbed.[33]

Physical therapists should recognize in planning therapy that several medications, such as SAARDs, may take weeks or months before maximum relief is obtained.

Adverse Effects and Drug Interactions Although similar adverse effects (Table 9-9) occur with all gold therapy, the incidence does differ depending on the formulation. The most common adverse effects, up to 60–80%, of intramuscular gold therapy are mucocutaneous in nature, ranging from erythema to exfoliative dermatitis.[34] Stomatitis may occur and will sometimes be preceded by a metallic taste. With oral gold therapy the most common adverse effect, up to 40%, is diarrhea, while 16% will experience GI irritation in the form of nausea, vomiting, or abdominal cramping.[35] Skin complications will occur in about 25% of patients on auranofin.[35] Exposure to sunlight or artificial ultraviolet light may exacerbate any skin rashes.[6]

All gold compounds can cause renal and liver toxicities. Renal effects, if recognized early, are usually mild and reversible. However, if gold therapy is continued the renal effects can become serious and chronic.[6] Bone marrow suppression is the most serious complication of chrysotherapy and may present as leukopenia, thrombocytopenia, agranulocytosis, or aplastic anemia in 1–3% of patients.[36] Up to 40% of patients may develop eosinophilia, which often accompanies or precedes other toxic reactions.[37] Vasomotor (or nitritoid) reactions consisting of flushing, weakness, dizziness, sweating, and hypotension may occur with gold sodium thiomalate.[6] If this occurs, aurothioglucose, which is absorbed more slowly, may be used.[6]

Gold compounds may be used safely in conjunction with salicylates, NSAIDs, or corticosteroids. Often one of these anti-inflammatory agents is used concomitantly to alleviate symptoms while waiting for the therapeutic effects of the gold compounds (3–4 months) to occur. Penicillamine, antimalarials, and the cytotoxic drugs cyclophosphamide, azathioprine, and methotrexate should not be used with the gold compounds. The safety of auranofin with high doses of corticosteroids or other gold compounds has not been determined.[3]

Availability and Administration Gold sodium thiomalate (Myochrysine[R] in USA and CAN) and aurothioglucose (Solganal[R] in USA and CAN) are both approved for adult and juvenile RA. Auranofin (Ridaura[R] in USA and CAN) is only approved for use in adults with RA as its safety in children has not yet been established. Auranofin may be preferred by some because it can be administered orally and has a more favorable adverse-effect profile. However, others prefer the injectable preparations, as they may be more effective than the oral product; they require patients to come to the physician's office regularly for follow-up and injections.[11] Efficacy of therapy appears to be affected by duration of disease, as those who have had RA less than 5 years respond better to gold therapy than those who have had the disease longer.[38] Gold has been administered intra-articularly; however, it does not appear to offer any therapeutic advantage over corticosteroids.[27]

Therapeutic effects may require at least 3–4 months of therapy. Chrysotherapy can be continued as long as the patient responds favorably to therapy and does not experience intolerable or toxic adverse effects. Baseline urinalysis and blood counts should be obtained prior to initiating therapy and regularly thereafter before each injection or monthly with oral therapy.[6] Patients should report to their physician if they notice any pruritus, skin rashes, stomatitis, fever, sore throat, or unusual bruising. If any toxicity is noticed, gold therapy should be discontinued, and once it has resolved, the patient should be reevaluated for reinstitution of therapy.

Gold Compounds: Considerations for Physical Therapy

- Gold therapy is a SAARD and so may not provide relief for up to 3–4 months.
- If patients complain of rashes, stomatitis, pruritus, fever, sore throat, or easy bruising they should be referred to their physician, as these symptoms may be indicative of more serious toxicities.

Penicillamine

Pharmacology and Pharmacokinetics Penicillamine, although a degradation product of penicillin, has no antibacterial activity. It is believed to work in the treatment of RA through both immunosuppressive and anti-inflammatory activities.[36] Penicillamine is well absorbed following oral administration, with peak concentrations occurring within 1 hour.[6]

Adverse Effects and Drug Interactions Penicillamine has a high incidence of adverse effects (Table 9-10), with the common adverse effect being skin rashes, occurring in up to 50% of patients.[36] Rashes occurring early in therapy may require discontinuation of penicillamine. Once the rash resolves, the drug can usually be restarted at a lower dose without any further problems.[6] Rashes with pruritus, occurring 6 months or more after the onset of therapy, do not resolve as easily. The rash may persist for weeks after the drug is discontinued and may recur if penicillamine is restarted.[6]

The commonest hematologic effects seen with penicillamine therapy are thrombocytopenia and leukopenia. They usually occur during the first year of treatment, often after 6 months.[36] The most common renal effect is proteinuria, seen in up to 32% of patients. Protein greater than 2 g/day in the urine is an indication to discontinue the drug.[36] Penicillamine has been associated with inducing the autoimmune syndromes of myasthenia gravis and SLE.[36]

Administration of penicillamine may cause GI irritation in the form of nausea, vomiting, diarrhea, and epigastric pain. Some patients will complain of blunted taste perception, especially for salt and sweets. This is usually self-limiting, resolving after 2–3 months of therapy.[6]

Table 9-10. Adverse Effects of Penicillamine*†

Adverse effects
Allergic/immunological effects
Pruritis
Lupus
Drug eruptions
Urticaria
Exfoliative dermatitis
Thyroiditis
Myasthenia gravis
Gastrointestinal effects
Anorexia
Nausea
Vomiting
Epigastric pain
Diarrhea
Hematological effects
Leukopenia
Thrombocytopenia
Bone marrow suppression
Agranulocytosis
Aplastic anemia
Hepatic effects
Hepatic dysfunction
Jaundice
Toxic hepatitis
Mucocutaneous effects
Skin rash
↑ skin friability
Excessive skin wrinkling
Oral ulcerations
Blunted taste perception
Renal effects
Proteinuria
Hematuria
Glomerulopathy

*Data from McEvoy GK (ed): AHFS Drug Information. Bethesda, American Society of Hospital Pharmacists, Inc, 1993.[6]

†This list is not all-inclusive; it includes effects that are most likely to occur, or if do occur, may be serious.

Due to similar hematologic and renal effects, penicillamine should not be used with gold therapy, antimalarials, phenylbutazone, or cytotoxic agents. The absorption of penicillamine will be decreased by the co-administration of iron salts, antacids, and food. Penicillamine may cause a decrease in serum digoxin levels, thereby potentially decreasing its pharmacological effects.[3]

Availability and Administration Penicillamine available as Cuprimine[R] 125- and 250-mg capsules in both the USA and CAN is approved for the treatment of RA in adults. It is not currently approved for use in children with JRA, as its safety and efficacy have not yet been established.[6] Therapy is started with 125–250 mg/day, which may be increased by 125–250 mg/day at 1- to 3-month intervals, to a maximum of 500–750 mg/day. It should be taken on an empty stomach so its absorption is not affected by food or other medications. As with other SAARDs, symptomatic relief may not occur for 8–12 weeks; an adequate trial is required as long as the drug is tolerated by the patient.[6] Baseline blood counts and urinalysis should be performed and repeated every 2 weeks for the first 4–6 months of therapy and monthly thereafter.[6]

Penicillamine: Considerations for Physical Therapy

- Penicillamine is a SAARD and so may not provide relief for 8–12 weeks.
- Patients complaining of fever, sore throat, or easy bruising should be referred to their physician, as these symptoms may be indicative of more serious toxicities.
- Monitor presence of skin rashes.

Sulfasalazine

Pharmacology and Pharmacokinetics Sulfasalazine (SZ), a conjugate of a sulfonamide antibiotic and a salicylate, was originally synthesized for the treatment of RA in the 1940s, when the disease was thought to be caused by an infectious organism. A high incidence of adverse effects with minimum efficacy led to its disuse.[39] There has recently been renewed interest in, and use of, the drug in the treatment of RA, using lower doses that cause fewer adverse effects. The exact mechanism of action of SZ in RA remains unclear, but the drug may have anti-inflammatory and immunomodulatory activities.[40] Sulfasalazine is poorly absorbed in the GI tract following oral administration. In the colon, SZ is broken down into its two components and the sulfonamide is absorbed. Most of the salicylate stays in the colon.[41]

Adverse Effects and Drug Interactions Adverse effects occur in up to 21% of patients receiving SZ, and can be divided into dose-related and idiosyncratic (Table 9-11).[42] Dose-related adverse effects tend to occur at doses greater than or equal to 4 g/day, and early in the course of therapy. Patients often experience nausea, vomiting, anorexia, headache, arthralgias, cyanosis, and tachycardia. These adverse effects can be minimized by an initial low dose and a slow increase in dosage. The idiosyncratic reactions, although rare, are much more serious and toxic. These adverse reactions include such effects as agranulocytosis, skin rashes, hepatic toxicities, and lung diseases.[42]

Absorption of SZ can be reduced by concomitant administration of ferrous sulfate or cholestyramine. Sulfasalazine may interfere with folic acid absorption and may decrease digoxin concentrations by up to 25%.[42] Warfarin and oral hypoglycemic agents may compete with sulfapyradine for its protein binding sites. Methotrexate may be displaced, thus increasing the risk of toxic effects.

Table 9-11. Adverse Effects of Sulfasalazine*†

Adverse Effects
Dose-Related Effects
Hematological effects
Heinz body anemia
G-6-PD deficiency hemolytic anemia
Leukopenia
Megaloblastic anemia
Other effects
Nausea
Vomiting
Anorexia
Headache
Fever
Arthralgia
Cyanosis
Reversible male infertility
Tachycardia
Neonatal kernicterus
Idiosyncratic Effects
Dermatological effects
Skin rash
Exfoliative dermatitis
Gastrointestinal effects
Colitis exacerbation
Hepatotoxicity
Pancreatitis
Hematological effects
Agranulocytosis
Hemolytic anemia
Pulmonary effects
Bronchospasm
Eosinophilia
Pulmonary infiltrate
Other effects
SLE
Raynaud's phenomenon

*Data from Dukes GE. In Koda-Kimble MA, Young LY (eds): Applied Therapeutics, The Clinical Use of Drugs, 5th ed, pp 220–1-20–14. Vancouver, Applied Therapeutics Inc, 1992.[42]

†This list is not all-inclusive; it includes effects that are most likely to occur, or if do occur, may be serious.

Availability and Administration The enteric-coated formulation of SZ (Salazopyrin EN-Tab® in CAN) is approved for the use of RA in adults. The USA product, Azulfidine EnTabs® is not officially approved for the treatment of RA. Therapy is initiated at 500 mg/day and increased by 500 mg/day at weekly intervals to a maximum of 2 g/day. Like other SAARDs, the onset of effect will not occur for several weeks to months; an adequate trial is necessary.[11] Baseline blood counts should be obtained and repeated periodically during therapy.

Sulfasalazine: Considerations for Physical Therapy

- Sulfasalazine is a SAARD, so it may not provide relief for several weeks to months.
- Patients may experience dose-related adverse effects (i.e., nausea, vomiting, headache, arthralgias) early in the course of therapy.
- Patients complaining of rashes, sore throat, or easy bruising should be referred to their physician, as these symptoms may be indicative of more serious toxicities.

Cytotoxic Agents

Methotrexate

Pharmacology and Pharmacokinetics Methotrexate (MTX) is an antimetabolite that has been used in the treatment of RA since the 1950s.[9] As an antimetabolite it acts as a folic acid antagonist, thus decreasing the production of a coenzyme vital to the cell life cycle—without this coenzyme the result is cell death. In the treatment of RA its exact mechanism of action is unclear, but it is believed to act primarily as an immunosuppressive agent. It also may have some anti-inflammatory activity.[36] Methotrexate is well absorbed following oral administration, with peak concentrations occurring within 1–4 hours.[6]

Adverse Effects and Drug Interactions The most frequent adverse effects with MTX therapy include nausea, vomiting, diarrhea, and dizziness (Table 9-12). These effects usually occur on the days that MTX is administered. As MTX affects rapidly dividing cells, it also can cause mouth and GI ulceration, dermatitis, alopecia, leukopenia, and thrombocytopenia.[9] Methotrexate may cause acute and chronic liver toxicity. Dry nonproductive cough, dyspnea, fever, and chest pain may be indicative of pulmonary toxicity and the drug should be discontinued. Some of the common adverse effects of MTX therapy, such as nausea, mouth ulceration, and anorexia, also are indicative of folic acid deficiency. This has led to the supplementation of folic acid 1 mg daily or folic acid 5 mg once weekly. This has been shown to reduce these adverse effects without altering the efficacy of MTX.[43]

Patients receiving MTX should avoid all alcohol, as this will increase the risk of developing chronic hepatotoxicity. Drugs that may displace MTX from its protein-binding site and therefore increase the risk of toxicity should be used cautiously. Examples include salicylates, SZ, sulfonamides, sulfonylureas, phenytoin, phenylbutazone, tetracyclines, and chloramphenicol. The risk of toxicity also may increase with concomitant use of NSAIDs.

Availability and Administration Methotrexate (Rheumatrex[R] in USA and CAN) therapy, approved for adults with RA, is started with 7.5 mg once weekly given as a single dose or in three divided doses spaced every 12 hours. This "pulse" type of therapy has been carried over from the MTX regimen used in the treatment of psoriasis and appears to be less toxic.[44] The dose may be increased by 2.5 mg/week every 6 weeks, to a maximum of 25 mg/week if no response is seen in 6–8 weeks. A response to therapy may be seen as early as 3 weeks.[28] Baseline and periodic blood counts, urinalysis, renal and liver function tests, and chest x-rays should be obtained to monitor for adverse effects.[1]

Table 9-12. Adverse Effects of Methotrexate*†

Dermatological effects
Rashes
Dermatitis
Urticaria
Acne
Gastrointestinal effects
Gingivitis
Gossitis
Stomatitis
Enteritis
Ulcerations
Anorexia
Nausea
Vomiting
Diarrhea
Hematological effects
Leukopenia
Thrombocytopenia
Anemia
Hemorrhage
Hepatic effects
↑ liver enzymes
Hepatic fibrosis
Hepatic cirrhosis
Pulmonary effects
Pneumonitis
Pulmonary fibrosis
Fever
Dry, nonproductive cough
Dyspnea
Chest pain
Hypoxemia
Other effects
Headache
Drowsiness
Blurred vision
Fatigue
Dizziness
Alopecia

*Data from McEvoy GK (ed): AHFS Drug Information. Bethesda, American Society of Hospital Pharmacists, Inc, 1993.[6]

†This list is not all-inclusive; it includes effects that are most likly to occur, or if do occur, may be serious.

Methotrexate: Considerations for Physical Therapy

- Methotrexate is a SAARD, so it may not provide relief for up to 3–6 weeks.
- On the day (or days) the patient is taking MTX they may experience nausea, vomiting, diarrhea, and dizziness—it might be best to avoid scheduling PTy on these days.
- Patients complaining of nonproductive cough, dyspnea, fever, chest pain, or easy bruising should be referred to their physician, as these symptoms may be indicative of more serious toxicities.

Azathioprine

Pharmacology and Pharmacokinetics Azathioprine is an immunosuppressive agent approved for the treatment of RA in adults. Although its exact mechanism of action in RA is unclear, it does provide symptomatic relief, probably through its immunosuppressive activities.[36] Following oral administration it is rapidly absorbed from the GI tract.[9]

Adverse Effects and Drug Interactions The frequent adverse effects with azathioprine are GI and hematologic. Gastrointestinal irritation in the form of nausea, vomiting, and diarrhea may be reduced by taking with food and dividing the doses.[9] Hematologic effects, such as leukopenia and thrombocytopenia, may occur with higher doses.[28] Use of azathioprine may increase the risk of malignancies, but this risk appears to be relatively low with the doses used in the treatment of RA.[9] Azathioprine also may increase the risk of infection. Liver toxicity and hepatitis may occur.

The dose of azathioprine may need to be reduced in patients also receiving allopurinol. Patients receiving azathioprine and other bone marrow suppressive agents should be monitored carefully for signs of toxicity.

Availability and Administration Azathioprine (Imuran[R] in USA and CAN) is approved for the treatment of RA in adults. Therapy should be started with a low dose of 1 mg/kg/day and increased by 0.5 mg/kg/day in patients who do not respond in 6–8 weeks.[9] A 12-week trial is needed to determine effectiveness of therapy.[9] Patients should have baseline and periodic blood counts throughout the course of therapy to monitor for adverse effects.

Azathioprine: Considerations for Physical Therapy

- Azathioprine is a SAARD, so it may not provide relief for up to 12 weeks.
- Patients may experience GI irritation—this can be reduced by taking with food and dividing the doses.
- Patients complaining of infections, sore throat, or easy bruising should be referred to their physician, as these symptoms may be indicative of more serious toxicities.

Cyclophosphamide and Chlorambucil

Cyclophosphamide (Cytoxan[R] in USA and CAN) and chlorambucil (Leukeran[R] in both the USA and CAN) are both immunosuppressive agents that have been used in the treatment of RA. Neither of these agents are approved for use in the treatment of RA but may be used as a last resort for patients who have active disease unresponsive to other treatment modalities.[20] As with other cancer chemotherapeutic agents, adverse effects may be toxic and very serious. The common adverse effects are bone marrow suppression and GI irritation in the form of nausea and vomiting. These agents also may cause malignancies, particularly leukemias. Therefore, if these drugs are used in the treatment of RA, patients should be informed of all potential toxicities and monitored very carefully for adverse effects.

Cyclosporine

Cyclosporine, an immunosuppressive agent, has been used for several years in organ and bone marrow transplantation. It also has been evaluated in the treatment of RA. Cyclosporine has been shown to improve symptoms of arthritis. In studies, doses less than 10 mg/kg/day have been shown to be successful at providing symptomatic relief.[20] The role in slowing the disease progression or inducing a remission is not yet known.

The major disadvantage to the routine use of cyclosporine is its high incidence of serious adverse effects, which range from hypertension to nephrotoxicity. Patients receiving this medication need to be monitored carefully and at regular intervals. Although cyclosporine may prove to be a very useful addition to therapy for RA, currently benefits of therapy must be weighed carefully against the known risks and toxicities associated with this agent.

Colchicine

Pharmacology and Pharmacokinetics Colchicine is used in both the prophylactic and acute treatment of gout. Although its exact mechanism of action is unknown, it does provide symptomatic relief by reducing the body's inflammatory response to the deposition of urate crystals in the affected joint. Colchicine also decreases lactic acid production, thereby interfering with urate deposition. Colchicine is absorbed from the GI tract following oral administration and is partially metabolized in the liver. Peak plasma concentrations of colchicine occur within 1–2 hours. Colchicine has a short plasma half-life of only 20 minutes following IV administration.[6]

Adverse Effects and Drug Interactions The common adverse effects from colchicine are nausea, diarrhea, abdominal pain, and vomiting. Bone marrow suppression (agranulocytosis, thrombocytopenia, leukopenia, and aplastic anemia), loss of body and scalp hair, rashes, peripheral neuritis or neuropathy, myopathy, renal damage, and increased liver function tests may occur with long-term use of colchicine. Swelling, redness, and pain may occur at the injection site when colchicine is administered IV.[6,7]

Elderly patients may be more susceptible to toxic effects of medications. They should be monitored carefully and referred to their physician when unexplained symptoms are present.

With chronic administration or high doses, colchicine may impair the absorption of vitamin B_{12}. Colchicine should be used cautiously with any drug that may cause GI toxicities or blood dyscrasias due to the possible potentiation of adverse effects. Concurrent use of alcohol also may increase the risk of GI toxicities. As well, alcohol is known to increase serum uric acid levels.

Availability and Administration Colchicine is available only in tablet form in Canada, and in both tablet and IV formulations in the United States. When used to treat acute attacks of gout, colchicine is most effective when started as soon as an attack is suspected. Pain and swelling should begin to subside within 12 hours and are usually gone within 48–72 hours. With IV administration, relief should be apparent within 6–12 hours.[45]

Colchicine: Considerations for Physical Therapy

- Patients presenting with an inflamed joint characteristic of gout (a constant squeezing pressure type of pain of increasing intensity usually of one joint) should be referred immediately to the physician as therapy (with colchicine) is most effective when given as soon as possible.
- Severe diarrhea, nausea, and vomiting may be early signs of toxicity—patients should be referred to their physician.
- Elderly patients may be more susceptible to toxicity and should be watched carefully for adverse effects (i.e., GI symptoms, unusual bruising, or prolonged bleeding).

Allopurinol

Pharmacology and Pharmacokinetics Allopurinol is used in the treatment of gout. It works by inhibiting an enzyme involved in the synthesis of uric acid. It effectively decreases serum and urine concentrations of uric acid.[45] Allopurinol is well absorbed following oral administration, with peak plasma levels occurring within 2–6 hours. Serum uric acid concentrations usually begin to fall within 24–48 hours, with the maximum effect seen in 1–3 weeks. Improvement in clinical symptoms, such as a decrease in the size of tophi, may take up to 6 months.[45]

Adverse Effects and Drug Interactions Allopurinol is generally well tolerated, with fewer than 1% of patients experiencing an adverse effect.[6] However, adverse effects may occur (Table 9-13). Allopurinol may exacerbate symptoms of acute gout during the first 6–12 months of therapy as uric acid is released from the tissues into the blood. Often patients will receive colchicine concurrently

Table 9-13. Adverse Effects of Allopurinol*†

Adverse effects
Central nervous system effects
Peripheral neuropathy
Headache
Somnolence
Dermatological effects
Rash
Severe dermatitis
Gastrointestinal effects
Nausea
Vomiting
Diarrhea
Abdominal pain
Gastritis
Dyspepsia
Hematological effects
Bone marrow suppression
Hepatic effects
↑ liver enzymes
Hepatitis
Hepatocellular damage
Hypersensitivity effects
Fever, chills
Leukopenia or leukocytosis
Eosinophilia
Arthralgia
Rash
Pruritus
Nausea
Vomiting
Exfoliative dermatitis

*Data from McEvoy GK (ed): AHFS Drug Information. Bethesda, American Society of Hospital Pharmacists, Inc, 1993.[6]

†This list is not all-inclusive; it includes effects that are most likely to occur, or if do occur, may be serious.

for the first 3–6 months of allopurinol therapy to alleviate these symptoms.[6]

The risk of bone marrow suppression is increased if patients are on allopurinol and a cytotoxic agent, such as azathioprine or cyclophosphamide. Alcohol and diuretics may increase serum uric acid levels, thus decreasing the effectiveness of allopurinol. Patients on captopril and other similar agents may be predisposed to severe hypersensitivity reactions. An increased incidence of dermatologic reactions occur in patients taking ampicillin or amoxicillin with allopurinol.[6,45]

Availability and Administration Allopurinol is available in tablets for oral administration in 100-mg and 200-mg strengths in the USA, and 100-mg, 200-mg, and 300-mg strengths in Canada. Patients are often started on 100 mg/day for 2 weeks, and then the dose is increased to whatever is needed to lower serum uric acid levels to below 6.5 mg/100 ml. The higher the dose of allopurinol, the greater the effect on the serum uric acid levels. Maintenance doses will vary from 200–600 mg/day.[45]

Allopurinol: Considerations for Physical Therapy

- GI irritation can be reduced by taking allopurinol with food.
- Maximum effectiveness may not be seen for up to 6 months.
- Patients noticing a rash or complaining of infections, sore throat, or unusual bruising should be referred to their physician, as these may be indicative of more serious toxicities.

Uricosuric Agents

Probenecid (Benemid[R] in USA and CAN), sulfinpyrazone (Anturan[R] in USA and CAN), and large doses (>4 g/day) of ASA are all uricosuric agents. They all work in the kidney to enhance the urinary excretion of uric acid. Therapy is usually initiated slowly, as excretion of a large amount of uric acid increases the risk of urate stone formation in the kidney. Initiation of uricosuric therapy also has been associated with acute gout attacks. Therefore, colchicine is often used concurrently to alleviate symptoms of acute gouty attacks.

The common adverse effects with probenecid therapy are nausea, vomiting, and anorexia, occurring in approximately 8% of patients.[27] Rash and hypersensitivity reactions occur in up to 5% of patients.[27] Sulfinpyrazone is an analogue of phenylbutazone but has no anti-inflammatory activities.

Compliance and Cost Issues

Compliance with therapeutic drug regimens is often a problem with chronic diseases and is often a concern of many health professionals in the treatment of arthritis. Medications used in treatment are often quite expensive. The drug itself may be costly, and cost may increase with number of doses needed per day, and with those that require routine monitoring of laboratory parameters. If the patient does not have insurance to cover these costs, doses may be skipped in an attempt to make the prescription last longer, or the prescription may never be filled. Generic versions of aspirin and many of the NSAIDs are now available, which helps to lower the costs. However, most of the SAARDs have no generic equivalents and they are generally quite expensive. Exact costs of medications can be obtained by calling a local pharmacy in the area.

As mentioned previously, many of these drugs have bothersome and often intolerable adverse effects. These are just some of the factors that may outweigh any benefits patients derive from the medications and may lead to noncompliance. Studies in patients with RA have found a compliance rate with medications ranging from 51–78%.[46] This may be due to the factors mentioned previously, and/or other patient-specific factors, such as lack of understanding of the disease and unrealistic expectations of the drug therapy.

Solutions to compliance problems are not easy due to the many factors that may be involved.[47] It is important that the health care provider listen to the patient to determine the possibility of noncompliance and the reasons for it. These should be discussed with the patient and possible solutions identified. Any instructions should be clear and easy to understand. If complexity of drug therapy is a problem alternatives should be sought. It may be possible to simplify regimens, or compliance aids such as medication calendars may be used. If financial difficulties are contributing to noncompliance, generic equivalents may be available. It may be possible to switch patients to drugs that do not require routine, costly laboratory monitoring.

Compliance with long-term therapy for chronic conditions, such as is seen with arthritis, is important. Health care professionals working together can help patients understand their disease and therapies and, it is hoped, address and overcome any difficulties with compliance.

The PT should create an environment in which the patient is comfortable discussing use of over-the-counter medications and possible noncompliance with prescribed medications.

Iontophoresis

As discussed, most drugs used in the treatment of arthritis are given primarily by the oral route of administration. Gold is given intramuscularly, while corticosteroids often are injected directly into the inflamed tissue. Another mode of administration, although not widely used, is iontophoresis.[48] This involves the topical administration of active drug ions that pass through the skin with the aid of a continuous direct current. Dexamethasone, a corticosteroid, applied in this manner has given relief of pain and other symptoms in the treatment of various musculoskeletal inflammatory conditions such as arthritis, bursitis, and tendonitis.[48] There is renewed interest in this type of drug delivery system for the treatment of many of the inflammatory conditions, as the technique is sterile, painless, and noninvasive.[48] Physical therapists may see a resurgence in the use of iontophoresis as new technology and more clinical data become available.

Topical NSAID preparations may be used as couplants during ultrasonic treatment and, theoretically, enhance skin penetration of the NSAID and improve drug efficacy while avoiding the GI irritative effect.[49]

Areas of Research

- Does PTy combined with anti-inflammatory drug therapy improve patient outcomes in rheumatoid arthritis?
- Do adverse reactions to medications impact the patient's ability to participate in and respond to PTy?
- What is the cost effectiveness of intra-articular therapy compared with iontophoresis and phonophoresis?

Summary

Patients may have to try several drugs before they find the one most effective for them, and they may be on a combination of drugs. The physical therapist should be knowledgeable about the following aspects of a client's drug therapy:

- what drug(s) are being taken?
- frequency of dosage
- speed of action (minutes, days, weeks?)

- physiologicial effects
- side effects

The therapist has a responsibility to understand potential interactions between a client's drugs and their response to PTy, both in a general sense and to specific modalities. Appropriate modifications should be made to the delivery of therapy; for example, aggressive mobilization or strengthening should not be performed at the peak period of pain relief or in the presence of active inflammation. It also is the PT's responsibility to advise the client to see their physician, and/or to contact the physician themselves, if adverse effects of drug therapy are suspected.

References

1. Krogh CME (ed): CPS, 29th edition. Ottawa, Canadian Pharmaceutical Association, 1994.
2. Zurich DB (product manager): Physicians' Desk Reference. Montvale, Medical Economics Data Production Company, 1993.
3. Olin BR (ed): Facts and Comparisons. St Louis, Facts and Comparisons, Inc, 1992.
4. Payan DG, Shearn MA: Nonsteroidal antiinflammatory drugs; nonopioid analgesics; drugs used in gout. In Katzung BG (ed): Basic and Clinical Pharmacology, 4th edition, pp 431–450. Norwalk, Appleton & Lange, 1989.
5. Boh LE: Osteoarthritis. In DiPiro JT, Talbert RL, Hayes PE, et al (eds): Pharmacotherapy: A Pathophysiologic Approach, 2nd edition, pp 1330–1342. New York, Elsevier Science Publishing Co, 1992.
6. McEvoy GK (ed): AHFS Drug Information. Bethesda, American Society of Hospital Pharmacists, 1993.
7. Halperin JA (executive director): USPDI, Drug Information for the Health Care Professional, vol 1. Rockville, The United States Pharmacopeial Convention, Inc, 1993.
8. Reynolds JEF (ed): Martindale, The Extra Pharmacopoeia. London, The Pharmaceutical Press, 1993.
9. Schuna AA, Coulter L, Lee SS: Rheumatoid arthritis and the seronegative spondyloarthropathies. In DiPiro JT, Talbert RL, Hayes PE, et al (eds): Pharmacotherapy, A Pathophysiologic Approach, pp 1313–1329. Norwalk, Appleton & Lange, 1993.
10. Amadio P, Cummings DM, Amadio P: Nonsteroidal antiinflammatory drugs. Tailoring therapy to achieve results and avoid toxicity. Postgrad Med 1993; 93(4):73–97.
11. Dahl SL: Rheumatic disorders. In Koda-Kimble MA, Young LY (eds): Applied Therapeutics, The Clinical Use of Drugs, 5th edition, pp 75-1–75-21. Vancouver, Applied Therapeutics Inc, 1992.
12. Henrich WL: Nephrotoxicity of nonsteroidal antiinflammatory agents. Am J Kidney Dis 1983; 2(4): 478–484.
13. Clive DM, Stoff JS: Renal syndromes associated with nonsteroidal antiinflammatory drugs. N Engl J Med 1984; 310(9):563–572.
14. Altman RD: Salicylates in the treatment of arthritic disease. How safe and effective? Postgrad Med 1988; 84(6):206–210.
15. Roth SH: Merits and liabilities of NSAID therapy. Rheum Dis Clin North Am 1989; 15(3):479–498.
16. Simon LS, Mills JA: Nonsteroidal antiinflammatory drugs. (second of two parts). N Engl J Med 1980; 302(22):1237–1243.
17. Gums JG: Disorders of the adrenal gland. In DiPiro JT, Talbert RL, Hayes PE, et al (eds): Pharmacotherapy, A Pathophysiologic Approach, pp 1168–1182. Norwalk, Appleton & Lange, 1993.
18. Flower RJ, Blackwell GJ: Antiinflammatory steroids induce biosynthesis of a phospholipase-A2 antiinflammatory inhibitor which prevents prostaglandin generation. Nature 1979; 278:456–459.
19. Goldfien A: Adrenocorticosteroids and adrenocortical antagonists. In Katzung BG (ed): Basic and Clinical Pharmacology, 4th edition, pp 479–492. Norwalk, Appleton & Lange, 1989.
20. Arnold M, Schrieber L, Brooks P: Immunosuppressive drugs and corticosteroids in the treatment of rheumatoid arthritis. Drugs 1988; 36:340–363.
21. Empire Rheumatism Council: Multicentre controlled trial comparing cortisone acetate and acetyl salicylic acid in the long term treatment of rheumatoid arthritis. Ann Rheum Dis 1957; 16:277–289.
22. Harris ED, Emkey RD, Nichols JE, et al: Low dose prednisone therapy in rheumatoid arthritis: a double blind study. J Rheumatol 1983; 10:713–721.
23. Medical Research Council and Nuffield Foundation on Clinical Trials: A comparison of cortisone and aspirin in the treatment of early cases of rheumatoid arthritis. Br Med J 1955; 1:695–700.
24. Spruill WJ, Wade WE: Other connective tissue disorders and the use of glucocorticoids. In Koda-Kimble MA, Young LY (eds): Applied Therapeutics, The Clinical Use of Drugs, 5th edition, pp 76-1–76-15. Vancouver, Applied Therapeutics Inc, 1992.
25. Myles AB, Schiller LFG, Glass D, et al: Single daily dose corticosteroid treatment. Ann Rheum Dis 1976; 35:73–76.
26. Docken WP: Low-dose prednisone therapy. Rheum Dis Clin North Am 1989; 15(3):569–576.
27. Schumacher HR Jr (ed): Primer on Rheumatic Diseases, 10th edition. Atlanta, Arthritis Foundation, 1993.
28. Hartnett M: DMARDs in rheumatoid arthritis. On Contin Pract 1989; 16(2):11–14.
29. Sigler JW: Parenteral gold in the treatment of rheumatoid arthritis. Am J Med 1983; 75(Suppl 6A): 59–62.
30. Lipsky PE: Remission-inducing therapy in rheumatoid arthritis. Am J Med 1983; 76(Suppl 4B):40–49.

31. Bluhm GB: The mechanisms of action of conventional chrysotherapy. J Rheumatol 1982; 9(Suppl 8): 10–17.
32. Delafuente JC, Osborn TG: Review of auranofin, an oral chrysotherapeutic agent. Clin Pharm 1984; 3: 121–127.
33. Blocka K, Furst DE, Landow E, et al: Single dose pharmacokinetics of auranofin in rheumatoid arthritis. J Rheumatol 1982; 9(Suppl 18):110–119.
34. Penneys NS, Ackerman AB, Gottlieb NL: Gold dermatitis: a clinical and histopathological study. Arch Dermatol 1974; 109:372–376.
35. Heuer MA, Pietrusko RG, Morris RW, et al: An analysis of worldwide safety experience with auranofin. J Rheumatol 1985; 12:695–699.
36. Pugh MC, Pugh CB: Current concepts in clinical therapeutics: disease-modifying drugs for rheumatoid arthritis. Clin Pharm 1987; 6:475–491.
37. Davis P, Hughes GRV: Significance of eosinophilia during gold therapy. Arthritis Rheum 1974; 17:964–968.
38. Luukkainen P, Kajander A, Isomaki H: Effect of gold on progression of erosions in rheumatoid arthritis. Scand J Rheumatol 1977; 6:189–192.
39. Anonymous: Sulfasalazine in rheumatoid arthritis therapy. Clin Pharm 1987; 6:921.
40. Pinals RS: Sulfasalazine in the rheumatic disease. Semin Arthritis Rheum 1988; 17(4):246–259.
41. Pullar T, Capell HA: Sulphasalazine: a "new" antirheumatic drug. Br J Rheumatol 1984; 23:26–34.
42. Dukes GE: Inflammatory bowel disease. In Koda-Kimble MA, Young LY (eds): Applied Therapeutics, The Clinical Use of Drugs, 5th edition, pp 20-1–20-14. Vancouver, Applied Therapeutics, Inc, 1992.
43. Chambers M: Rheumatoid arthritis. Pharm Pract 1993; 9(7)CE1:3–7.
44. Letendre PW, DeJong DJ, Miller DR: The use of methotrexate in rheumatoid arthritis. Drug Intell Clin Pharm 1985; 19:349–358.
45. Young LY: Gout and hyperuricemia. In Koda-Kimble MA, Young LY (eds): Applied Therapeutics, The Clinical Use of Drugs, 5th edition, pp 74-1–74-15. Vancouver, Applied Therapeutics Inc, 1992.
46. Deyo RA: Compliance with therapeutic regimens in arthritis: issues, current status, and a future agenda. Semin Arthritis Rheum 1982; 12(2):233–244.
47. Boza RA, Milanes F, Slater V, et al: Patient noncompliance and overcompliance. Postgrad Med 1987; 81(4):163–170.
48. Cummings J: Iontophoresis. In Nelson RM, Currier DP (eds): Clinical Electrotherapy, pp 317–329. Norwalk, Appleton & Lange, 1991.
49. Benson HAE, McElnay JC: Topical non-steroidal anti-inflammatory products as ultrasound couplants: their potential in phonophoresis. Physiotherapy 1994; 80(2):74–76.

CHAPTER 10

Orthotics, Splinting, and Lifestyle Factors

Barbara Hanes, BSc(OT)

This chapter describes how the client with arthritis should be involved in their treatment and take control of what is happening in their body. A client with arthritis can learn to think ahead and develop a positive, creative attitude to all daily activities, and at the same time protect inflamed joints and save energy. All of the principles outlined in this chapter can be incorporated into a person's life and can give any client with arthritis a new sense of control over their disease.

Orthotics/Splinting

Orthotics (splints) are externally applied devices that support a joint or enhance its function. In arthritis, orthotics are provided to stabilize joints, provide better positioning, reduce pain, prevent deformity, and improve function.

Historically, there is evidence of orthotic use dating back to the papyrus splint. The poliomyelitis epidemics of this century contributed to the development of better and more effective orthotic devices. Improved biomechanical designs and the introduction of lightweight, strong, low-temperature materials that are resistant to wear have provided the client with a wide array of orthotics. While the majority of devices have been developed for neuromuscular impairments, these advances have impacted the physical management of arthritis. Most publications on the management of arthritis include indications and descriptions for recommended orthotics. There is consensus that orthotics are helpful; however, there have been few controlled trials of their efficacy.[1]

Rheumatoid arthritis (RA) affects the peripheral joints of the hand, wrist, and foot in 90% of clients. Most deformities of these joints are caused by inflammation and proliferation of the synovial

PHYSICAL THERAPY IN ARTHRITIS, Joan M. Walker, PhD, PT, and Antoine Helewa, MSc(Clin Epid), PT, W.B. Saunders tissue in the joints. This, in turn, causes destruction of cartilage, erosion of bone, ligamentous laxity, muscle and tendon imbalance, and possibly tendon rupture. The end result can be instability, subluxation, or complete dislocation of joints.

Orthotic Assessment

On first contact with a client, an initial evaluation of the wrist, hand, and foot joints must be performed. Because the course of the disease is so variable for each client, subsequent reassessments are needed to monitor changes in the condition. Appendix III gives an example of hand and foot assessments; other detail is presented in Chapter 8.

Types of Orthoses

Only common types of orthoses recommended for clients with arthritis will be described. The occupational therapist and the orthotist are experts in the design and fabrication of specialized orthotics, which are not available from commercial stores.

Hand Orthoses

Resting Hand Splint

The orthosis most associated with arthritis is the resting hand splint, commonly called a *static wrist-hand orthosis* (WHO). This splint plays an essential role in treatment of acute wrist-hand synovitis. It helps relieve pain, reduce inflammation, and properly position joints.[2,3] Fabrication of resting splints requires a custom fit. Low-temperature thermoplastics are the preferred materials to use, as they are easy to work with, inexpensive, and durable.

Zoeckler and Nicholas[2] showed that 63% of the clients received moderate to great relief from pain and morning stiffness by using night resting splints. These investigators indicated that splints should be worn consistently at night when there is active inflammation in the hand joints.[2] Biddulph reported an improvement of 24% in grip strength, improvement in ability to perform activities of daily living (ADL), and reduction of pain in 22 clients with arthritis who wore a WHO for 10 days.[4]

The underlying pathology of arthritis must be taken into consideration when positioning the hand in a resting splint. Every joint has a maximum loose-packed position, or resting position, in which the joint capsule is most relaxed and the greatest amount of joint play is possible. The maximum loose-packed position is often adopted by inflamed joints, as the capsule then is able to accommodate the most fluid. This position is used for prolonged immobilization in casts or splints, in order to avoid damaging the joint when inflammation is present. There may be circumstances where it is difficult or impractical to use the maximum loose-packed position. When choosing an actual resting position for an inflamed joint it is important to balance the need for the "loosest" position possible with correction for deformity.[5]

The ideal resting splint will hold the wrist in 5–10 degrees of extension and the metacarpophalangeal (MCP) joints in 10–20 degrees of flexion, with ulnar drift corrected radially. The palmar arch should be maintained and the proximal interphalangeal (PIP) joints should be in 10–15 degrees of flexion. When the thumb is involved, it is best placed in midposition, halfway between opposition and flexion/extension, adduction/abduction. The design of this resting splint should assist in reduction of median nerve compression in the carpal tunnel (Fig. 10-1). The WHO should extend proximally two thirds of the forearm and distally to just past the MCP joints, allowing the interphalangeal (IP) joints to flex. If both thumbs are involved, the

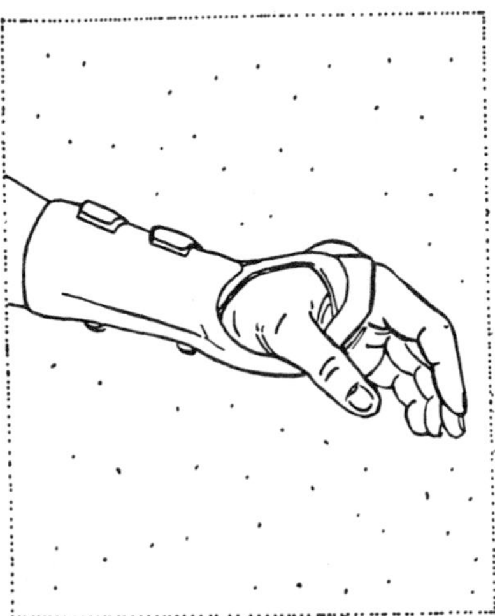

Figure 10-1. Resting splint: assists in pain relief, reduction of inflammation, and proper positioning of joints. (From The Arthritis Society: Think Ahead, How to Manage Pain and Fatigue. Ontario Division, Toronto, The Arthritis Society, 1990. With permission.)

most affected joint should be immobilized and pincer grasp allowed on the less affected hand. This facilitates a client wearing bilateral splints and is most likely to improve compliance.

Strap closures may need to be adapted to ensure independence in application and removal of the orthosis. It is important to ensure a client can apply and remove the orthotic and live safely (e.g., turn a light on and off).

Work Splint

A *static wrist orthosis* (WO) or work splint often is prescribed for a painful wrist to improve overall hand function. This splint keeps the wrist in a functional position and helps relieve wrist pain by supporting the joint. These splints are worn during the day to reduce wrist stress when performing heavier activities (Fig. 10-2). Work splints, which allow some wrist movement, have been shown to improve the client's grip strength at pain onset.[6] A minor drawback of this splint is that it may interfere with fine motor tasks.[7]

A rigid wrist orthosis worn continually can create compensatory stress on the MCP joints. If a client has acute wrist synovitis and active MCP synovitis, this stress can aggravate MCP arthritis. Education of the client is necessary so that they develop an on/off routine with the WO, using it for heavier activities but not for less stressful ones. This will enable the client to protect the wrist joint yet not compromise the MCP joints.

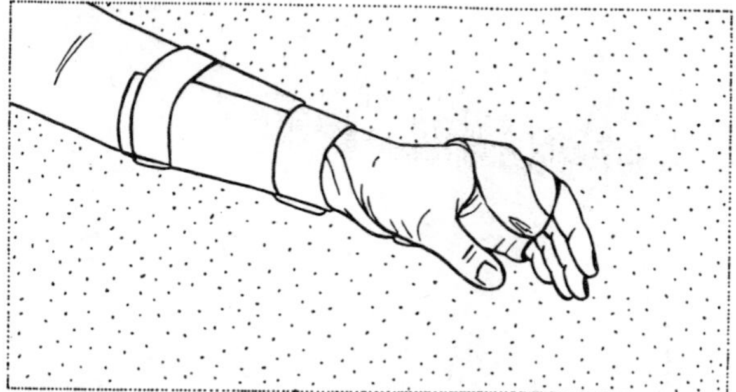

Figure 10-2. Working splint: maintains the wrist in a functional position and relieves joint pain through joint support. (From The Arthritis Society: Think Ahead, How to Manage Pain and Fatigue. Ontario Division, Toronto, The Arthritis Society, 1990. With permission.)

A work splint should hold the wrist between 0 and 10 degrees of extension to stabilize the wrist yet allow full mobility of MCP, PIP, and distal interphalangeal (DIP) joints, as well as the carpometacarpal (CMC) of the thumb. The volar support in the palm should not exceed the dorsal palmar crease.[6] The thenar eminence must be totally free to permit full excursion of the thumb (Fig. 10-3).

There are different types of prefabricated wrist orthoses on the market, available through medical/health supply companies and large drugstore chains. The fit of these splints is of utmost importance and must meet all of the above-mentioned criteria. There is, however, a place for custom-fabricated work splints by health care professionals using a number of different types of material, such as low-temperature thermoplastics, leather, or elas-

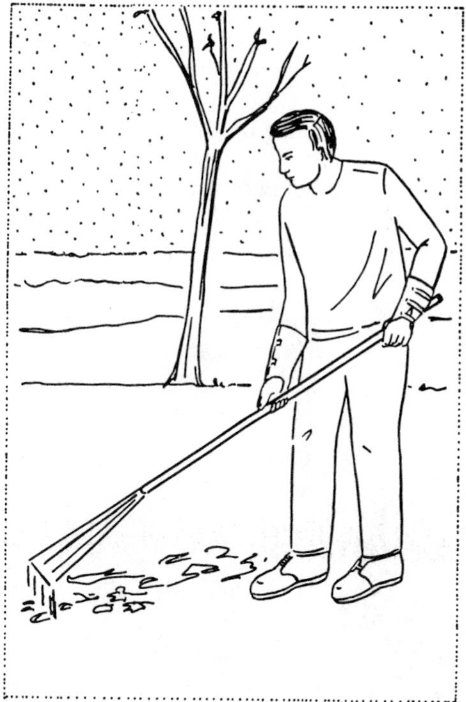

Figure 10-3. Working splint: the design and fabrication must stabilize the wrist but allow full mobility on MCP, PIP, and DIP joints, and the thumb CMC joint. (From The Arthritis Society: Think Ahead, How to Manage Pain and Fatigue. Ontario Division, Toronto, The Arthritis Society, 1990. With permission.)

tic. This choice is dependent on the availability, comfort, and appropriateness of an "off-the-shelf" product. There have not been any studies in which a custom-fitted WO was compared with an off-the-shelf WO as regards cost, compliance, and efficacy.

Finger Splint

Static and dynamic splints often are indicated when reducible deformities (e.g., swan-neck or boutonnière) occur in the fingers (see Fig. 3-8). Splints that apply force to the damaged rheumatoid joint may help correct the contractures caused by connective tissue shortening. "Prolonged passive stretch at moderate tension on a contracted joint may elongate tight soft tissues."[8, p 83]

Three-point pressure or a figure-of-eight splint will apply pressure to the PIP joint in either flexion or extension in an effort to reduce or prevent further joint contracture.[8] This type of splinting, however, does not resolve the predisposing condition, such as chronic synovitis, nor can it correct deformity caused by eroded cartilage or bony changes. These splints are designed to facilitate the client's use of a joint for specific hand functions by positioning in a mechanically advantageous position, in the presence of joint damage.[8]

For a swan-neck deformity, a PIP *double-ring flexion splint* could be fabricated. This splint (ring) is designed to prevent the hyperextension of the PIP joint (Fig. 10-4*A*). Fingertip prehension is increased and, as a result, there may be improvement in grip strength, thumb and finger opposition, function in ADL, and cosmesis.

For a boutonnière deformity a PIP *double-ring extension splint* could be fabricated (Fig. 10-4*B*). This splint is designed to prevent further flexion of the PIP joint. The design of this splint will not enhance fingertip prehension, but it does assist in maintaining both flexion and extension in that joint.

These types of double-ring splints can be fabricated from different types of materials. Low-temperature thermoplastics, custom fitted by a therapist, is often indicated because of the low cost and easy accessibility. When required, permanent custom-fabricated silver rings may be used. Precise measurements by a health professional are sent to a company that fabricates the permanent silver ring splints (see Appendix I). While a drawback to this type is the increased cost, many insurance companies are now covering this cost. The benefits of the silver ring splints are the slim fit that allows several to be worn on each hand, the cosmetic appeal of looking like jewellery, and the ease of removal. The silver ring custom fitted orthoses provide an aesthetic option for long-term management of swan-neck and boutonnière deformities.[9]

A

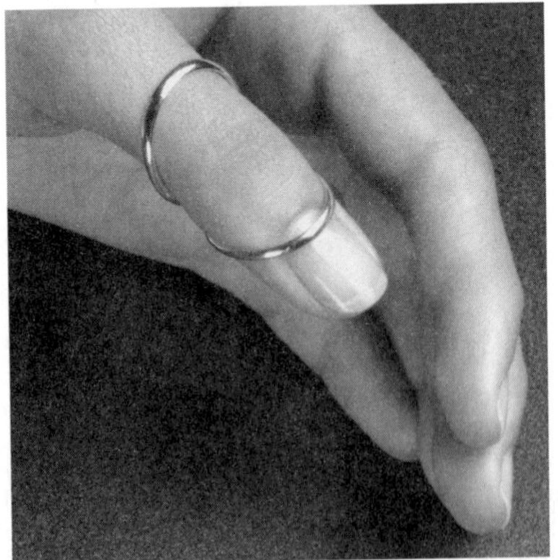

B

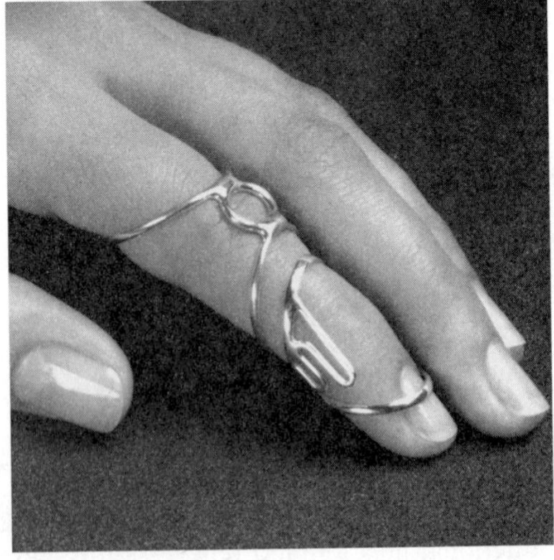

Figure 10-4. *A*, A double silver ring splint (*Siris swan neck*) blocks hyperextension of the IP joint of the thumb. By stabilizing the joint, power and prehension are improved. *B*, Double-ring splints (*Siris boutonnière and lateral support*) can stabilize and correct for more complicated deformity. (Courtesy of the Silver Ring Splint Company, Charlottesville, VA.)

Dynamic Hand Splinting

Dynamic splinting is very specialized and must be done by only those therapists with in-depth knowledge and expert splinting skills. The common type of dynamic splint that is fabricated for clients with arthritis is a *postsurgical wrist-MCP* orthosis, as used following MCP joint arthroplasty. The orthosis supports the wrist and controls position and alignment of the fingers, while allowing active flexion. The goal of management is to apply controlled low-amplitude force over a prolonged period to influence the organization and synthesis of new scar tissue forming in and around the joint capsule, the encapsulation process.[9,10]

Dynamic splinting is a specialized area and is usually done following surgery. This is usually performed by an occupational therapist or an orthotist. (See "Additional Readings" for more comprehensive resources.) A therapist's involvement in this type of splinting would be dependent on the surgical intervention performed at the medical center.

Compliance

Belcon et al estimated that about 50% of patients with arthritis are noncompliant, regardless of the nature of the intervention.[11] These authors reviewed 19 reported studies to assess the compliance to medications, physical therapy, and splint prescription. They observed drug compliance to range from 16–84%, physical therapy from 39–65%, and splint use from 25–65%. Studies of splint compliance have shown that use of resting hand splints is less than optimal.[12–14] In a study to identify psychological factors related to compliance or noncompliance of splint use in clients with RA, Moon et al reported that only one third of clients complied (n=46).[12]

Feinberg demonstrated that the health care provider's attitude and behavior can influence client compliance with splint wearing.[15] Forty subjects were randomly assigned to a standard treatment group or to a compliance-enhancing group. The experimental therapy consisted of the use of learning principles, sharing of expectations, and use of a positive affective tone and behavior by the therapist; additionally, clients were encouraged to assume responsibility for their care. Results showed that the experimental group wore their resting hand splints more often and had better disease outcomes as exhibited by a shorter duration of morning stiffness (p=.01).[15]

Client compliance with splint wearing improves when a daily record of wearing time, amount of morning stiffness, grip strength, and number of painful joints is recorded. This assessment involves the client in their own monitoring system, and clients are able to see the benefits of using the splint(s). The client then becomes a willing and active participant in the use of a modality.

Comfort and proper fit of an orthosis is another factor that will increase compliance with splint wearing. It is important that a therapist with knowledge of joint positioning in arthritis and good splinting skills be the fabricator of these types of orthoses. Compliance also is improved when the client can apply and remove the splint(s) independently. The type of strapping used, and the ability to make a pincer grasp, is of utmost importance.

Foot Orthoses

Pathomechanics

Valgus deformity of the hindfoot is common in clients with RA.[16] Changes in the forefoot often are the presenting complaint and are commonly discussed in the literature. Studies, however, have shown that, as the duration of the disease increases, hindfoot deformities are a greater determinant of disability.[17] Any derangement of the subtalar joint has major implications on foot function.[16]

In healthy gait, the line of weight bearing begins in the lateral part of the heel and advances medially toward the forefoot. During this, the head of the talus locks into the navicular cavity and the midtarsal joints become rigid. As the foot moves into toe-off, the forces pass through plantar surfaces of the medial metatarsals and the hallux, creating maximal load and stress on the plantar soft tissues.

Possible causes of valgus deformity of the hindfoot include cartilaginous changes in subtalar and midtarsal joints, laxity of joint capsules and ligaments secondary to constant inflammation and swelling, rupture of the tendon of tibialis posterior, equinus contracture of the ankle, and weakness of the calf muscles.[18] Keenan et al suggested that valgus deformity of the hindfoot results from exaggerated pronation forces on the weakened and inflamed subtalar joint. These forces are caused by alterations in gait secondary to symmetrical muscular weakness and the effort of the client to minimize pain.[16] The authors reported that clients who had valgus deformity of the hindfoot had more pain in the forefoot.

In clients with RA, the foot is everted while weight bearing, and the axes of motion in the talonavicular and calcaneocuboid joints are more parallel than normal which, in turn, causes an unlocking of the midtarsal joints.[19] This prevents early heel rise in the stance phase and decreases pressure over the painful heads of the metatarsals.[16] It is common for clients with pain in the forefoot to walk with limbs in lateral rotation, which shortens the lever arm of the foot and decreases the pressure on the painful metatarsal heads. In addition, calf muscles are weak and less effective, resulting in a shuffling gait that characterizes the functional disability of these clients. This abnormal gait pattern is due to delayed heel rise, decreased stride length, and a slow gait velocity.[16]

Spiegel and Spiegel observed that there was very little hindfoot pronation in clients during the early stages of the disease, but that as time went on the valgus deformity became more marked.[17] The effect of time on the development of valgus deformity of the hindfoot indicates that this is an acquired deformity in clients with RA.[16] This raises the possibility that early preventive measures may be effective.

Pain in the forefoot or ball of the foot (*metatarsalgia*) results from repeated stress to the soft tissues. As IP joint ligaments become stretched by inflammation, the weight-bearing stresses during stance causes extension of the toes. The metatarsal (MT) heads begin to drop and their fat pads are forced forward, leaving the bony heads unprotected. This results in painful callosities. The MT heads will begin to erode, leaving sharp bony spicules that produce the sensation of "walking on marbles."[20] The forefoot splays due to weak intrinsic muscles with lax and ineffective collateral ligaments.

As the disease progresses, toe deformities develop. Hallux valgus, deviation of the first ray laterally, occurs as the result of ligamentous laxity and joint instability. As the forefoot abducts, weight bearing encourages lateral angulation. Improper footwear will aggravate the deformity.[21]

Hammer toes are the dislocation of the MTP joints. There is a loss of balance between the flexors and extensors of the toes resulting in hyperextension at the MTP joints, flexion at the PIP joints, and extension at the DIP joints. Shoe wearers develop callosities, usually over the second and third PIP joints.[22]

Claw toes occur as the result of overpull of the extensor tendons and weakness of the intrinsics. All joints of the toes become flexed and the tip of the toes comes in contact with the ground.[22]

Foot Management

Since studies indicate that valgus foot deformities in arthritis are acquired over time, early preventive interventions are shown to be of prime importance. The objectives are to relieve pain, align the foot, and prevent further changes. The goal is to improve function by controlling the structural abnormalities, specifically hindfoot pronation, and loss of longitudinal and transverse arches. Client education is essential, with emphasis on the importance of pain relief and supportive footwear to maintain alignment.[23]

Assessment

A full foot assessment must be completed first to determine management strategies (Appendix III). Assessment includes inspection for signs of flattening; tarsitis; presence of "ankle pain" which, in fact, often proves to be midtarsal pain; pain provocation by pronation and supination motions; and valgus hindfoot.[24] A count of active and damaged joints should be conducted to evaluate the inflammatory status of the ankle, subtalar, midtarsal, and all the joints of the metatarsus. Active and passive range of movement (ROM) should be assessed at the ankle, subtalar, and midtarsal joints. The presence or absence of callosities, nail changes, fungal infections, tenosynovitis, and deformities should be noted. The integrity of the transverse and longitudinal arches should be determined in terms of height and flexibility. The thickness and condition of the skin also must be noted.[23] These observations are essential for treatment planning.

Footwear

Supportive footwear is the mainstay of foot management in arthritis. While there is a great variety of shoes on the market from which the client may choose, not many are shaped to accommodate RA deformities. Guidelines for selection of a suitable shoe are:

- wide and deep enough to allow room for toe deformities
- a lace-up type of shoe to provide support through the arch
- a shock-absorbing sole and a low heel to decrease stress on the MT heads
- has a removable insole that allows replacement with an orthosis if necessary
- a heel counter firm enough to provide support yet narrow enough to grip the foot and stay in place during walking
- where hand involvement also exists, Velcro fastening may be used; however, this may not hold the foot firmly in the shoe. Velcro is recommended only where the client is unable to use modification, such as elastic laces, and has no other persons available to assist (i.e., lives alone).

Top-quality running shoes will accommodate the feet of clients with RA provided they do not have severe deformity. These shoes are available, less expensive, and more acceptable. They need to have (1) a soft upper toe box that is rounded, (2) a wide width, and (3) a removable insole and a shock-absorbing sole (Fig. 10-5). Velcro closure may be preferred by clients with hand involvement.

Extra depth shoes (or in-depth) are required for the more involved foot. This shoe is deep and wide and will accommodate many deformities. The upper is made of soft leather, such as deerskin, to decrease pressure on deformed structures.

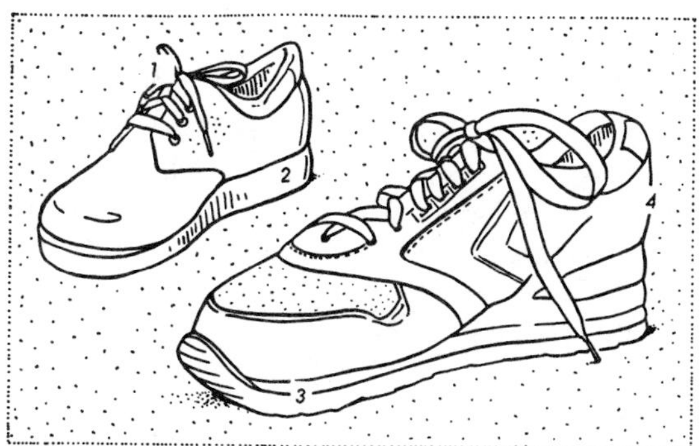

Figure 10-5. Appropriate, supportive footwear. Shoes must have adequate width and depth to accommodate foot changes. (From The Arthritis Society: Think Ahead, How to Manage Pain and Fatigue. Ontario Division, Toronto, The Arthritis Society, 1990. With permission.)

Sandals, such as Birkenstock or NAOT brands, may be another alterative, provided the footbed is wide enough, arch support is provided, and cupping around the heel is present to control the hindfoot.

Modification of the shoe can be made in the heel, shank, or sole area, depending on the foot problem, and may include metatarsal pads, arch supports, and wedges. They provide support and alignment to bones during gait and dissipate weight-bearing stresses from painful areas of the foot. Many top-of-the-line running shoes have their own removable insert that adequately cups the hindfoot and supports the longitudinal arch. A metatarsal pad is needed to relieve pressure on metatarsal heads.

In addition to selection of appropriate accommodative shoes, orthotics may be required to give firmer support to unstable joints and relieve pain by stress reduction. Orthotics can be fabricated from materials as soft as plastazote to more rigid types, such as leather, PPT, and fiberglass. When no control of the hindfoot is required, the orthotics often are fabricated with heat-moldable polyurethanes or neoprene closed-cell rubber, which provide softness and cushioning. These types of insoles often are fabricated by an occupational therapist. Firmer controlling, corrective type of orthotics are made by an orthotist, chiropodist, or podiatrist.

Insoles are intended to unload the metatarsal heads during the initial to midstance phase of gait, provide shock absorption, and reduce friction under the MT heads during terminal stance. Custom-made insoles are made from a plaster mold of the client's foot and are more expensive than the temporary off-the-shelf products. They last many years, however, and can be used in different shoes and some insurance plans cover the cost of these orthoses.

Heel pain due to plantar fascitis, subcalcaneal spurs, or rheumatoid nodules also can be a common problem. Rubber heel cups have been used to alleviate painful heel syndrome. A heel cup supports the foot and arch, relieves the tender area, and has a cushioning effect. These products are available from health supply companies and large drugstore chains.

Custom-made shoes are fabricated to reduce pain that prevents ambulation in the client with severe foot changes. The insole of the shoe conforms to these changes and distributes the pressure over the entire foot sole. Shoemakers who specialize in making custom-made shoes for arthritis clients should be used.[25]

The ultimate goal is to educate the client with arthritis about the importance of supportive footwear and to motivate them to take responsibility for care of their feet. If the client is unable to manage nail and skin care, a referral should be given to a chiropodist or nurse trained in this area. Inappropriate fashions do not offer appropriate support, and the client must recognize the importance of relieving stress on affected joints. Painful feet make walking difficult and greatly reduces their function.

Summary

It is important to remember that orthotics are only a part of a comprehensive management program. Splinting programs will be most effective when combined with anti-inflammatory therapy, client education in joint protection and energy conservation, proper use of the orthotic, pain reduction techniques, and maintenance of ROM and muscle strength. Orthoses, therefore, must be evaluated within the context of a total program.

More controlled clinical studies of orthosis usage are required. Specifically, a clarification of the effects of orthotics on inflamed joints, including their effects on specific and overall client function, is needed.[1]

Lifestyle Factors

Arthritis will cause pain and fatigue in most people. Inflammation and damaged joints are primarily responsible for the pain. The excess energy the body uses during performance of ADL is the main source of fatigue. Clients with arthritis must develop a sense of control over their disease, by learning to protect inflamed joints and to save energy for priority tasks. This sense of control is achieved when the client adopts principles of joint protection and energy conservation outlined in this chapter.

Principles and Goals

The objectives of energy conservation and joint protection principles are to:

- conserve energy
- reduce stress
- reduce inflammation and pain
- preserve the integrity of the joint structures

These principles have become the basis of occupational therapy (OT) intervention with arthritis clients. The client should identify his/her needs and prioritize with the assistance of appropriate health professionals which methods will work best. While there are no published studies on the efficacy of joint protection techniques, the effectiveness of these principles can be easily demonstrated in the treatment setting (home, health facility). A randomized clinical trial of home occupational therapy that included these principles in clients with RA showed statistically significant and clinically important improvement in function with reduction in disease activity.[26]

While a positive impact of OT has been demonstrated, no studies were located demonstrating physical therapy (PT) impact in this area.

Clients should be taught to look for the signs and symptoms of inflammation so that they are better able to monitor improvements in function resulting from these methods. When the techniques are used correctly and combined with anti-inflammatory therapy, there will be gains in efficiency and reduction of pain.

There are many methods for teaching energy conservation and joint protection. Silwa, an occupational therapist, developed guidelines that emphasize the value of individualized instruction and the teaching of concepts rather than standardized rules.[27] These guidelines for client education include the following:

- explanation of the value of joint protection based on the inflammatory process
- recognition and monitoring of the signs and symptoms of inflammation (e.g., warmth, swelling, pain)
- establish awareness for the need to modify tasks based on disease activity level
- establish awareness that ignoring pain and pursuing some activities may aggravate joint damage
- understand what proper joint alignment is and the consequence of prolonged malalignment
- learn the importance of pacing by balancing activities with rest periods
- understand that the condition can be exacerbated by ignoring fatigue

For these guidelines to be effective, educational material must be specific to the client's need and at their level of understanding.

Energy Conservation

Fatigue is a symptom of arthritis. Managing fatigue involves new ways of organizing time, tasks, and rest periods. Clients with inflammatory arthritis must pace themselves and determine the physical demands of a task. They should determine whether a task can be done in sitting, since sitting generally requires 25% less energy compared to standing. Work areas are more accessible when all objects needed are within easy reach (Fig. 10-6). As use of proper body mechanics saves energy, correct work heights should be used (Fig. 10-7). It should be emphasized that good posture is not simply a matter of standing or sitting tall, but the correct use of the body at all times, since this facilitates muscle action and minimizes energy consumption.

Avoiding joint strain should become a way of life that the client practices in all positions used in both leisure and work activities. Advice should be given to change positions, at least hourly. For example, changing from standing to sitting or lying will be restful because the level of muscle activity is changed, circulation is improved, and stiffness is prevented.

Energy-Saving Strategies

Such strategies are numerous. Basic strategies involve planning, prioritizing, and delegating tasks. Clients should plan ahead so that all necessary daily activities can be managed, including rest, exercise, and leisure. Clients should preplan and organize their week in terms of essential home and work activities (Fig. 10-8). *Elimination of unnecessary tasks* is important; for example, drip-dry clothing may save ironing; air drying dishes may save towelling. *Delegation of tasks* is another important rule for clients to adopt. Recruiting family or friends for heavier household tasks will allow the client to save valuable energy. *Reduction in task repetition* will be helpful; for example, laundry could be done once a week and vacuuming once every 2 –3 weeks. *Simplification of tasks* is another key to saving energy. Meal preparation is reduced when a client increases the ingredients and prepares enough for three or four meals, freezing some.

Clients need to learn to *rest before an activity* causes exhaustion. Frequent rest periods of 5–10 minutes can help increase the energy reserve (Fig. 10-9).[28] A moderate work pace consumes the least energy. Clients should learn to work at a constant relaxed pace, using easy flowing movements.

Performing tasks efficiently is another method of saving energy. The client should be well organized and use the easiest method possible to get things done. Tips for clients include:

- Frequently used equipment should be stored in drawers or on shelves that are between waist and shoulder level, to decrease the amount of stooping and reaching needed.

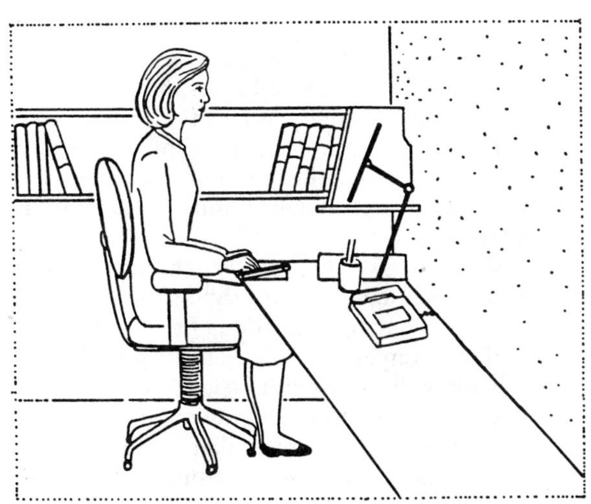

A

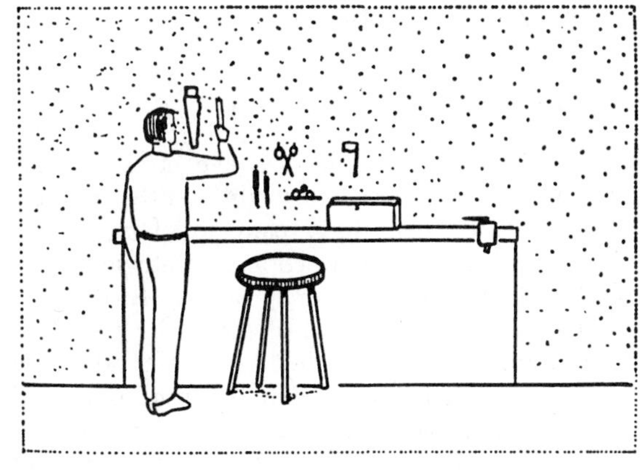

B

Figure 10-6. *A* and *B*, Organized work space. (From The Arthritis Society: Think Ahead, How to Manage Pain and Fatigue. Ontario Division, Toronto, The Arthritis Society, 1990. With permission.)

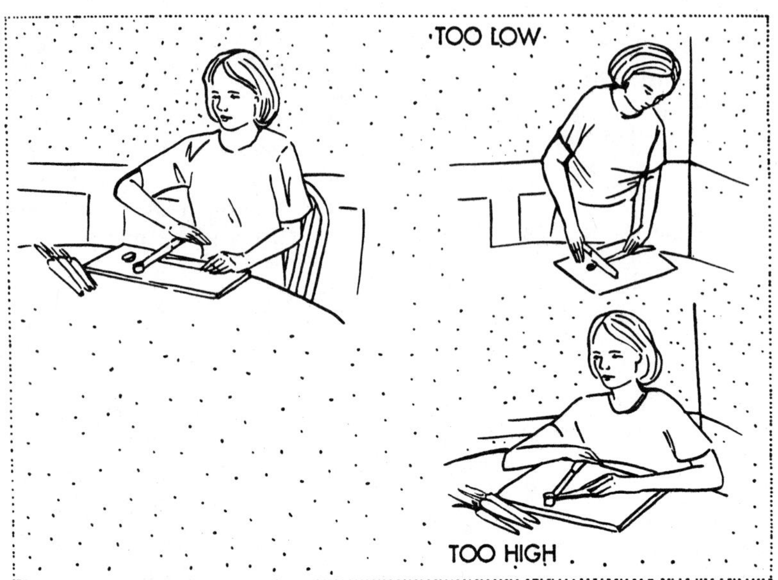

Figure 10-7. Correct work height encourages the use of proper body mechanics. (From The Arthritis Society: Think Ahead, How to Manage Pain and Fatigue. Ontario Division, Toronto, The Arthritis Society, 1990. With permission.)

- Seldom-used items should be stored on less accessible shelves.
- Maximum use should be made of all space. Use of items, such as "Lazy Susans," pull-out bins, and racks will keep equipment organized and within each reach.[29]

Clients will learn that by employing energy-saving steps, they can accomplish more using less energy, and improve the quality of their lives.

Principles of Joint Protection

Joint protection techniques relieve stress on affected joints. Everyone reacts differently to their arthritis. Most clients have pain and fatigue, but individuals differ in their coping strategies. Pain and damage to the joints may lead to further inactivity, with resultant loss of strength. This loss greatly impacts on the client because adequate muscle strength is essential to support damaged joints. Pain, however, should not be ignored, as doing so can lead to further damage and discomfort.

Daily activities stress painful and swollen joints, which are then more vulnerable to damage and, with instability, may become malaligned.

Clients must be made aware that pain occurring during an activity is an important warning.

Performance of an activity that causes pain lasting more than 1–2 hours indicates the joints have been overstressed. Advice should include maintaining muscle strength to support inflamed joints that may be stressed during movement, and to wear their work splint when muscle strength is inadequate.

Excess body weight greatly increases joint stresses. Clients that are overweight should consult a nutritionist to plan a nutritious but low-fat diet. A general, low-impact aerobic exercise program for stable clients will assist with weight loss.

Advice should include the protection technique of using larger rather than smaller joints. For example, a client could push up from a chair with the forearms and use a shoulder purse, knapsack, or fanny pack instead of a hand purse, thus using the larger shoulder joint instead of small hand joints. The body weight should be used to push large objects instead of hands (Fig. 10-10).

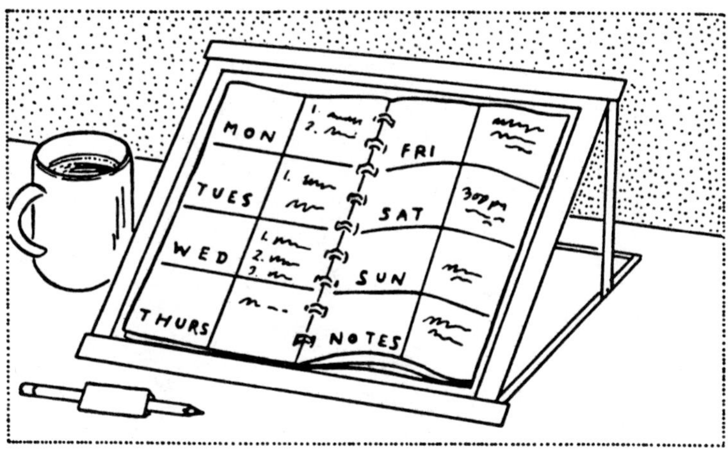

Figure 10-8. Use of a weekly schedule allows clients to plan all necessary daily activities including rest, exercise, and leisure. (From The Arthritis Society: Think Ahead, How to Manage Pain and Fatigue. Ontario Division, Toronto, The Arthritis Society, 1990. With permission.)

Clients should be advised that the easiest methods are often the best to protect joints. Examples include:

- Tip to pour rather than lifting the tea/coffee pot and slide pots between the sink and the stove.
- Maximize the effect of gravity (e.g., use a laundry chute to eliminate carrying and stairs).
- Use convenience food (e.g., cake mixes, frozen vegetables, premade pastry).
- Decrease clothing care by using modern fabrics, such as Permapress.

There are many ways of improving the hand function of clients with arthritis. Clients must learn how to protect their hands and use them effectively. Tips include:

- Larger objects are easier to grip. Handles or utensils can be enlarged with foam, which reduces the tendency to ulnar drift when gripping objects (Fig. 10-11).
- The best grip for the hands is straight across the palm.
- Two hands should be used whenever possible to distribute the weight and improve stability (Fig. 10-12).
- Static holding should be avoided.
- Use of suction cups or clamps to hold objects will free both hands to perform the task.
- Assistive devices should be used whenever possible, such as a book stand instead of holding a book, or a cutting board with stainless steel rails to stabilize vegetables.
- Levers help make work much easier. Levered

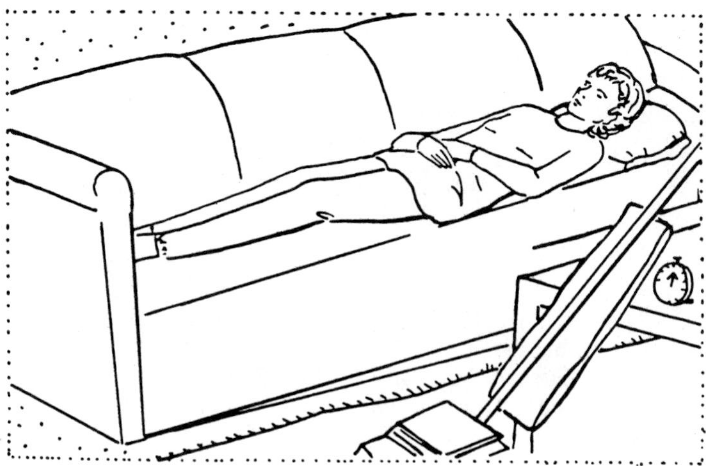

Figure 10-9. Client's energy reserves can be increased by frequent rest periods. (From The Arthritis Society: Think Ahead, How to Manage Pain and Fatigue. Ontario Division, Toronto, The Arthritis Society, 1990. With permission.)

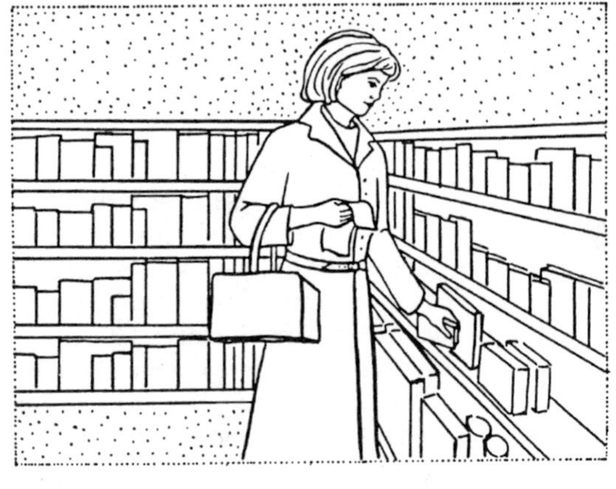

A

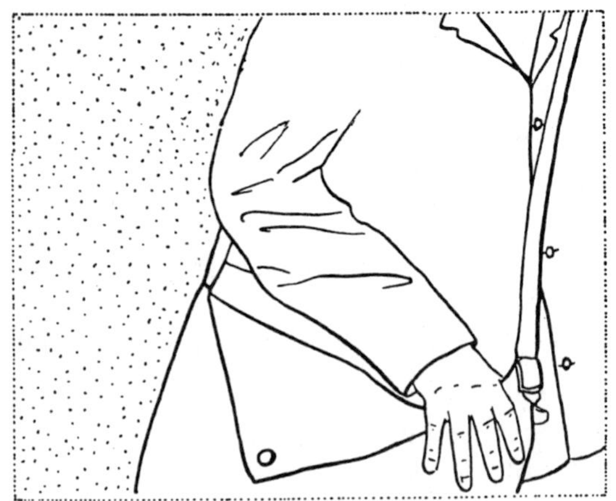

B

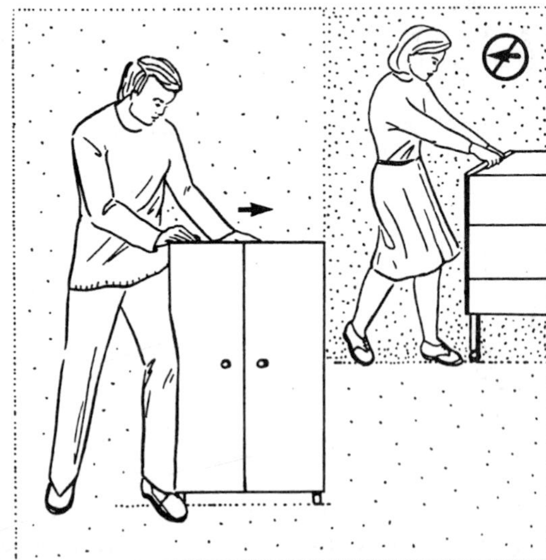

C

Figure 10-10. *A* to *C*, Clients must learn to use large joints and body weight to achieve tasks. (From The Arthritis Society: Think Ahead, How to Manage Pain and Fatigue. Ontario Division, Toronto, The Arthritis Society, 1990. With permission.)

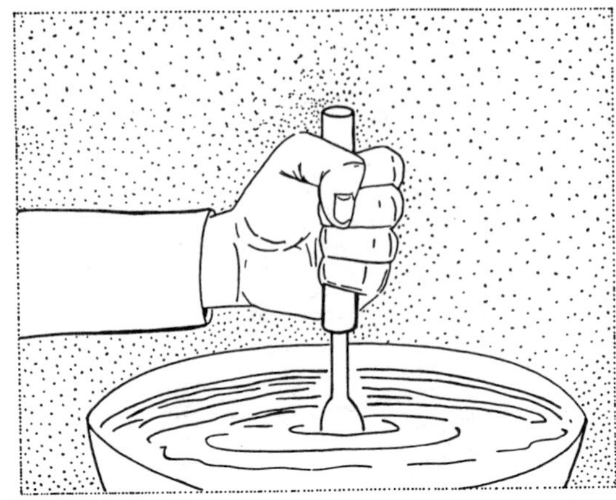

Figure 10-11. Larger objects are easier to grip and reduce the tendency to ulnar drift. (From The Arthritis Society: Think Ahead, How to Manage Pain and Fatigue. Ontario Division, Toronto, The Arthritis Society, 1990. With permission.)

taps take much less effort than regular ones and also protect joints (Fig. 10-13).

- Long-handled equipment increases the range of hand function and decreases the amount of bending required.
- Electrical equipment can make most jobs easier (e.g., a food processor or blender saves hand energy) (Fig. 10-14).

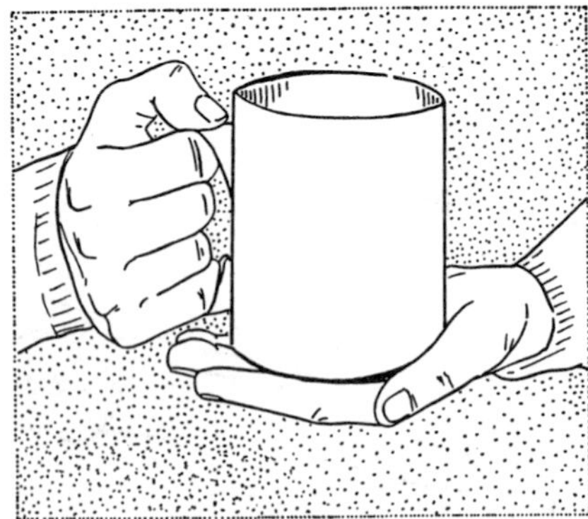

Figure 10-12. Distribute weight by using both hands. (From The Arthritis Society: Think Ahead, How to Manage Pain and Fatigue. Ontario Division, Toronto, The Arthritis Society, 1990. With permission.)

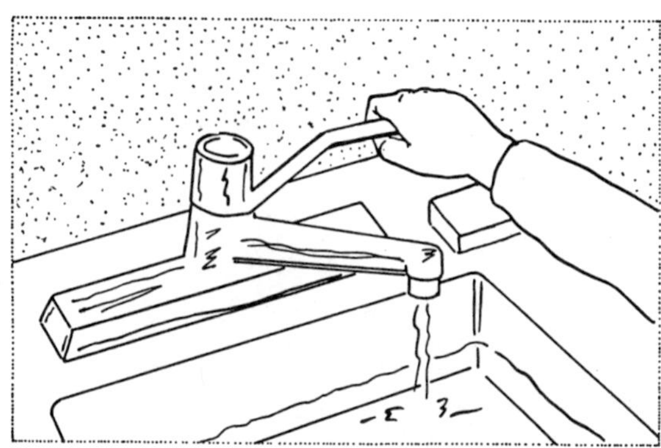

Figure 10-13. Use of levers makes work easier. (From The Arthritis Society: Think Ahead, How to Manage Pain and Fatigue. Ontario Division, Toronto, The Arthritis Society, 1990. With permission.)

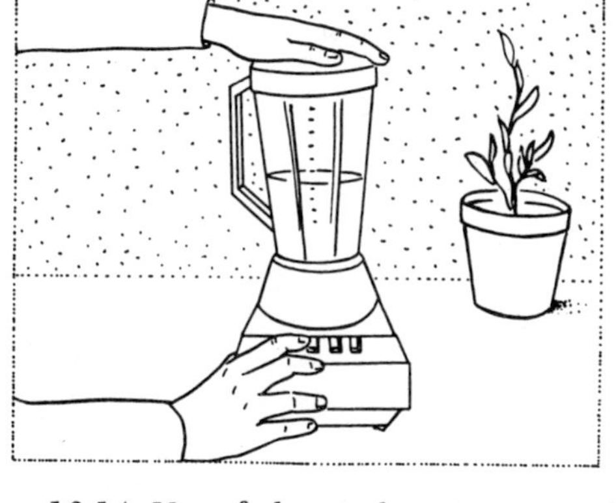

Figure 10-14. Use of electrical equipment makes most jobs easier. (From The Arthritis Society: Think Ahead, How to Manage Pain and Fatigue. Ontario Division, Toronto, The Arthritis Society, 1990. With permission.)

- Lightweight equipment reduces load on hand joints (e.g., plastic mixing bowls instead of glass, melmac dishes instead of china or pottery).

It also is important that the client wears their prescribed splints when performing tasks, since these splints are designed to protect wrist and hand joints and decrease pain on activity.[29]

Assistive devices (equipment specifically designed to increase independence) may be needed by some clients. In the bathroom, devices such as a raised toilet seat and grab bars will increase safety and independence. A bath bench and a hand-held shower attachment will eliminate the need to get into a bathtub (Fig. 10-15). A raised cushion placed in an appropriate chair will ease standing up and decrease stress at hip and knee joints (Fig. 10-16).

Additional advice that may benefit the client with arthritis is to use wheels or casters to reduce stress on joints. Furniture with casters is moved more easily when vacuuming. A trolley in the kitchen helps with all aspects of meal preparation (Fig. 10-17). Bundle buggies assist shopping and a

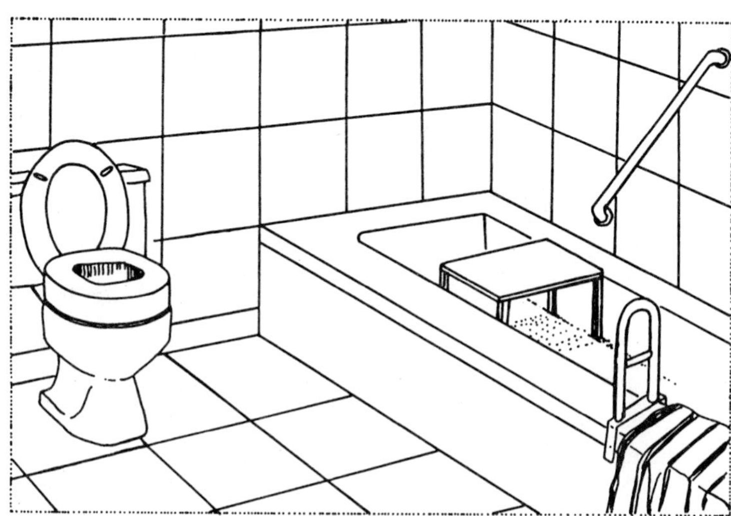

Figure 10-15. Use of assistive devices in bathroom can increase independence. (From The Arthritis Society: Think Ahead, How to Manage Pain and Fatigue. Ontario Division, Toronto, The Arthritis Society, 1990. With permission.)

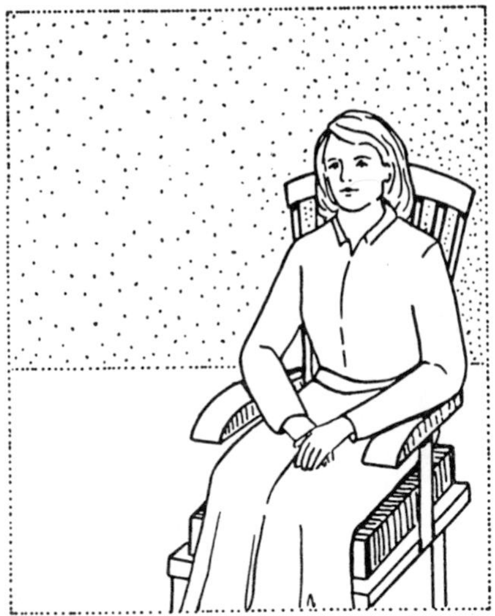

Figure 10-16. Use of a raised cushion will decrease the stress at hip and knee joints. (From The Arthritis Society: Think Ahead, How to Manage Pain and Fatigue. Ontario Division, Toronto, The Arthritis Society, 1990. With permission.)

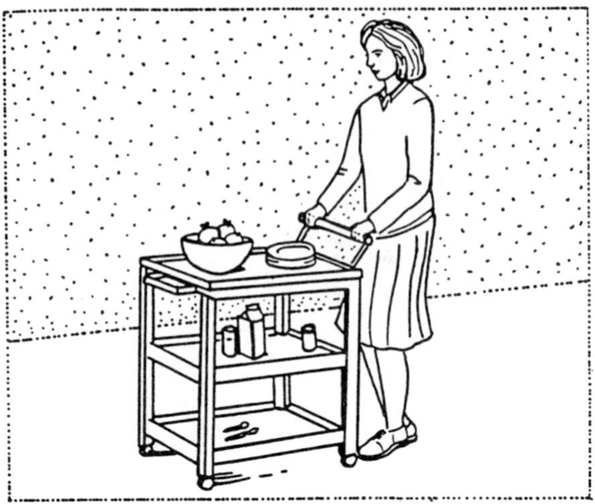

Figure 10-17. Use of wheels reduces stress on joints. (From The Arthritis Society: Think Ahead, How to Manage Pain and Fatigue. Ontario Division, Toronto, The Arthritis Society, 1990. With permission.)

wagon can greatly assist garden activities. When traveling, luggage on wheels is a necessity.

Conclusion

It is very important for clients to become involved and take responsibility for management of their arthritis. Arthritis can be controlled in most individuals; however, the search for a cure continues. Our research, however, has shown that clients, by incorporating the principles in this chapter, can help themselves and develop a sense of control over their disease. Consultation with appropriate health care professionals is of utmost importance for the client who wants to enhance their quality of life. The physical therapist should work closely with the occupational therapist to reinforce recommended lifestyle changes, the wearing of orthoses, and appropriate footwear.

Case Study

Mrs K is a 33-year-old right-handed homemaker who was diagnosed in 1990 with rheumatoid arthritis. She lives in a two-storied house with her husband and 4-year-old son. Her chief complaints were constant tiredness, pain in her feet, difficulty looking after her son, and doing housework.

Assessment

On evaluation, she had 26 active joints with 12 effusions involving hands, feet, and knees. The damaged joint count was three. Grip strength was reduced: R, 120 mm Hg; L, 130 mm Hg. Morning stiffness was consistently 1.5 hours. Sensation was intact.

There was moderate limitation of both active and passive ROM of the elbows, shoulders, hips, and knees attributed to pain. Functional limitations included the following: difficulty lifting heavy objects such as pots and pans, opening jars, peeling and chopping, dressing hygiene and child care due to pain, and decreased strength. Heavy housework, such as vacuuming, also was a problem. Walking farther than a block was limited by foot pain. Constant fatigue interfered with her functional abilities.

Goals of Treatment

Goals were discussed with Mrs K and mutually agreed upon. They were to improve hand function, increase walking tolerance, decrease the fatigue level, and improve her functional capabilities.

Treatment Strategies

Bilateral work splints were provided to increase grip strength and decrease pain in wrists on activity. Bilateral resting splints were fabricated to place the joints of the wrist and fingers in loose-packed position while providing proper positioning and reducing the amount of morning stiffness.

A foot assessment was completed and Mrs K given a prescription for supportive footwear. (In Ontario, Canada, running shoes are an orthopedic prescription; client pays no tax.) When appropriate running shoes were purchased, metatarsal pads and longitudinal arch supports were added under the converter insole. This provided relief of pain in the ball of the foot, and walking tolerance increased.

Energy conservation and joint protection techniques were reviewed and practiced while the therapist was in the home. Emphasis was placed on working out a balance between rest and activity. Since finances were not a concern and her husband did not have time to help with the heavier tasks, domestic help was hired for 2 days/week. Structural changes were made to the house to facilitate ADL. A laundry chute was installed to decrease stair usage. The tub in the master bathroom was replaced with a walk-in shower. A hand-held shower head and a shower seat were added to facilitate safety and protect her joints. Mrs K was provided with built-up grips for cooking utensils, a jar opener, a book rest, and a wide-handled potato peeler. Levered taps were installed in the kitchen and bathroom.

Without the heavier tasks to do, Mrs K was able to pace herself and have time for her son and his activities. She was now able to fit in her own interests. She enrolled in a modified aquatics program and joined a gardening club to learn more about hydroponics. At the 6-month follow-up, Mrs K had 12 active joints and three effusions and no further change in the damaged joint count. Grip strength was increased (R, 180 mm Hg; L, 190 mm Hg) and morning stiffness had decreased to 30 minutes. Mrs K reported she had increased energy and could walk for 1 hour without foot discomfort. Improved hand function enabled her to lift her son and open jars while wearing her work splints.

This case study demonstrates the value of appropriate orthotics, energy conservation, and joint protection techniques, with the client accepting responsibility for effective management of the disease process.

References

1. Merritt J: Advances in orthotics for the patient with rheumatoid arthritis. J Rheumatol 1987; 14(Suppl 15):62–67.
2. Zoeckler AA, Nicholas JJ: Prenyl hand splint for rheumatoid arthritis. Phys Ther 1969; 49:377–379.
3. Fess EE, Philips CA: Hand Splinting: Principals and Methods, 2nd edition, pp 309–324. St Louis, CV Mosby Co, 1987.
4. Biddulph SL: The effect of the Futuro wrist brace in pain conditions of the wrist. S Afr Med J 1981; 60: 389–391.
5. Eyring EJ, Murray WR: The effect of joint position on the pressure of intra-articular effusion. J Bone Joint Surg 1964; 46A(6):1235–1241.
6. Nordenskiold U: Elastic wrist orthosis. Reduction of pain and increase in grip force for females with rheumatoid arthritis. Arthritis Care Res 1990; 3:158–162.
7. Backman CL, Deitz JC: Static wrist splint: its effect on hand function in three women with rheumatoid arthritis. Arthritis Care Res 1988; 1:151–160.
8. Falconer J: Hand splinting in rheumatoid arthritis. A perspective on current knowledge and directions for research. Arthritis Care Res 1991; 4:81–86.
9. Melvin JL: Orthotic treatment for arthritis of the hand. In Rheumatic Disease in the Adult and Child: Occupational Therapy and Rehabilitation, 3rd edition, pp 379–418. Philadelphia, FA Davis Co, 1989.
10. Swanson AB: Flexible Implant Resection Arthroplasty in the Hand and Extremities, pp 171–183. St Louis, CV Mosby, 1973.
11. Belcon MC, Haynes RB, Tugwell P.: A critical review of compliance studies in rheumatoid arthritis. Arthritis Rheum 1984; 27:1227–1233.
12. Moon M, Moon B, Black W: Compliance in splint-wearing behavior of patients with rheumatoid arthritis. N Z Med J 1976; 83:360–365.
13. Feinberg J, Brandt KD: Use of resting splints by patients with rheumatoid arthritis. Am J Occup Ther 1981; 35:173–178.
14. Nicholas JJ, Gruen H, Weiner G, et al: Splinting in rheumatoid arthritis. I. Factors affecting patient compliance. Arch Phys Med Rehabil 1982; 63:92–94.
15. Feinberg J: Effect of the arthritis health professional on compliance, with use of resting hand splints by patients with rheumatoid arthritis. Arthritis Care Res 1992; 5:17–23.
16. Keenan MA, Peabody TD, Gronley JK, et al: Valgus deformities of the feet and characteristics of gait in patients who have rheumatoid arthritis. J Bone Joint Surg 1991; 73A:237–247.
17. Spiegel TM, Spiegel JS: Rheumatoid arthritis in the foot and ankle—diagnosis, pathology and treatment. The relationship between foot and ankle de-

formity and disease duration in 50 patients. Foot Ankle 1982; 2:318–324.
18. Jahss MH: The subtalar complex. In Jahss MH (ed): Disorders of the Foot, vol 1, pp 727–763. Philadelphia, WB Saunders Co, 1982.
19. Mann RA: Biomechanics. In Jahss MH (ed): Disorders of the Foot, vol 1, pp 37–67. Philadelphia, WB Saunders Co, 1982.
20. Giannestras N: Foot Disorders: Medical and Surgical Management, 3rd edition. Philadelphia, Lea & Febiger, 1980.
21. Inman VT: Hallux valgus: a review of etiologic factors. Orthop Clin North Am 1974; 5(1):59–63.
22. Thomas WH: Reconstructive surgery and rehabilitation of the ankle and foot. In Kelley WM, et al (eds): Textbook of Rheumatology, vol 2, pp 1999–2013. Philadelphia, WB Saunders Co, 1981.
23. The Arthritis Society B.C. Division: Principles of Arthritis Management—The Team Approach, pp 87–88. The Arthritis Society, B.C. Division, 1984.
24. Bouysset M, Tebib J, Noel E, et al: Rheumatoid metatarsus. The original evolution of the first metatarsal. Clin Rheumatol 1991; 10(4):408–412.
25. Deland JT, Wood B: Foot Pain. In Kelley WM, Harris ED, Ruddy S, et al (eds): Textbook of Rheumatology, 4th edition, vol 1, pp 457–469. Philadelphia, WB Saunders Co, 1993.
26. Helewa A, Goldsmith CH, Lee P, et al: Effects of occupational therapy home service on patients with rheumatoid arthritis. Lancet 1991; 337:1453–1456.
27. Silwa J: Performance objectives for joint protection instruction. AHP Newsletter Arthritis Foundation, 1978; 12(4).
28. Arthritis Society: Think Ahead: How to Manage Pain and Fatigue. The Arthritis Society, Ontario Division 1990, 16 pp.
29. Gilbert D: Energy expenditures for the disabled homemaker: review of studies. Am J Occup Ther 1965; 19:321–328.

Additional Readings

Brand P: Clinical Mechanics of the Hand. St Louis, CV Mosby Co, 1985.

Fess E, Philips CA: Hand Splinting: Principles and Methods, 2nd edition. St. Louis, CV Mosby Co, 1987.

Ziegler E: Current Concepts in Orthotics: A Diagnosis-Related Approach to Splinting. Rolyan Medical Products, 1984.

Malick M: Manual on Static Hand Splinting, 2nd edition. Pittsburgh, Hammarville Rehabilitation Center, 1972.

Malick M: Manual on Dynamic Hand Splinting with Thermoplastic Materials. Pittsburgh, Hammarville Rehabilitation Center, 1974.

CHAPTER 11

Cardiovascular Health and Physical Fitness for the Client with Multiple Joint Involvement

Marian A. Minor, PhD, PT

Prolonged inactivity and poor fitness are clearly associated with increased mortality and morbidity. Inactivity is an independent risk factor in all causes of mortality. Inactivity is as important as smoking, obesity, and elevated cholesterol in increasing the likelihood of coronary artery disease, atherosclerosis, hypertension, diabetes, and some types of cancer.[1] Whether inactivity is due to a self-selected sedentary life style or the diagnosis of arthritis, the threat to health and longevity is similar and clear. In addition, for the person with multiple joint involvement, the consequences of prolonged inactivity add dramatically to the problems of pain, stiffness, loss of motion, weakness, functional limitation, and disability.

The purpose of this chapter is to provide information relevant to exercise, physical fitness, and health for the person with multiple joint involvement. The impact of inactivity and the benefits and

PHYSICAL THERAPY IN ARTHRITIS, Joan M. Walker, PhD, PT, and Antoine Helewa, MSc(Clin Epid), PT, W.B. Saunders Company feasibility of exercise for the person with arthritis will be described. The role of the health professional in promoting successful exercise behaviors will be discussed, as well as methods of appropriate physical fitness assessment and exercise prescription. The discussion of exercise program implementation will include program content and structure.

Inactivity and Exercise in Arthritis

The presence of arthritis can create serious health problems in ways other than direct consequences of disease and side effects of therapy. Arthritis is the primary cause for limitation in physical activity in adults. In persons over 65, 12% report limitation in physical activity due to arthritis.[2] Heart disease is a close second. Persons with a diagnosis of rheumatoid arthritis (RA) have reported that one of the first adaptations they make is to give up leisure and recreational activities, a primary source of physical activity for adults. In addition to the threat of prolonged inactivity to general health, inactivity produces many of the same signs and symptoms traditionally attributed to the arthritis disease process, namely: muscle weakness and atrophy, decreased flexibility, cardiovascular deficit, fatigue, incoordination, osteoporosis, depression, and lowered pain threshold (see Chapter 3).

It is well documented that many persons with arthritis are deconditioned and less fit than their peers without arthritis. Cardiovascular deficits in persons with RA and osteoarthritis (OA) have been measured at 40% and 20%, respectively.[3] Increased oxygen uptake, heart rate, and ventilation, indicative of increased energy expenditure and early-onset fatigue, have been reported during submaximal exercise performance.[8] Figure 11-1 displays measurements of fitness and functional tasks in persons with RA and OA compared to noninvolved peers.

Are people with arthritis in poor physical condition due to the disease process itself? Do we think to ourselves, "Of course she's in bad shape, she has arthritis"? In recent years, this widespread assumption has been challenged by a growing number of persons with arthritis and arthritis health professionals who have engaged in studies of the efficacy of conditioning exercise programs to improve health and fitness.

Stationary bicycle, walking, aquatic exercise, and low-impact aerobic dance have been investigated.[4–11] Some protocols also included resistance exercise for muscle strengthening, and all included flexibility exercise. Intensity of the aerobic stimulus has been reported at 60–80% of age-predicted maximal heart rate for durations of 15–30 minutes. Frequency generally has been three to four times a week for 8–16 weeks. The majority of persons with either RA or OA, between the 20th and 80th decades, participating in the exercise research were living independently in their own community. Results of these studies have shown 12–21% improvement in cardiovascular performance, 0–55% increase in muscle strength, as well as significant increases in flexibility. Traditional measures of arthritis disease activity, such as grip strength, 50-ft (15.24 m) walking time, and articular index have demonstrated either improvement or no change in disease activity/severity. Measurements of function and health status also showed significant improvement in areas of physical and social activity, depression, anxiety, and self-concept. The findings of these studies demonstrated that although many people were deconditioned when they began an exercise program, most were able to exercise at levels necessary to produce a training effect and made significant gains in fitness, health status, and function. Table 11-1 displays results of exercise studies in arthritis.

Role of the Health Professional in Exercise Adoption and Maintenance

The person with arthritis can exercise to maintain or improve health and physical fitness. Information to guide development of successful exercise programs is now becoming available to both health professionals and persons with arthritis (see Table 11-2). *Knowledge itself, however, is not sufficient to ensure adoption and maintenance of safe and healthy exercise behaviors.*

Beliefs and Barriers

Positive beliefs about the usefulness of exercise and minimal barriers to the performance of exercise are necessary for a person to begin and maintain new exercise behaviors. The health professional must believe that exercise for health and fitness is important and feasible and be willing to explore the beliefs of the client in the process of making exercise recommendations. In addition, work and home roles and responsibilities, socioeconomic

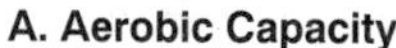

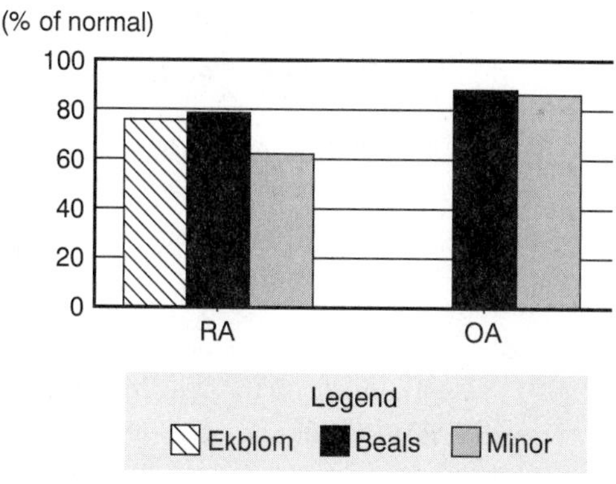

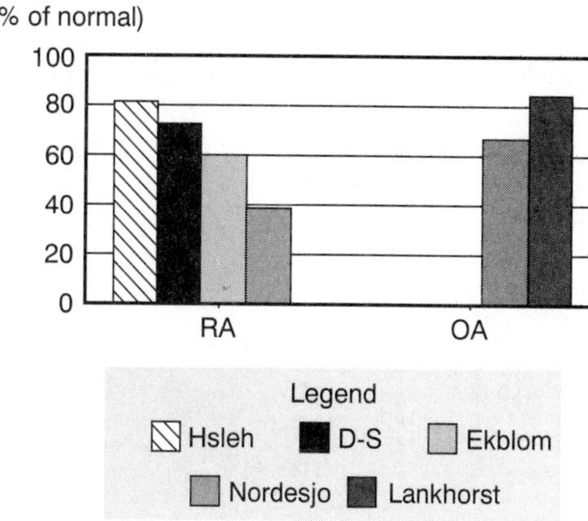

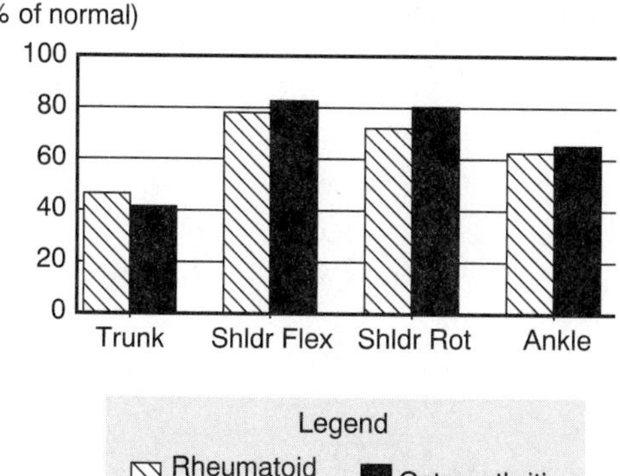

D. Functional Tasks
(Ekblom et al., 1974)

Task	Deficit
Walk	42%
Stairs (up and down)	40%
Step height	24%

Figure 11-1 Comparative physical function in arthritis. Measurements of: (*A*) aerobic capacity,[8,22,23] (*B*) muscle strength,[22,24–26] (*C*) flexibility,[8] and (*D*) functional performance[22] of persons with rheumatoid arthritis (RA) and osteoarthritis (OA) compared to controls or published norms. Results are expressed as a percentage of normal (100%) of each measurement. Shldr Flex, shoulder flexion; Shldr Rot, medial and lateral shoulder rotation; Ankle, dorsiflexion. (From Minor MA: Physical activity and management of arthritis. Ann Behav Med 1991; 13[3]:117–123. With permission.)

considerations, and client preference must be taken into consideration to eliminate as many barriers as possible.

Self-Efficacy for Exercise

One of the most important factors in the willingness to adopt and subsequently maintain a new behavior is a positive belief in the ability to perform that behavior—self-efficacy. This is particularly true in exercise and affects both willingness to begin participation and ability to maintain the habit. Self-efficacy for a particular activity can change. Self-efficacy increases with personal, successful experiences and that of others in the activity, as well as having a positive interpretation of sensations surrounding the activity.[12]

The health professional plays a key role in helping the person with arthritis build self-efficacy for exercise. Setting realistic goals, including previously successful experiences, offering peer groups, and designing periodic assessments to reinforce the efficacy of the exercise are only a few strategies that can be used to build self-efficacy for exercise.

Table 11-1. Efficacy of Physical Conditioning Exercise in Rheumatoid Arthritis and Osteoarthritis*†

Variable	Ekblom et al[4]	Harkcom et al[6]	Danneskiold-Samsoe et al[7]	Minor et al[8]	Perlman et al[9]
Sample					
No. subjects/Dx	23/RA	20/RA	8/RA	40/RA:80/OA	43/RA
Age (yrs)	38–63	27–68	35–66	21–83	27–81
Intervention					
Length (wks)	5	12	8	12	16
Frequency	bid	3x/wk	2x/wk	3x/wk	2x/wk
Duration (mins)	20–40	15–30	45	60	60
Intensity	NR	70% MHR	NR	60–80% MHR	60–70% MHR
Mode	Bicycle; strength	Bicycle	Pool; strength	Pool; walk	Low-impact aerobic dance
Physical Results					
Aerobic capacity	21% inc	32% inc	12% inc	20% inc	NR
Endurance	50% inc	39% inc	NR	26% inc	NR
Strength	27–55% inc	NSD	9–38% inc	NR	NR
Flexibility	NR	NR	NR	25% inc	NR
Physical activity	NR	NSD	NR	27% inc	16% inc
Psychosocial Results					
Depression	NR	NR	NR	23–37% dec	25% dec
Anxiety	NR	NR	NR	19% dec	NSD
Pain	NSD	NSD	NR	13–23% dec	17% dec
Disease Results					
Joint involvement	NSD	41% dec	NR	40% dec	25–40% dec
Grip strength	NR	NSD	NR	22% inc	NR
50-ft walk time	NR	NSD	NR	12% dec	17% dec

*From Minor MA: Physical activity and management of arthritis. Ann Behav Med 1991; 13(3):117–123. With permission.

†Review of published intervention studies, 1975–1990.

Dx, diagnosis; NR, not reported; NSD, no significant difference from mean baseline value ($p \geq .05$); MHR, maximal heart rate; inc, increase; dec, decrease.

Exercise for Health and Fitness

Physical fitness is a useful concept in the assessment and recommendation of exercise for all persons. Physical fitness has five components:

1. Cardiovascular status
2. Muscle strength
3. Muscle endurance
4. Flexibility
5. Body composition

A comprehensive exercise evaluation and prescription should consider current capacity and needs in all five areas. To achieve improved fitness, an effective and safe exercise prescription incorporates current status and abilities of the individual in a training program that supplies physiologic overload to produce adaptation and improve cardiovascular and musculoskeletal function.

The exercise prescription should incorporate current levels of fitness, abilities, and preferences of the exerciser in a program that supplies physiologic overload to achieve adaptation and improvement in cardiovascular and musculoskeletal function.

Table 11–2. Exercise Tips for the New Exerciser

Walking
- Start on flat, level surface. Use cane if helpful.
- Stretch out heel cord and calf muscles before and after.
- Warm up and cool down with a stroll.
- Choose a comfortable pace. Sing or talk as you go along.
- If knees get sore, walk more slowly and swing your arms to get the briskness you want.
- Wear supportive shoes with good soles. Athletic (shock absorbing) insoles can help increase comfort and reduce shock on feet, knees, hips, and spine.

Swimming
- Swim only with life guard present.
- Vary strokes for comfort and overall conditioning.
- Use mask and snorkel if head turning is a problem.
- Begin and end at a slower pace.
- If water is cool, finish up with a warm shower or soak.

Water Aerobics
- Protect your feet with water shoes or slippers.
- Don't get chilled. Take a warm shower or bath afterward.
- Wear tights, t-shirt, disposable latex gloves to retain body heat in the water.
- Use flotation device to add buoyancy if knees and hips are painful.
- Regulate exercise intensity by changing the speed, arc of movement, and length of lever arm. Going more slowly, through a smaller arc, or with flexed elbows or knees lessens your exertion and joint stress.

Bicycle (outdoors or stationary)
- Start and end with no resistance or on flat ground.
- Pedal with ball of your foot.
- Make sure seat height allows your knee to be comfortably straight at the bottom of the pedal stroke.
- Don't lean on or over handlebars.
- Feet should be able to swivel freely within pedal straps.
- Keep speed of pedalling at or below 60 rpm. Use gears if applicable to protect knees.

Low-Impact Aerobic Dance
- Wear shoes and exercise on a hard floor or firm carpet.
- Don't bounce, lunge, or do low squats.
- Control your movements. Don't move too fast at the outer range of your movements.
- Change movements frequently if you start to feel muscle fatigue or joint soreness.
- Avoid prolonged exercise with arms, especially with arms above shoulder level.

It is important to recognize the distinction between exercise training to improve physical fitness and exercise habits to improve or maintain health. Early investigations in the field of exercise science often studied healthy young men who were also athletes. The focus was generally to improve competitive performance in persons who were already fit. Therefore, much of the information about prescribing exercise to improve fitness indicated that fairly intense exercise regimens were needed. Recent epidemiologic studies of health risk factors and exercise research in less fit populations, however, reveal important information. These findings are relevant to the health and fitness of persons with musculoskeletal impairments and limitations in mobility.

It is not necessary for a person to participate in an intense, highly regimented exercise program or attain a high level of athletic fitness to improve health status. Even persons with low fitness levels who engage in low-intensity but regular physical activity are at significantly less risk for a number of degenerative and potentially fatal conditions. Increased activity improves health status even in the presence of other risk factors.

A routine that includes 20- to 30-minute sessions of low- to moderate-intensity exertion in an aerobic activity three to five times a week is necessary for health maintenance and is sufficient to significantly reduce the probability of cardiovascular illness. Such a routine would be comparable to a comfortable but somewhat brisk walk, bicycle ride, swim, or household tasks such as mowing the yard or raking leaves.

Persons who are extremely deconditioned can achieve significant improvements in cardiovascular capacity, muscle strength, and endurance when they participate in regular exercise at low levels of intensity. Regular walking, swimming, or bicycling at moderate levels of intensity can result in significant improvement in cardiovascular health and muscular strength and endurance in older and deconditioned persons.

Obesity is also associated with inactivity. A healthy proportion of lean to fat body mass is necessary for good health, as well as for physical fitness. In addition to the medical problems associated with obesity, obesity is also associated with knee OA in women.[13] Healthy levels of body fat for men and women are 20% and 30%, respectively.

In addition to dietary manipulations restricting total calories and fat, a successful weight management program requires a regular exercise program. From early childhood, obesity is more closely related to low levels of physical activity than to excessive caloric intake. Low- to moderate-intensity aerobic activities performed at least three to four times a week for at least 30 minutes a session improves weight loss and maintenance. This type of exercise not only increases total energy expenditure during and for some period of time following the exercise, but also improves fat oxidation and raises metabolic rate over the long term. Inefficient oxidation of fat appears to be a major discriminator between obese and nonobese people. A daily program that increases energy expenditure by 100 calories (equivalent to walking or jogging 0.6 km) and decreases caloric intake by 100 calories (one slice of bread with pat of butter) can result in the loss of 4.5 kg in 6 months.

Body composition also can be improved by muscle strength training that produces muscle hypertrophy. The increased muscle mass and increased percentage of metabolically active tissue serve to increase the resting metabolic rate and reduce the proportion of fat stores in the body.

Studies of resistance training for muscle strengthening in persons with RA and OA have indicated that increases in strength, muscle hypertrophy, and lean body mass are possible and associated with improved function and decreased pain.[3,5,6,9–11]

Persons with arthritis are a heterogenous population, ranging widely in age, disease, impairments, functional goals, and interests. Some are interested in and capable of performing exercise programs with a goal to improve physical fitness. Other persons may need instruction and support to participate in cardiovascular or pulmonary rehabilitation programs (see Table 11-2). Others may not be candidates for fitness training programs, but can be educated and encouraged to adopt appropriate exercise habits to improve or maintain health and reduce the risk of inactivity-related illness.

Low- to moderate-intensity aerobic activities performed at least three to four times a week, for at least 30 minutes a session, improve weight loss and maintenance.

Physical Fitness Assessment

Assessment of physical fitness and exercise status, in addition to disease-related considerations, is the foundation for the prescription of safe and effective exercise. Assessment also provides a baseline from which to monitor for harm and measure progress. The multidimensional, holistic concept of physical fitness is particularly appropriate for assessment and exercise recommendation for persons with arthritis. Physical fitness is a comprehensive look at musculoskeletal and cardiovascular function. This comprehensive yet categorical perspective allows specificity and grading of the exercise program as required by current need and changes in disease status. Physical fitness also provides a popular health- and wellness-oriented framework into which therapeutic exercise can be incorporated. This can be especially important for the acceptance and adoption of healthy exercise behaviors by the person with arthritis.

Assessment measures should be chosen to meet client and professional needs. There are a variety of assessments of the components of fitness that have been standardized and allow comparison to age- and gender-matched peers without arthritis.[14–17] Other measures, such as grip strength, 13.5-m (50-ft) walking time, isokinetic knee extension, and aerobic capacity have been used in arthritis and exercise research and reported in the scientific literature. These measures have proven validity and safety for use by persons with arthritis. Research needs require the use of such measures to allow meaningful comparison and communication of results. Assessment for clinical documentation and personal information can be met by more individualized approaches guided by functional needs and program goals. A comprehensive test of physical fitness must include assessment of all five components.

Cardiovascular Assessment

Cardiovascular fitness or aerobic capacity is primarily a function of the body's capacity to transport and use oxygen to sustain physical exertion. Good cardiovascular fitness requires an efficient heart, healthy pulmonary and vascular systems, and aerobically conditioned muscle.

Cardiovascular assessment prior to exercise can be performed for two reasons: *diagnosis of cardiovascular disease* and *assessment of current aerobic fitness*. Some information about current cardiovascular fitness is necessary for the prescription of an individualized exercise program. This information can be obtained by self-report or by a submaximal test of exercise performance. The assessment of current fitness by these means, however, does not supply information about possible cardiovascular disease. Thus, safety for increased activity must be addressed by other means. The Physical Activity Readiness Questionnaire (PAR-Q) (Fig. 11-2)[14] is frequently used for initial screening in nonmedical settings prior to beginning an exercise program.

Cardiovascular Disease

Opinions vary regarding the necessity of a physician-supervised exercise stress test with 12-lead electrocardiograph (ECG) before beginning an aerobic exercise program. At this time, the American College of Sports Medicine (ACSM) recommends that risk factors, symptoms, and the intensity of the exercise to be performed should be considered in determining the need for a physician-supervised exercise stress test.[18] Guidelines for exercise testing recommendations appear in Table 11-3.

Other sources suggest self-report screening, such as the PAR-Q or clearance by medical history.

For persons with a history of systemic inflammatory disease with the potential for cardiovascular or pulmonary involvement, a careful history and medical review is necessary before any marked increase in physical activity. The choice of a submaximal or symptom-limited stress test, with or without physician supervision or gas exchange analysis, should be based on medical considerations and institutional policy.

Aerobic Capacity

Aerobic capacity can be assessed by a variety of methods. Self-reports of intensity, duration, and frequency of current physical activity can be useful. Submaximal clinical and field tests of exercise performance estimate aerobic fitness by comparing the intensity of the exercise (speed or distance traveled or workload achieved) and the heart rate response. Results can be expressed as levels of fitness or as aerobic capacity by rate of oxygen consumption (in milliliters per kilogram per minute). Choice of an assessment measure should be based on the following considerations: need to compare to normative data, research or clinical use of data, current ability, and joint status of the client. Follow-up testing to evaluate effectiveness of the exercise program will provide the most meaningful information if the assessment mode matches the training mode (e.g., bicycle exercise/bicycle ergometer; walking exercise/treadmill or walking field test).

Muscle Strength

Muscular strength is the force generated by muscular contraction. Strength can be improved and measured by isometric, isotonic, or isokinetic contractions. Muscle strength is associated with strength in tendons and ligaments, as well as increased muscle mass. To achieve functional gains, muscle strengthening programs must consider the principle of specificity of training. Therapeutic assessment of muscle strength is traditionally by manual muscle test, determination of a maximum load (1RM), and more recently the use of a dynamometer to quantify torque and work. Fitness assessments of muscle strength also have been developed for use in field settings and are generally performance based. Grip strength and pull-ups are examples of these tests. The choice of muscle strength assessment (type, speed, and range of contraction) should consider the following: muscle groups that will be trained, muscle groups that could be expected to improve as a result of the general exercise routine, and muscle strength important to function.

Muscle Endurance

Muscle endurance is the capacity of muscle to sustain force over time. Endurance can be measured and trained in all types of contractions and can be either aerobic or anaerobic. Muscle endurance is associated with the ability to sustain a level of per-

Physical Activity Readiness Questionnaire - PAR-Q (revised 1994)

PAR - Q & YOU

(A Questionnaire for People Aged 15 to 69)

Regular physical activity is fun and healthy, and increasingly more people are starting to become more active every day. Being more active is very safe for most people. However, some people should check with their doctor before they start becoming much more physically active.

If you are planning to become much more physically active than you are now, start by answering the seven questions in the box below. If you are between the ages of 15 and 69, the PAR-Q will tell you if you should check with your doctor before you start. If you are over 69 years of age, and you are not used to being very active, check with your doctor.

Common sense is your best guide when you answer these questions. Please read the questions carefully and answer each one honestly: check YES or NO.

YES	NO		
☐	☐	1.	Has your doctor ever said that you have a heart condition and that you should only do physical activity recommended by a doctor?
☐	☐	2.	Do you feel pain in your chest when you do physical activity?
☐	☐	3.	In the past month, have you had chest pain when you were not doing physical activity?
☐	☐	4.	Do you lose your balance because of dizziness or do you ever lose consciousness?
☐	☐	5.	Do you have a bone or joint problem that could be made worse by a change in your physical activity?
☐	☐	6.	Is your doctor currently prescribing drugs (for example, water pills) for your blood pressure or heart condition?
☐	☐	7.	Do you know of any other reason why you should not do physical activity?

If you answered

YES to one or more questions

Talk with your doctor by phone or in person BEFORE you start becoming much more physically active or BEFORE you have a fitness appraisal. Tell your doctor about the PAR-Q and which questions you answered YES.

- You may be able to do any activity you want — as long as you start slowly and build up gradually. Or, you may need to restrict your activities to those which are safe for you. Talk with your doctor about the kinds of activities you wish to participate in and follow his/her advice.
- Find out which community programs are safe and helpful for you.

NO to all questions

If you answered NO honestly to all PAR-Q questions, you can be reasonably sure that you can:

- start becoming much more physically active — begin slowly and build up gradually. This is the safest and easiest way to go.
- take part in a fitness appraisal — this is an excellent way to determine your basic fitness so that you can plan the best way for you to live actively.

DELAY BECOMING MUCH MORE ACTIVE:

- if you are not feeling well because of a temporary illness such as a cold or a fever — wait until you feel better; or
- if you are or may be pregnant — talk to your doctor before you start becoming more active.

Please note: If your health changes so that you then answer YES to any of the above questions, tell your fitness or health professional. Ask whether you should change your physical activity plan.

Informed Use of the PAR-Q: The Canadian Society for Exercise Physiology, Health Canada, and their agents assume no liability for persons who undertake physical activity, and if in doubt after completing this questionnaire, consult your doctor prior to physical activity.

You are encouraged to copy the PAR-Q but only if you use the entire form

NOTE: If the PAR-Q is being given to a person before he or she participates in a physical activity program or a fitness appraisal, this section may be used for legal or administrative purposes.

I have read, understood and completed this questionnaire. Any questions I had were answered to my full satisfaction.

NAME ______________________

SIGNATURE ______________________ DATE ______________________

SIGNATURE OF PARENT ______________________ WITNESS ______________________
or GUARDIAN (for participants under the age of majority)

continued on other side...

Supported by:  Health Canada Santé Canada

Figure 11-2. Physical Activity Readiness Questionnaire (PAR-Q) (revised 1994), for people aged 15–69. (From Canadian Standardized Test of Fitness Operations Manual, 3rd edition. Fitness Canada, 1986; revised 1994 Canadian Society for Exercise Physiology, Gloucester. With permission.) *Illustration continued on opposite page*

...continued from other side

PAR - Q & YOU

Physical Activity Readiness Questionnaire - PAR-Q (revised 1994)

We know that being physically active provides benefits for all of us. Not being physically active is recognized by the Heart and Stroke Foundation of Canada as one of the four modifiable primary risk factors for coronary heart disease (along with high blood pressure, high blood cholesterol, and smoking). People are physically active for many reasons — play, work, competition, health, creativity, enjoying the outdoors, being with friends. There are also as many ways of being active as there are reasons. What we choose to do depends on our own abilities and desires. No matter what the reason or type of activity, physical activity can improve our well-being and quality of life. Well-being can also be enhanced by integrating physical activity with enjoyable healthy eating and positive self and body image. Together, all three equal VITALITY. So take a fresh approach to living. Check out the VITALITY tips below!

Active Living:

- accumulate 30 minutes or more of moderate physical activity most days of the week
- take the stairs instead of an elevator
- get off the bus early and walk home
- join friends in a sport activity
- take the dog for a walk with the family
- follow a fitness program

Healthy Eating:

- follow Canada's Food Guide to Healthy Eating
- enjoy a variety of foods
- emphasize cereals, breads, other grain products, vegetables and fruit
- choose lower-fat dairy products, leaner meats and foods prepared with little or no fat
- achieve and maintain a healthy body weight by enjoying regular physical activity and healthy eating
- limit salt, alcohol and caffeine
- don't give up foods you enjoy — aim for moderation and variety

Positive Self and Body Image:

- accept who you are and how you look
- remember, a healthy weight range is one that is realistic for your own body make-up (body fat levels should neither be too high nor too low)
- try a new challenge
- compliment yourself
- reflect positively on your abilities
- laugh a lot

Enjoy eating well, being active and feeling good about yourself. That's VITALITY®

FITNESS AND HEALTH PROFESSIONALS MAY BE INTERESTED IN THE INFORMATION BELOW.

The following companion forms are available for doctors' use by contacting the Canadian Society for Exercise Physiology (address below):

The **Physical Activity Readiness Medical Examination (PARmed-X)** - to be used by doctors with people who answer YES to one or more questions on the PAR-Q.

The **Physical Activity Readiness Medical Examination for Pregnancy (PARmed-X for PREGNANCY)** - to be used by doctors with pregnant patients who wish to become more active.

References:

Arraix, G.A., Wigle, D.T., Mao, Y. (1992). Risk Assessment of Physical Activity and Physical Fitness in the Canada Health Survey Follow-Up Study. **J. Clin. Epidemiol.** 45:4 419-428.

Mottola, M., Wolfe, L.A. (1994). Active Living and Pregnancy, In: A. Quinney, L. Gauvin, T. Wall (eds.), **Toward Active Living: Proceedings of the International Conference on Physical Activity, Fitness and Health**. Champaign, IL: Human Kinetics.

PAR-Q Validation Report, British Columbia Ministry of Health, 1978.

Thomas, S., Reading, J., Shephard, R.J. (1992). Revision of the Physical Activity Readiness Questionnaire (PAR-Q). **Can. J. Spt. Sci.** 17:4 338-345.

***To order multiple printed copies of the PAR-Q**, please contact the*

Canadian Society for Exercise Physiology
1600 James Naismith Dr., Suite 311
Gloucester, Ontario CANADA K1B 5N4
Tel. (613) 748-5768 FAX: (613) 748-5763

The original PAR-Q was developed by the British Columbia Ministry of Health. It has been revised by an Expert Advisory Committee assembled by the Canadian Society for Exercise Physiology and Fitness Canada (1994).

Disponible en français sous le titre «Questionnaire sur l'aptitude à l'activité physique - Q-AAP (revisé 1994)».

Supported by: 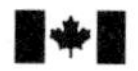 Health Canada Santé Canada

Figure 11-2. *Continued*

Table 11-3. Guidelines for Exercise Testing*

Purpose
Screen for silent ischemia
Basis for exercise prescription

Coronary Artery Disease Risk Factors (≥ to 2 = at risk)
Hypertension, BP ≥160/90 mm Hg
Serum cholesterol ≥240 mg/dl (6.2 mmol/L)
Cigarette smoking
Diabetes mellitus
Family history

Perform Supervised Exercise Stress Test for
1. Apparently healthy: men ≥40 yrs; women ≥50 yrs for *vigorous* exercise only
2. Persons at risk with no symptoms: all ages for *vigorous* exercise only
3. Persons at risk with symptoms and with disease: all ages for moderate and vigorous exercise

*Data from Gordon NF, Kohl HW, Scott CB, et al: Reassessment of the guidelines for exercise testing. Sports Med 1992; 13(5):293–302.

formance without fatigue. It is closely related to functional ability and strength. Energy-efficient maintenance of good posture requires endurance in postural muscles at a low intensity of isometric contraction. Endurance is tested easily with timed maximum repetition tests of submaximal muscular effort (sit-ups, leg extensions) or functional tasks (sit to stand, toe raises). Using this strategy, a greater number of repetitions accomplished within the time period represents improved muscle endurance. Endurance testing also is possible on most of the computerized muscle testing and rehabilitation equipment. Meaningful measures of muscle endurance are those that simulate functional needs and are specific to the muscle groups responsible for the performance.

Flexibility

Flexibility is the component of fitness measured by the active range of motion of the spine and extremities. Flexibility, affected by joint structure, as well as periarticular tissue extensibility, is a measure particularly relevant for persons with arthritis. Disease processes, inactivity, and pain converge to produce decreased joint range of motion and general inflexibility. Goniometry of selected joints and field tests, such as the sit-and-reach test (Canadian Standardized Test of Fitness), provide useful information upon which to base the exercise prescription and provide baseline information. Progress in client-selected functional tasks that are limited by lack of flexibility also may be used to assess progress (reaching over head, kneeling, putting on shoes).

Meaningful measures of muscle endurance should simulate functional needs and be specific to the muscle groups responsible for the performance.

Body Composition

Body composition is the proportion (percentage) of lean to fat body mass. Body composition is a better gauge of health and fitness than is weight. Although definitions of obesity vary, 20% and 30% body fat are considered upper limits of body fat for men and women, respectively. Body fat can be influenced successfully by weight management programs that include dietary and exercise changes. Exercise programs that increase muscle mass, stimulate fat oxidation, and/or increase energy expenditure can reduce the percentage of body fat.

Body composition can be assessed adequately by measurement of skin folds and use of appropriate tabled norms or formulae.[16,17] Computerized bioelectrical impedance methods also are available. Calculation of waist/hip girth ratio can be used to assess changes in body fat distribution. Fat deposits in chest and abdomen are associated with greater risk for cardiovascular disease. A waist/hip girth ratio greater than 0.9 is considered a health risk.

Assessment Tools

Selecting appropriate measurement tools to measure physical fitness in persons with multiple joint involvement requires a consideration of physical ability and disease status. The three sources listed below contain a variety of measurement tools from which to choose.

Sources of Fitness Measurement Tools

1. Cole B, Finch E, Gowland C, Mayo N: In Basmajian J (ed): Physical Rehabilitation

Outcome Measures. Toronto, Ontario, Canadian Physiotherapy Association, 1994.
2. Neiman DC: Fitness and Sports Medicine. Palo Alto, CA, Bull Publishing Company, 1990.
3. Pollock ML, Wilmore JH: Exercise in Health and Disease, 2nd edition Philadelphia, WB Saunders Co, 1990.

Exercise Program Components

A comprehensive fitness program has three parts: a warm-up, an aerobic exercise period, and a cool-down. Within this framework it is possible to include exercises to improve or maintain flexibility, range of motion, muscle strength and endurance, and cardiovascular fitness and health. Specific therapeutic goals and disease-related considerations for disease activity, joint protection, progressive grading, and self-management strategies also are easily accommodated.

This compartmentalized approach to the exercise prescription gives the health professional and the person with arthritis an easily individualized and modified exercise program. For example, an extremely deconditioned person may require an initial program to increase flexibility and strength to prepare for more vigorous and weight-bearing activities. In this case, the health professional and client design an appropriate flexibility and strengthening program with goals to increase strength and flexibility, improve function, manage pain, and prepare for the addition of an aerobic component. When the client is able to perform eight to ten repetitions of these exercises within a 15-minute period, the client will be able to add a short aerobic component, such as 5 minutes of walking or stationary bicycling, gradually progressing to 20–30 minutes. A brief cool-down follows this more vigorous activity. If a disease flare occurs or there is increased joint pain, the client can reduce aerobic activity and perform only the warm-up routine until the acute episode subsides. In this way, the exercise habit is maintained and the client gains the knowledge and experience to self-manage exercise and activity.

Warm-Up or Preaerobic Component

This component provides a neuromuscular and cardiovascular warm-up and is essential to the exercise routine. During this time, exercises are done for range of motion, flexibility, and to prepare the body for more vigorous activity. Some strengthening exercise also can be performed at this time. This warm-up is needed for exercise safety by all exercisers, and is particularly important for the person with arthritis. The warm-up routine can be designed to incorporate individualized range of motion and strengthening exercises and serve as the traditional home exercise program.

The warm-up can be progressed in number of exercises and repetitions to include 12–15 exercises performed five to ten repetitions each. It is extremely important to include pelvic stabilization and trunk rotation exercises in the warm-up to minimize the chances for low back pain with the increased activity. The goal can be 15 minutes of continuous low-intensity exercise, which is an indication of readiness to proceed to an aerobic stimulus activity.

Aerobic Exercise

The aerobic exercise component provides the stimulus for adaptation and training of cardiovascular efficiency, muscular endurance, and activity tolerance. It is this dynamic, repetitive exercise requiring the use of large muscle groups that also appears to benefit general health, emotional status, weight management, self-concept, and fatigue.

The aerobic component can be designed to meet individual needs and variations in disease activity. Experience with and availability of a variety of aerobic activities gives the exerciser freedom to alternate modes. A flexible prescription of intensity, duration, and frequency that the client understands and can adjust to meet daily needs promotes self-management skills and appropriate activity levels. The utilization of *interval training techniques* (i.e., alternate bouts of brisk and low-intensity activity) and *additive bouts of exercise* (i.e., add four 5-minute exercise bouts during the day for 20 minutes of exercise) enable even the most deconditioned and sedentary person to safely engage in health-promoting physical activity.[19] Alternating exercise intensity within an exercise session or performing several short sessions during the course of the day also provides the person who has vulnerable joints and fluctuating disease activity with a method to establish a health-promoting exercise program.

Exercise success and maintenance appear to be enhanced by using time rather than distance as the aerobic exercise goal. For example, 20 minutes of walking, biking, or swimming is easier to maintain successfully than set mileage or number of laps.

Using alternate forms of exercise that vary weight bearing and joints involved also fosters maintenance of the exercise habit. A stationary bicycle is a good alternate for walking on days when knees are sore; a walk may be a better choice of exercise than swimming on a day when hands, wrists, and shoulders are painful. These strategies are particularly useful to the person with arthritis who has "good and bad days" and needs to regulate, but not omit, exercise.

Cool-Down Component

Once the client is performing 10 minutes or more of aerobic activity at an intensity of 70% or more of age-predicted heart rate (moderate intensity), a 3- to 5-minute cool-down period is necessary. During this time, exertion is reduced to a low intensity and gentle, static stretching of exercised muscles is performed. The goal of the cool-down period is to allow the cardiovascular response to safely adjust to less demand and to gently stretch muscle to minimize the possibility of delayed-onset muscle soreness.

As with the warm-up routine, low-intensity cool-down activities can be designed and used in a daily program that provides general as well as therapeutic benefit. The warm-up and cool-down may be combined to form a 25- to 30-minute exercise routine for flexibility, strength, and pain management without the more intense aerobic period. These routines can be used on days when aerobic exercise is not done.

Resistance Training

Recommendations for physical fitness for the general population now include guidelines for muscle strengthening. Maintaining muscle mass and strength is considered an important part of good health and fitness. Appropriate resistance training in persons with RA and OA can result in muscle strengthening, improved function and independence, and increased lean body mass without increased joint pain or disease activity.

Knowledge of disease process, biomechanics, and joint protection principles must form the foundation for any weight training program for the client with multiple joint involvement. Eight to ten exercises, at 8–12 repetitions, each performed at least twice a week, is the basic recommendation for health-related strength training.[20]

The principles of circuit resistance training appear to be appropriate for the person with arthritis. This mode of exercise, designed to improve upper and lower body strength and provide a cardiovascular training effect, employs low resistance with high repetition and is easily graded and progressed.

Exercise Prescription

The exercise prescription derives from the physiologic principles of overload and specificity of training. *The **overload principle** states that a physiologic stress greater than that to which the organ or organ system normally is subjected is necessary to produce physiologic adaptation and increased capacity.* The exertion required to overload cardiac function of a 70-year-old woman who has been inactive for the last 10 years will be much less than that required to produce improved cardiovascular fitness in a 25-year-old recreational athlete. ***Specificity of training** means that gains in capacity and performance are greatest when the training activities correspond closely to the desired outcome.* If you want to swim faster you must train by swimming fast. If you want to improve walking speed you must train by walking faster. General improvement of muscle strength and endurance is desirable. The most functional improvement can be obtained, however, when muscle conditioning uses the muscles in the same sequence, velocity, and range required by the task.

Physiologic overload and specificity of training are addressed in the exercise prescription through recommendations for: (1) modes of exercise, (2) intensity, (3) duration, and (4) frequency. Manipulation of these variables in accordance with results of a fitness assessment and personal exercise goals produces an individualized exercise prescription. For the person with arthritis, this prescription also takes into account disease-related needs and may incorporate therapeutic and recreational exercise.

> **Exercise success and maintenance appear to be enhanced by using time rather than distance as the aerobic exercise goal.**

Exercise recommendations for the person with arthritis must include education regarding response to joint inflammation and adaptation of physical activity to reduce joint stress. For example, swimming or stationary bicycling may be substituted for walking when there is knee, hip, or ankle inflammation. Graded progression of return to vigorous or resistive exercise following immobilization is necessary to protect weakened cartilage, bone, and periarticular structures.

The client must be educated for self-management so he or she can adjust the exercise routine as needed for changes in disease activity, pain, weather, availability of exercise resources, schedule conflicts, and interests.

The concept of physical fitness and the prescription of distinct components of the exercise program are particularly useful in helping the individual understand how to wisely select and modify activities.

Arthritis-Related Considerations

As a group, people with arthritis tend to be at high risk for undetected coronary disease, osteoporosis, and musculoskeletal injuries. Effects of disease, consequences of therapy, and long periods of inactivity contribute to the problem list.

Extra-articular Manifestations

Extra-articular manifestations of systemic inflammatory diseases should be assessed and considered in the exercise prescription. Systemic involvement in many of the arthritides requires that a careful history and physical examination precede any conditioning exercise program. Pericarditis, nephritis, and vasculitis *preclude* increased activity. Pulmonary fibrosis may limit ventilation and safe exertion at high intensity. Signs of active, systemic disease should be heeded and the initiation of more vigorous exercise delayed awaiting effective medical control. Cardiovascular and pulmonary complications may limit exercise capacity, particularly in diseases with a major systemic component, such as systemic sclerosis, systemic lupus erythematosus, and RA. The seronegative spondyloarthropathies (ankylosing spondylitis and psoriatic arthritis) may be associated with heart involvement and conduction defects. In general, the limitations do not interfere except during high-intensity exercise. However, elderly, deconditioned, and biomechanically inefficient people expend considerably more energy than younger, fit, and agile people to accomplish the same task. Even walking at a slow speed (2 mph) requires significantly greater exertion than might be expected.

Articular Mainfestations

Articular manifestations of arthritis should be considered in terms of active inflammation and joint integrity. Inflamed joints are particularly vulnerable to injury. Overuse of an actively inflamed joint may aggravate the inflammatory process and increase joint damage. Synovial tissue ischemia, increased intra-articular temperature and pressure, and the presence of immune complexes are associated with joint inflammation. Although the effects of gentle active or passive range-of-motion exercise are not yet defined and may be useful, current findings caution against vigorous activity in the presence of active inflammation. It appears, however, that activity as tolerated does not produce damage.

Active Inflammation

Painful, swollen joints need to be protected from deforming forces and unnecessary joint stress. Acute joint inflammation should be controlled prior to conditioning levels of exercise. This may require a course of drug therapy and/or joint aspiration. Joint effusion increases intra-articular pressure during joint motion and may lead to joint damage.

Control of inflammatory disease processes and joint swelling should be achieved prior to a conditioning exercise program.

Rest in the form of protective splints and activity modification also may be recommended. For a disease flare in one or a few joints, it is often possible to alternate modes of exercise so that the exercise habit is maintained and joints are protected. For example, a painful and swollen knee may be protected by a change from a 30-minute walking routine every other day to 10 minutes daily on the stationary bicycle with no resistance.

Joint Integrity

Joints with loss of joint space, damaged cartilage, laxity or tightness in periarticular tissue, chronic effusion, or malalignment are highly susceptible to activity-related injury. Joint pain and swelling following activity should be treated as an "overuse" or athletic injury. Preventive steps should be taken to strengthen the joint in preparation for a return to activity. If joint integrity or stability is not amenable to change, activity modifications can decrease the amount of joint stress incurred. A clinical knowledge of biomechanics is essential. For example, intra-articular pressure in the hip can be reduced up to 50% by use of a cane in the contralateral hand during ambulation. Biomechanical stress at the knee joint increases with faster walking speed. Stair climbing produces the greatest hip joint pressures of any locomotor activity.

Exercise recommendations for the person with arthritis must include education regarding response to joint inflammation and adaptation of physical activity to reduce joint stress.

Table 11-4. Definitions of Exercise Intensity*

Moderate Exercise
- 40–60% max $\dot{V}O_2$ = 60–75% max heart rate
- Well within current capacity
- Sustainable comfortably for 60 minutes
- Slow progression
- Noncompetitive

Vigorous Exercise
- >60% max $\dot{V}O_2$ = >75% max heart rate
- Substantial challenge
- Fatigue within 20 minutes

*Data from Gordon NF, Kohl HW, Scott CB, et al: Reassessment of the guidelines for exercise testing. Sports Med 1992; 13(5):293–302.

Intensity

Intensity is prescribed by the exertion or effort expended during the aerobic stimulus portion of the exercise program. The recommendation for intensity is based on the preexercise fitness assessment. Persons who are deconditioned or who have not exercised for 3 months or more should begin at a low intensity. In persons with low initial capacity, intensity of 50–60% maximal heart rate (MHR) is both safe and adequate to produce a training effect. For persons with average levels of fitness, intensity of 60–80% MHR will be appropriate and probably well tolerated. Intensity of exercise is relative to the individual, and also can be described in terms of the exerciser's ability to maintain the activity (Table 11-4).

Intensity during exercise sessions most often is monitored by heart rate response or self-report of perceived exertion. It is useful to prescribe an exercise range with a lower intensity as the threshold for training and the higher intensity as the "not to exceed" level. Individuals can learn to regulate activity successfully within the range, modifying exertion as desired.

Heart rate response may not be an appropriate measure of intensity if the person is taking medications to regulate heart rate, or if the economy of effort is poor and heart rate is not a meaningful indicator of actual energy expenditure. For these reasons, it is often desirable to prescribe and teach exercise intensity regulation with the rating of perceived exertion scale. For some persons, the simple "talk test" may be the most useful way to make sure that exercise intensity does not exceed a moderate level. The talk test only requires that the person be able to speak normally and converse while exercising. If the exerciser is short of breath, or cannot speak in comfortable sentences, the exercise is too intense and effort should be decreased.

High-intensity exercise is clearly associated with increased injury and relapse. For the person with arthritis, maintaining intensity at a safe and satisfying level is a challenge for both the exerciser and the health professional. It is often the younger client who presents the greatest challenge. Balancing joint health, intensity, and socially desirable activities is necessary to produce age-appropriate, enjoyable, and safe exercise opportunities.

Duration

Duration of the exercise session is highly variable and can be manipulated with intensity to provide the desired exercise stimulus. Duration of the aerobic portion of the exercise period probably needs to be at least 30 minutes of continuous activity at a level of intensity above normal daily activity to produce changes in fitness. Minimal requirements for health, however, suggest that 20 minutes of even low-intensity activity may be protective. Two modifications in duration may provide particular benefit to persons with arthritis unable to safely exercise vigorously for 30 minutes.

The first modification is *interval training*. This method incorporates alternate bouts of high- and low-intensity exercise during the exercise session. For example, the runner may alternate 30 seconds of sprinting with 30 seconds of jogging. This scheme delays fatigue and allows a greater total exertion and work over a period of time than a continuous high-intensity activity. For the person with arthritis who may not be able to sustain a continuous 15 minutes of brisk walking without knee swelling and fatigue, a regimen of slow and brisk walking could be combined as follows: slow walk 3 minutes/brisk walk 3 minutes; slow 2 minutes/brisk 3 minutes; slow 2 minutes/brisk 3 minutes; slow 2 minutes for a total of 18 minutes of continuous activity. A gradual increase in the periods of brisk walking provides a conditioning period and a safe progression to longer duration and greater intensity. A second modification of the duration component is the use of *additive bouts* of exercise. The total duration of exercise may be increased by performing several short bouts of exercise throughout the day. If a person is unable to perform 20 minutes of continuous walking, he or she may wish to walk for 10 minutes in the morning and 10 minutes in the afternoon, or for 5 minutes four times a day for a total duration of 20 minutes. Additive bouts of exercise appear to be sufficient to fulfill the requirements for exercise for health but probably do not provide the stimulus necessary for improving cardiovascular fitness. Some persons who initially use additive bouts, however, can lengthen and combine these short bouts as endurance and strength improve, and eventually perform a longer continuous session. Other persons may continue to obtain the health-related benefits of regular activity in the form of several short sessions during the day.

Frequency

Frequency of exercise depends on the exercise goal and mode of exercise. A frequency of three to four times a week for an aerobic stimulus appears to produce optimal results in terms of cardiovascular benefit with a minimal risk of injury or fatigue. A frequency of 5 days per week is safe and effective when the intensity is low. Similarly, resistance training to improve strength should be performed no more often than 2–3 days a week to allow the muscle time to repair and adapt.

Stretching and Flexibility

On the other hand, stretching and flexibility exercises are most effective when performed at least once daily. Flexibility exercise performed in the morning may reduce morning stiffness and pain in preparation for the day's activities. Flexibility exercise performed in the afternoon, when motion may be greatest, can maintain or increase range with a minimum of pain and stretching. Flexibility exercise performed in the evening may significantly reduce stiffness the next morning.

By taking advantage of the exercise program component system (warm-up, aerobic exercise, and cool-down), an exercise program can be designed that allows for a different frequency of each component.

Exercise Choices

The choice of exercise modalities depends upon client preference, exercise goals, musculoskeletal impairment, and available resources. It is wise to help the client identify and learn to be comfortable in performing at least two activities that require rhythmic, repetitive muscular work of large muscle groups. These activities should vary in requirements for weight bearing and joints used to perform the activity. Other considerations might be activities for both indoors and outdoors, for changes in weather, and for solitary or group exercise. Table 11-5 presents an exercise prescription for health (see Table 11-2 for exercise tips for the *new exerciser*).

Disease-Specific Considerations in Aerobic Exercise

Osteoarthritis

Protection of articular cartilage is the basis of early OA management and a key consideration in exercise. Cartilage health requires motion and the mechanical action of repetitive loading and unloading (rest) for nutrition and stimulation of normal remodeling. Hyaline cartilage failure can be caused by either excessive loading of normal cartilage or physiologic loading of abnormal cartilage. Hyaline cartilage also responds pathologically to prolonged periods of nonweight bearing and/or immobilization. The changes that occur with immobilization are similar in many respects to those characteristic of OA (see Chapter 3).

The therapeutic exercise regimen should supply loading and motion to compromised cartilage to promote nutrition and normal remodeling without exacerbating the disease process. This can be

Table 11-5. Exercise Prescription for Health

Exercise mode Activities that involve large muscle groups, entire body if possible, in dynamic, repetitive motion. Examples: walk, swim, dance, bicycle, row, aquatic exercise, calisthenics.
Frequency Three to four times a week for moderate intensity. Daily for low intensity.
Duration Accumulation of 20–40 minutes per exercise day.
Intensity Low to moderate intensity: 50–75% of age-predicted heart rate; 3–5 METs; 1,100–3,000 kcal/wk.
Self-Monitoring Strategies Exercise heart rate per exercise prescription. Scale of perceived exertion (0–10): 3–5 exercise exertion. Talk Test: able to converse comfortably during exercise.

achieved by altering duration and/or intensity of joint loading. It has been suggested that continual weight bearing should last no longer than a maximum of 2–4 hours, followed by at least 1 hour of nonweight bearing to allow the cartilage to decompress.[27]

Muscular strength and endurance are important for joint protection, particularly at the knee. The major mechanism within the body for absorbing the shock of impulsive loading occurs through reflexly controlled neuromuscular mechanisms and eccentric contraction (active lengthening of muscle while maintaining tension). Weakness, fatigue, and unskilled motion interfere with this mechanism and increase the risk of injury.

Furthermore, joint stability and alignment are improved by strong and extensible ligaments, tendons, and muscles crossing the joint. Exercise to improve muscle strength and endurance is mandatory when the knee joint is involved.

Stretching exercises that include the knee should be carefully selected. Joint laxity is common. If this is the case, further stretching of posterior structures (hamstring stretching), rotation with a fixed foot, or pressure on medial and lateral joint structures is contraindicated. Many popular fitness routines contain such exercises (i.e., long sitting stretches, hurdler's stretch, lunges).

OA in one joint is a multijoint problem. Assessment of strength; range of motion; and functional performance at the hip, knee, and ankle bilaterally should be performed and deficits addressed in the exercise program. Generally, weakness, stiffness, and pain in one knee is associated with limited motion and strength in the contralateral knee, hips, and ankles.

Osteoarthritis in one joint is a multijoint problem.

Rheumatoid Arthritis

In RA, three areas in which synovitis, pain, and instability frequently occur and often are overlooked in exercise planning are: hands and wrists, feet, and cervical spine. Activities that require a tight grasp, vigorous repetitive motion, or weight bearing by hands and wrists may be contraindicated in a person with active or chronic hand and wrist involvement. Often, activities can be adapted to protect these vulnerable joints: upright rather than racing style handlebars on bicycles, weight bearing on forearms rather than on hands and wrists during mat and calisthenic exercises, adapting aquatic exercises to avoid the need to grip the side of the pool or exercise equipment.

Foot

Hindfoot instability, clinically expressed as calcaneal valgus, often is associated with collapse of the medial longitudinal arch, midfoot and metatarsal subluxation and pain, and digit deformities. Involvement of foot and ankle can occur quite early in the disease process and severely limit daily activities and the ability to bear weight. Foot and ankle symptoms often are overlooked and undertreated. Early attention to hindfoot position and stability, and support and maintenance of mid- and forefoot alignment is essential. Semirigid and rigid orthoses that supply biomechanical correction or support can significantly decrease foot, ankle, and knee pain and protect joints.

Spine

Forty to 80% of people with RA have cervical spine involvement. These joints are the second most commonly involved joints in RA. Subluxation and erosions may occur leading to possible nerve root and/or spinal cord compression. Excessive motion, upper extremity or occipitally radiating pain, and tenderness to pressure over involved vertebrae are early signs of cervical spine disease. Exercise should be geared toward maintaining adequate flexibility (but not hypermobility) in the cervical region, and muscular strength and endurance to promote proper head and upper body posture. Isometric exercise and proper head and upper body posture, during activity and rest, help improve tone and strength of periarticular structures and reduce mechanical impingement of cord or nerve roots.

Extreme flexion or extension or any position that places pressure on the base of the skull or cervical spine should be avoided (i.e., plough position, extreme bridging). Neck pain may be a problem in curl-ups for abdominal strengthening. This difficulty also may occur in OA of the cervical spine. It is possible to perform abdominal strengthening and keep the head and neck supported by maintaining a pelvic tilt against resistance provided by weight of the lower extremities (leg raises from supine).

Ankylosing Spondylitis and Psoriatic Arthritis

These seronegative spondyloarthropathies are characterized by inflammatory involvement of the spine, ribs, sacroiliac, peripheral joints, and enthesopathies. Exercise-related management includes particular attention to range of motion, flexibility, posture, and chest expansion. Enthesopathies may cause pain and stiffness and at the same time make the site of ligament insertion vulnerable to injury during exercise. Gentle, static stretching performed daily to prevent tightness and contracture is safer and more effective than remedial stretching.

In AS, special attention must be paid to maintaining good posture, strengthening hip and back extensors, and maintaining ventilatory function. A properly prescribed and performed exercise program is extremely effective in preserving function with this disease. Some time spent prone daily helps to avoid hip and trunk flexion contractures. Low-impact activities, good musculoskeletal and cardiovascular fitness, and good shoes with shock-absorbing insoles can help maintain an active life style. Swimming, with mask and snorkel to reduce the need for cervical rotation, has proved to be an extremely effective and well-accepted form of fitness exercise for people with AS.

Systemic Lupus Erythematosus (SLE)

Exercise-related issues are fatigue, often compounded by inactivity and deconditioning; intermittent arthralgias and myalgias; systemic deficits that may affect activity choice; and protection from overexposure to the sun. Regular moderate activity has been shown to decrease fatigue and improve mood in women with SLE.[28] Use of corticosteroids to control disease activity increases the risk of osteoporosis, stress fractures, and avascular necrosis of the femoral head. *Complaints of pain in back or lower extremities should be considered as serious.* People at risk for these problems should engage in low-impact activities and carefully increase exercise duration in conjunction with general muscle strengthening when disease is under control.

Fibromyalgia

Attention to proper posture and conditioning exercise regimens may be useful in managing this disorder. Regular participation in dynamic, low- to moderate-intensity exercise is known to enhance slow wave sleep, aerobically condition muscle, reduce exercise-induced muscle microtrauma, raise pain threshold, and promote muscular relaxation. McCain et al showed moderate improvement in subjects who participated in conditioning exercise (flexibility and bicycle ergometer).[21] Heat, cold, massage, relaxation training, and postural exercises in combination with a gradually progressive low- to moderate-intensity aerobic exercise program often are recommended.

Sample Exercise Program

Client

A 21-year-old woman college student has had RA for 2 years. Her medical management consists of oral methotrexate and injectable gold salts. She has limited motion and pain of all upper extremity joints with chronic effusions in elbows, wrists, and metacarpophalangeal joints. There is knee, midfoot, and forefoot pain with some swelling and loss of motion in both knees. Knee and foot pain is aggravated by weight-bearing activities. Her gait is slow with limited motion in knees and ankles. In standing, her posture demonstrates a forward head, rounded shoulders, mild kyphosis, and slight flexion at hips and knees.

Exercise Goals

Her exercise goals are to (1) improve general flexibility, strength, and endurance; (2) improve posture; and (3) develop exercise habits for maintenance of physical fitness through life.

Exercise Plan

Phase I: Daily Preaerobic Conditioning Program

Flexibility exercise with emphasis on hips, knees, ankles, shoulders, and spine. Strengthening (isometric and gravity resisted) for hip, knee, ankle, trunk extensors, and posterior shoulder girdle. Start with three to five repetitions of 12 exercises and increase repetitions and exercises to tolerance. She may continue to build to a 30-minute regimen if desired, and may add an aerobic component when 15 minutes is well tolerated.

Phase II: Aerobic Component

Add three times a week, alternating aerobic activities as desired.

1. Ride a stationary bicycle starting with 5–10 minutes pedalling at 50–60 rpm with no resistance. This may be performed in two or three bouts per day. Gradually increase resistance and speed as tolerated, always beginning with 5-minute warm-up. Use additive bouts to reach goal of 30 minutes per exercise day.
2. Initiate a walking program with 5–10 minutes of walking at a comfortable pace, in supportive shoes, and on level ground. Regulate speed and distance to avoid post-exercise knee pain and swelling. Use additive bouts of walking to reach goal of 30 minutes per exercise day.

Phase III: Total Physical Fitness Program

1. Daily flexibility routine of 15–30 minutes.
2. Aerobic exercise of choice three to four times per week. Also explore swimming, water aerobics, walking, and outdoor bicycling as alternate forms of aerobic activity.
3. Add resistive exercise component of eight to ten exercises, progressing to ten repetitions, two or three times a week. Use free weights, elastic bands, or equipment. Use wrist weights or equipment that does not require gripping to avoid hand and wrist stress.

Important Questions

Exercise Physiology and Therapeutic Effects

1. Are there physiologic effects of an acute bout of exercise or chronic adaptation to the exercise stimulus that may affect the disease process?
2. Why do a number of the aerobic exercise studies show up to a 40% decrease in joint swelling for subjects who participate in regular aerobic exercise of moderate intensity? Is this clinically important event due to improved vascularization or lymphatic circulation; mechanical pumping; some neurochemical effect on the inflammatory process, or improved joint health and decreased biomechanical stress?

Exercise and the Immune System

1. What are the links between exercise physiology and psychoneuroimmunology?
2. What is the connection between neuro-musculoskeletal and immune function? Research in the areas of growth hormone levels, neuropeptide levels, and the effects of overtraining on the immune system give clues that important linkages exist.

Therapeutic Benefits of Exercise

Are there differential effects of exercise on specific symptoms and for specific diagnoses? For example, if aquatic exercise consistently produces decreased morning stiffness and walking is associated with improvements in social activity, it may be possible to recommend forms of exercise that best address individual and disease-related needs.

References

1. Blair SN, Kohl HW, Paffenbarger RS, et al: Physical fitness and all-cause mortality. A prospective study

of healthy men and women. JAMA 1989; 262:2395–2401.

2. Yelin EH, Felts WR: A summary of the impact of musculoskeletal conditions in the United States. Arthritis Rheum 1990; 33:750–755.
3. Minor MA: Physical activity and management of arthritis. Ann Behav Med 1991; 13(3):117–124.
4. Ekblom B, Lovgren O, Alderin M, et al: Effect of short-term physical training on patients with rheumatoid arthritis. Scand J Rheumatol 1975; 4:87–91.
5. Nordemar R, Ekblom B, Zachrisson L, et al: Physical training in rheumatoid arthritis. A controlled long-term study. I. Scand J Rheumatol 1981; 10:17–23.
6. Harkcom TA, Lampman RM, Banwell BF, et al: Therapeutic value of graded aerobic exercise training in rheumatoid arthritis. Arthritis Rheum 1985; 28:32–39.
7. Danneskiold-Samsoe B, Lynberg K, Risum T, et al: The effect of water exercise therapy given to patients with rheumatoid arthritis. Scand J Rehabil Med 1987; 19:31–35.
8. Minor MA, Hewett JE, Webel RR, et al: Efficacy of physical conditioning exercise in patients with rheumatoid arthritis or osteoarthritis. Arthritis Rheum 1989; 32:1397–1405.
9. Perlman SG, Connell KJ, Clark A, et al: Dance-based aerobic exercise for rheumatoid arthritis. Arthritis Care Res 1990; 3:29–35.
10. Stenström CH, Lindell B, Swanberg E, et al: Intensive dynamic training in water for RA functional class II—a long-term study of effects. Scand J Rheumatol 1991; 20:358–365.
11. Kovar PA, Allegrante JP, MacKenzie CR, et al: Supervised fitness walking in patients with osteoarthritis of the knee. A randomized, controlled trial. Ann Intern Med 1992; 16:529–534.
12. Holman H, Mazonson P, Lorig K: Health education for self-management has significant early and sustained benefits in chronic arthritis. Trans Assoc Am Phys 1989; 102:204–208.
13. Felson DT, Zhang Y, Anthony JM, et al: Weight loss reduces the risk for symptomatic knee osteoarthritis in women: the Framingham study. Ann Intern Med 1992; 116:535–539.
14. Canadian Standardized Test of Fitness Operations Manual, 3rd edition. Fitness Canada, 1986.
15. Cole B, Finch E, Gowland C, et al: In Basmajian J (ed): Physical Rehabilitation Outcome Measures. Toronto, Ontario, Canadian Physiotherapy Association, 1994.
16. Neiman DC: Fitness and Sports Medicine. Palo Alto, CA, Bull Publishing Company, 1990.
17. Pollock ML, Wilmore JH: Exercise in Health and Disease, 2nd edition. Philadelphia, WB Saunders Co, 1990.
18. Gordon NF, Kohl HW, Scott CB, et al: Reassessment of the guidelines for exercise testing. Sports Med 1992; 13(5):293–302.
19. Blair SN, Kohl HW, Gordon NF: How much physical activity is good for health? Ann Rev Publ Health 1992; 13:99–126.
20. American College of Sports Medicine Position Stand: The recommended quantity and quality of exercise for developing and maintaining cardiorespiratory and muscular fitness in healthy adults. Med Sci Sport Exerc 1990; 22:265–274.
21. McCain GA, Bell DA, Mai FM, et al: A controlled study of the effects of a supervised cardiovascular fitness training program on the manifestations of primary fibromyalgia. Arthritis Rheum 1988; 31: 1135–1141.
22. Ekblom B, Lovgren O, Alderin M, et al: Physical performance in patients with rheumatoid arthritis. Scand J Rheumatol 1974; 3:121–125.
23. Beals CA, Lampman RM, Banwell BF, et al: Measurement of exercise tolerance in patients with rheumatoid arthritis and osteoarthritis. J Rheumatol 1985; 12:458–461.
24. Danneskiold-Samsoe B, Grimby G: Isokinetic and isometric muscle strength in patients with rheumatoid arthritis. The relationship to clinical parameters and the influence of corticosteroids. Clin Rheumatol 1986; 5:459–467.
25. Lankhorst GJ, Van de Stadt RJ, Van der Korst JK, et al: Relationship of isometric knee extension torque and functional variables in osteoarthritis of the knee. Scand J Rheumatol 1982; 14:7–10.
26. Nordesjo L-O, Nordgren B, Wigren A, et al: Isometric strength and endurance in patients with severe rheumatoid arthritis or osteoarthrosis in the knee joints. Scand J Rheumatol 1983; 12:152–156.
27. Bland JH: Joint, muscle and cartilage physiology as related to exercise. Arthritis Care Res 1988; 1:99–108.
28. Robb-Nicholson LC, Daltroy L, Eaton H, et al: Effects of aerobic conditioning in lupus fatigue: a pilot study. Br J Rheumatol 1989; 28:500–505.

CHAPTER 12

Physical Therapy Management of the Child and Adolescent with Juvenile Rheumatoid Arthritis

F. Virginia Wright, MSc(Clin Epid), PT
Elaine Smith, MSW

Juvenile rheumatoid arthritis (JRA) belongs within a large group of connective tissue disorders that occur in children and adolescents.[1] The inflammatory process can affect the dense connective tissue structures within and surrounding the joints, as well as the diffuse connective tissue network throughout the body. While many of these connective tissue disorders also occur in adults, their clinical prognosis and presentation may be vastly different in children. Disorders such as seronegative JRA, the focus of this chapter, are essentially unique to childhood.[2]

PHYSICAL THERAPY IN ARTHRITIS, Joan M. Walker, PhD, PT, and Antoine Helewa, MSc(Clin Epid), PT, W.B. Saunders Company

Diagnosis

Therapists should recognize that there are three JRA onset types as determined by the clinical course in the first 6 months of the disease: pauciarticular, polyarticular, and systemic. Criteria for diagnosis and classification of JRA are presented in

Chapter 4 with the medical management. While the majority of children with JRA will be rheumatoid factor (RF) –negative (seronegative), 10% of children will have later-onset RF-positive polyarticular disease, which has the same aggressive course as adult RA.[2]

Relevance of Disease Course and Prognosis

It is important that the physical therapist (PT) recognize the differences between the various subtypes of JRA with respect to manifestations and prognosis. Seronegative JRA is characterized by soft tissue swelling, early connective tissue contracture in response to joint stiffness and pain,[3] rapid loss of muscle strength,[4] juxta-articular osteoporosis, local growth disturbances, and later joint destruction. There is a tendency for ankylosis, particularly at cervical spine apophyseal, carpal, and tarsal joints.[5] The primary manifestations of JRA are summarized in Table 12-1. Changes in seronegative JRA differ from the proliferative synovitis, ligamentous laxity, and rapid destructive patterns and thus the prognosis seen in adult RA or rheumatoid factor–positive JRA. There is evidence that the thickness and growth potential of the young cartilage offers resistance to deep erosions into bone, and there is a possibility of healing in JRA.[6]

Table 12-1. Manifestations of JRA

- Joint pain and stiffness
- Muscle spasm and atrophy
- Joint contractures
- Systemic manifestations (i.e., rash, pericarditis, lymphadenopathy)
- Skeletal growth disturbances
- General failure to grow (primary or as a result of drug therapy)
- Eye involvement (chronic iridocyclitis in pauciarticular JRA)
- Nutritional deficiencies
- Fatigue
- Fibrositis
- Aerobic deconditioning
- Osteoporosis (primary or as a result of drug therapy)

Up to 80% of children with JRA will be in complete remission by late adolescence[1]; however, their ultimate functional status is extremely variable.[7] Losses in joint mobility and bony damage that remain at the time of remission will persist as primary and significant limiting factors of functional mobility. Reconstructive surgery may be indicated once bone growth is nearing completion in late adolescence (i.e., joint replacements[8,9]).

Prognosis is generally considered excellent for regaining full joint mobility and functional ability in children with pauciarticular onset before 5 years of age,[1] although iridocyclitis may occur as a serious ocular complication.[7] Prognosis is more guarded with seronegative polyarticular JRA; poor functional outcomes are related to hip involvement or a persistent and prolonged disease course,[8] and up to 20% of individuals may continue to have active disease as adults.[7] Children with systemic-onset disease have a poorer prognosis,[1] particularly in conjunction with extensive visceral involvement and long-term corticosteroid use.

Goals and Components of Overall Management

Table 12-2 presents management objectives and components.[1,2,4,10–13] When a child is the central focus, the management team will consist of a large group of individuals with diverse health care and educational backgrounds. These individuals likely represent the child's community, school, and local hospital, as well as the tertiary care center's rheumatology program (Fig. 12-1). They may vary in understanding and experience with children with chronic diseases, such as JRA. In small communities, the child may be the only one with JRA. Service providers have to develop strong communication strategies between themselves and with the child, family, and any other caregivers to ensure coordinated and effective care (see Case History #1).

Drug Management and Implications

Pharmacologic agents are used in JRA to decrease and control overall inflammation and systemic manifestations, and to relieve pain. Early use of medications is advocated. They act in tandem with physical management efforts to reduce or prevent joint contractures, damage, and disability. The

Table 12-2. Overall Management of JRA*

Objectives	Management Components
• Decrease inflammation • Control/reduce pain	• Drug management • Pain management strategies • Exercise/modalities/hydrotherapy
• Increase and maintain ROM (prevent/reduce deformity) • Increase and maintain strength • Maintain and optimize function	• Rest/joint protection/splinting positioning • Orthopedic surgery interventions (tendon releases, osteotomies, joint replacement)
• Encourage independence in daily activities • Encourage positive psychosocial and emotional development • Increase child's and family's understanding of JRA and its management	• Guidance/adaptations regarding functional activities, school, and recreation • Psychological and psychosocial support/counseling • Education about JRA

*Data from Cassidy and Petty 1990,[1] Shore 1988,[2] Scull et al 1986,[10] Erlandson 1989,[11] Donovan 1979,[12] Boone et al 1974.[13]

drugs prescribed also are used in adult rheumatic diseases (see Chapter 9). The critical issue for a PT in relation to drug management is a current awareness of the child's medication profile. There must be a clear understanding of the goals of this management and the expected timelines, and patterns of change. This necessitates close reciprocal communication with the child's rheumatologist for information and feedback.

Assessment and treatment protocols should be strongly influenced by the drug management program. For example, a child who starts on methotrexate requires a thorough physical therapy (PTy) assessment at baseline, followed by identical sequential assessments at 3- to 4-month intervals for the first year[14] to determine efficacy. A child scheduled for intra-articular steroid injections will require preinjection assessment with emphasis on the physical and functional status of the joints to be injected. This should be followed by postinjection assessments, initially at close intervals (i.e., 2, 6, and 12 weeks after injection), and then at more extended intervals as dictated by other aspects of the child's management. There also should be a 3- to 6-week period of intensive therapy following injection to work at resolution of joint contractures and improvements in strength and function.

Assessment and treatment protocols should be strongly influenced by the drug management program.

The PT should be alert to the child's response to anti-inflammatory and disease-modifying drugs to ensure that overly intensive PTy is not administered in the presence of overt inflammation.

Assessment Approaches

The focus of this section is on the selection and adaptation of assessment techniques from adult rheumatology. In some cases adaptation is not appropriate, and tools for pediatrics or JRA are necessary.

Identification of an Active Joint

Criteria to identify an active joint in a child with confirmed JRA are similar to those used in an adult, discussed in Chapter 8 (Fig. 12-2). Joints should be examined bilaterally for comparative

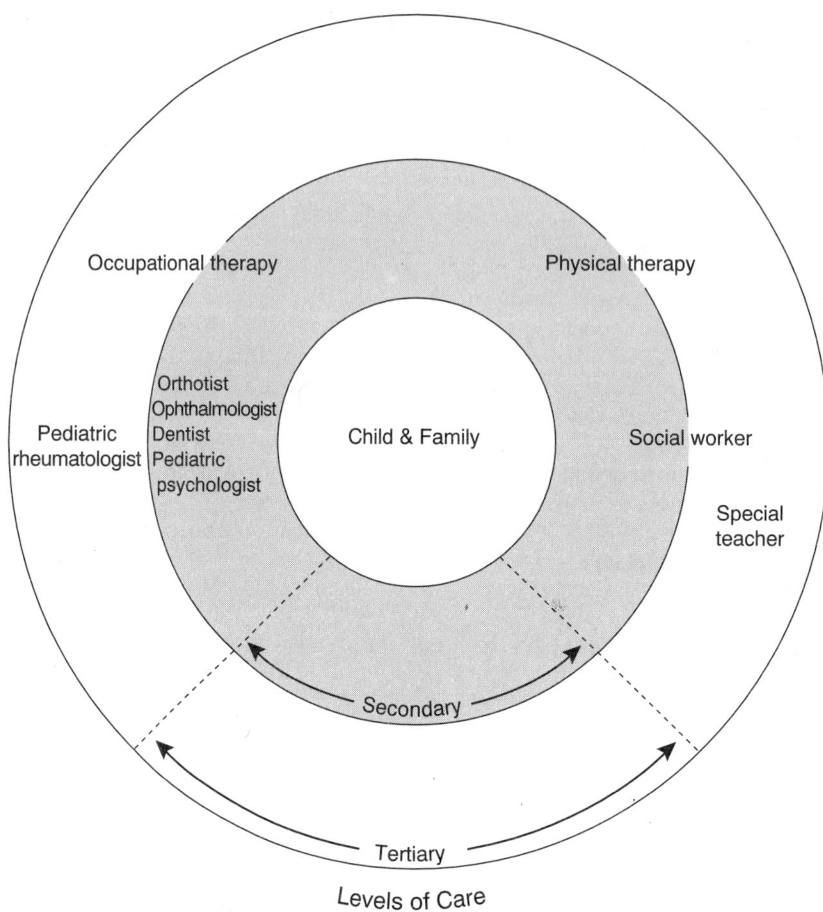

Figure 12-1. The arthritis team. Three levels of care are shown. Primary care providers are the family members/personal caregivers, family physician, and teacher. Team members in secondary and tertiary care may be located in a hospital, clinic, home, or school. Tertiary care members may be located only in large urban centers where specialist care is provided.

symmetry, contour, muscle wasting, deformity, and ligamentous stability.[2] Occasionally there will be a dry synovitis[11] in which range of movement (ROM) will be restricted and stress pain evident even though there is no sign of an effusion.

Nonverbal cues in a young child, such as subtle withdrawal of the limb or slight facial grimace during stress pain testing may provide more information about active joint pain than direct questioning about whether a movement hurts.[3] In some circumstances a child may have a fear of telling the team about pain or functional losses because of anticipation of health professionals' reactions. The consequences of admitting to pain may include recommendations for inpatient hospitalization or increased outpatient therapy appointments, possibility of intra-articular injections, or restriction of normal peer activities and sports. Consequently, the child's subjective comments sometimes may not agree with observational findings.

Nonverbal cues in a young child during stress pain testing may provide more information about active joint pain than direct questioning about whether a movement hurts.

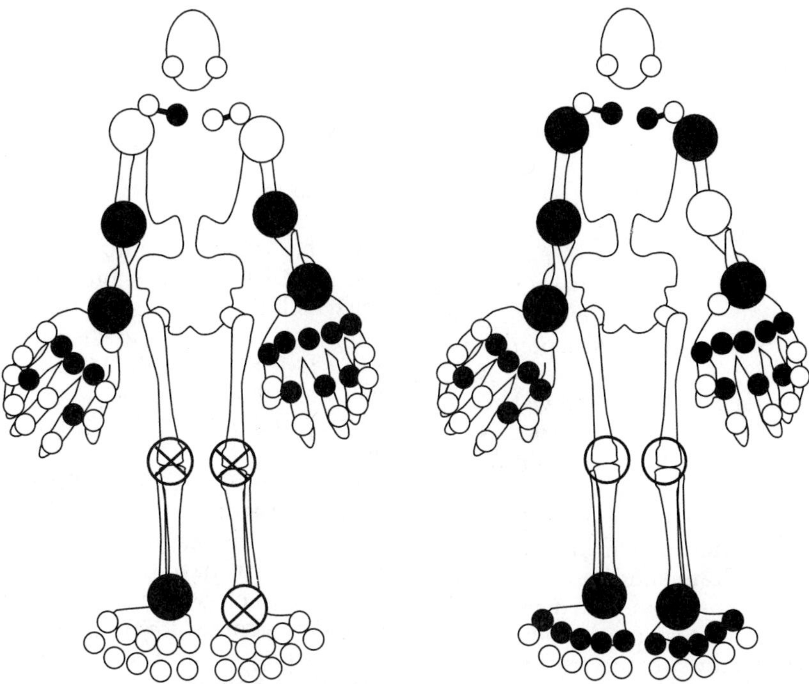

Figure 12-2. Example of active joint count in a child with polyarticular disease. There are 38 active joints. The left figure shows 22 with an effusion (●) or soft tissue swelling (X). The right figure shows joints with stress pain or tenderness (●).

Impact of Hypermobility

During assessment it is important to recognize that up to 10% of all children are hypermobile.[15] The tendency to hypermobility will mask an early joint contracture and adds to the difficulty in early diagnosis. Bilateral comparisons of joint ROM and an overall check for signs of hypermobility are important aspects of joint assessment in pediatrics.[15] For example, a child with pauciarticular JRA may be hypermobile and have 15 degrees of hyperextension of the right elbow while the left elbow has extension only to neutral. While there is no stress pain or effusion in the left elbow, the difference in ROM and radiologic evidence of overgrowth at the left radial head strongly suggests a previously active joint.

Suggestions for the Assessment Process

The child's PT and occupational therapist (OT) may find that working together during the assessment process will reduce the assessment burden on the child and family and provide a more cohesive and integrated assessment of the child. Following the establishment of the child's medical history and the subjective details (obtained from child and parent), the PT and OT should proceed together with the active joint count. Use of the joint man (homonculus) should become a standard way of recording the information on effusions, stress pain, damage, and deformity for each joint (see Fig. 12-2). The joint count should be completed before any other aspects of the physical assessment are undertaken, to put subsequent findings into an appropriate perspective.

Comprehensive assessment of ROM, strength, gait, fine and gross motor skills, and functional abilities may require several assessment sessions over a couple of weeks, particularly in a child with multiple joint involvement.[4] Assessment sessions also can be integrated with initial therapy to work on primary problem areas. The assessment time provides an excellent opportunity for education of the child and parent about the findings and any changes since the last assessment. Diagrams of muscles and joints and use of a skeleton are helpful to explain the assessment information to the child and family.

Assessment periods can be profitably used also for education of the child and the parents.

Outcome Measures for JRA

Many of the objective PTy outcome measures used in JRA have been imported directly from adult rheumatology and are presented in Chapter 8 (i.e., active joint count, ROM, muscle strength testing, gait or footprint analysis,[16,17] and timed walk). The main difference in their use in pediatrics is the need for modifications of the instructions provided to the child, and for interpretation of results using pediatric normative values where available.

The measures that will differ in JRA are those that are self-report in nature and those that reflect function or quality of life. Given the emergence of a strong emphasis on client-centered practice, self-report measures have come to the forefront as a way to enlist the client's viewpoint. Since the mid 1980s there has been tremendous interest in developing self-report measures with content validity for children. These measures have been developed according to physical and psychosocial developmental perspectives to ensure a focus relevant to a child's priorities and capabilities in the home, school, and community settings.[18]

JRA self-report measures for children who are at least 8 years of age include simple visual analogue scale ratings (i.e., pain, overall status, change since last assessment), and indices of pain, functional abilities, psychosocial status, and quality of life. There is evidence that children's self-report responses are reliable[19,20] and valid.[21]

Evaluation of Function

Changes in functional capabilities often are far more important to a child than the gains in ROM and strength that underlie these improvements. The self-report functional or quality of life scales that have been developed or adapted for JRA since the mid 1980s include the Juvenile Arthritis Functional Assessment Report (JAFAR),[21] the Child Health Assessment Questionnaire (CHAQ),[22] the Juvenile Arthritis Functional Status Index (JASI),[23,24] and the Juvenile Arthritis Quality of Life Questionnaire (JAQQ).[25] Test-retest reliability has been established to varying degrees for these measures when children are the respondents.[21,24,25] Work is underway evaluating validity and responsiveness to change.

Evaluation of Priority Functions

Evaluation of a child's individual functional priorities can be added to a functional evaluation. Two measures that address priority activities are the MACTAR patient preference questionnaire,[26] for which the wording has been adapted for use by children,[23] and the Canadian Occupational Performance Measure (COPM).[27] The functional priority lists are valuable for client-centered treatment goal setting and may prove responsive to change in status.

Parents will need to be the respondents on self-report questionnaires when the child is too young to answer (<8 years). Some of the JRA functional measures that have been designed for school-aged children, such as the JASI,[23] do not have age-appropriate content for a young child. Instead, consider using other pediatric functional measures that have been designed for evaluation of young children with physical disabilities. One such measure is the Pediatric Evaluation of Disability Inventory (PEDI), which is a developmentally based functional questionnaire.[28] The PEDI can be completed by the parent(s) or health care professional(s) as they reflect on the child's abilities to perform self-care, mobility, and social function tasks. Ratings are separately obtained for the extent of caregiver assistance required to complete these activities. There is preliminary evidence of the PEDI's discriminant validity when used with children with JRA.[29]

The Developmental Sequence and Function

The delayed acquisition of complex fine and gross motor skills (i.e., cutting with scissors, pouring from a pitcher, hopping on one leg, one-handed ball catching) sometimes observed in young children with JRA may be due to physical inability to perform the task because of restriction and pain. This delay should not introduce concern; improvement in the child's physical status probably will lead to rapid learning of these skills. Useful ideas on the impact of JRA on acquisition of age-appropriate skills are given by Atwood.[30]

There may be occasions in which acquired skills are lost and effort is required to ensure that they are regained. For example, a child may have achieved dressing independence at age 6, and then temporarily be incapable of performing these tasks because of a disease flare. In some situations, the regaining of independence from this dependent situation may require considerable effort and problem-solving skills on the part of the team and family.[30]

Evaluation of Pain

Until recently, the prevailing viewpoint has been that children with JRA experience little pain.[31,32] A new understanding of pain in JRA has emerged with the advent of assessments that permit a child's rating of pain and discomfort in words and colors that are meaningful at their cognitive stage.[19,33] Thorough assessment of pain should cover its multidimensional nature. This might include body diagram outlines that the child colors in to identify the location and intensity of pain.[19,33] The use of word check lists allows description of the affective, sensory, and evaluative dimensions of pain.[19,33–35] The following are examples of words used in these pediatric assessments that do not appear in an adult scale, such as the McGill Pain Questionnaire: "awful," "pin-like," "stiff," "scary," "itching," "like a sharp knife," "hitting," "screaming," "uncontrollable."[34] Visual analogue scales can be employed either to indicate the magnitude of pain at selected joints during various activities and at rest, or to rate global pain.[32,36]

Children can reliably describe and score their pain on pediatric pain assessments.

The Pediatric Pain Questionnaire (PPQ)[19] is one self-report measure well suited for use in JRA. It incorporates the multifaceted approach to pain assessment using components of the combinations described above and has been validated in children (4–16 years) with JRA. There also is strong evidence verifying children's ability to reliably describe and score their pain on other similar multimodal pediatric pain assessments.[33,35,37] These pain scales require between 30 and 45 minutes for a school-aged child to complete, following an initial explanation from the therapist. Validation studies of their specific use in JRA have yet to be published.

Psychosocial Issues that Influence Management

Initial Reactions to Diagnosis

The inherent difficulty in diagnosing JRA often causes delays in the initiation of appropriate management. The weeks during diagnosis may have been spent on an acute-care ward with others with life-threatening diseases (i.e., leukemia), and families may have fears associated with this experience. While the diagnosis of JRA will at least relieve concerns about a life-threatening illness, the fact that JRA is unpredictable in its course and prognosis may put parents and children on an emotional roller coaster. This makes it difficult to assimilate the extensive information provided by the health care team[38] and families may initially have difficulty following recommendations. New information must be provided in small sections and reiterated to facilitate easier understanding and acceptance.

Stages of Grief

A child and their family will go through various stages of grief following the diagnosis of JRA: shock and disbelief, isolation, anger, resentment and bargaining, self-blame, depression, and then, it is hoped, acceptance.[39] The response to the illness will vary between and within families, further intensifying family stress.[11] Grief often reemerges with each new complication, with new life experiences, and with transition through the developmental stages.

JRA may have its greatest disruptive effect on the child's life in the first year following diagnosis.[40] The child and family may find life styles altered in social, financial, time, energy, emotional, and behavioral areas, thereby increasing family stress.[41] In some cases this precipitates a crisis. Coping mechanisms previously used within the family may be inadequate, and external support from the arthritis team is necessary for identification of solutions. Table 12-3 provides a list of family-related factors to assist direct decisions about the extent of involvement of team members, particularly the social worker.[41–43]

Impact on the Family

Having a child with JRA will bring about changes in the family life style and dynamics[44] that must

Table 12-3. Family-Related Factors that May Affect Coping with JRA*

- Nature of the relationships within the family (parent with child with JRA, marital, siblings)
- Physical and emotional strengths and weaknesses of the child and other family members
- Family members' level of sharing of care responsibilities
- Physical dependence of the child and associated care burden on parents/caregiver
- Availability of extended family supports
- Parenting skills
- Communication skills within and beyond the family unit
- Problem-solving skills of child and family members
- The family's belief system (spiritual, cultural, and relating to illness)
- Life experiences concerning illness and medical care
- Financial impact of the care requirements
- Availability and level of specialization of local health care resources

*Data from McCormick et al 1986,[41] Leventhal 1984,[42] Stein and Jessop 1984.[43]

be recognized when planning the rehabilitation program[45] (Table 12-4). Demands on time, energy, and finances will increase in various ways.

Parenting Issues

One key concept in parenting and caring for a child with JRA is that discipline must be maintained as close to the family's usual routine as possible.[46] In some families there may be overprotection of a child with JRA, while in others unrealistic demands may be placed on the child to achieve physical gains (i.e., several hours of therapy every day).

The issue of dependence versus independence, which is difficult in most families as a child develops, may become an arena for parent-child conflict. Noncompliance issues also are a potential parent-child conflict involving a number of emotions for both parties. If parents ignore the child's inappropriate behaviors making special concessions, the child quickly learns that people behave differently towards him/her and may take advantage of this. Behavioral limits still must be

Table 12-4 Potential Impact of JRA on the Family*

- One parent giving up their job to meet increased care requirements
- Changes in caregiver roles and responsibilities
- Rearrangement or elimination of social activities and interests causing family isolation
- Increased transportation requirements for appointments and travel to school
- New set of expenses for drugs, splints, and transportation that compound the effects of lost salary
- Treatment and appointment time requirements
- Home therapy time demands
- Loss of time for family activities
- Lack of sleep (both parent and child) in response to illness demands
- Emotional stress of dealing with a child's behaviors and compliance
- Need to develop strategies to manage pain
- Challenges of splinting regimens and compliance
- Physical demands on parent to assist with child's mobility
- Handling of issues related to the child's emerging independence

*Data from Atwood 1989,[44] Allaire et al 1992.[45]

set regardless of chronic disease[47] with some choices to allow the child a sense of personal control.

Developmental Considerations

It is essential to recognize the many changes that may occur simultaneously in the life of a child with JRA. In addition to developmental maturation, there will be changes related to the child's arthritis over time and in the family's responses to both.[43]

The process of continuous developmental change (physical, cognitive, and psychosocial) always must be carefully considered when PTy treatments are planned, implemented, and evaluated. For example, an approach that worked well when the child was 5 years old may be met with resistance once the child is 6 and in grade 1 and begins to assert independence by questioning and refusing previously accepted treatment. Issues that must be addressed include the child's resistance to wearing wrist splints to school, unhappiness about having to leave school several days per week to attend therapy, and fatigue from spending an entire day at school. If these issues are not recognized and handled promptly, the therapy program is susceptible to failure.

The impact of JRA on psychosocial development and well-being has been the object of considerable research, but conclusions on the existence and extent of psychosocial problems remain controversial because of methodologic limitations in the studies.[48] Despite this lack of consensus, it is important for the PT to be aware of the potential impact of a chronic disease on a child's developing socialization, independence (locus of control), and self-concept. There may be limited opportunities to explore new skills, excel at physical tasks, interact with peers outside of the home, make decisions, or take responsibility for oneself.[30]

The severity of the arthritis does not necessarily correlate with the child's ability to adapt. Some children with severe JRA adapt quite well, whereas others with "mild" pauciarticular involvement demonstrate greater adjustment problems.[48] In the latter case, there may be considerable fear of deterioration and difficulties in fitting in with a peer group. The child may perceive himself/herself as belonging to neither the group of children who are severely physically disabled nor with non–physically challenged peers.

Reactions to the disease may be very difficult to read in an adolescent. A tough and cynical exterior or an overly accepting attitude may mask great concern about the disease and the future, regardless of the severity of the disease. Awareness of this helps the health care team members to be sensitive to potential problems.

Communication with the Child and Family

Open and frequent communication with the child and family is essential so that potential difficulties can be anticipated or dealt with quickly. The child or family members may require psychosocial counseling to facilitate adjustment to the disease and its impact, to encourage expression of feelings, and to assist in development of coping strategies.

The Child's Response to the Disease

Through the course of the disease, the child's mood and ability to comply and work hard during therapy will fluctuate in response to any number of factors. Overall, the child may feel a lack of control over life, as many decisions and intrusive treatment procedures become a daily and unavoidable experience. Episodic behavioral changes, in which the child becomes demanding or manipulative, may appear to the child to be the only avenue to exert some control over the environment.

The variable nature of the arthritis may be particularly confusing and disturbing, where recurrent periods of pain and restriction are difficult to cope with and understand.[11] For example, dramatic and rapid physical improvement often occurs following multiple intra-articular steroid injections. These gains may be followed several months later by a sudden return of the symptoms, pain, and limitations. At the time of injection, the child and family must be warned of this possibility so that appropriate goal setting, follow-up, and support can be anticipated.

Potential emerging fears, emotions, and behaviors seen as a result of any of the above are outlined in Table 12-5. Lack of mobility, time, or energy for peer activities may increase isolation and sadness, and reduce self-confidence. One contributor to stress, anxiety, and sadness is the child's perception of being a burden on the family by causing major life style changes. For example, the need for an accessible school and regular access to medical care may actually necessitate a family move to a different city even when it means that one parent has to stay behind to continue at a job.

Table 12-5. Emotions and Behaviors that May Occur in a Child with JRA

Anxiety about:
Long-term dependence on family
Outcome of the disease
Academic success and future career planning
Severe illness or death
Handling of chronic pain
Intrusive and painful medical procedures
Potential resultant behaviors and emotions:
Anger
Depression
Withdrawal and isolation
Low energy
Sadness
Passivity
Inferiority
Low self-esteem

Consequences of a Child's Fears and Anxieties

The child needs to develop a way of dealing with feelings of fear and anxiety. If unexpressed, these may emerge as negative behaviors, emotional insecurity, or poor adjustment to the disease and its management. Defiance and hopelessness have been identified as a child's ways of fighting back against lack of control over the disease.[47] These may manifest as a refusal to take medications, participation in activities that are physically risky, failure to attend PTy sessions, demonstration of profound apathy during PTy, or lack of compliance with home programs.

Suggestions for Helping a Child to Deal with Feelings

The team can provide a forum for a child's or adolescent's expression of these fears and stresses. Play activities utilizing doll houses, puppets, or stories; individual counseling; music; and art can all facilitate the expression of feelings. Role playing may be of particular value for adolescents. The adolescents we work with have initiated role-playing topics, such as physician, patient, and parent at clinic, injections and blood work, or the demanding or protective parent/therapist/teacher, and have played these scenes out in graphic detail. Group format (exercise, discussion) will reduce the sense of isolation, provide sense of belonging, shared goals, and a safe environment of expression of feelings and effective problem solving.

Team Considerations

The child's adjustment may be strongly influenced by the reactions of others close to them, and by their ongoing experiences.[11,49] Differences in beliefs and value systems of arthritis team members also will affect the care of the child with JRA. The team must be aware of their feelings about the disease process, potential outcomes, and the attitudes they project. Staff may see complex cases where the successes are slow in coming, gains barely visible, and the disease process unpredictable with flare-ups and regression. Staff and families may at times feel helpless and discouraged about a particular child's condition.

Occasionally, the family's frustration about unpredictability of the arthritis is expressed as anger towards various team members, often the ones they see the most frequently. Team members should retain their objectivity. Issues behind the anger should be recognized and managed. The team should acknowledge the difficulties associated with temporarily aggravating pain during exercise sessions, sharing difficult information, and the effect of these on the relationship with the family.

Team members should be aware of setting realistic expectations not only for the child but also for themselves.[50] Prevention of deterioration of a child's physical capabilities is often a major accomplishment when disease is aggressive and persistent. It is essential to recognize the work of the child, parents, and team and give credit! Respect should be given to the disease process and its ability to frustrate the best treatment plan. The team, the child, and the family should remember they cannot work miracles.

Conversely, team members who have close association with a child over a number of years should not underestimate the positive impact they can have through their actions and suggestions on the child's development and perceptions. Open communication between team members and the family is essential to share different viewpoints, to gain a full understanding of the child's and family's progress, and to identify accomplishments.

Respect should be given to the disease process and its ability to frustrate the best treatment plan. The team, the child, and the family need to remember they cannot work miracles.

Treatment Principles

Physical therapy for children must be relevant to the age and developmental and emotional maturity of the child. Differences between JRA and adult RA dictate a very different physical management strategy, in terms of the nature and goals of treatment. PTy and OTy exercise and splinting approaches in JRA emphasize stretching of soft tissue contractures, strengthening of surrounding musculature to regain or maintain joint mobility, encouragement of optimal positioning of joints that are susceptible to fusion, and facilitation of the highest level of function.

The PTy assessment and treatment approach should be proactive. Contractures often can be anticipated based on an understanding of the typical patterns of restriction and overgrowth in JRA (Table 12-6) and preventative treatment programs instituted. The use of joint endfeels[13,51] and radiograph review are key factors in guiding the treatment program decisions. While the course of JRA is difficult to predict, a child's disease pattern may establish itself over time[1] (i.e., recurrent joint inflammation at hips and knees while other joints and systemic disease remain quiet). An understanding of the child's pattern and type of disease helps therapists focus on the primary goals of treatment.

It is essential also to recognize and treat secondary contractures (i.e., those that arise in a joint adjacent to one with arthritis). For example, a hip flexion contracture may occur secondary to a knee flexion contracture in a child with knee arthritis only. The knee synovitis and flexion contracture will likely respond to treatment, but unless attention also is directed to the hip, a permanent hip flexion contracture and compensatory lumbar hyperlordosis may remain.

Pain Management

Pain in JRA has a considerable impact on the overall quality of life of the child and family. Pain assessment and management in these children merits further attention.[32] The influence of pain and stiffness on the child's ability to cope with and participate in daily activities (school and recreational) should be considered carefully. Fatigue, reluctance to walk, irritability, interrupted sleep at night and muscle tenderness all may originate from uncontrolled or chronic pain and synovitis,[3,52] and translate into reduced quality of life. A dramatic positive change in affect is often noted once the child's pain is controlled. Despite awareness of the impact of pain, it is not unusual for team members and families to be extremely surprised when the child experiences this positive behavioral change in response to reduction of pain.

Responses Towards Pain

The child and family may find it difficult to push through the day's activities and therapy demands when pain is present. An important consideration is the parents' and child's fears of what the pain means.[49] They may question whether further damage occurs by encouraging the child to perform the painful exercises or activities. Timko et al[53] observed that parental stress intensifies when the child is experiencing increased physical functional limitations or when pain is a primary concern. They recommended the teaching of pain management and coping skills that will enhance the control that the child and parent have over the situation. Therapists also may have difficulty working a child through pain that occurs during treatment; some may make exceptions and offer special privileges because of sympathy for the child.

Teaching pain management and coping skills will enhance the child's and family's control over the disease process.

Problem Solving Related to Pain

It is essential to be aware of the child's pain before, during, and after PTy treatment, and also to identify the aggravating and relieving factors. This identification should facilitate interpretation of the source of pain, and allows clinical judgment to determine whether the particular treatment should be continued as is or modified. It also should help to reduce the child's and parents' concerns about

Table 12-6. Clinical Manifestations, Patterns of Contracture and Restriction[*†]

Clinical Manifestations	Restriction/Adaptation
Cervical Spine	
• In polyarticular and systemic JA	• Loss of extension, rotation, and side flexion
• Narrowing then fusion of apophyseal joints, specifically C2,3	• May develop torticollis
• Dysplasia of vertebral bodies	• Eye movements compensate for lack of neck ROM
• Odontoid process instability (less common than in adult RA)	
Temporomandibular Joint	
• Undergrowth (micrognathia) and altered occlusion of teeth	• Restriction of mouth opening, pain, and difficulty when chewing
• Mandibular asymmetry if unilateral	• Greater functional restriction when cervical spine involved and extension is restricted
• Less common in PA-JRA	
Shoulder Region	
• Overgrowth of humeral head with irregular shape, shallow glenoid fossa	• Insidious loss of GL-H ABD, and FLEX, tightening of pectorals and protractors
• Subluxation may occur	• More dysfunction when elbow and wrist involved
Elbow	
• Occurs in all subtypes	• Extension lost early
• Overgrowth of radial head restricts ROM	• Shoulder ROM initially compensates for supination $\downarrow$
• Ulnar nerve entrapment possible	• Wrist involvement accentuates pronation, supination losses
Wrist	
• All subtypes, starts early	• Rapid loss extension
• Accelerated carpal maturation	• Marked weakness extensors
• Undergrowth of ulnar styloid, with severe changes may migrate dorsally	• Tend to rest in flexion and ulnar deviation with notable spasm of wrist flexors
• Radio- and intercarpal fusion	• Distal R-U disease causes loss of pronation and supination
• Carpal tunnel syndrome	
Hand	
• Premature epiphyseal fusion and growth abnormalities	• PIP (especially fourth) more common than DIP contractures
• Flexor tenosynovitis may be dramatic	• Loss of MCP flexion (especially second), loss of MCP hyperextension
• Involvement later in PO and S-JRA than in PA-JRA	• Marked $\downarrow$ grip strength
• MCP and CMP subluxation	• Boutonnière < swan neck deformities
Thoracolumbar Spine	
• Unusual site in JRA	• Kyphosis in association with neck and shoulder involvement
• Steroid drug therapy may cause osteoporosis, wedging vertebral bodies, small compression fractures	• Lumbar lordosis secondary to hip flexion contractures
	• Scoliosis secondary to lower limb asymmetries

Table continued on opposite page

Table 12-6. Continued

Clinical Manifestations	Restriction/Adaptation
Hip	
• Femoral head overgrowth • Osteoporosis • Trochanteric growth changes • Shallow acetabulum and reduced femoral-neck angle, specially if weight bearing limited	• Flexion contracture-may be masked by lumbar lordosis • Marked spasm of ADDs and FLEXs • Loss of ABD and rotations, eventually flexion
• Lateral subluxation of femoral head aggravated by tight ADDs	• May have marked pain on weight bearing
• Potential for protrusio acetabuli, avascular necrosis • Primary cause of ROM ↓ and dysfunction • Occurs in PO and S-JRA after few years	• Secondary deformities of contralateral hip, knees, lumbar spine
Knee	
• Most common joint involved in all subtypes, involved early	• Rapid development of flexion contracture
• Distal femoral overgrowth (medial)—may cause leg length discrepancy in unilateral disease	• Rapid atrophy of quadriceps • Loss of patella mobility due to adhesions
• Knee valgus aggravated by tight hamstrings, iliotibial band • Posterior tibial subluxation secondary to prolonged joint involvement or excessive correction of knee flexion contracture	• Risk of femoral fracture associated with falling due to flexion loss and osteoporosis • Loss of flexion (often only 90 degrees) • Secondary development of hip flexion contracture
Ankle/Foot	
• Altered growth produces bony changes in tarsals, potential fusion	• Early loss of inversion, eversion
• Hindfoot valgus/varus due to ankle involvement or secondary to knee valgus • MTP subluxation	• Later loss of dorsiflexion and plantar flexion, specifically in minimally ambulatory children • Altered gait, loss of MTP hyperextension affects toe-off
• Hallux valgus	• Overlapping of IPs (specially with hallux valgus)
• IPs-growth changes due to premature epiphyseal closure	

*Data from Ansell 1992,[95] Atwood 1989,[30,44] Cassidy and Petty 1990,[1] Emery 1993,[4] Libby et al 1991,[96] Reed and Wilmot 1991,[5] Rhodes 1991,[55] White 1990.[97]

†The listing is not inclusive; features characteristic of juvenile arthritis are given.

PA, pauciarticular; PO, polyarticular; S, systemic; IP, interphalangeal; MCP, metacarpophalangeal; DIP, distal interphalangeal; GL-H, glenohumeral; CMP, carpometacarpal-phalangeal; MTP, metatarsophalangeal; ↓, decreased; ↑, increased; ABD, abduction/abductors; ADD, adduction/adductors; FLEX, flexion, flexors.

the implications of pain and allow them to work through it.

A careful line of questioning must be adopted when the child indicates pain. The child should be asked to pinpoint the site and duration of pain, (i.e., "use your index finger to point to the place where your pain is, and tell me as soon as it has disappeared"). Frequently the pain that a child with JRA experiences during therapy is muscular in nature and resolves immediately following the stretching or strengthening exercise. Many children need help to differentiate between pain and stiffness,[46] and between muscle and joint pain. Other types of pain are typical of embarking on a higher level physical activity and are usually temporary (i.e., severe foot pain in a child who has been minimally ambulatory prior to multiple joint corticosteroid injections and who has just started to walk greater distances).

Management of Pain

The use of pharmacologic and PTy pain relieving modalities in children has been covered extensively in Chapters 9 and 13, and does not differ markedly from those used with adults with RA.

In our clinical experience, the majority of children tolerate and sometimes even prefer ice to heat as long as it has been introduced positively and gradually with clear explanation as to its purpose. It is important in the use of any electrotherapy modality for which the dosage depends on the child's feedback that the child be old enough to be able to appreciate and describe sensations associated with the modality (i.e., at least 6 years of age).

Other Pain Management Techniques

Recently, there has been recognition of other techniques, such as guided imagery, meditative breathing, and progressive muscle relaxation[32] that may provide the child with a means to personally control or handle their pain[49]; these may permit a more full and happy participation in daily life. Simple relaxed breathing techniques may be possible for a child as young as 4 years of age. The other strategies listed above are more cognitively advanced and are best reserved for school-aged children and adolescents.[54]

Effectiveness of these nonpharmacologic methods has yet to be rigorously evaluated in clinical trials. Wider use of validated pain questionnaires, such as the PPQ,[19] may yield greater understanding.

Basic Concepts About Exercise in JRA

Grading of Exercise Based on Disease Activity

Detailed guidelines are presented in the JRA literature for the type of exercise appropriate to the stage of disease activity[10,12] (i.e., acute, subacute, or chronic). Unless a child has severe systemic illness or is experiencing an acute episode of generalized joint spasm and pain, bed rest and immobilization of joints should be avoided.

If inflammation is subacute or chronic, the treatment program is progressed to include active and strengthening exercises, functionally based gross motor activities, and conditioning exercises.[12,55] Daily exercise programs that take each joint through a full active ROM are advocated,[56–58] since routine activity does not always require that a joint move to its limit.[11]

It is essential to recognize that different levels of disease activity may exist within various joints at any one time. In the presence of acute synovitis, recommended therapy consists of gentle active-assisted and passive exercises for the targeted joints with an emphasis on the concurrent use of modalities such as ice, hot packs, or wax for relief of pain and swelling.[1]

While it is generally agreed that exercise must not be so vigorous as to aggravate inflammatory activity or to encourage joint instability, the causal relationship between levels of physical activity and inflammation is unclear. Recent studies on exercise in JRA[59–62] emphasized limitations in muscle performance and aerobic capacity associated with JRA rather than on PTy efficacy. For lack of other empirical evidence, conclusions from the RA studies still form the basis of exercise protocol decisions in JRA (see Chapter 13). Ultimately, decisions regarding the appropriate intensity of exercise and physical activity rely on the PT's judgment and clinical experience and on careful monitoring of the child's response to therapy.

Management of Specific Joints

Details on restriction and adaptation of the various joints are presented in Table 12-6 in association with the typical patterns of contracture and bony change. Surgical interventions, covered in Chapter 6, usually are a later-stage management strategy. The primary exception to this rule is the use of soft tissue releases at the hip joint. Since about 33% of children with JRA will eventually develop hip involvement, surgical lengthening of contracted hip flexors and adductors may be important in children (≥6 years old).

PTy for Young Children

The greater soft tissue flexibility and hypermobility in children under 8 years of age[15] and the earlier stage of disease of younger children point to the need for intensive therapy at this early age.[1] This need for concentrated work with young children results in a dilemma. Are young children able to cope with the exercise, stretching, and splinting regimens that are advocated to alleviate contractures when they are unable to comprehend the rationale behind these efforts?

It may be tempting to allow the focus of therapy for young children to be on play-directed, developmentally based activity versus treatment focusing on joint ROM and strengthening. The lack of joint-specific mobilization and stretching, however, may result in the establishment of very resistant contractures that subsequently require soft tissue releases or reconstructive surgery. In our clinical experience, young children (2–5 years old) can participate in and enjoy JRA group pool and gym therapy sessions (Fig. 12-3) and tolerate soft tissue stretches and splinting. Age-appropriate compliance-enhancing strategies (i.e., stickers and games) should be built into all aspects of their program.

PTy for Children with Pauciarticular JRA

There may be a tendency to regard the joint involvement of a child with pauciarticular JRA as less serious than multiple joint involvement in a child with polyarticular disease. Deformity of even one or two joints in a child with pauciarticular JRA is a serious long-term sequela of the disease. Early intensive rehabilitation efforts are needed for these "mildly involved" children. For example, a knee flexion contracture of 15 degrees with associated knee valgus deformity of 10 degrees, and compensatory hindfoot varus of 5 degrees in a young child invites concern about abnormal growth pressures across open epiphyses. This altered growth situation is compounded by hyperemia (increased blood flow) that may occur at the distal femur and proximal tibia in conjunction with knee synovitis.[5] Research in adult subjects has suggested that the increased intra-articular pressure that occurs in the presence of muscle imbalance and shortening may encourage osteoarthritic changes.[63]

Age-appropriate compliance-enhancing strategies must be built into all aspects of children's programs.

Hydrotherapy

All publications reviewed on JRA rehabilitation mention hydrotherapy as a means to relieve pain

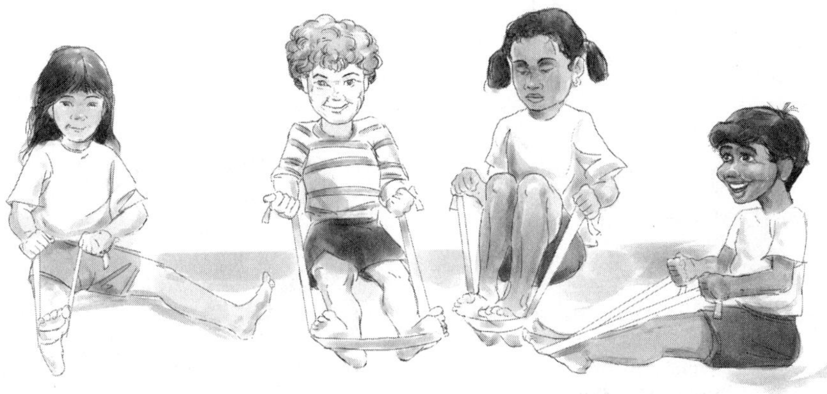

Figure 12-3. Group exercise session.

and encourage joint ROM.[1,10–13,55,57] Although hydrotherapy is favored by many PTs to increase joint mobility and strength in adult and pediatric practice, there have been few published efficacy studies on the topic.[64] Incorporation of active exercise during hydrotherapy should increase blood flow and facilitate a rise in muscle core temperature. This mild heating of muscle may facilitate maximal contractions due to reduced muscle viscosity, and increased biochemical reactions.[65]

Value of Hydrotherapy in JRA

The buoyancy and weight-relieving properties of water are of great importance for children with JRA, allowing painful and stiff joints to move with little force. The pool may be the only place in which a child with severe lower extremity involvement is able to tolerate walking. It also is of great value in early postoperative stages or following an acute disease flare. Since lower extremity joints are minimally loaded in shoulder-deep water in the pool, it is a safe environment within which to work on aerobic conditioning.

Effectiveness of Hydrotherapy in JRA

In an effort to evaluate the specific effects of pool therapy (stretching, ROM, and strengthening exercises), Bacon et al[59] conducted a one-group pre- and post-test study of 11 children with JRA. Only statistically significant improvements were shown for several hip ROM measures and for heart rate recovery. Insufficient sample size and the reduced validity of a one-group design drastically limited conclusions.

The pool is a safe environment for work on aerobic conditioning.

Overview of Hydrotherapy Techniques

Skillful use can be made of water's turbulence, surface tension, and viscosity to safely and comfortably provide varying degrees of resistance.[66] Bad Ragaz lower extremity mobilization and strengthening techniques are highly suitable for children with JRA.[67] This technique has combined the principles of proprioceptive neuromuscular facilitation with hydrotherapy so that movement and muscular work are facilitated in a controlled manner. Various inner tubes or rings are used to support the child during Bad Ragaz techniques. Manual techniques and the buoyancy and turbulence of the water are used to produce the desired movement patterns. The child ultimately has control of how much work she or he exerts during these techniques.

In general, the incorporation of water wings and other flotation devices to either assist or resist movement adds variety and interest,[66] and provides free and secure movement for children with very restricted mobility. This freedom of movement deserves special notice. Observers watching pool groups of children with JRA often remark that it is hard to believe that these children who demonstrate such ease of movement in the water are the same ones who had such difficulty changing for the pool and walking into the water. The freedom of movement also does not go unobserved by the children. Many in our clinical practice have remarked that their mobility problems would be solved if they could just live in a water-covered environment!

Group Pool Sessions

The pool is an ideal medium for group exercise therapy sessions.[59] Group membership may consist of children of diverse ages (3–16 years old) and varying disease activity. A group session integrates ROM, strengthening, aerobic, and swimming activities. Individual variation in performance according to age and physical ability is taken into account. Children and adolescents who have attended the group for a long time or are a little older act as role models and "peer educators" for the newer or younger members.

Group sessions also are a way to foster leadership skills. The participants may take turns "running" the group, which provides a chance to feel competent physically, cognitively, and socially. They also are an opportunity for fun, lively peer interactions, and water sports/games. This may be the one time for children of all ages with JRA in a particular community to be together. A large number of children can participate in several group pool sessions per week within the constraints of the PT staff time, thus using the PT's time more efficiently.

Group pool sessions are an easy way to get a younger child to work hard. Quality movement should not be expected from a young child. The child can be expected to follow along with a sequence of movements as long as she or he feels securely supported in the water. As the child matures, familiarity with the hydrotherapy protocol will allow a focus on achieving the optimal range and repetition speed for each exercise.

Stretching of Soft Tissue Structures

In children, lengthening of muscle needs to occur in tandem with skeletal growth if ROM and flexibility are to be maintained. Shortening of muscle and tendon and the resulting joint contractures are early problems of primary importance in JRA. The resulting contractures, which are initially flexible, may persist through the course of the disease and remain as a major cause of disability. The holding and use of joints in positions of physiological flexion may to some extent mimic the effects of actual immobilization of the joint, and result in decreased length of muscle fibers.

Table 12-7 lists the joints of greatest concern for flexion contractures in JRA. Resolution of contractures is possible if attended to early on in conjunction with local control of synovitis. There is little evidence, however, on which stretching methods are most efficacious. Studies provide evidence that muscle and tendon respond to brief stretching with improved immediate post-treatment flexibility, and that heat may facilitate stretching.[68–71] In JRA there should be leeway for gain in extensibility in restricted muscle because of opportunities for growth and healing. Conversely, there may be considerable risk of adverse effects including damage to immature epiphyseal areas in the proximity of tendinous attachments.

Suggested Approaches to Brief Stretching

The two main types of stretching to consider in JRA are brief stretch (i.e., 60-second hold during PTy) and prolonged low-load stretch for several hours (i.e., night splints for hands, elbows, or knees; night hip traction, wrist working splints for day wear).

Brief stretching may gently mobilize the joint, temporarily extend muscle fibers, and prepare the tissues for their lengthened position in the splint. This active stretching is necessary to assist in gradual breakdown of scar tissue, adhesions, and fibrotic contractures that may be present in an inflammatory tissue disease.[72]

Stretching pain should be minimized whenever possible so that reflex spasm in response to pain does not sabotage results. For example, passive stretches and gentle grade 1 mobilizations of finger joints are best undertaken in a warm pool after the child has exercised for about 20 minutes. Research indicates that ideally a static stretch should be maintained for as long as tolerated (i.e., at least 2 minutes) to permit the plastic deformation of connective tissue rather than just a temporary lengthening of elastic myofibrils.[73,74] The child must learn to relax during the stretch. One way to facilitate this is to encourage deep breathing. Active and active-assisted exercises always should be used after the stretch to promote use of the joint and muscles within the newly acquired range.

Stretching sessions often are tolerated better if children feel that they are doing the same warm-up exercises that some of their heroes do every day, such as hockey and baseball players, ballet dancers, wrestlers, Superman. Naming a stretch after a child's hero (i.e., the Superman knee stretch), may be a very simple and effective way of increasing the child's compliance with the stretch. Similarly, before and after stretch measurement using a tape measure gives a child tangible feedback on immediate gains and marks progress over the weeks.

Table 12-7. Joints Susceptible to Flexion Contractures in JRA

Joints
Elbows
Wrists
Metacarpophalangeal
Proximal interphalangeal
Distal interphalangeal
Hips
Knees

Splinting: An Approach to Prolonged Low-Load Stretching

Rationale for Use of Splints

If the connective tissue needs elongation to facilitate permanent lengthening,[75] use of a prolonged low-load stretch via night resting splints is an appropriate option. An additional concern in JRA emphasizing the importance of night splints is the extent of morning stiffness experienced.[52] If allowed to sleep without splints, the position of comfort usually will be flexion—consequently, the first hours of the day are spent in the counterproductive activity of actually getting the limb "straight" again.

A child's compliance to stretching can be enhanced by naming a stretch after one of their heroes, such as "the Superman knee stretch."

Types of Splints

The splints fabricated for children with JRA are similar to those provided in adult RA as far as their design, materials, and purpose (Chapter 10). Resting splints for elbows, wrists and hands, knees, and occasionally ankles are provided to ensure optimal positioning through the night and a prolonged low-load stretch. Neck collars, specially designed cervical pillows, and Buck's skin traction for the hips are other devices used to promote an optimal "extended" sleeping posture and encourage relaxation of muscle spasm.

Splints that may be prescribed to support, protect, and optimally position joints during daily activities include wrist working splints, neck collars, and foot orthoses (Fig. 12-4). Occasionally dynamic splints are indicated for resolution of contractures (i.e., dynamic finger splints). Extreme care should be taken to guard against joint subluxation and epiphyseal damage that may occur secondary to overzealous corrective force.

Manufacture of Splints

Given the frequency of alteration required for many splints, it may be most expedient and cost-effective for therapists to be responsible for their fabrication and adjustment. Prefabricated splints are not ideal, since they do not conform to joint angles and may not provide the correct support.

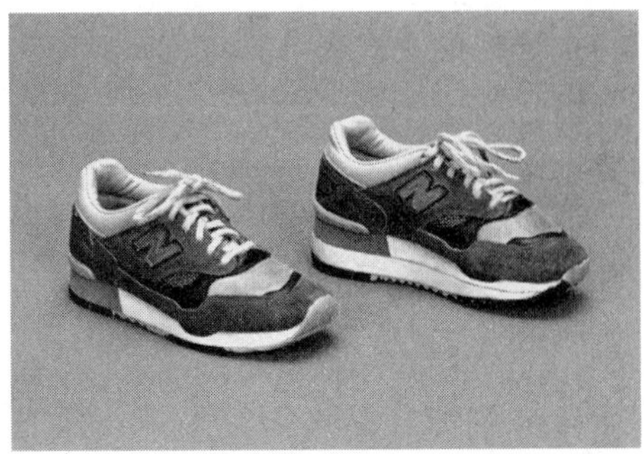

Figure 12-4. Shoe with lift.

A splinting session is ideally preceded by a pool therapy treatment in which the soft tissue structures are heated and stretched so that slight reduction of the contracture is achieved prior to splinting. In other situations when a permanent splint is being fabricated following contracture resolution or when molding to the contracture is difficult, collaboration with an orthotist may be advised. Issues related to splinting materials are given in Chapter 10. While standard guidelines for positioning of the joint(s) are a helpful starting point, the child's individual contracture pattern, soft tissue extensibility, and radiographic findings always should direct the splinting process.

Characteristics of a Good Splint

The splint should contain the joint well, providing up to two thirds circumferential support along the long bones. This may prevent the child from inadvertently pulling out of the splint during use. For example, shallow wrist working splints allow a child to pull over the lateral splint border into ulnar deviation. Overcorrection of contractures should be avoided—a straight knee splint used for a bent knee will not provide adequate support posteriorly to allow the spasm in the soft tissue structures to relax. Furthermore, forcing a knee straight into a splint that employs a three-point pressure system may simply encourage posterior tibial subluxation.

Serial Splints

The use of serial splinting allows a gradual correction of a flexion contracture. Three or four serial splints over a period of about 20 weeks may gain resolution of a stubborn flexion contracture. The first splint would be molded to conform exactly to the contours of the existing contracture. Subsequent remoldings should permit reduction of the splint angle in accordance with improvements of the underlying joint angle as soft tissue structures lengthen.

Initial improvement in flexion contractures may occur surprisingly quickly in response to an intensive rehabilitation effort. This is particularly the case when splinting immediately follows intra-articular joint injections that have permitted substantial reduction of joint inflammation and associated muscle spasm. Frequent monitoring and adaptation, possibly every 1–2 weeks, is needed for splints that have been made to reduce contractures.

Serial Casting

There may be times when serial casting using plaster or hexcelite is preferable to serial splinting with thermoplastic materials. The main drawback to serial splinting is that the splints can be removed by the child. The most that can be expected is an 8- to 10-hour period per day when the low-load stretch is maintained. Serial casting, on the other hand, ensures that the child will wear the cast and maintain the soft tissue lengthening until the cast is removed by the PT, OT, or orthotist. Joints that are particularly amenable to serial casting procedures are the wrist, knee, and ankle.

One approach to serial casting that does not place undue burden on the child and family is to cast the child's joint at the end of the week, leave the cast on over the weekend, and bivalve the cast on the following Monday afternoon. This provides about 72 hours of gentle soft tissue stretch, support, and accompanying relaxation of the periarticular structures. The child then daily wears the bivalved cast for 18–24 hours, for 1–2 weeks, at which point a second cast is applied and the entire procedure repeated. Pool therapy (with cast removed) is essential during this interim period to allow the child to actively work the muscles in the new range. The 1- to 2-week time interval in between castings is important to allow the soft tissue structures to accommodate to their new length.

As long as there are no adverse effects (i.e., aggravation of joint inflammation), three to four serial casts may be appropriate within the cycle. A thermoplastic splint then is fabricated to maintain the joint in the corrected position. The splint-wearing schedule depends on the joint, the type of splint (resting versus day time), and the child's tolerance.

It is better to gradually introduce splints, to gain compliance with one before the next splint is introduced.

Methods to Enhance Splint-Wearing Compliance

Compliance issues are paramount when considering resting and working splints. A splint that is not worn cannot be effective no matter how well it is designed! Table 12-8 presents a summary of potential reasons for noncompliance with splinting.

Table 12-8. Reasons for Noncompliance with Splints*

- Discomfort due to inadequate fit
- Restriction of function when in splint
- Increased stiffness associated with use
- Uneasiness/self-consciousness about peers' reactions to splint
- Insufficient understanding (child or parent) about reasons for wearing splint
- Unrealistic splint wearing schedule
- Lack of positive reinforcement/recognition for splint wear
- Lack of improvement in joint position or function despite previous compliance

*Data from Reed et al 1993,[81] Rapoff et al 1985,[86] Wynn and Eckel 1986.[87]

A child may be prescribed a full set of splints (wrist working, hand, and knee resting splints) during a single clinic visit along with a rigorous wearing schedule. The difficulty of suddenly being expected to simultaneously tolerate several splints through the night should be recognized. From our clinical experience, it is better to gradually introduce the various splints, gaining compliance with one for several weeks before the next is introduced. The decision as to which splint to start with should be based on the priority therapy goals. For example, if knee contracture resolution is a primary goal, knee splint wear would be started first followed by addition of other splints as tolerated.

Many children are keen to participate in fabricating their splints (i.e., cutting out and adhering straps, choosing the color of splinting material and straps, and decorating the splint). Companion splints may be made at the same time for the child's favorite stuffed animal (Fig. 12-5). The child then takes on the responsibility of ensuring that their stuffed friend *also* wears the splint every night!

Positive feedback recognizing compliance is imperative since gains in ROM may be intangible to the child. Acknowledgment of splint wear can take the form of stickers for the splints or a reward point system. Splint wear needs to be encouraged for the entire night (i.e., until the child gets out of bed in the morning). Otherwise, parent-child confrontations can arise around when the splints can be removed (i.e., 2 AM versus 5 AM versus 7 AM).

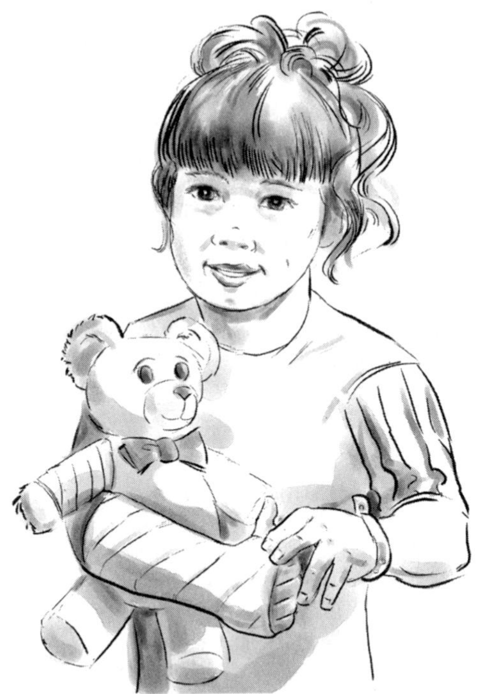

Figure 12-5. Compliance with splint wearing can be enhanced by making a splint for the child's favorite toy.

For young children it may be advisable for parents to put splints on after the child has fallen asleep.

Some children have difficulties coping with the immobility associated with splint wear at night. A child with polyarticular disease who has difficulty turning in bed without splints may be dramatically restricted once the splints are on. Simple abilities, such as getting out of bed to go to the bathroom, may be completely limited. Therapists need to help parents work out a system so that assistance to reposition or get up is readily available (i.e., two-way voice monitor in child's room, bell to ring for assistance).

During times in which contracture reduction is being undertaken, splints should be worn every night so that there is no opportunity for back-sliding. When the joint status is stable and disease relatively quiet, a program of alternate-night splint wear may be considered. Guidelines should be clear and compliance monitored closely to ensure that splints are not abandoned altogether.

A child may have great concern about the profound morning stiffness associated with wear of night resting splints. This will occur when a joint is maintained in one position all night as a result of the gelling phenomenon often present. Children's anxiety about this stiffness and reluctance to wear the splint or hip traction may be reduced if they are warned of the sensation in advance and given measures to help the discomfort resolve (i.e., morning tub bath, gentle ROM exercises after splint removal, or a sling suspension set-up over the bed that is used prior to getting up).

A frequent reason for noncompliance relates to the fit of the splint. Children grow quickly and a splint may be too short or tight within several months of fabrication. The parent and child need to be warned of this at the time the splint is fabricated and instructed to bring it back for adjustments should any of the borders become snug.

Muscle Strengthening

Mechanisms of muscle atrophy in JRA are undefined, but are likely similar to those of adult RA. Disuse atrophy, reflex inhibition due to effusion and pain, nonspecific myositis, ultrastructural muscle fiber damage due to the disease process, and drug-induced myopathy have been observed as frequent muscle changes in adult RA.[1,76] All JRA publications reviewed recommend isometric exercise as the safe way to increase strength.[10,13,55,62] While studies in RA provide an indication of isometric exercise effectiveness,[76] parallel evidence in JRA is unavailable.[62] There may be greater potential for strength improvement in JRA than in adult RA, given a child's potential for growth and healing and the less destructive nature of the disease.

Muscle Strengthening Protocols

A child with JRA whose muscle weakness has been present for several months may be unable to elicit maximal effort from targeted muscles. Patterns of compensation for certain muscle groups, such as the hip abductors and extensors, often are well established. Some children may be fearful of attempting an antigravity hold due to anticipation of pain or joint damage. For weak musculature (i.e., marginally grade 3), an active-assisted antigravity lift and gentle support during the isometric hold will reduce the child's fears of the limb painfully dropping and encourage active contraction of the targeted muscle group.

At the beginning of training, methods of providing muscle feedback should facilitate the re-learning of maximal muscle activation. Biofeedback via a simple hand-held unit in conjunction with isometric exercise may be useful at this stage.[4] It serves as a comfortable alternative to neuromuscular electrical stimulation which probably gives more sensory than motor input given the low intensities that children tolerate.

When using progressive resistance exercises (PRE), evaluation of the child's repetition maximum (RM) should be done frequently at the beginning of training (i.e., every week), and then determined as appropriate as training progresses. An example of an initial isometric PRE program for children with quadriceps weakness might consist of two sets of six isometric contractions each using a weight that equals a 75% RM for the first set, followed by a 50% RM for the second set.

The RM program lends itself well to home programs both in terms of time required and the ease with which the child can document and see their gains. The RM strengthening program can be adapted for use with sling and spring set-ups where the resistance of the spring is used in computation of the RM. This approach encourages active ROM at large joints, such as the hip, offering light spring resistance at the end of range to facilitate contraction of the target muscle group. Resistive nonelastic webbing materials can be an inexpensive alternate to use of weights for an isometric home program.[4]

Aerobic Capabilities and Training

Exercise recommendations in current PTy literature provide little mention of aerobic exercise.[60] In a comparative study of the aerobic capacity of 16 children with JRA and 16 nondisabled age- and sex-matched controls, computerized gas analysis was used to measure aerobic capacity during a bicycle ergometer test.[60] As hypothesized, aerobic capacity of children with JRA was clinically and statistically lower ($p<.001$) than the control group. A limitation in interpretation of results was the difficulty in differentiating between reduced aerobic capacity and pathophysiologic factors associated with JRA (i.e., pain, stiffness, and decreased ROM).

Until the results of studies of aerobic exercise in JRA are available, parallel studies in adults with RA provide the most appropriate information on the influence of aerobic programs on inflamed joints and on levels of conditioning. There is evidence that the aerobic walking and aquatic programs can be undertaken without aggravating joint inflammation.[77,78] Generalizability of results, however, to JRA should not be assumed, since disease processes and prognosis are distinctly different.

The pool may be the best place to conduct group aerobic exercise programs,[76,79] since weight bearing and impact are reduced by buoyancy. The standard stationary bicycle or arm ergometer are other impact-reducing options, although these are less appealing than the pool. A child's interest and motivation is heightened if given access to a computerized bicycling system (available in health club facilities) that provides a video course to ride with feedback on speed and distance. There also may be some exciting and creative possibilities for use of virtual reality exercise-adapted equipment in the future.

Cross-Training

The concept of cross-training, which incorporates a combination of strengthening and endurance activities, recently has been introduced into the rehabilitation field.[76] If efficacious, this approach should enhance the individual's functional strength and capabilities. A simple version of cross-training in JRA that would minimize joint stresses might be a weekly program consisting of bicycling/use of the arm ergometer, swimming and water aerobics, isotonic exercises in the pool, and isometric exercises on land. This type of cross-training program was studied in ten children with JRA who participated in a training program over a 3-month period.[80] Type II fibers in the quadriceps muscle did demonstrate a tendency to a more normal electromyographic (EMG) response pattern after training, although endurance and strength were unchanged. Lack of improvement probably was related to an inadequate sample size to detect a signficant difference.

Implications of Osteoporosis

Varying degrees of osteoporosis are commonly seen in JRA, particularly in children who have required prolonged corticosteroid use or who have had periods of restricted mobility.[5] There is an increased likelihood of pathologic fractures in the presence of limited ROM (i.e., femoral fracture when knee flexion is less than 90 degrees and the child falls).[1] This potentially serious complication provides a compelling reason for recommendation of exercise and weight-bearing activities to increase bone density, encourage growth at epiphyses, and improve flexibility and muscle strength.[81,82] When weight bearing on land is difficult because of lower extremity weakness or pain, a walking program in the therapy pool may be the only means to maintain ambulatory abilities. This should be emphasized until the disease symptoms subside sufficiently to permit standing with use of a walker or crutches on land.

Work on standing balance (i.e., use of balance boards) has been recommended as a way to reduce the risk of falling.[4] Innovative motor strategies are needed to accommodate for joint restriction and muscle weakness. Children who have had arthritis from early years may have inadequate development of equilibrium responses.

Despite all efforts to maintain or increase a child's ambulatory abilities, it still may be necessary to provide the child with an alternate means of mobility for long distances in the community or at school. Available options include tricycles/bicycles (Fig. 12-6), battery powered scooters, or wheelchairs (manual or electric). One advantage of scooters over wheelchairs is that the child is likely to leave a scooter at the door of the classroom and walk to his or her desk. With a wheelchair, there is a reduced tendency to get in and out of it during the day, and consequently the opportunities for short-distance weight bearing are greatly reduced.

Options for Therapy within the Community

There is a need for long-term vigilant follow-up for children with JRA. The PTy program must be flexible and correspond with changes in disease activity. Caution should be observed when including a child with JRA in a group pool or gym session that consists of older adults with arthritis. Unless the differences in disease are clearly explained and understood, new fears about prognosis may arise in the child's mind. It is better to schedule children together to provide a supportive and similar peer group.

While it is optimal to set up therapy within the child's community, there may be a lack of appropriate facilities/services in many outlying and rural areas. Even within urban areas it may be difficult to find clinicians (even among those experienced in adult rheumatology) who feel comfortable working with children with JRA. Furthermore, the policy of many acute care hospitals may limit the length of outpatient treatment (i.e., 6–8 weeks). Clearly, this does not address the capricious nature of the disease in JRA nor the importance of maximizing ROM and function during the child's

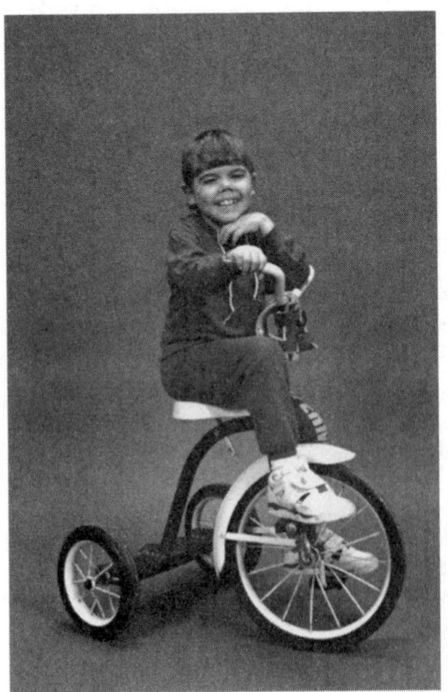

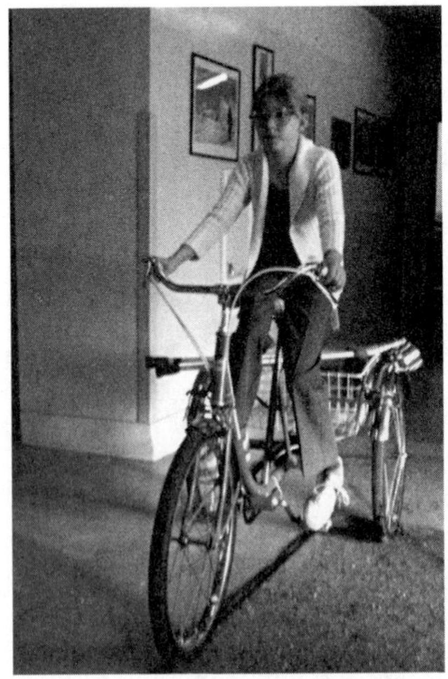

Figure 12-6. Tricycles and bicycles offer an alternate means for mobility over long distances when ambulation is restricted.

growing years. As discussed earlier, change is not always in a positive direction. Sometimes tremendous effort must be expended for the child to maintain ROM and ambulatory status. This apparent lack of progress often is used as a reason for not considering a child as meriting continued outpatient intervention.

It is crucial that the pediatric rheumatology team from the tertiary care centers forge strong links with the identified treatment team in the child's community and work out the best method of support both for the local team's needs and for the child and family. Letters of support from the child's rheumatologist with rationale for the need for long-term follow-up often are very effective in encouraging extended outpatient care. Methods of communication, such as teleconferences, computer linkages, or videotapes of therapy assessment and treatment sessions, are effective ways of sharing information.

Home Programs

Melvin and Atwood[46] suggested that a child's daily home exercise program should include not more than seven simple exercises. Careful evaluation of the child's *specific* exercise requirements, coupled with a current understanding of the literature on the effectiveness of these techniques, and sensitivity to the family's home situation will help in developing a working plan for exercise that should at least stand a chance of success. The idea of a daily exercise home program of 20–30 minutes may be appealing to the PT. Factors such as fatigue after a lengthy school day, the demands of homework, opportunities to spend time after school with friends, and family time constraints, however, may make this impossible. This does not mean that the health care team's principles and better judgment need to be compromised. Flexibility and problem-solving skills should be employed so that a feasible home and community therapy plan can be created and undertaken.

Goal-Setting and Compliance Enhancement

One of the greatest challenges in designing the rehabilitation program for a child with JRA is the multitude of goals on which to work during the child's already limited school and extracurricular time. This is particularly the case for children with polyarticular JRA, where 20 or more joints may be identified as problems at any one time. There is always a sense that gains must be made as early and quickly as possible. This, however, must be tempered by a consideration of what the child and family can actually cope with at any one point in time and within their life style.

There is evidence that older children and adolescents are interested and capable of participating in decision making in relation to their care, and that compliance with treatment may be enhanced when this process is allowed.[83] The problems and goals identified by the child, team, and parent(s) may not always correspond with each other in terms of content, priority, or expression. Noncompliance may result if a child and parent(s) do not understand how the goals are attained.[84] It is important to take the time to listen to, understand, and respond to a child's viewpoint.[85]

Barriers to Compliance

The extended months or years over which the child and family are expected to adhere to treatment regimens can lead to boredom and indifference, and ultimately may wear down child and family compliance.

Realistic, achievable goal setting is important to both the family and team to avoid negative reactions.

Frustration is encountered in situations where progress that was anticipated does not materialize even after complying with the prescribed treatments and recommended life style changes. The family may ask many questions pertaining to the perceived failure. Was there not more that could have been done by staff or family? Were the decisions that were made about medications the right ones? Lack of improvement often translates into a reduction in compliance.[84] The PT needs to help child and family understand that in some circumstances maintaining the status quo is an accomplishment in itself. This relates to the importance of realistic goal setting to avoid setting-up the family and team for despair, guilt, and anger.

Importance of Positive Reinforcement

The PT must recognize the importance of feedback during therapy. An honest, positive comment always can be found even when change is not happening as anticipated. The PT may be one of the few people who will actually remark on the effort put forth by the child and family. Parents may not be fully comfortable with recognizing their child's efforts.

Use of goal-specific contracts with a meaningful incentive at the end do not have to be equated with bribery; rather, the physical gains gradually achieved from improved compliance in splint wear or exercise may mean very little to the child, necessitating a tangible reward from time to time.

Methods to Enhance Exercise Compliance

Factors that influence compliance and simple ways to enhance exercise adherence are outlined in Tables 12-9 and 12-10.[84,86,87,89] Parents who are actively involved in encouraging their child's compliance with medications and exercise enhance their child's adherence to the regimens.[84] Reported compliance may be greater for the medication component of the treatment regimen than for the complimentary exercise program.[84] A decrease in the reported compliance for adolescents was observed that appeared to correspond with the shift of personal responsibility from the parent to the adolescent.[84] While transfer of responsibilities to the adolescent is recommended, it should occur gradually along with individualized compliance strategies, support, education, and follow-up.

Table 12-9. Factors that May Influence Compliance*

Parental Factors
- Level of awareness of the importance of different aspects of the child's care
- Attitudes towards the individual or facility providing the care
- Belief in the efficacy of treatment

Therapist Factors
- Level of sensitivity to child's/family's lifestyle and belief system
- Ability to set realistic short- and long-term goals
- Ability to provide positive reinforcement
- Flexibility to changes in child's status
- Willingness to explain/provide education during assessment and treatment sessions

Child/Adolescent Factors
- Time restrictions due to school, work, and social life
- Discouragement/boredom with long-term treatment programs
- Emerging independence and autonomy

*Data from Wynn and Eckel 1986,[87] Mayo 1978.[88]

Table 12-10. Compliance-Enhancing Strategies for Exercise Programs*

- Incentives such as stickers, and cumulative rewards after several weeks of sticker acquisition
- Clearly written, age-appropriate home exercise programs
- Daily journals to track exercise compliance
- Child participates in design and writing of own exercise program and exercise calendar
- Child allowed to make choices within exercise program regarding order of exercises, selection of exercises, number of repetitions, and so forth
- Personalized exercise videotapes
- Regular phone calls by PT/OT to children in remote areas to support/encourage/reduce isolation
- Opportunities to participate in JRA/pediatric orthopedic exercise groups
- Inclusion of sibling or friend in exercise session at therapy facility or home
- Short-term admissions to rehabilitation facility for "tune-up" from time to time
- Participation in JRA summer camps

Education About JRA

A child's individual understanding of disease and treatment must be evaluated rather than assuming comprehension levels on the basis of the child's age, length of time since diagnosis, and previous educational interventions.[88] Misconceptions about JRA and its treatment may be held despite previous exposure to JRA education in the clinic setting. These misconceptions may have serious implications when it comes to a child's willing participation in therapeutic regimens. It is essential that time be taken with each child to ascertain their level of understanding of the disease and to offer appropriate education.

The child's ability to handle uncomfortable questions from peers and others may depend on understanding of the disease, its manifestations, and its management. There should be opportunities to attend group and individual education sessions. The clinic may not be the best setting for provision of education about their disease and its management. The stress and anxiety of the clinic visit and any treatment decisions made may interfere with processing of this information. Repetition of information presented at clinic, and review of treatment choices, should occur at follow-up sessions. Families may be more inclined to ask questions and retain valuable information in this more relaxed environment.

Discussion of treatment priorities and accomplishments can be easily built into each therapy assessment and treatment session. This provides informal education and review of the child's understanding, compliance with [illegible]se, and splinting [illegible]

Educatio[illegible]

The langu[illegible]A may be too abst[illegible] choose age-approp[illegible] materials carefully to explain concepts to a child. Recently, arthritis organizations (Canadian and American) have recognized the need for an individualized, consumer-friendly teaching approach. Several fun workbooks are available to facilitate a child's interest in learning more about their arthritis (i.e., *JRA and Me—A Fun Workbook*[90]). These booklets also may be helpful for the siblings of the child with arthritis who are easily overlooked in terms of their importance in the family unit. Siblings may have unspoken fears about what is happening to their brother or sister. Materials directed towards parents with a self-help focus are given in Appendix I. Parents may want to share these materials with other family members, such as grandparents, whose perception may be that arthritis is an elderly person's disease that inevitably leads to permanent and severe disability.

> **It is essential to select age-appropriate words and materials carefully to explain concepts to a child.**

Participation in School Activities

There is considerable interest in identifying the challenges that children with JRA face in the school setting. This focus is appropriate given that school is the occupation of childhood and is an essential contributor to academic and psychosocial development.[91] Difficulties encountered by a child with JRA include writing problems,[91] mobility restrictions and limitations in participation in physical education,[92] functional restrictions, and problems with self-esteem and peer relationships.[93]

In middle childhood, the peer group exerts a strong influence on a child; feedback from friends is essential for a child to gain independence from parents.[94] In JRA there is a conflicting situation where the illness itself creates a dependence. Therapists can help to devise strategies that will encourage maximum and realistic independence at home and school according to the child's capabilities. Interactions with a peer group also have a strong impact on self-image and expectations and provide an opportunity to receive feedback on accomplishments. The child has a need to be the same as others and will be apprehensive about obvious differences from peers. Changes in abilities and appearances (i.e., short stature, cushingoid features due to prednisone use) may invite comments from peers. The child may need assistance from the arthritis team in learning to handle questions and difficult situations.

Suggestions for Adaptations within the School Environment

Children with JRA require understanding and support in the school system if they are to succeed academically and keep pace with their peer group developmentally and socially. Decreased attendance at school due to illness and medical/therapy appointments[91] often creates a number of realistic fears about academic accomplishment and future career planning. A child with JRA may be the only one with the disease in their school.

Misconceptions about the disease and its prognosis are plentiful. Therapists often have a strong role within the school to provide support and education (written materials and in-service session) to school personnel, and can share information about JRA with the child's class.[91]

Specific physical problems of a child with JRA can be identified using a school check list, such as the 39-item list described by Atwood.[44] The child indicates whether or not each of the items pertains to him/her. Items in the list include rating of ability to get to and from school, the impact of stiffness of various activities, mobility within the school, tolerance of the school day, writing and activity of daily living skills, and the extent of understanding and empathy of classmates and teachers. The child and PT can share the completed list with the teacher to assist in the problem solving process.

Adaptations may be required for children with mobility limitations to ensure safe and full access to the school's key facilities (i.e., cafeteria, washrooms, library, gymnasium). Ideas to ease the physical stress of the child's day are listed in Table 12-11. Children with mild disease may simply need slight modification of gym class content to allow full participation in the day. Children with more severe disease may require an assistant to help them in the washroom or to assist in getting from the school bus to class, in addition to physical modifications to the school environment.

Table 12-11. Suggestions for Reduction of Stress during Child's School Day*

- Modifications to the child's school schedule (i.e., altered course load, timetable, classroom location)
- Provision of a place to lie down for a rest during lunch or recess
- Opportunity to do own exercises during gym class
- Environmental modifications
- Permission to use the school elevator
- Assignment of a classroom buddy to help with carrying books
- Physical assistance by a teacher's assistant
- Provision of notes for classes missed
- Availability of a computer for note taking in the classroom
- Frequent opportunities to stand/walk in classroom to counteract lower extremity stiffness

*Data from Erlandson 1989,[11] Atwood 1989.[44]

Splint Wear at School

Daytime splints (i.e., wrist working splints, neck collars) may meet with marked resistance, since they are designed to be worn during school and extracurricular hours. The child may feel that a splint draws tremendous attention to their physical disability. For some children with mild disease it may be the only visible sign of arthritis. The team should be aware of these issues when providing splints, and make sure that appropriate support is in place to lessen the anxiety. This support may take the form of the PT or OT going to the child's school to talk to the class about JRA and splints. In other circumstances the teacher or parent may want to give a talk to the class. For children who are not comfortable with sharing information about JRA, it may be appropriate for the therapist just to inform the teacher about the purpose and wearing schedule for the splints. In all cases, it is important for the person who provides the splint to the child to ask the child and parent(s) what type of support is needed to make splint wear more acceptable.

The child may find that wearing a daytime splint restricts movement to the extent that functional activities such as writing are difficult. In some cases splint adjustment may be required, whereas in others time and practice should be advocated to reduce the functional difficulty.

Barriers to Academic Achievement

One potential obstacle to academic achievement is the amount of time that a child with JRA misses from school due to medical and therapy appointments. Wherever possible, therapy appointment times should be kept to after school hours or occur at the beginning or end of the school day. A family may have a difficult time deciding when it is appropriate to keep their child home from school (i.e., does prolonged morning stiffness necessitate a day at home?), and guidance from the health care team often is warranted. A letter from the child's rheumatologist to school personnel may clarify questions on health issues relating to participation in physical education, recess activities, and attendance at school.

Absence from school, poor health, occasional difficulty concentrating due to pain, and low energy levels during class time may cause some gaps or delays in the child's academic performance. Children having difficulty at school may benefit from psychological assessment reviewing the child's strengths and weaknesses. The information gained then can be used to provide support to the child and guidelines for the school in establishing academic programs. One concern is that the child who is academically capable may be slotted into a lower stream at school because of being behind due to poor attendance. It is important that a child who might ultimately be physically restricted has the opportunity to achieve full academic potential so that career paths are not further limited.

For high school students, a lower course load may be necessary to avoid high levels of stress and anxiety that actually incapacitate the student. The team may be helpful to school personnel during a student's early high school years to assist in career planning in conjunction with realistic goal setting related to the arthritis and its prognosis.

Recreational and Extracurricular Activities

Time should be made available for the child to participate in recreational and extracurricular activities along with the peer group. Activities that are minimally affected by the physical limitations imposed by JRA such as music, art, crafts and hobbies, drama, swimming, and computer activities will give the child greater opportunity to excel. Health professionals can assist the family, child, and teachers identify such activities.

Individuals with JRA are generally encouraged to participate in all activities within their capability and tolerance.[1] This assumes, however, that children are capable of limiting their own activities. While the intent of this guideline is to encourage the child with JRA to have as normal a life as possible, there may be a problem with the concept.[11] A child who has had prolonged early-onset JRA with marked restriction may never be tempted to try activities beyond their tolerance. Activity modification, however, will be particularly difficult for an older child with recent onset JRA, or one who was previously extremely athletic. The child may be willing to take the risk of temporary postactivity pain that they anticipate might happen, but in fact may be immobilized by pain for several days.

The PT has a role in helping the child to better gauge their activity tolerance, and to learn how to grade participation in potentially demanding school and extracurricular activities. A meeting between the PT and the school's physical education teacher often helps to dispel myths about the child's potential activity level. It also allows the setting of clear guidelines for physical activity so that the child feels supported in decisions to participate or refrain from specific gym and recess activities. Self-management strategies should be provided to assist the child manage mild stiffness and pain, since these will inevitably occur following some activities.

Future Research Directions

There is a lack of published clinical research evaluating the effectiveness of the various rehabilitation interventions for children and adolescents with JRA. This research is now possible and essential, given the advent of validated functional outcome measures that have direct relevance to the goals of rehabilitation.

Summary

Despite the stresses and difficulties, children with JRA and their parents often demonstrate a positive spirit to continue despite the challenges. Strong personal attributes such as determination, courage, and resilience often develop through the course of treatment. Certain characteristics may be heightened (i.e., empathy, caring, sense of humor), and frequently adolescents with JRA express career goals that are within the helping professions (i.e., nurse, social worker, teacher).

It is important to remember that the needs of children with JRA are extremely different from those of adults with RA. Management must be sensitive to the particular needs of a child and the family and respond to changes resulting from both the disease and the developmental process. The majority of children will reach adulthood without arthritis. The impact of the disease during childhood and any persisting contractures, joint damage, and functional loss will have a dramatic impact on quality of life as an adult. A strong partnership between the child, family, and the extended rheumatology team is imperative if therapy goals are to be realized.

Case History #1

History Michelle is a 13-year-old girl of French/Italian background. She lives in the northern part of the province in a rural community with few resources. She is flown out to an acute care pediatric hospital 700 miles away when ill.

She has had polyarticular systemic-onset arthritis since 3 years of age. While the disease was relatively quiet for the last 4 years, Michelle experienced a serious flare 6 months ago involving 40 joints. She also had a recurrence of her systemic rash and experienced marked fatigue, generalized muscle pain, and acute hip pain. With this flare, there was a marked deterioration in her physical condition with loss of independence in functional abilities and a sudden loss of her walking abilities for distances beyond 20 ft (10 m).

Michelle has missed 50 days of school since the exacerbation of her arthritis. She has always been a good student and attempts at home to keep up with the grade 8 work. Home tutoring is available for only 3 hours per week.

She lives about 30 minutes away from the school by school bus. With the recent disease flare and her need to use a manual wheelchair for mobility, she has not been able to use the regular school bus. The school lacks full accessibity, but Michelle is currently the only student with impaired mobility. A ramp has been built for Michelle to allow wheelchair use of one of the outside doors. Once inside the school, the classroom areas are accessible but the library and gymnasium-cafeteria only can be reached by stairs. Michelle is isolated from her peer group in school during breaks, gym, and assemblies, since she cannot access these areas.

Psychosocial Status Michelle is depressed and angry about her arthritis and its recurrence after several years of minimal disease activity.

Michelle's mother is overwhelmed with added physical and emotional demands. She is unemployed, a quiet and shy person who is not accustomed to large cities, medical systems, or making decisions. Father is a laborer and is often away from home for weeks at a time. Both parents had difficult childhoods with significant losses. Both experience many fears about the future and are grieving for Michelle who is dependent and requires significant care. Her father worries a lot about Michelle's future but does not like to show emotion and does not share feelings or fears with his wife or two daughters. He presents as very practical.

The other daughter, Renee, is 8 years of age. She worries about Michelle and her parents but also feels jealous and sad. She is often left behind with extended family for several weeks when Michelle is flown out to the hospital.

Her mother acts as the primary caregiver due to the father's extended time away from home. She feels torn in several directions: she has to be with Michelle but also wants to be with her husband and Renee. The father initially resisted the decision to fly out for treatment, so the final decision was made by the local doctor.

There is some extended family support within the community but few resources for therapy. Most of the buildings in the community are not accessible to someone who requires mobility devices such as scooters or wheelchairs. Michelle's house is not accessible, and the family cannot afford the major renovations that are required.

The family has great difficulty in planning financially for needs. Social Services (SS) is assisting with costs of medical needs and transportation and hospitalization in the pediatric rheumatology treatment center, but cannot reimburse retroactively. Because the family is uncomfortable asking for help, they often do not initiate requests until after the fact (i.e., money for food or lodging). Requests to SS often are made too late to get approval for funding.

Plan, 4 Weeks After Admission A new medication regimen was established (methotrexate) and intra-articular steroid injections given to shoulders, wrists, hips, knees, and ankles to relieve the marked synovitis and pain. The orthopedic consultation revealed that Michelle has had extensive damage to her hip joints and will likely require total hip replacements in about 5 years.

During the hospital stay, Michelle and her mother were initially overwhelmed by the entire situation. Her mother cried when approached by staff, and Michelle took her anger out on her mother. Counseling was provided to engage mother in expressing feelings, dealing with the grief process, and gaining more self-confidence.

Progress Following the intra-articular injections, Michelle was admitted to the affiliated pediatric rehabilitation facility for intensive therapy. With this transfer, Michelle's mother needed living and food arrangements for at least a 3-month period. The center's social worker liased with home community social services and was able to arrange funding for residence and mobility needs.

Michelle responded quickly to the intra-articular steroid injections with a marked decrease in the synovitis in all joints that had been injected and a dramatic relief of her severe hip pain. She received daily 1-hour pool therapy sessions, during which hip ROM and strength, and walking in shoulder deep water were emphasized.

With a decrease in hip pain and improved strength and ROM (40-degree hip flexion contractures reduced to 20 degrees), she progressed to walking on land with a walker fitted with trough crutches. The primary complaint during ambulation was of ankle pain when weight bearing, although this gradually subsided as Michelle's tolerance and endurance improved. *At discharge* 12 weeks later, Michelle was able to walk with trough crutches only and was able to manage distances of 500 ft (200 m) before needing a rest. Michelle was eventually able to manage a flight of stairs using her crutches.

Therapy and nursing staff helped Michelle become more independent (e.g., dressing), although she still required much prompting to initiate these activities rather than rely on her mother's help. A sock aid and a reaching device were provided to maximize Michelle's independence.

OT sessions also focused on hand mobility and function. Wrist cock-up splints were fabricated for daytime wear, although compliance with these was still only marginal at the time of discharge. Michelle had not worn daytime splints before and was very self-conscious about her appearance in them. Hand resting splints also were fabricated and Michelle was very consistent in wearing these every night.

Michelle attended the center's school, and by the end of the admission (12th week) had caught up on four of her grade 8 courses. Her academic program for grade 9 will require close evaluation on her return to her home school. Michelle attended recreation programs every evening at the center, and demonstrated continually increasing levels of confidence, self-image, and leadership abilities. She discovered that she had a talent for drama and puppetry, and the recreation staff were able to locate a drama club in her home town so that she could pursue this interest.

Michelle was seen by the social worker for individual counseling regarding separation, adjustment to disability, dependence on others for self-care and mobility, fears, depression, family dynamics, and peer interaction. The social worker was able to address upcoming issues, identify concerns, problem solve, and guide Michelle in assuming responsibility for the future. She participated in arthritis discussion groups with several other adolescents with JRA—this was the first time that she had the opportunity to meet with others with similar challenges.

Formal and informal education sessions were provided by nursing, OT, PT, and social workers about arthritis and its treatment (i.e., medications, stretchings, steroid injections, and possible future surgical procedures). During the admission, her mother became less terrified of the city and became comfortable in the rehabilitation center, in residence and community. She connected with the local church, as religion was important to her. A volunteer in the parish was available to take her out, and helped in arrangements that allowed the sister to come to the city and attend the local school.

Her father visited after Michelle and her mother had been at the center for 2 months. A team/family meeting was held (and included the rheumatologist from the acute-care center) to answer his questions and gain his support. As time passed on the new medication and intensive PT/OT regimens, Michelle and her mother noted gradual progress in her mobility and independence levels. Her father appeared to have a somewhat difficult time acknowledging Michelle's progress.

Discharge Planning A 1-hour teleconference meeting was held between the local school teacher and principal and the rehabilitation center's teacher, OT, PT, and social worker. Accessibility and mobility needs were reviewed with school personnel in Michelle's community and with the local social services staff. Early in Michelle's admission to the center, the OT had sent information to the school regarding suggestions for improving accessibility and mobility. During the teleconference, the local school indicated that they had been able to accommodate a few of the inexpensive suggestions (i.e., grab rail in the washroom); however, the problem of the stairs within the school and on the school bus had not yet been resolved. As

Michelle can now manage stairs with crutches, the lack of elevator or ramps will not restrict her mobility at school in the short term. Fortunately, the high school that she will be attending next year is all on one level.

Michelle's timetable was modified slightly to provide her with more time to transfer between classes, and she was given a second set of school books so that she would not have to carry them to and from school. While Michelle was encouraged to walk in the classroom and for 20- to 30-m distances in the corridor, she could use the scooter for longer distances in and outside the school. She was given permission to do her therapy exercises in the nurse's office rather than attending daily gym classes.

Since the nearest hospital and PT department is 90 km (50 miles) away from Michelle's house, a community care nurse will visit Michelle at school twice weekly to help with her therapy exercises. Ongoing counseling and support also have been arranged through the local social services agency. Michelle's parents set up a basic sling and pulley system above her bed so that she could do her hip ROM exercises every morning before rising.

It was evident that long-distance mobility at school and in the community would continue to be a problem. A mobility scooter was purchased to allow Michelle to manage these distances and keep up with her peers. Social services and a community club were able to share the portion of its cost that was not covered by the province's assistive devices program.

The center's social worker and PT arranged to call Michelle and her mother on a 3-weekly basis to provide support and monitor progress with exercises, splints, and walking. The local physician will monitor blood levels on current medications and send results via facsimile each week to Michelle's rheumatologist. Michelle will return to the acute-care rheumatology clinic in 4 months for follow-up. She then will be admitted to the rehabilitation center for a 2- or 3-week intensive therapy "tune-up," with particular emphasis on her hips and her walking.

Case History #2

History Five-year-old Maria was recently diagnosed with pauciarticular JRA. She initially felt unwell, with complaints of lower extremity joint pain and a mild limp when walking. The family doctor initially suggested that Maria had growing pains. However, Maria's physical activity level continued to decrease. Her parents noted that she was very stiff in the morning, often taking up to 30 minutes to get out of bed. Her right knee and left ankle developed profound swelling and heat. Her right knee rapidly developed a 35-degree flexion contracture. The parents requested further assessment and were referred to the rheumatology department of the acute-care pediatric hospital in their city. Diagnosis was made after numerous tests.

Maria was started on a nonsteroidal anti-inflammatory drug (NSAID) and referred to a nearby children's rehabilitation center for PT assessment. Because the family lived within a 30-minute drive of the center, she could attend outpatient PT sessions there.

On assessment, it was evident that the greatest physical priority was to reduce the right knee flexion contracture as quickly as possible. A leg length discrepancy of 0.5 cm had developed at the right knee in conjunction with medial femoral condyle overgrowth. There also was a right hip 10-degree flexion contracture, although there was no sign of arthritis at the hip. This contracture was likely secondary to the right knee flexion contracture. Left ankle and midfoot involvement was causing some loss of supination; Maria had a tendency to walk with a very pronated left midfoot and valgus hindfoot.

Reaction to the Diagnosis and Implementation of Treatment Parents felt guilty that the diagnosis was not made earlier and that they may not have initially believed or understood their daughter's complaints. They were shocked with the diagnosis of JRA, seeing arthritis as a disease of people over 60. They were keen to obtain reading material on JRA, and expressed intense anxiety regarding treatment, particularly medications and possible side effects. They wanted the medications to provide a quick miracle, and believed that more PTy (i.e., several hours per day) would make Maria better faster.

The parents went through the stages of grieving (i.e., shock, denial, anger, why us?). They wondered if they did or didn't do something that caused disease (i.e., went to Florida and left children with grandparents; perhaps the stress of this separation caused arthritis). They wanted some assurance that the arthritis would be gone in several months. The parents also had a difficult time dealing with the pain associated with the therapy stretches and the blood work. The parents, extended family, and peers tended to be overprotective out of sympathy for Maria. The rules at home changed, with fewer expectations and limits. Maria's brother, Michael, became concerned, sad, and worried that he too might get arthritis. He also felt jealous of the attention that Maria was getting, and also sometimes felt angry and guilty.

With the need to attend PTy three times per week, medical appointments for blood work, and do exercises at home, there were additional demands on the parents' time and energy. Maria's mother has had a difficult time emotionally and physically with back pain and had to take 8 weeks off work last year. She became worried about her job security now that she once again has to ask for time off from work to take Maria to her therapy and medical appointments.

Maria was initially scared and knew that her parents and extended family were worried, which must mean that the condition was serious. She did not know what was going on or why it was happening to her; she felt she was the only person in the world with arthritis. Her behavior deteriorated, and she became clingy and experienced severe anxiety when separated from her parents. She needed to be held during therapy and when having blood work. Within a couple of weeks of starting the PT home program, the exercises became an arena for parent/child conflict.

Intervention Plan Maria was registered at the children's rehabilitation center for the outpatient pool and gym PT program. In addition to PT, she attended a children's JRA education group. In an effort to regain full extension at Maria's right knee, the PT fabricated a knee resting splint (molded to Maria's knee after pool therapy, hot pack, and stretching). This splint was to be upgraded on a weekly or biweekly basis to accommodate the gradual improvement in knee extension. The work on knee extension was facilitated by use of intra-articular steroids that were injected into the right knee by the rheumatologist 2 days prior to the first PT session. The knee contracture was reduced to 25 degrees (a 10-degree change) within 2 days.

A left shoe orthosis was fabricated in the orthotics department to bring the hindfoot closer to neutral alignment and to allow the forefoot to rest in less pronation. A shoe lift of 0.5 cm was added to the sole of the left shoe to accommodate the leg length discrepancy caused by the synovitis at Maria's right knee.

The social worker initially met with the parents, Maria, and Michael to identify specific goals and to assess strengths, concerns, and fears. Biweekly sessions were scheduled with the mother to provide ongoing discussion and supportive counseling. These sessions occurred when Maria was attending pool or gym therapy. On alternate weeks, Michael met with the social worker to discuss his fears and other feelings. Maria had the opportunity to talk about her arthritis in a group format with three other children (ages 5–11) with JRA. They meet biweekly before the group pool session. A team conference with Maria's kindergarten teacher was planned because mother was unsure that they were aware of what to do with her, since they had never had a child with JRA in the school before.

Progress After 2 Months of Rehabilitation During the 2 months of outpatient care at the rehabilitation center, her mother met other parents, received emotional support, and her feeling of isolation was reduced. Maria met other children in pool therapy, social work, and education sessions, and saw others wearing splints. These experiences reduced her anxiety, and increased her self-confidence and her understanding regarding arthritis and the reasons for medications, stretches, and so forth. Both parents learned the therapy routine and watched the team's interactions with Maria. When they encountered resistance at home with Maria's exercises they were able to discuss this with the PT and social worker. To reduce some of the tensions and resistance, the home program was modified in terms of scope and a change in the type of rewards offered to Maria for complying. Exercise was selected as one of the topics for discussion in the children's social work group.

Future Plans Maria's disease activity is minimal with only mild soft tissue swelling at her left ankle and no stress pain. Maria's knee contracture resolved in 7 weeks, and her final knee resting splint is in full extension. This splint will continue to be worn every night until all signs of synovitis at the right knee are gone. Then, the splint will be weaned off gradually (i.e., one night per week without, two nights without, etc). The hip flexion contracture proved resistant to stretching and is still at about 10 degrees. Maria will need to continue with prone lying and hip flexor stretchings until it resolves. The mobility at her left hindfoot and midfoot have improved, and the orthotic requires adjustment to accommodate this gain in motion. Her gait has improved dramatically and the limp has totally resolved. She is able to run and skip again without pain, and has no further difficulty with sitting cross-legged on the floor at school.

Maria's treatment sessions at the center have been reduced to once weekly, and coincide with the day that the social work discussion group is held. She will see the rheumatologist on a 3-monthly basis. The PT will continue to reassess Maria's status on a monthly basis making sure that she does a thorough joint screening assessment to detect promptly any new joints that might have synovitis. Maria has returned to her full activity level and is able to keep up with her peers in all kindergarten activities.

References

1. Cassidy JT, Petty RE: Juvenile rheumatoid arthritis. In Cassidy JT (ed): Textbook of Rheumatology, pp 113–219. New York, Churchill Livingstone Inc, 1990.
2. Shore A: Arthritis in childhood. Med North Am 1988; 26:4869–4877.
3. Truckenbrodt H: Pain in juvenile chronic arthritis: consequences for the musculoskeletal system. Clin Exp Rheumatol 1993; 11:S59–S63.
4. Emery HM: The rehabilitation of the child with juvenile chronic arthritis. Balliere's Clin Pediatr 1993; 1:803–823.
5. Reed MH, Wilmot DM: The radiology of juvenile rheumatoid arthritis: a review of the English language literature. J Rheumatol 1991; 18(S31):2–22.
6. Brewer EJ, Giannini EH: Juvenile rheumatoid arthritis. Clin Rheum Dis 1983; 9:629–640.
7. Ansell BM: Chronic arthritis in childhood. Ann Rheum Dis 1978; 37:107–120.
8. Swann M: Juvenile chronic arthritis. Clin Orthop 1987; 219:38–49.
9. McCullough CJ: Surgical management of the hip in juvenile chronic arthritis. Br J Rheumatol 1994; 33: 178–183.
10. Scull SA, Dow MB, Athreya BH: Physical and occupational therapy for children with rheumatic diseases. Pediatr Clin North Am 1986; 33:1053–1077.
11. Erlandson DM: Juvenile rheumatoid arthritis. In Logigian MK, Ward JD (eds): A Team Approach for Therapists—Pediatric Rehabilitation, pp 195–227. Boston, Little, Brown & Co, 1989.
12. Donovan WE: Physical measures in the treatment of JRA. In Miller JJ (ed:) Juvenile Rheumatoid Arthritis, pp 209–227. Littleton, MA, PSG Publishing Co, 1979.
13. Boone JE, Baldwin J, Levine C: Juvenile rheumatoid arthritis. Pediatr Clin North Am 1974; 21:885–915.
14. Fife RZ: Methotrexate use in juvenile rheumatoid arthritis. Orthop Nurs 1993: 12(1):32–36.
15. Gedalia A, Person DA, Brewer EJ, et al: Hypermobility of the joints in juvenile episodic arthritis/arthralgia. J Pediatr 1985; 107(6):873–876.
16. Lechner DE, McCarthy C, Holden MK: Gait deviations in patients with juvenile rheumatoid arthritis. Phys Ther 1987; 67:1335–1341.
17. Falconer J, Hayes KW: A simple method to measure gait for use in arthritis clinical research. Arthritis Care Res 1991; 4:52–57.
18. Lovell DJ: Newer functional outcome measurements in juvenile rheumatoid arthritis: a progress report. J Rheumatol 1992; 19(S33):28–31.
19. Varni JW, Thompson KL, Hanson V: The Varni/Thompson pediatric pain questionnaire. I. Chronic musculoskeletal pain in juvenile rheumatoid arthritis. Pain 1987; 28:27–38.
20. Wright V, Law M: An evaluation of the reliability of observational and self-report measures used in paediatric rheumatology (abstr). Physiother Can 1993: 45(2):S2.
21. Howe S, Levinson J, Shear E, et al: Development of a disability measurement tool for juvenile rheumatoid arthritis. The juvenile arthritis functional assessment report for children and their parents. Arthritis Rheum 1991; 34:873–880.
22. Singh G, Athreya B, Fries J, et al: Measurement of health status in children with juvenile rheumatoid arthritis. Arthritis Rheum 1994; 37:1761–1769.
23. Wright V, Law M, Crombie V, et al: Development of a self-report functional status index for juvenile rheumatoid arthritis. J Rheumatol 1994; 21:536–544.
24. Wright V, Law M, Longo Kimber J, et al: Validation of a functional status index for juvenile rheumatoid arthritis. Physiother Can 1992; 44(2):S6.
25. Duffy CM, Arsenault L: Juvenile arthritis quality of life questionnaire (abstr). Arthritis Rheum 1992; 35: S222.
26. Tugwell P, Bombardier C, Buchanan WW, et al: The MACTAR patient preference disability questionnaire. J Rheumatol 1987; 14:446–451.
27. Law M, Baptiste S, McColl MA, et al: An outcome measure for occupational therapy. Can J Occup Ther 1990; 57(2):82–87.
28. Haley SM, Coster WJ, Ludlow LH: Paediatric functional outcome measures. Phys Med Rehabil Clin North Am 1991; 2:689–723.
29. Feldman AB, Haley SM, Coryell J: Concurrent and construct validity of the Pediatric Evaluation of Disability Inventory. Phys Ther 1990; 70:602–610.

30. Atwood M: Developmental assessment and integration. In Melvin J (ed): Rheumatic Disease in Adult and Child: Occupational Therapy and Rehabilitation, 3rd edition, pp 188–214. Philadelphia, FA Davis Co, 1989.
31. Vandvik IH, Eckblad G: Relationship between pain, disease severity and psychosocial function in patients with juvenile chronic arthritis (JCA). Scand J Rheumatol 1990; 19:295–302.
32. Lovell D, Walco GA: Pain associated with juvenile rheumatoid arthritis. Pediatr Clin North Am 1989; 36(4):1015–1027.
33. Savedra MC, Tesler MD, Holzemer WL, et al: Pain location: validity and reliability of body outline markings by hospitalized children and adolescents. Res Nurs Health 1989; 12:307–314.
34. Tesler M, Savedra M, Ward JA, et al: Children's language of pain. In Dubner R, Gebhart GF, Bond MR (eds): Proceedings of the 5th World Congress on Pain, pp 350–351. New York, Elsevier Science Publishers, 1988.
35. Wilkie DJ, Holzemer WL, Tesler MD, et al: Measuring pain quality: validity and reliability of children's and adolescents' pain language. Pain 1990; 41:151–159.
36. Badley EM, Papageorgiou AC: Visual analogue scales as a measure of pain in arthritis: a study of overall pain and pain in individual joints at rest and on movement. J Rheumatol 1989; 16:102–105.
37. Van Cleve LJ, Savedra MC: Pain location: validity and reliability of body outline markings by 4 to 7 year old children who are hospitalized. Pediatr Nurs 1993; 19(03):217–220.
38. Brewer EJ, Angel KC: Parenting a Child with Arthritis. Los Angeles, Lowell House, 1992.
39. Sabbeth B: Understanding the impact of chronic childhood illness on families. Pediatr Clin North Am 1984; 31(1):47–69.
40. Timko C, Stovel KW, Moos RH: Functioning among mothers and fathers of children with juvenile rheumatic disease: a longitudinal study. J Pediatr Psychol 1992(b); 17(6):705–724.
41. McCormick MC, Stemmler MM, Athreya BH: The impact of childhood rheumatic diseases on the family. Arthritis Rheum 1986; 29:872–879.
42. Levanthal JM: Psychosocial assessment of children with chronic physical disease. Pediatr Clin North Am 1984; 31:71–86.
43. Stein REK, Jessop DJ: General issues in the care of children with chronic physical conditions. Pediatr Clin North Am 1984; 31(1):189–198.
44. Atwood M: Treatment considerations. In Melvin J (ed): Rheumatic Disease in Adult and Child: Occupational Therapy and Rehabilitation, 3rd edition, pp 215–234. Philadelphia, FA Davis Co, 1989.
45. Allaire SH, DeNardo BS, Szer IS, et al: The economic impact of juvenile rheumatoid arthritis. J Rheumatol 1992; 19:952–955.
46. Melvin JL, Atwood M: Juvenile rheumatoid arthritis. In Melvin JL (ed): Rheumatic Disease in Adult and Child: Occupational Therapy and Rehabilitation, 3rd edition, pp 135–187. Philadelphia, FA Davis Co, 1989.
47. Adams DW, Deveau EJ: Coping with Childhood Cancer—Where Do We Go From Here? Reston, VA, Reston Publishing Co, 1984.
48. Quirk ME, Young MH: The impact of JRA on children, adolescents, and their families: current research and implications for future studies. Arthritis Care Res 1990; 3:36–43.
49. McGrath PJ, McAlpine L: Psychologic perspectives on pediatric pain. J Pediatr 1993; 122(5):2–8.
50. Kurland R, Salmon R: When problems seem overwhelming: emphases on teaching, supervision, and consultation. Social Work 1992; 37(3):240–244.
51. Cyriax J: Textbook of Orthopaedic Medicine. Volume 1—Diagnosis of Soft Tissue Lesions. London, Balliere Tindall, 1975.
52. Simmons BP, Nutting JT: Juvenile rheumatoid arthritis. Hand Clin 1989; 5(2):157–168.
53. Timko C, Stovel KW, Moos RH, et al: Adaptation to juvenile rheumatic disease: a controlled evaluation of functional disability with a one-year follow-up. Health Psychol 1992; 11(1):67–76.
54. Davis M, Eshelman ER, McKay M: The relaxation and stress reduction workbook. Oakland, CA, New Harbinger Publications Inc, 1988.
55. Rhodes V: Physical therapy management of patients with juvenile rheumatoid arthritis. Phys Ther 1991; 71:910–919.
56. Barkley E, Brewer EJ: Home treatment program. In Brewer EJ (ed): Juvenile Rheumatoid Arthritis, pp 132–155. Philadelphia, WB Saunders Co, 1970.
57. Jarvis RE: Physiotherapy for children and young adults with arthritis. Physiotherapy 1978; 64:143–145.
58. Ansell BM: Rehabilitation. In Arden GP, Ansell BM (eds): Surgical Management of Juvenile Chronic Polyarthritis, pp 202–215. London, Academic Press, 1978.
59. Bacon MC, Nicholson C, Binder H, et al: Juvenile rheumatoid arthritis: aquatic exercise and lower extremity function. Arthritis Care Res 1991; 4:102–105.
60. Giannini M, Protas EJ: Exercise response in children with and without juvenile rheumatoid arthritis. Phys Ther 1992; 72:365–372.
61. Klepper SE, Darbee J, Effgen SK, et al: Physical fitness levels in children with polyarticular juvenile rheumatoid arthritis. Arthritis Care Res 1992; 5:93–100.
62. Giannini JM, Protas EJ: Comparison of peak isometric knee extensor torque in children with and without juvenile rheumatoid arthritis. Arthritis Care Res 1993; 6(2):82–88.
63. Barrie HJ: Unexpected sites of wear in the femoral head. J Rheumatol 1986; 13:1099–1104.
64. Toomey R, Grief-Schwartz R, Piper MC: Clinical evaluation of the effects of whirlpool on patients

with Colles' fractures. Physiother Can 1986; 38: 280–284.

65. Walmsley RP, Swann I: Biomechanics and physiology of muscle strengthening. Physiother Can 1976; 28: 197–200.
66. Jamison L, Ogden D: Aquatic therapy using PNF patterns. Tucson, AZ, Therapy Skill Builders, 1994.
67. Boyle A-M: The Bad-Ragaz ring method. Physiotherapy 1981; 67(9):265–268.
68. Etnyre BR, Abraham LK: Gains in range of ankle dorsiflexion using three popular stretching techniques. Am J Phys Med 1986; 65:189–196.
69. Condon SM, Hutton RS: Soleus muscle electromyographic activity and ankle dorsiflexion range of motion during four stretching procedures. Phys Ther 1987; 67:24–30.
70. Wessling KC, DeVane DA, Hylton CA: Effects of static stretch versus static stretch and ultrasound combined on triceps surae extensibility in healthy women. Phys Ther 1987; 67:674–679.
71. Henricson AS, Fredericksson K, Persson I, et al: The effect of heat and stretching on the range of hip motion. J Orthop Sports Phys Ther 1984; 6:110–115.
72. Magyar E, Talerman A, Mohacsy J, et al: Muscle changes in rheumatoid arthritis. Virchows Arch [A] 1972; 373:267–278.
73. Bohannon RW: Effect of repeated eight-minute muscle loading on the angle of straight leg raising. Phys Ther 1984; 64(4):491–497.
74. Godges JJ, MacRae PG, Engelke KA: Effects of exercise on hip range of motion, trunk muscle performance, and gait economy. Phys Ther 1993; 73:468–477.
75. Williams PE: Use of intermittent stretch in the prevention of serial sarcomere loss in immobilised muscle. Ann Rheum Dis 1990; 49:316–317.
76. Galloway MT, Jokl P: The role of exercise in the treatment of inflammatory arthritis. Bull Rheum Dis 1993; 42:1–4.
77. Harkcom TM, Lampman RM, Banwell BF, et al: Therapeutic value of graded aerobic exercise training in rheumatoid arthritis. Arthritis Rheum 1985; 28:32–39.
78. Minor MA, Hewett JE, Webel RR, et al: Efficacy of physical conditioning exercise in patients with rheumatoid arthritis and osteoarthritis. Arthritis Rheum 1989; 32:1396–1405.
79. Kircheimer JC, Wanivenhaus A, Engel A: Does sport negatively influence joint scores in patients with juvenile rheumatoid arthritis. Rheumatol Int 1993; 12 (6):239–242.
80. Oberg T, Karsznia A, Gare BA, Lagerstrand A: Physical training of children with juvenile chronic arthritis. Effects of force, endurance and EMG response to localized muscle fatigue. Scand J Rheumatol 1994; 23:92–95.
81. Reed AM, Haugen M, Pachman LM, et al: Repair of osteopenia in children with juvenile rheumatoid arthritis. J Pediatr 1993; 122(5):693–696.
82. Vargo MM, Gerber LH: Exercise strategies for osteoporosis. Bull Rheum Dis 1993; 42(5):6–9.
83. Taylor L, Adelman HS, Kaser-Boyd N: Perspectives of children regarding their psychoeducational decisions. Prof Psychol Res Prac 1983; 14(6):882–894.
84. Hayford JR, Ross CK: Medical compliance in juvenile rheumatoid arthritis. Arthritis Care Res 1988; 1: 190–197.
85. Petr CG: Adultcentrism in practice with children. Fam Soc 1992; 73(7):408–416.
86. Rapoff MA, Lindsley CB, Christopherson ER: Parent perceptions of problems experienced by their children in complying with treatment for juvenile rheumatoid arthritis. Arch Phys Med Rehabil 1985; 66: 427–429.
87. Wynn KS, Eckel EM: Juvenile rheumatoid arthritis and home physical therapy program compliance. Phys Occup Ther Pediatr 1986; 6:55–63.
88. Mayo NE: Patient compliance: practical implications for physical therapists—a review of the literature. Phys Ther 1978; 58:1083–1090.
89. Berry SL, Hayfors JR, Ross CK, et al: Conceptions of illness by children with juvenile rheumatoid arthritis: a cognitive developmental approach. J Pediatr Psychol 1993; 18:83–97.
90. Falco JL, Block DV, Vostrjs MD, et al: JRA and ME—A Fun Workbook. Atlanta, GA, Rocky Mountain Juvenile Arthritis Center. Arthritis Foundation, 1987.
91. Whitehouse R, Shop JT, Sullivan DB, et al: Children with juvenile arthritis at school—functional problems, participation in physical education. Clin Pediatr 1989; 28:509–514.
92. Stoff E, Bacon MC, White PH: The effects of fatigue, distractibility, and absenteeism on school achievement in children with rheumatic diseases. Arthritis Care Res 1989; 2:54–59.
93. Taylor J, Passo MH, Champion VL: School problems and teacher responsibilities in juvenile rheumatoid arthritis. J School Health 1987; 57:186–190.
94. Weitzman M: School and peer relations. Pediatr Clin North Am 1984; 31:59–69.
95. Ansell BM, Rudge S, Schaller JG: Color Atlas of Pediatric Rheumatology, pp 13–75. London, Wolfe Publishing Limited, 1992.
96. Libby AK, Sherry DD, Dudgeon BJ: Shoulder limitation in juvenile rheumatoid arthritis. Arch Phys Med Rehabil 1991; 72:382–384.
97. White PH: Growth abnormalities in children with juvenile rheumatoid arthritis. Clin Orthop 1990; 259:46–50.

CHAPTER 13

Physical Therapy Management of Patients with Rheumatoid Arthritis and Other Inflammatory Conditions

Antoine Helewa, MSc(Clin Epid), PT

Rheumatoid arthritis (RA) and other related syndromes are characterized by inflammation of the synovium and connective tissues of diarthrodial joints and, to a lesser extent, the related tissues—tendons and their sheaths; bursal and periarticular subcutaneous tissues. The systemic and extra-articular manifestations suggest use of the term rheumatoid disease; however, these are less frequent and severe than lesions in the joints.[1]

The joint inflammation of RA is, with minor variation, similar in its effects to that found in other inflammatory arthritis syndromes, such as juvenile arthritis (JA or JRA), ankylosing spondylitis (AS), Reiter's syndrome, and psoriatic arthritis.

PHYSICAL THERAPY IN ARTHRITIS, Joan M. Walker, PhD, PT, and Antoine Helewa, MSc(Clin Epid), PT, W.B. Saunders Company © 1996.

While systemic disease is the chief problem in systemic lupus erythematosus (SLE), the features of joint inflammation, although seen less frequently, are similar to those of RA.

The physical therapy (PT) management of JRA and AS is covered extensively in Chapters 12 and 15. This chapter will focus primarily on the PT management of RA, and since the joint inflammation in RA shares common features with that of Reiter's syndrome, psoriatic arthritis, and SLE, by extension, the PT management of these conditions also will be covered. Distinctions in the PT management of the other syndromes, where they exist, will be noted.

The chapter will begin with a description of PT elements in the management of inflammatory joint disease, followed by management objectives, goal setting, and contracts. Aspects of PT management then will be discussed under the following broad strategies: analgesic PT, rest and activity, therapeutic exercise, restoration of function, and goal setting and contracting.

The chapter will conclude with one case history and a discussion of research questions important to physical therapists.

Elements of Physical Therapy

PT is an essential treatment strategy for patients with RA and other inflammatory arthritic syndromes. Any patient with inflammatory joint disease must receive PT at one time or another regardless of disease stage and severity, but preferably in the early stages of the disease. As early medical diagnosis is frequently difficult to reach, patients often are referred to PT after joint manifestations and problems with physical function have become established. There also is a misconception that PT can do little for these patients in the early stages of the disease, or when the inflammation is raging, which ignores the important early treatment strategies designed specifically to reduce impairment and disability.

It is preferable that patients with inflammatory joint disease receive PT in the early stages of the disease.

It is exposure of patients with RA to PT as a health discipline that is important and not necessarily any of its individual modalities in isolation. Best results are achieved when PT is delivered as a package, custom tailored to the patient's needs and encompassing elements of disease education, counseling, assessment, treatment, and independence in activities of daily living. Three basic elements form the core of PT practice for patients with RA. PT should:

- help nature restore normal physical function, such as the application of therapeutic exercise to restore muscle strength
- ensure that the body's own healing processes do not become a source of the difficulty (e.g., scarring, contracture, pannus and degenerative changes)
- in a chronic, unrelenting lifelong disease, apply strategies that will prevent further deterioration of function

PT techniques are seldom applied singly, but usually in combination. For example, therapeutic exercise could be preceded by the application of cold packs to antagonistic muscle groups to enhance the response of the agonists. Disease education and its impact on dysfunction would precede training in joint protection and energy conservation where appropriate. PT should be applied in association with some medical therapies, such as anti-inflammatory medications, analgesics, and surgery.

Management Objectives

To achieve success, PT management in patients with RA must be accompanied by an accurate diagnosis; quantitative assessment of disease activity, impairment, and function; effective anti-inflammatory therapy; and in the presence of joint deformities and destruction, judicious rheumatoid surgery. Chapters 3 and 4 cover extensively disease features and diagnosis of RA. Chapter 8 deals exclusively with assessment strategies, and Chapter 6 covers surgical interventions.

Generally, the objectives of PT in the management of patients with RA are to control pain, increase and maintain joint mobility and muscle strength, maintain cardiopulmonary fitness, protect joints, conserve energy, and preserve function.[2] To accomplish these objectives, PTs use a variety of treatment techniques. Central to all these techniques is the judicious application of therapeutic exercise, tailored to the patient's needs. Most other techniques used are primarily adjuncts to therapeutic exercise and include heat, cold, and electrical muscle stimulation.[2] Table 13-1 provides a summary of the techniques commonly used in the treatment of patients with RA, listed by objective and physiological effects sought. Table 13-2 outlines general principles to follow when planning a treatment program. PT objectives are to:

- control pain
- increase and maintain joint mobility and muscle strength
- maintain cardiopulmonary fitness
- protect joints
- conserve energy
- preserve function

Analgesic Physical Therapy

Analgesic PT modalities alone are not effective in the management of the acutely inflamed joints of

Table 13-1. Summary of Physical Therapy Techniques for Rheumatoid Arthritis*

Modality	Effects	Objective	Comments
Analgesics			
Cold	Inhibits nerve conduction	Controls pain and muscle spasm	Best for active joints[†] Applied to muscles in spasm (flexors)
Heat	Increases nerve conduction	Controls pain and muscle spasm	Best for chronic joints Applied to muscles in spasm (flexors)
TENS	Inhibits nerve conduction	Controls pain	Limited to one or two sites
Facilitatory			
Electrical muscle stimulation or ice massage	Facilitatory	Preserves or restores muscle strength	Precedes strengthening exercises
Therapeutic exercise			
Mobilizing	Elasticity of joint and soft tissue structures	Preserves or restores joint range	Active joint: exercise to pain tolerance
Strengthening (isometric/isotonic)	Facilitatory	Preserves or restores muscle strength	Active joint: submaximal isometric
Conditioning (aerobic)	Muscle endurance, cardiopulmonary fitness	Preserves or restores physical fitness	Low-impact or water aerobics

*From Helewa A, Smythe HA: Physical therapy in rheumatoid arthritis. In Wolfe F, Pincus T (eds): Rheumatoid Arthritis. Pathogenesis, Assessment, Outcome and Treatment, pp 415–433. New York, Marcel Dekker, 1994. With permission.

[†]Exercise should not be applied to joints anesthesized by cold.

TENS, transcutaneous electrical nerve stimulation.

uncontrolled RA. Only determined anti-inflammatory therapy will offer relief of pain due to raging disease. In general, pain-relieving PT modalities offer short-term relief of pain lasting 1 or 2 hours, serving as warm-up or to relieve muscle tightness and spasm in preparation for therapeutic exercise or certain activities of daily living. Given alone, they serve a very limited purpose and raise unduly a patient's hopes of obtaining the sought after, long-lasting relief of chronic pain. Two forms of analgesic PT are commonly used: thermal applications and electrical stimulation.

Thermal Applications

The two most commonly applied thermal techniques in patients with RA (and by consensus the most sensible) are the application of simple hot or cold packs. Heat in general, when applied to actively inflamed RA joints, has been known to increase nerve conduction. In view of that, it can increase pain sensation in active joints. For mildly inflamed joints, moist heat has the advantage of relieving the "gel phenomenon."

Cold, on the other hand, has opposite physiological effects, and therefore can be beneficial to intensely inflamed joints. Cold pain relief is due to counterirritant effects and endorphin release.[3–5] Other known effects of cold include reduction of edema formation and joint swelling.[3–6] The anti-inflammatory effects of cold are mediated through vasoconstriction, reducing hyperemia,[7] as well as direct effects on abnormal metabolic processes by reducing the activity of collagenase in the inflammatory reaction.[8] Cold also reduces muscle spasm by decreasing the conductivity of the muscle spindles; the stimulus threshold for firing is raised, thus decreasing the afferent firing rate.[3,6]

In contrast, the application of ice cubes, using a few short strokes over a muscle belly, can stim-

Table 13-2. General Principles in Physical Therapy Management of Rheumatoid Arthritis*

1. Treatment plans must be based on an accurate diagnosis and assessment of disease activity and dysfunction.
2. The selection of treatment techniques and dosage specifications must be supported by scientific evidence. If this evidence is unavailable, then the treatment and dosage should make biological sense. Careful assessment and periodic review of treatment results is essential.
3. Treatment techniques should be brief and simple to apply (preferably by the patient) and adapted for home use.
4. Treatment techniques should be pain free and safe. If joint swelling or pain lasts 2 hours or more after treatment, the therapy should be reviewed or its intensity reduced.
5. Therapeutic exercise has many objectives and is central to PT management; all other techniques are largely treatment adjuncts.
6. Strategies to improve patient compliance, in addition to principles 3 and 4, should be based on patient instruction about the disease and its treatment.

*From Helewa A, Smythe HA: Physical therapy in rheumatoid arthritis. In Wolfe F, Pincus T (eds): Rheumatoid Arthritis. Pathogenesis, Assessment, Outcome and Treatment, pp 415–433. New York, Marcel Dekker, 1994. With permission.

ulate muscle response by facilitating alpha motoneuron discharge.[9,10] This facilitatory response is very effective when applied to muscles inhibited by joint pain or swelling.

In patients with inflamed joints, hot or cold applications are not interchangeable, because they have opposite physiological effects. However, an uncontrolled study of patients with RA with chronic knee problems showed that there was no difference in pain or stiffness between hot or cold packs applied over a 5-week period.[5] In another study of patients with RA (30 active knee joints in all), 15 were allocated at random to a control group and 15 to an ice treatment group. All patients were stabilized on bed rest for 1 week and both groups received therapeutic exercise during the experimental period. After 5 days of therapy, there was no difference between the groups in joint circumference or thermographic measurement of skin temperature. The small sample size and the possibility of a type II error may have contributed to these results.[11] Another randomized trial of 18 patients with RA and with shoulder pain showed no difference between results from use of hot or cold packs. But, again the sample size was inadequate.[12]

At first glance these studies would suggest that hot or cold applications are interchangeable, and that patient choice should determine the application of one technique or another. However, a closer analysis showed that the three studies were fraught with methodological problems, such as a lack of a control group in one, and small sample sizes in the other two. Therefore, the question of the interchangeability of hot or cold modalities in RA has not been addressed properly in randomized controlled trials.

Paraffin Wax

Another form of heat applied to the hands of patients with RA is melted paraffin wax heated to 48°C. As its most useful effect is in the relief of morning stiffness, it should be applied by the patients in their own homes. However, home wax applications are fraught with danger, and unless the wax is heated in a double boiler, it can cause a fire. A safer alternative is to apply mineral oil to the hands, wear rubber dish washing gloves, and soak in hot water from the tap for 5–10 minutes (also see Chapter 16).

Short-Wave Diathermy (SWD)

This modality was used frequently in the past for its purported deep heating effects. A randomized clinical trial of 131 patients with RA and osteoarthritis (OA) showed no difference in range of movement (ROM), walking, and stair climbing time between patients who received exercise and one of SWD, sham SWD, or infrared and electrical muscle stimulation. The improvement seen in all patients was probably the result of the treatments received, plus the encouragement obtained.[13] *A recent study showed that by raising intra-articular temperature by 2.4°C, SWD can potentially cause harm.*[14]

In light of these results and the fact that SWD is a very expensive modality (>$10,000 per unit), is likely to aggravate joint pain, and can cause slow healing skin burns if not applied carefully, there is consensus that overall hot packs by far are safer, cheaper, and equally effective when compared to

SWD. Furthermore, SWD's unwieldy bulk and costs make it impractical for home use by patients.

Ultrasound

A Medline search of the literature revealed no controlled studies of ultrasound on patients with RA. The lack of well-performed controlled studies leads to uncritical and inappropriate application of a modality that may at times be harmful and an unnecessary expense.[7]

Applying Thermal Packs

On balance, the simple application of hot or cold packs is the most appropriate form of thermal modality in the treatment of RA. Hot or cold packs are usually applied for 15–20 minutes, the material wrapped in a damp towel to permit even conduction of thermal energy. Ice should never be applied directly to the skin (ice massage excepted), nor should the weight of a limb or torso rest on the pack, as this may burn the cold, anesthetized skin.[2] In a clinical setting, crushed ice can be obtained from special ice-making machines. In the home it can be obtained in the form of ice cubes, crushed ice, or use of a pack of frozen peas, depending on availability. The crushed ice is usually placed in the middle third of a regular bath towel forming a rectangle of about 18 × 8 inches, depending on the part to be cooled. The towel is then folded longitudinally, at which point the crushed ice will adhere to the wet towel, preventing its escape. The ends of the towel free from ice are held tightly in a knot with rubber bands to prevent escape from either end. The pack is then applied to the skin overlying the area to be cooled, leaving one layer of toweling between the crushed ice and the skin surface. Other forms of cooling body surfaces that are commercially available are local sprays and cryowraps.[15]

Ice, with the exception of ice massage, should never be applied directly to the skin.

Cold Rx Protocols

There are two commonly used cold treatment protocols in RA, illustrated by the following examples. The first involves the treatment of a knee with moderate synovitis, spasm of the knee flexors, and quadriceps muscle atrophy. Treatment begins with a cold pack application to the skin overlying all knee flexors (hamstrings, popliteus, and gastrocnemius) for 15–20 minutes. This will decrease muscle spasm by reducing muscle spindle activity. This is followed with ice massage, given in short strokes for 1 minute, to the skin overlying the quadriceps muscles to stimulate muscle response by facilitating alpha motoneuron discharge in muscles inhibited by pain and swelling. This sets the stage for the application of specific therapeutic exercise techniques to enhance this effect, such as hold relax, slow reversals, or slow isometric reversals.

The second protocol would involve the management of a severely inflamed knee joint, held in about 30 degrees of flexion (the position preferred by the knee with excess synovial fluid). Cold would be applied on the skin surfaces surrounding the knee joint, reaching proximally to the upper end of the suprapatellar pouch and distally below the tibial tubercle. Cold over a joint surface will increase the pain threshold by directly reducing the activity of pain-conducting fibers and receptors, and by supplying competitive sensations, as suggested by the gate-control theory.

It also will reduce inflammation by decreasing the activity of collagenase in the inflammatory reaction. As this may result in cold anesthesia, immediate rigorous isotonic exercise to already inflamed and distended ligamentous structures may result in a competing inflammatory response and lead to further pain and ligamentous laxity. Ideally, gentle slow isometric reversals should be applied, followed by one or two free active movements in the pain-free range.

Cold should not be used in patients with Raynaud's phenomenon, cold hypersensitivity, cryoglobulinemia (presence in blood of a protein that forms gels at low temperatures), or paroxysmal cold hemoglobinuria (presence of hemoglobin in the urine following local or general exposure to cold). It also should be avoided if it proves uncomfortable.[16]

A practical homemade hot pack can be made by placing a wet facecloth or small towel in a plastic freezer bag and heating it in a microwave oven for 1 minute. The heated pack is then wrapped in a damp towel and applied to the affected area for 15–20 minutes. Hot packs should not be applied to inflamed joints, as this may potentially cause harm by increasing the intra-articular temperature of a joint.[8,14] Localized heat also may be hazardous in conditions involving impaired arterial circulation, impaired sensation, local hemorrhage, malignancy, or inflammation.[17]

Electrical Stimulation

Analgesic electrical stimulation plays a limited role in the management of patients with RA, but can be useful in the treatment of intractable regional pain. The two modalities in common use are transcutaneous electrical nerve stimulation (TENS), and interferential currents.

Transcutaneous Electrical Nerve Stimulation

TENS application results in release of endorphins in the spinal cord due to increased stimulation of large myelinated nerve fibers, which tend to override the nociceptive inputs from unmyelinated C and small myelinated A delta fibers.[18,19] Portable TENS devices lend themselves well for home use and application by the patient. To determine response to TENS, three trials are first attempted—one at rest, another during walking, and a third during normal manual activities. The pain visual analogue scale is used to determine response under these conditions. The TENS is usually applied for a period of 30–45 minutes. Criteria for success are 3 hours pain relief, improved sleep, and reduced intake of pain medications. Altogether, 25 randomized trials of TENS have been published; of these, only two involved patients with RA. The first was double blind and involved 32 subjects allocated to active TENS and placebo TENS to the wrist, and who were stabilized on "anti-inflammatory analgesics."[20] Resting pain and gripping pain were measured by a visual analogue scale. The experimental group had a statistically significant reduction in both resting and gripping pain; however, the observation period lasted only 3 weeks, and patients were not followed-up longer. Also, sample size estimates were not given. The second trial also was double blind and involved 33 patients allocated to TENS and placebo TENS. The results showed no statistically significant difference between the two groups. Sample size was not justified.[21]

The remaining 23 studies of patients without RA also show conflicting results, with about half showing that TENS is not better than placebo.[7] In view of this, TENS continues to be a controversial modality and its effects on patients with RA must be investigated more rigorously.

Interferential Currents

This is a special modification of middle-frequency currents (>1,000 Hz), which tend to avoid the sensory disadvantage of lower frequency currents such as TENS (80–120 Hz) by passing through the skin without being felt.[7] Interferential currents are impractical for patients with RA with multiple joint involvement, and the high cost of these devices (>$10,000) diminishes their importance as a therapeutic choice. More importantly, there are no randomized clinical trials assessing treatment efficacy in patients with RA. An unpublished randomized trial of interferential current efficacy on patients with OA of the knee showed no difference between active and placebo therapy.[22]

The effects of TENS on patients with RA require further investigation.

Effects of Systemic Rest

The systemic manifestations of RA, reflected in fever, weight loss, anemia, and visceral involvement, suggest that a period of physical bed rest may rapidly improve an acute episode. Total bed rest is rarely advisable, as it can lead to deconditioning. Some patients also have expressed fears of becoming crippled if confined to bed. Younger patients also fear that prolonged bed rest may threaten income and job security.[23] On the other hand, hyperactive patients and those with stressful life styles who have systemic disease and multiple joint involvement can benefit from a short period of complete bed rest. The value of rest has been attributed to a slowing down of metabolic demand during joint use, which may reduce the level of microinfarctions of synovial villi, the source of rice bodies found in severely involved joints.[24] The prohibitive cost of hospitalization to patients, government, and third-party payers makes total bed rest unattractive in today's climate of cost constraints. Two randomized clinical trials comparing total bed rest with activity showed no significant overall anti-inflammatory effect on the bed rest groups, and the benefits shown were marginal.[23,25] This is not to be confused with hospitalization for RA where inpatient therapy was shown to be superior to intensive outpatient therapy.[26]

As RA can put a tremendous strain on both physical and emotional resources, bed rest for 1–2 hours once or twice daily may prevent fatigue and improve recuperation.[23,27]

Therapeutic Exercises

Muscle wasting is a common feature of patients with RA, and cannot be attributed to disuse alone. The leading causes of muscle atrophy have been attributed to deposition of inflammatory cells in the muscles of patients with RA (myositis); inflammation of the endothelial layer of blood vessels supplying muscle spindles, muscle fibers, and nerves of skeletal muscles (vasculitis); deposition of inflammatory cells in peripheral nerves leading to demyelination (neuropathy); reflex inhibition induced by pain and swelling; and finally disuse atrophy. Movement loss and immobility also may lead to fixed contractures of periarticular and intra-articular soft tissue structures, through shortening of collagen, which also may cause loss of articular cartilage.

For a therapeutic exercise program to succeed, the factors leading to atrophy of muscle fibers, listed above, must be eliminated first. Hence, determined anti-inflammatory therapy in any form is at the core of exercise management. Therapeutic exercise for patients with RA serves many purposes, and usually only one purpose is achieved optimally by any specific exercise.[28] For example, exercises to increase ROM cannot be substituted for exercises designed to strengthen muscles, and these in turn are not a substitute for endurance or conditioning exercises.

Anti-inflammatory therapy is the basis of exercise management. Causes of muscle atrophy first must be controlled.

The main objectives of therapeutic exercises are to:

- preserve motion or restore lost motion, increase muscle strength, and increase endurance
- provide cardiovascular conditioning
- increase bone density
- enhance a feeling of well-being
- provide active recreation[2]

For patients with controlled disease but residual impairment, exercise is by far the most important aspect of their therapy; however, exercise is given at all stages of RA and must be tailored to suit the patient's disease state.[2]

To date, there is strong evidence that patients with inflammatory arthritis will benefit from regular supervised exercise without aggravation of their joint symptoms.[29–36] Machover and Sapecky have shown that patients with RA can increase the strength in their quadriceps muscles with isometric exercise.[37] Other investigators also demonstrated that patients with RA can increase both type 1 and type 2 muscle fiber size, as well as their strength and aerobic capacity, after performing endurance training on treadmills or bicycles. This also correlated with improvements in activities of daily living.[29,32,33,38] These findings were supported by more recent studies using similar design and treatment maneuvers.[31,39] The intense but recent drive to prescribe aerobic exercise for endurance training must be tempered by other sobering effects of exercise. Excessive use of limbs affected by erosive arthritis affects the degree of joint destruction, indeed it has been shown that loss of limb use due to paralysis appears to confer a degree of sparing in patients with RA.[40–42] This leaves unanswered the question whether the ameliorating effect of a unilateral neurologic lesion is simply a lack-of-use phenomenon, or whether the presence of fully functioning nerves is necessary for the development of arthritis.[43]

For RA, four types of exercise by objective exist:

- active mobilizing exercise to maintain or restore joint movement and the flexibility of soft tissue structures
- strengthening exercise to maintain or restore muscle strength
- conditioning exercise to maintain or restore endurance and aerobic capacity
- passive techniques of joint mobilization

Mobilizing Exercise

The objectives of mobilizing exercises are to increase joint mobility and therefore relieve joint stiffness, and to enhance the flexibility of soft tissue structures that may be compromised by immobility, abnormal posture, or pathological changes triggered by the inflammatory process.

Before embarking on a mobilizing regimen, a thermal modality should be applied to improve connective tissue flexibility in targeted structures. Cold is the modality of choice for actively as well as chronically inflamed joints, and moist heat may be used for inactive or stiff and damaged joints. However, the typical patient with RA may require mobilization of multiple joints, where the local application of cold or hot packs may be inefficient. In these cases, localized cold immersion bath for limbs, a warm shower, or a swim in a warm pool may be preferable. Some of the mobilizing exercises prescribed can be carried out in the shower or pool.

Mobilizing Techniques

Actively inflamed joints should be moved gently through the possible range by the patient or with assistance from a PT. Three repetitions for each joint, once or twice daily, are recommended. Due to the possibility of pain and ligamentous stretching, the limbs should be handled with extreme care. As joint inflammation subsides, the joints should continue to be moved as above, but through full range possibly with assistance at the end of range, to ensure that shortened joint structures and tendons are fully stretched. Special proprioceptive neuromuscular facilitation (PNF) techniques could be applied early on for selected muscle groups, moderated by the extent and severity of the inflammation.[44] As these involve the use of manual resistance to muscle contraction, the amount of resistance can be varied according to the patient's tolerance, and inflammatory activity. In patients with joint laxity, these techniques should be applied with caution. Two techniques are in common use for actively inflamed and painful joints: hold-relax and slow reversal-hold-relax.

Special PNF techniques should be applied with caution and moderated by the extent and severity of the inflammation.

Hold-relax involves applying moderate manual resistance to an isometric contraction. Since no joint motion is involved, the technique achieves relaxation where muscle spasm is accompanied by pain.[44] For example, in a patient with RA with tightness of knee flexors limiting extension range, the part may be taken passively to the limit of extension; at that point the operator applies slowly moderate manual resistance to the knee flexors, by instructing the patient to hold that position, allowing no movement. The operator then instructs the patient to relax the knee flexors. As tension is released, the part may be taken passively into extension to the limit of the range or limit of pain. The process is repeated again, a number of times to patient tolerance, each repetition gaining further extension range. The underlying principle in hold-relax is that an isometric contraction of the flexors is followed by flexor inhibition and extensor facilitation due to the Golgi tendon organ effect.[44]

Slow reversal-hold-relax using the above example involves an isotonic contraction of knee extension, followed *without relaxation* by an isometric contraction of the knee flexors, followed by voluntary relaxation of the flexors, followed by isotonic contraction of extensors. Again, the maneuver is repeated to patient tolerance. Maximal isometric resistance to the flexors is applied to the rotation component to achieve maximal voluntary relaxation and facilitation of the extensor muscle group. As this technique involves more vigorous isotonic and isometric muscle contractions, it would be more suitable for patients whose joint inflammation is controlled but who are left with residual muscle tightness. The techniques *should not be used* on patients with joint pain or joint laxity.

Physical therapists with knowledge of PNF movement patterns should apply these techniques to selective muscle groups in their respective diagonal spiral patterns. A sensation of full muscle stretch accompanies these techniques, but their application should be pain free. Pain following their application lasting more than 1 hour should be a warning to be cautious, less vigorous, or not to use the technique.

Passive stretching techniques used by athletes should be applied with extreme caution on patients with RA, as they may lead to an inflammatory response in otherwise controlled joints, or lead to further laxity in compromised joint structures. Muscle groups and joints targeted for mobilizing exercise are shown in Table 13-3. *Water* is an excellent medium for free active mobilizing exercises, through regular swimming or structured group exercises. As patients with RA may be sensitive to cold, the water temperatures should be about 30°C (86°F). Buoyancy in water diminishes joint loading by reducing the effect of gravity. Water also provides generalized relaxation and enhances pain-free motions.[45] Patients who live at home could join a biweekly YMCA or YWCA swim program or another community pool program to help maintain their mobility and function. Unfortunately, some of these pools do not have sufficient heat and may not be accessible to disabled patients with RA. Swimming also can be a very effective means to build endurance in the extremities. This

Table 13-3. Muscle and Joints Targeted for Strength Training and Stretching*

	Muscle group	
Joints	*Strengthen*	*Stretch (ROM)*
Head and neck	Extensors, retractors	All muscle groups[†]
Scapulo/humeral	Scapular retractors and depressors Shoulder flexors, abductors, and rotators	Scapular protractors and elevators Shoulder adductors and rotators
Elbows	All muscle groups	All muscle groups
Forearm, wrist, and hands	Supinators, pronators, adductors and abductors of wrist and fingers, flexors and extensors of wrist and fingers	Supinators, pronators Wrist and finger flexors and adductors Hand intrinsics
Hips	Abductors, extensors, rotators	Flexors, rotators, and adductors
Knee	Extensors, flexors	Flexors (hamstrings, gastrocnemius)
Foot and ankle	All muscle groups	All muscle groups
Trunk	Flexors, extensors	All muscle groups

*From Helewa A, Smythe HA: Physical therapy in rheumatoid arthritis. In Wolfe F, Pincus T (eds): Rheumatoid Arthritis. Pathogenesis, Assessment, Outcome and Treatment, pp 415–433. New York, Marcel Dekker, 1994. With permission.

[†]Contraindicated in subluxed atlantoaxial joints.

also is a useful form of socialization, for otherwise homebound individuals.

Manual Therapy

Mobilizing techniques to peripheral joints are rarely used in inflammatory arthritis, due to underlying joint laxity and damage. Mobilizing exercises controlled by the patient's active movement in normal movement patterns are always preferred.

> **Aquatherapy is useful, as the buoyancy in water reduces the effect of gravity and thus loading on joints; however, patients with RA require higher water temperatures than usual.**

Strengthening Exercise

The objective of strengthening exercises is to restore and maintain optimal strength in muscles that support affected joints. More often than not these muscles have residual atrophy, brought on by the inflammatory process, reflex inhibition, and disuse. The ultimate objective is the recovery of function rather than the restoration of normal muscle morphology.

In planning a strengthening exercise program the following principles must be kept in mind:

- the joint condition should not be worsened by the exercise
- the muscles should not be exercised to fatigue, and any resistance offered to isotonic or isometric contractions must be submaximal
- actively inflamed joints should not be put through many repetitions and movement should not be resisted
- muscles acting on actively inflamed joints should be exercised isometrically for both strength and endurance
- the appearance of joint swelling and pain that exceeds 1 hour in duration following exercise are indications of excessive exercise, especially if symptoms increase overnight

The choice of a therapeutic exercise program should be related to the patient's normal activities, and the patient should be encouraged to keep this in mind. Therefore, in planning a program a number of questions should be asked:

- Is the object to concentrate on isolated muscle action or isolated joint movement, or is the object to encourage mass muscle action and functional multiaxial movement patterns?
- Should the exercises for a particular muscle group be isometric or isotonic?
- What starting position should be used?
- Should resistance be applied, and, if so, how much resistance and by what means?

Isolated Movements versus Mass Patterns

Since the ultimate object of therapeutic exercise is to restore or maintain function, functional mass movement patterns are the technique of choice. Mass movement patterns should be based on those developed by Voss and colleagues,[44] as they confer several advantages:

- the mass movement patterns are based on observed normal activities, incorporating three-dimensional movements
- in keeping with Beevor's axiom, the brain knows nothing of individual muscle action but knows only of movement; hence, the movement patterns, being natural, are easier to learn
- in managing a complex and widespread joint disease like RA, mass movement patterns, especially those performed bilaterally, are less time consuming and provide for normal and coordinated group action of muscles as well as integrated joint mechanics[44]

In contrast, isolated muscle work and simple joint movements take longer to learn and longer to perform. Isolated movements can be useful for specific regional impairments, where mass movement patterns may be contraindicated due to joint damage or deformity.

Isometric versus Isotonic

The choice between these two types of muscle contractions depends on the inflammatory status of the joints on which these muscles are acting and on the object of exercise. Isometric exercise at submaximal effort offers greater protection for inflamed or unstable rheumatoid joints. At maximal effort, a study of patients with RA showed that three maximal isometric contractions of the quadriceps, in full extension and at 90 degrees of flexion, held for 6 seconds, produced a 27% increase in strength in the exercised leg, and 17% in the quadriceps of the contralateral limb.[37] While isometric training has been shown to improve performance of isotonic tasks, clinically important improvements also have been noted for both types of tasks regardless of type of contraction.[46]

Isometric exercise at submaximal effort is preferred for inflamed or unstable rheumatoid joints.

In contrast, isotonic work is best for isotonic tasks, and if applied judiciously with submaximal resistance to noninflamed joints, it can enhance muscle performance and improve function. However, it must be tailored to the needs of the patient with RA, taking into consideration factors related to age, severity, strength, amount of joint destruction, and the patient's special functional needs.[47] One session a day is recommended, increasing the number of repetitions and resistance to tolerance.

Isometric or isotonic muscle work, combined with mass muscle contractions using normal patterns, may provide the greatest potential for improvements in functional performance.[44] Techniques such as isometric reversals, slow reversal, or slow reversal hold, superimposed over mass patterns using submaximal manual resistance, provide adequate facilitation, particularly in the early stages of recovery.[44] Manually resisted isometric reversal techniques can be applied in functional postures, such as sitting, standing, or a variety of ambulation stances. In the absence of joint inflammation, the resistance and the repetitions can be increased, and the use of external resistance, such as weights or weight-and-pulley systems can be encouraged. Self-resisted isometric exercises also can be applied by the patient using an unyielding strap.

Starting Positions

A number of positions can be used, varying from lying to sitting and standing. For mass movement patterns, the lying position provides the greatest stability. Sitting and various stances in standing are ideal functional positions for enhancing the stability of upright postures.

Resisted Muscle Work

Repetitive muscle overloading results in hypertrophy and increased functional capacity, whereas lack of use produces atrophy.[48] Type II muscle fibers respond to techniques that employ high resistance and a low number of repetitions. Increases in the cross-sectional area of these fibers are predominantly responsible for the observed hypertrophy.[48] In applying resistance, extreme care should be exercised. Isometric manual resistance in the subacute stage progressing to isotonic work confers many advantages over mechanical resistance. More specifically, the operator can:

- handle the limb with care, avoiding painful regions
- gauge and vary the amount of resistance the patient can sustain throughout the range without stressing the joints
- gauge better the patient's power output, particularly when compliance is a problem
- vary more readily the point where resistance is applied
- resist more readily opposing muscle groups during reciprocal motion or during postural stabilization
- apply more effectively facilitatory techniques such as pressure on the muscle belly, traction, approximation, and the stretch response

In most situations the point of resistance should not cross a joint, but preferably be applied to one joint at a time. The amount of manual resistance for isometric work should not exceed the patient's ability to maintain the position, and in the subacute stage should be submaximal. Patients with acutely inflamed joints should perform free active isometric work with minimal or no outside resistance. In order to obtain a training effect, resistance to isotonic work must not exceed 80% of the patient's maximal effort, and in all cases movement should not be impeded. *Mechanical resistance* can take the form of weights, or materials with elastic properties. Weights have the disadvantage of offering constant resistance throughout the range in isotonic work, placing the muscles at a mechanical disadvantage due to the changing angle of pull. Elastic materials such as springs, dental, or rubber dam offer greater resistance the more they are stretched, putting muscles again at a disadvantage as it shortens, due to the decreasing angle of pull and shortening of muscle fibers. Weight and elastic resistance are best suited for muscle work in the outer to middle range. Muscle groups and joints targeted for strengthening exercises are shown in Table 13-3.

Conditioning Exercises

Conditioning exercises through endurance training can have two major purposes:

- to improve the maximal aerobic capacity (i.e., to increase the maximal mechanical power output that can be maintained aerobically)
- to increase aerobic capacity (i.e., to increase the capacity to sustain a given workload for a longer time)[7]

Patients with RA often are limited in their activities by pain or fear of pain, disability, fatigue, and a belief that strenuous physical activities are to be avoided.[2] These limitations lead to lower physical work capacity, low muscle strength, and low cardiovascular capacity and endurance.[49] *The value of rest as a way to control disease and prevent deformities, has been increasingly challenged by investigators who recommend early activity and fitness training.*[30,31] This trend towards early activity also is seen in other disease categories, such as cardiovascular and respiratory diseases, as a valuable part of recovery. Early control of disease activity through (1) aggressive drug management, lessening the need for rest and joint protection techniques; (2) the increased cost of hospitalization and its debilitating effects; and (3) greater public preoccupation with physical fitness, all may have contributed to that trend.[2] More important are findings that patients with RA have a low level of cardiopulmonary fitness and that conditioning exercises to improve endurance help these patients resume optimal function.[32,34]

For detailed discussion of this form of training, and description of fitness assessments and training program components, the reader is referred to Chapter 11.

Manual Therapy

Techniques of manual therapy to peripheral joints, as recommended by Maitland, Kaltenborn, and others, have a very limited role to play in the management of RA. As most RA joints are unstable due to ligamentous laxity, accessory passive movements could only add insult to injury. One exception might be the shoulder joint, where grade I or II mobilization may be attempted, provided the joint is not *inflamed*. Manipulation techniques have no role to play in the management of peripheral or spinal RA joints, as the laxity often encountered in spinal ligaments, especially of the upper cervical vertebrae, when subjected to a sudden manipulative thrust, could lead to tragic consequences. Passive mechanical traction to the spine is rarely used in patients with RA due to ligamentous laxity and potential danger of subluxation or dislocation.

Reeducation of Gait

The mobility and ambulatory activities of patients with RA are hampered by pain and the effects of joint inflammation and destruction. The restrictions are not only limited to lower limb structures, but also involve all weight-bearing joints including those of the upper limbs when walking aids such as canes, crutches, or a walker are required. In preparation for gait activities, patients should have proper footwear as described in Chapter 10.

A review of the biomechanical and pathophysiological status of joints should determine whether the patient should ambulate independently, with aids, or navigate in a wheelchair. Acutely inflamed weight-bearing joints should not be unduly stressed and flail destroyed joints may not provide sufficient stability to ambulate safely. Under these conditions, walking aids must be considered. For severely involved patients, a walker with or without wheels may be required. Alternately, axillary crutches with additional gutter support for the forearms (to avoid weight bearing on hands and wrists) may be advisable. Less involved patients may manage with canes (two are always better than one) that have contoured handles. Patients who are unable to stand may have to resort to motorized scooters. Further discussion of use of walking aids and safety measures for ambulation are found in Chapter 16.

Therapists should ensure that acutely inflamed weight-bearing joints are not unduly stressed and that flail destroyed joints have sufficient stability for safe ambulation.

Techniques of rhythmic stabilization will be very helpful in the reeducation of upright posture and a sense of balance.[44] Propulsion forward, backward, or sideways can be initiated with the assistance of the PT, actively by the patient or against resistance. Walking then can be progressed from parallel bars to crutches, canes, and free walking.

Posture

Patients with RA frequently have problems maintaining correct posture, whether in lying, sitting, standing, walking, or during the performance of a variety of activities. Incorrect postures can lead to contracture of soft tissue structures, poor balance, and increased energy expenditures; all are factors that can be detrimental to the rehabilitation outcomes of these patients.

Postural awareness and correction with mirror feedback in sitting, standing, and walking is a useful approach and increases the patients' perceptions of their body position in space. Proper balance and posture can be taught by applying judiciously techniques of rhythmic stabilization in a variety of starting positions as discussed earlier.[44]

During prolonged periods of sitting and lying, special attention to correct posture and positioning is critical if contractures and deformities are to be avoided. Correct positioning must be tempered with patient comfort. A PT's unrealistic expectations often can lead to poor patient compliance with the recommended postures. For example, insistence on maintaining a straight knee in bed if the joint is inflamed leads to extreme pain and discomfort. The joint effusion forces the knee into about 30 degrees of flexion, a position that permits the joint to hold a maximal amount of fluid. Indeed, it would be desirable for the acutely inflamed knee to be held in flexion to maintain the integrity of vulnerable and possibly lax collateral ligaments. Achievement of 0 degrees at the knee is a goal, as knee flexion contracture increases the energy cost of gait, pressures across the joint, and contributes to hip flexion contractures.[50]

Whether in sitting or lying, the guiding principle is the maintenance of well-supported functional positions, patient comfort, and frequent changes of position.

Physical Therapy for Surgical Candidates with RA

Patients with RA with irreversible joint destruction in key joints may be suitable candidates for rheumatoid surgery. Pre- and postoperative physical therapy is of critical importance for successful surgical outcomes. Chapter 6 describes the common surgical procedures used in patients with arthritis and the surgical criteria applied by orthopedic surgeons, rheumatologists, and physical therapists to determine a candidate's suitability for a particular surgical procedure.

Patients with RA considered for surgery often have advanced disease with clear evidence of joint destruction, manifested by joint instability, cartilage destruction, gross limitation of movements with ankylosis, and torn and damaged soft tissue structures. The patient's condition may be further complicated by intractable pain and gross limitation of function. For example, it is not uncommon for patients with damaged hips or knees to be confined to a wheelchair. The pain and functional limitations often lead to poor aerobic fitness and muscle wasting. Therefore, successful postoperative outcomes are dependent on the extent of preoperative preparation and conditioning.

Presurgical Management

At the outset, the risks and benefits of surgery are explained to the patient by the surgeon, anesthetist, and physical therapist, each presenting a different perspective. The patient then can make an informed decision about proceeding with surgery, balancing the risks and benefits against their own personal goals. The value of presurgical physical conditioning is explained to the patient, and a structured, individualized program, designed by the PT, is offered at least 2 weeks prior to surgery. A three-pronged approach is at the core of presurgical management: determined anti-inflammatory therapy, general physical conditioning, and strengthening of muscles that will be directly compromised by the surgery. Control of joint inflammation prior to surgery, especially weight-bearing joints, will make mobility, transfers, and ambulation easier postoperatively.

General conditioning will involve a modified aerobic training program, preferably in a pool. The object is to increase endurance and cardiovascular conditioning. As RA is a systemic disease that may compromise cardiac and pulmonary function, surgical candidates must be taught preoperative breathing exercises and abdominal muscle strengthening exercises to help with coughing and expectoration.

A program to strengthen muscles that are directly compromised is very important for successful surgical outcomes. If joint surgery is contemplated (e.g., for a knee replacement), isometric resisted exercises to the quadriceps and hamstring muscles will be required to strengthen muscles that may be reflexly inhibited by pain.

Postsurgical Management

Following surgery, the patient with RA and the physical therapist face unique challenges, due to the articular and extra-articular manifestations of the disease. Other factors such as age, gender, compliance, type of surgery, prosthesis used, surgical site (i.e., upper or lower limb), the surgeon's objectives, and the ambulatory status of the patient influence the rehabilitation process.

The articular and extra-articular manifestations of rheumatoid disease uniquely challenge postoperative rehabilitation.

The overall objective is to return the patient to their optimal level of function in the shortest possible time, without compromising the surgical outcomes.

Early Systemic Management

The patient with RA, more than any other surgical candidate, is susceptible to severe deconditioning, and vascular and cardiopulmonary complications. Those confined to bed in the immediate postoperative period (e.g., lower limb surgical patients) must begin the day following surgery, in bed, a general activity program designed to minimize muscle atrophy, joint contractures, demineralization of long bones, vascular obstructions, and chest complications. This can be accomplished by a program of general free active or resisted active exercise, to the nonsurgical sites, lasting about 10 minutes, performed three times a day, for as long as the patient is confined to bed. Where possible, isotonic/isometric presses taught to the patients can be a very useful and practical approach to management, as the PT may not be available that frequently, and the patient can participate in their own management at an early stage. Upon returning from the recovery ward, breathing exercises and coughing routines are very important in the first 3 days, to enhance the cough reflex inhibited by the action of the general anesthetic and clear airways.

Another important early management objective is to prepare the patient for ambulatory activities and transfers from lying to sitting to standing with assistance. This will involve trunk exercises, strengthening of antigravity muscles of the other lower limb, and strengthening of upper limbs, as the use of walking aids is inevitable. For patients with lower limb surgery whose upper limbs are involved, this will present a unique challenge. Patients with upper limb surgery, who require a walking aid to ambulate, will be equally challenged.

Early Local Management

Management of structures close to the surgical site will depend on the type of surgery and the surgical objectives established by the surgeon. Generally, muscle tone and joint mobility must be restored as early as permissible. *Isometric setting exercises are by far the safest to perform when movements in the early stages are contraindicated.* Similarly, resisted exercises to the contralateral limb or other body segments, as well as providing conditioning, will produce stimulation of muscles at the surgical site, through overflow. Joint mobility in the early stages can be restored by means of active assisted exercise and the application of hold-relax PNF techniques. After the surgical wound is healed the patient may begin to exercise safely in a pool, well supported by water buoyancy.

Postsurgical Ambulation

More often than not, the patient with RA following surgery will ambulate with assistance or walking aids. Initially, the patient progresses from performing transfers in and out of bed or chair, followed by standing, non-weight bearing, or partial weight bearing. An excellent medium for early ambulation is a hydrotherapy pool equipped with parallel bars. Rhythmic stabilization exercises to the trunk and limbs, in sitting and standing with aids, are useful preparatory strategies that correct postures and provide patients with confidence. Ambulatory aids can range from walkers to crutches or canes depending on the patient's status. Platform walkers can be especially useful for those with lower or even upper limb surgery.

Late Postsurgical Management

The management objectives for the surgical site, following wound healing, are similar to those of postacute inflammatory disease. Specific PNF techniques can be employed using modified patterns of movement, with carefully applied manual resistance. Slow reversals combining isotonic/isometric muscle work would be the best universal techniques for building endurance, coordination, or muscle strength. Isometric reversals and hold-relax will be the techniques of choice for joint mobility. In the latter stages, mechanical resistance may be added to the program together with a home program on discharge from the hospital.

Goal Setting and Contracting

To maximize the benefits of physical therapy intervention, it is essential that the components of the proposed treatment program are acceptable to the patient and relate to the patient's complaints. The treatment goals should be negotiated based on what the patient and physical therapist identify as important, realistic, and achievable.

The patient requires sufficient information about the disease process and its potential effects to make informed choices of treatment strategies. The physical therapist needs to understand the impact of the disease on the individual patient's life style and function, in order to propose a treatment package that is likely to result in the desired outcome. The risks and benefits of the proposed treatment should be explained to the patient, as well as the risks of not adhering to the treatment regimen. Both parties, where possible, should agree to time frames and agree to the factors that will indicate that goals have been achieved or require modification.

A contract may be developed acknowledging the patient's responsibilities, as well as those of the physical therapist. An understanding should be reached that the contract is likely to succeed, but can be renegotiated if necessary.

An example of a goal-setting process is as follows:

- The patient identifies shoulder pain, an inability to reach the second shelf in the kitchen cupboard and to put on overhead garments. The physical therapist identifies the cause of the problem as active inflammation in the shoulder joint, reduced ROM due to soft tissue contracture, and decreased muscle strength. The physical therapist proposes ice to the shoulder followed by isometric strengthening exercises and five repetitions of active ROM exercises twice daily for 2 weeks.
- The patient expresses dislike for ice treatment, states that she cannot be sure to adhere to two sessions daily, but feels confident that she can apply heat and do three repe-

titions of ROM exercises, twice daily, 5 days/week.

- The indicators that the treatment objectives have been met may be a reduction of pain by 50%, and an ability to reach beyond the second shelf in the cupboard. These, in themselves, may be the rewards for effort expended by the patient. Other rewards could be a "day off" from treatment, or an outing.

While this negotiation process may seem onerous, it provides the patient with an element of control in the overall management process of their disease. It focuses the intervention on areas of importance to the patient and reduces the frustration inherent in imposing lengthy, complicated, unwanted or unnecessary protocols destined for failure due to noncompliance.

The Team Approach

The associations between functional loss and deformity, chronic pain and medications, self-concept and appearance are complex.[51] Different but comprehensive strategies are needed to treat all features of the disease. The core rehabilitation team consisting of physical and occupational therapists, and physicians (mostly rheumatologists), plays an important role in the care of patients with RA by teaching patients how to evaluate and solve problems pertaining to mobility, self-care, and psychosocial function.[51] Other team members include the rheumatologically trained nurses, psychologists, social workers, orthotists, physiatrists, orthopedic surgeons, and pharmacists. Except for nurses and pharmacists, these other health professionals are recruited on a consultation basis to deal with complex problems relevant to their specialty.

Patients with work-related problems can also benefit from job or vocational counselors. Determination of the patient's level of function, the ergonomics or energy requirements to perform work, and an evaluation of the work site with respect to physical barriers are important factors to consider in job counseling.

Research Questions

In the physical therapy management of patients with RA, there are many questions that remain unanswered. While there is information available on the beneficial effects of exercise and certain treatment adjuncts, few of the reported studies employed a randomized controlled design, and even fewer studies have looked at the long-term benefits or risks of physical therapy. Some research questions come to mind.

- Are the outcomes of patients with RA improved in the long term following a program of conditioning exercises?
- Are the outcomes of patients with RA improved in the long term following a structured, but custom-tailored, program of physical therapy?
- Are the outcomes of patients with RA improved in the long term with fewer joint complications (laxity, contractures, erosions, cartilage destruction) following exposure to physical therapy and determined anti-inflammatory therapy?
- Do patients with RA have fewer destroyed joints when exposed to energy conservation and joint protection techniques?
- Are the outcomes of patients with RA improved following a program of home physical therapy?
- Do PNF relaxation techniques confer greater benefits to patients with RA than passive stretching?
- Is a water aerobic training program better than recreational swimming in deconditioned patients with RA?

Case History

Family and Clinical History Mrs. G. is a 45-year-old woman, divorced with three children (14, 10, and 8 years old), and works as a full-time secretary. She attends fitness classes once a week. A year ago, she described onset of foot pain, after prolonged walking, relieved by a change in footwear. Wrists became swollen and stiff. Saw a general practitioner (GP) who diagnosed her problem as carpal tunnel syndrome. Wrist problems improved on nonsteroidal anti-inflammatory drugs (NSAIDs) and wrist support.

Three months later, Mrs. G. experienced general fatigue, increased foot pain, bilateral knee pain, and difficulty managing stairs. Wrists also were painful and swollen and several finger joints were swollen. She had difficulties gripping objects, as in turning a water tap. She continued to work full-time, but stopped fitness classes.

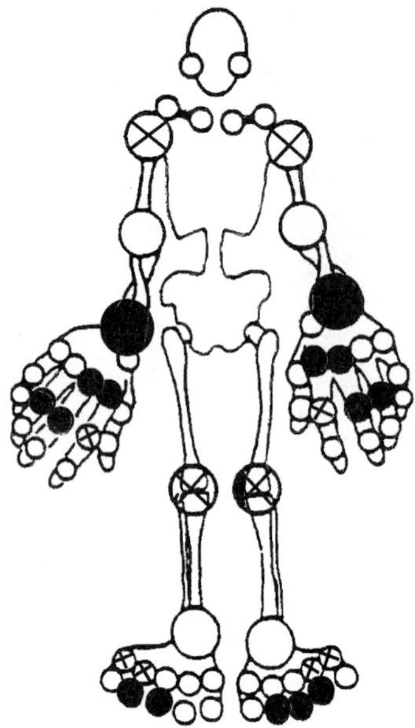

Figure 13-1. Mrs. G.'s joint count (●, active joint; ⊗, active joint with effusions).

At 6 months, Mrs. G. was exhausted, depressed, and additional joints were involved. She had difficulty sleeping due to pain, as well as increased difficulty with stairs and kitchen activities. She experienced morning stiffness lasting 90 minutes after waking up and moving around. She also had difficulty getting on or off a bus and doing general housework. At this time she revisited her GP, who told her she has "arthritis." NSAIDs were prescribed and Mrs. G. took time off work. She had a homemaker visit twice a week and was subsequently referred to a physical therapist and a rheumatologist.

Physical Therapy Mrs. G.'s chief complaints were: painful hands, wrists, shoulders, knees, and feet; swelling of wrists, MCPs, and knees. She had general difficulties with activities of daily living and was unable to go to work.

Initial PT Assessment

- morning stiffness: 90 minutes
- grip strength: R, 142/20, L, 138/20
- active joints: 25, of which 10 were effusions and no joint destruction (Fig. 13-1)
- extra-articular features; nodules: left olecranon, flexor tendon of R index finger
- muscle strength:
  quadriceps: R, 92/20; L, 104/20
  shoulder abductors: R, 86/2; L, 110/20
- ROM: see Table 13-4

Rx Plan

1. Education about disease, its effects, and its management
2. Resting and work splints for wrists, footwear modifications
3. Joint protection techniques—posture and work habits
4. Tips on how to conserve energy—general rest
5. Analgesic modalities: oil and glove routine to hands; ice to knees and wrists; warm shower AM with shoulder exercises
6. Therapeutic exercises: (1) ROM—knees, wrists, shoulders, and hands, three repetitions, two to three times daily and gradually increase as inflammation subsides; and (2) isometric presses to quadriceps, hip abductors, hip extensors, and all shoulder muscle groups, performed twice daily—increase repetitions and intensity as inflammation subsides

Table 13-4. Mrs. G.'s Range of Movement in Selected Joints

	Shoulders			Wrists			Knees	
	R	*L*		*R*	*L*		*R*	*L*
Fwd Flex	0–140	0–160	Flex	0–75	0–80	Flex	25–136	15–140
Abd	0–120	0–140	Ex	0–60	0–75			
LR*	0–60	0–75						
MR†	0–60	0–70						

*LR, lateral rotation; †MR, medial rotation.

Compliance The patient was very compliant with her rest program, application of analgesic modalities, and exercise programs. She practiced joint protection, wore splints as required, and used tap turner, jar opener, and so forth.

Rheumatologist The rheumatologist stressed importance of adequate NSAID dose; this advice was reinforced by the PT.

After 6 Weeks PT reassessment showed:

- less fatigue
- morning stiffness of 45 minutes
- 14 active joint count, 5 effusions
- grip strength R, 166/20; L, 154/20
- muscle strength:
  quadriceps: R, 124/20; L, 140/20
  shoulder abductors: R, 98/20; L, 124/20
- increased shoulder ROM
- full L knee extension, R knee flexion contracture of 10 degrees
- wrists:
  flexion R, 80 degrees; L, 90 degrees
  extension R, 70 degrees; L, 80 degrees
- able to do some light activities
- in the home—climbing stairs and getting on and off chairs was easier

PT Rx Progression

- increase muscle strength and endurance using slow reversal techniques for upper and lower limb patterns—combination of isometric/isotonic muscle work
- increase ROM in resistant joints by using hold-relax techniques to shoulders, wrists, and knees
- a water aerobics program in a local pool

The rheumatologist noted a decrease in inflammatory measures, but disease was still active, and recommended use of disease suppressant therapy; however, Mrs. G. was reluctant. Patient returned to work part-time and was able to continue with PT at home on her own.

After 6 Months She was able to continue with work, uses splints, but was tired at the end of the day; her children help with house chores. She attended pool program regularly, decreased use of analgesic modalities, and continues with exercise. She continues NSAIDs, but still has pain and swelling, especially of the hands. Shoulder ROM is still limited.

After 8 Months Generalized flare of the disease:

- 22 active joints, 8 effusions
- morning stiffness for 75 minutes
- grip strength: R, 148/20; L, 142/20
- losing ROM in shoulders
- knees swollen bilaterally
- difficulty with tasks such as dressing, grocery shopping etc.
- unable to go to work

Rheumatologist Mrs. G. agrees to disease suppressant therapy and was prescribed methotrexate, and was re-referred to PT.

PT Management

Goals

- pain relief, increase ROM in shoulders and knees
- increase strength and endurance
- restore activities of daily living

Rx

- increase rest periods
- modify wrist splint
- restart analgesic modalities
- restart gentle ROM
- increase strength and endurance
- gradually progress to PNF techniques as inflammation subsides

After 9 Months She responds to rest; however, long-acting disease suppressants are not effective. Active joint count is 16, with 4 effusions. She continues with PT as above, progressed in intensity.

After 12 Months Disease suppressant gradually takes hold with a substantial decrease in inflammatory activities. Active joint count is 4, with no effusions. Morning stiffness of 20 minutes. Patient continues on a decreased dose of disease suppressant therapy.

PT program intensified to gain full ROM, endurance, and strength, and she continues with the pool.

After 14 Months The patient returns to work full-time, with her disease well controlled. She continues with pool program and general conditioning exercises, and is discharged from PT.

References

1. Hough AJ Jr, Sokoloff L: Pathology of rheumatoid arthritis and allied disorders. In McCarty DJ (ed): Arthritis and Allied Conditions, 11th edition, pp 674–697. Philadelphia, Lea & Febiger, 1989.
2. Helewa A, Smythe HA: Physical therapy in rheumatoid arthritis. In Wolfe F, Pincus T (eds): Rheumatoid Arthritis, Pathogenesis, Assessment, Outcome and Treatment, pp 415–433. New York, Marcel Dekker, 1994.
3. Benson TB, Copp EP: The effects of therapeutic forms of heat and ice on the pain threshold of the normal shoulder. Rheumatol Rehabil 1974; 13:101–104.
4. Prentice WE: An electromyographic analysis of the effectiveness of heat or cold and stretching for inducing relaxation in injured muscle. J Orthop Sports Phys Ther 1982; 3:133–140.
5. Kirk JA, Kersley GD: Heat and cold in the physical treatment of rheumatoid arthritis of the knee. A controlled clinical trial. Ann Phys Med 1968; 9:270–274.
6. DonTigny R, Sheldon K: Simultaneous use of heat and cold in treatment of muscle spasm. Arch Phys Med Rehabil 1962; 43:235–237.
7. Schlapbach P, Gerber NJ (eds): Physiotherapy: Controlled Trials and Facts, Rheumatology, vol 14. Basel, Karger, 1991.
8. Harris ED Jr, McCroskery PA: The influence of temperature and fibril stability on degradation of cartilage collagen by rheumatoid synovial collagenase. N Engl J Med 1974; 290:1–6.
9. Hartviksen K: Ice therapy in spasticity. Acta Neurol Scand 1962; 38(Suppl 3):79–84.
10. Knutsson E, Mattsson E: Effects of local cooling on monosynaptic reflexes in man. Scand J Rehabil Med 1969; 1:126–132.
11. Bulstrade S, Clarke A, Harrison R: A controlled trial to study the effect of ice therapy on joint inflammation in chronic arthritis. Physiother Pract 1986; 2:104–108.
12. Williams J, Harvey J, Tannenbaum H: Use of superficial heat versus ice for the rheumatoid arthritic shoulder: a pilot study. Physiother Can 1986; 38:8–13.
13. Hamilton DE, Bywaters EGL, Please NW: A controlled trial of various forms of physiotherapy in arthritis. BMJ 1959; I:542–544.
14. Oosterveld FGJ, Rasker JJ, Jacobs JWG, et al: The effect of local heat and cold therapy on the intraarticular and skin surface temperature of the knee. Arthritis Rheum 1992; 35:146–151.
15. Olson JE, Stravino VD: A review of cryotherapy. Phys Ther 1972; 52:840–853.
16. Sutej PG, Hadler NM: Current principles of rehabilitation for patients with rheumatoid arthritis. Clin Orthop 1991; 265:116–124.
17. Lehmann JF, DeLateur BJ: Therapeutic heat. In Lehmann JF (ed): Therapeutic Heat and Cold, 3rd edition. Baltimore, Williams & Wilkins, 1982.
18. Ersek RA: Transcutaneous electrical neurostimulation: a new therapeutic modality for controlling pain. Clin Orthop 1977; 128:314–324.
19. Sjolund B, Terenius L, Eriksson M: Increased cerebrospinal fluid levels of endorphins after electroacupuncture. Acta Physiol Scand 1977; 100:382–384.
20. Abelson K, Langley GB, Sheppeard H, et al: Transcutaneous electrical nerve stimulation in rheumatoid arthritis. NZ Med J 1983; 96:156–158.
21. Langley GB, Sheppeard H, Johnson M, et al: The analgesic effect of TENS and placebo in chronic pain patients. Rheumatol Int 1984; 4:119–123.
22. Young SL, Woodbury MG, Fryday-Field K, et al: Efficacy of interferential current stimulation alone for pain reduction in patients with osteoarthritis of the knee: a randomized placebo control clinical trial. Phys Ther 1991; 71(Suppl):S52.
23. Alexander GJM, Hortas C, Bacon PA: Bed rest, activity and the inflammation of rheumatoid arthritis. Br J Rheumatol 1983; 22:134–140.
24. Cheung HS, Ryan LM, Kozin F, et al: Synovial origins of rice bodies in joint fluid. Arthritis Rheum 1980; 23:72–76.
25. Mills JA, Pinals RS, Ropes MW, et al: Value of bed rest in patients with rheumatoid arthritis. N Engl J Med 1971; 284:453–458.
26. Helewa A, Bombardier C, Goldsmith CH, et al: Cost-effectiveness of inpatient and intensive outpatient treatment of rheumatoid arthritis. A randomized, controlled trial. Arthritis Rheum 1989; 32:1505–1514.
27. Lee P, Kennedy AC, Anderson J, et al: Benefits of hospitalization in rheumatoid arthritis. Q J Med 1974; 43:205–214.
28. Swezey RL: Rheumatoid arthritis: the role of the kinder and gentler therapies. J Rheumatol 1990; 17(Suppl 25):8–13.
29. Nordemar R: Physical training in rheumatoid arthritis: a controlled long-term study. II. Functional capacity and general attitudes. Scand J Rheumatol 1981; 10:25–30.
30. Nordemar R, Ekblom B, Zachrisson L, et al: Physical training in rheumatoid arthritis, a controlled long term study I. Scand J Rheumatol 1981; 10:17–23.
31. Minor MA, Hewett JE, Webel RR, et al: Efficacy of physical conditioning exercise in patients with rheumatoid arthritis and osteoarthritis. Arthritis Rheum 1989; 32:1396–1405.
32. Ekblom B, Lovgren O, Alderin M, et al: Effect of short term physical training on patients with rheumatoid arthritis I. Scand J Rheumatol 1975; 4:80–86.
33. Nordemar R, Edstrom L, Ekblom B: Changes in muscle fibre size and physical performance in patients with rheumatoid arthritis after short-term physical training. Scand J Rheumatol 1976; 5:70–76.

34. Ekblom B, Lovgren O, Alderin M, et al: Effect of short term physical training on patients with rheumatoid arthritis. A six month follow-up study. Scand J Rheumatol 1975; 4:87–91.
35. Hicks JE: Exercise in patients with inflammatory arthritis and connective tissue disease. Rheum Dis Clin North Am 1990; 16:845–870.
36. Hsieh LF, Didenko B, Schumacher HR Jr, et al: Isokinetic and isometric testing of knee musculature in patients with rheumatoid arthritis with mild knee involvement. Arch Phys Med Rehabil 1987; 68:294–297.
37. Machover S, Sapecky AJ: Effect of isometric exercise on the quadriceps muscle in patients with rheumatoid arthritis. Arch Phys Med Rehabil 1966; 47: 737–741.
38. Nordemar R, Berg U, Ekblom B, et al: Changes in muscle fibre size and physical performance in patients with rheumatoid arthritis after 7 months physical training. Scand J Rheumatol 1976; 5:233–238.
39. Perlman SG, Connell KJ, Clark A, et al: Dance-based aerobic exercise for rheumatoid arthritis. Arthritis Care Res 1990; 3:29–35.
40. Thompson M, Bywaters EGL: Unilateral rheumatoid arthritis following hemiplegia. Ann Rheum Dis 1962; 21:370–377.
41. Glick EN: Asymmetrical rheumatoid arthritis after poliomyelitis. BMJ 1967; 3:26–28.
42. Bland JH, Eddy WM: Hemiplegia and rheumatoid hemiarthritis. Arthritis Rheum 1968; 11:72–80.
43. Vignos PJ: Physiotherapy in rheumatoid arthritis. J Rheumatol 1981; 8(1):173.
44. Voss DE, Ionta MK, Myers BJ (eds): Proprioceptive Neuromuscular Facilitation—Patterns and Techniques, 3rd edition. Philadelphia, Harper & Row, 1985.
45. Gerber LH, Hicks JE: Exercise in rheumatic disease. In Basmajian JV, Wolf SL (eds): Therapeutic Exercise, 5th edition, p 351. Baltimore, Williams & Wilkins, 1990.
46. DeLateur B, Lehmann J, Stonebridge J, et al: Isotonic versus isometric exercise: a double-shift transfer-of-training study. Arch Phys Med Rehabil 1972; 53: 212–217.
47. Semble EL, Loeser RF, Wise CM: Therapeutic exercise for rheumatoid arthritis and osteoarthritis. Semin Arthritis Rheum 1990; 20:32–40.
48. Galloway MT, Jobe P: The role of exercise in the treatment of inflammatory arthritis. Bull Rheum Dis 1993; 42:1–4.
49. Ekblom B, Lovgren O, Alderin M, et al: Physical performance in patients with rheumatoid arthritis. Scand J Rheumatol 1974; 3:121–125.
50. Perry J, Antonelli D, Ford W: Analysis of knee-joint forces during flexed-knee stance. J Bone Joint Surg 1975; 57A:961–967.
51. Gerber L: Rehabilitation of patients with rheumatic diseases. In Schumacher HR (ed): Primer on the Rheumatic Diseases, 10th edition, pp 314–319. Atlanta, Arthritis Foundation, 1993.

CHAPTER 14

Physical Therapy Management of the Patient with Osteoarthritis

Carolee Moncur, PhD, PT

The demographics, etiology, pathophysiology and assessment of persons with osteoarthritis (OA) have been introduced elsewhere in this textbook. It is important to recall this information, since OA is a common condition for which, in consultation with the patient, a realistic and feasible treatment plan is necessary. Often patients report they have been told nothing can be done for their OA except to learn to live with it and take analgesics. While much of the rationale for physical therapy (PT) of this condition is based on tradition and anecdotal data, this does not preclude the existence of sound alternatives to offer the patient to remediate some of their complaints and symptoms and to empower them to manage their arthritis with life style changes. For example, data generated by Felson et al[1] demonstrated that the greatest risk factor in developing OA of the knee is obesity, the prevention of which may require changing eating and exercise habits.

PHYSICAL THERAPY IN ARTHRITIS, Joan M. Walker, PhD, PT, and Antoine Helewa, MSc(Clin Epid), PT, W.B. Saunders Company © 1996.

Process of Clinical Decision Making

There are several ways to approach the design and implementation of a plan of care for the patient with OA; however, I will outline the process of clinical decision making that I find most expedient in practice. This may be called an algorithm for planning and implementing treatment (Fig. 14-1).[2–16] The algorithm works by asking a series of questions whose answers will construct a planning pathway for care of the patient. For the remainder of this chapter, I intend to lead you through these questions and then explain the rationale for the finished plan of care.

Treatment Planning: Using the Algorithm

Having reviewed Figure 14-1 carefully to determine how to proceed, consider the case of Mrs. G., who is a 73-year-old widow, slightly obese by 35 kg (77 lb), who has been referred for PT with a diagnosis of cervical spondylosis[17] at the levels of C5–C7. Using information from the assessment chapter in this text, the answers to the first five questions of the algorithm can be determined. Yes, osteoarthritis is present (Q.1); OA is located in the cervical spine (Q.2), and there is joint enlargement (Q.3).

The assessment process has revealed that the patient has pain in a radicular pattern over C5–C7, particularly at the extreme ends of rotation of the head to the left and right. Without seeing radiographs, this clinical sign may be due to osteophyte production. Furthermore, she demonstrates the following characteristics:

- decrease in all neck movements
- decreased strength in the neck muscles and abductors of the glenohumeral joint
- complains of fatigue and decreased endurance when holding her head in one position for an extended period of time
- audible joint crepitus as she rotates her head right and left
- forward head posture with a slight kyphosis of the thoracic spine
- point tenderness in the trapezius muscle in the suboccipital and suprascapular regions
- reports difficulty in looking over her right shoulder when she is backing her car out of the garage
- reports discouragement because she is unable to work at her computer for more than 10 minutes because of neck pain (during her history she reported that she is an avid genealogist and wears glasses with trifocal lenses)

This information will help formulate the answer to question four of the algorithm: *Is there functional impairment?* It is important to determine Mrs. G.'s beliefs about her spondylosis and her expectations and preferences regarding treatment. Mrs. G. agrees that she has functional impairment because she is less able to do the important things in her life.

It would appear that Mrs. G. does not have joint instability, decreased balance, comorbidity such as heart disease, or concerns about her socioeconomic status. However, she does demonstrate the following characteristics:

- joint deformity (forward head posture and kyphosis)

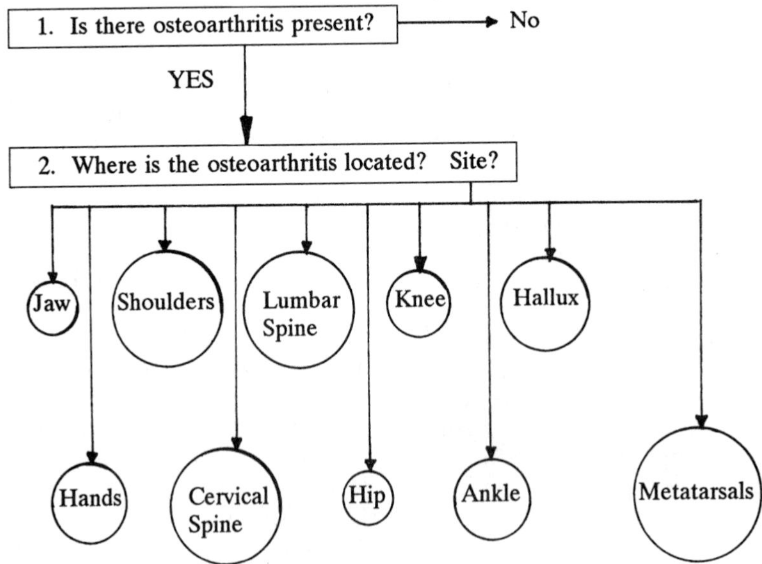

Figure 14-1. Algorithm for planning and implementing treatment of osteoarthritis. *Illustration continued on opposite page*

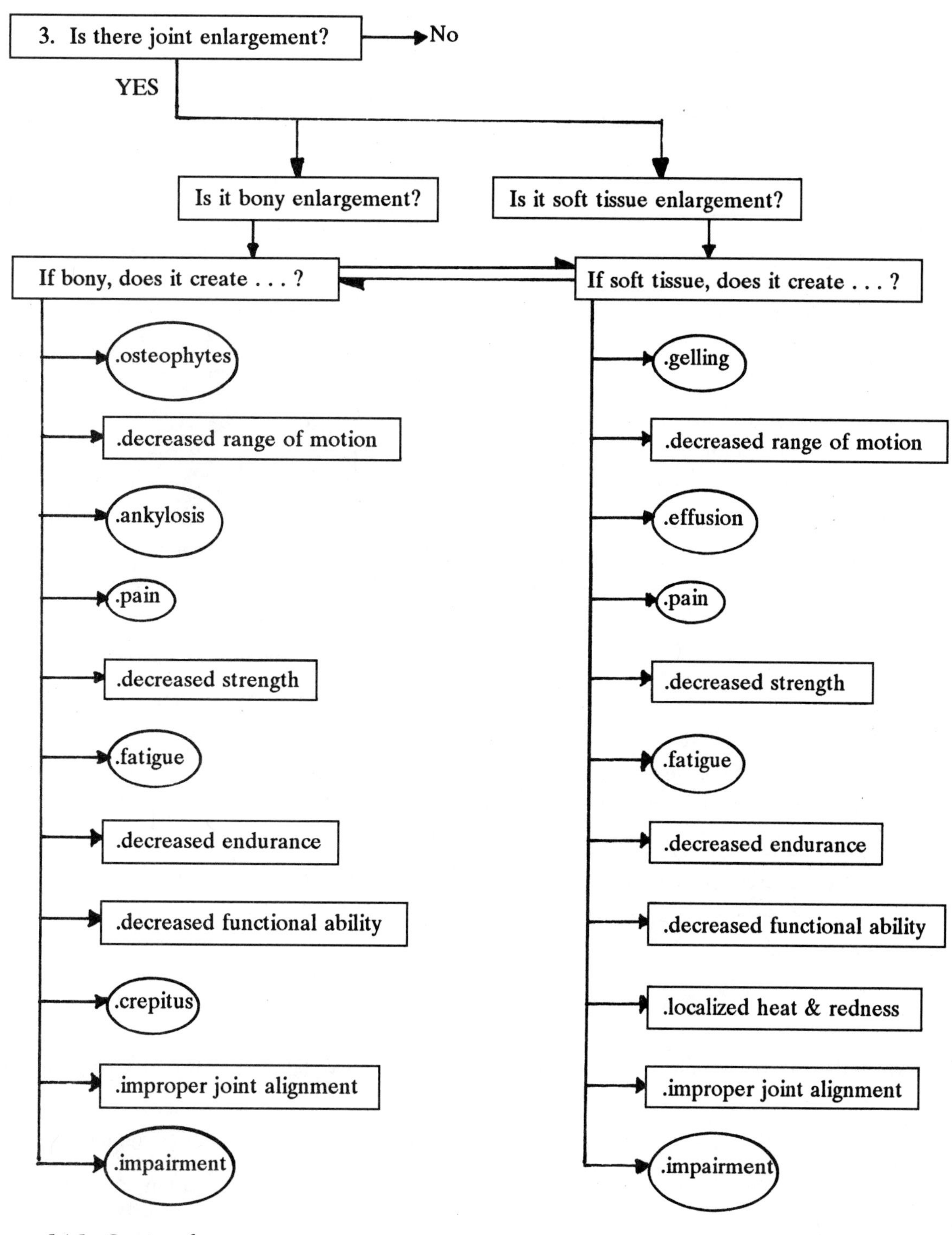

Figure 14-1. *Continued*

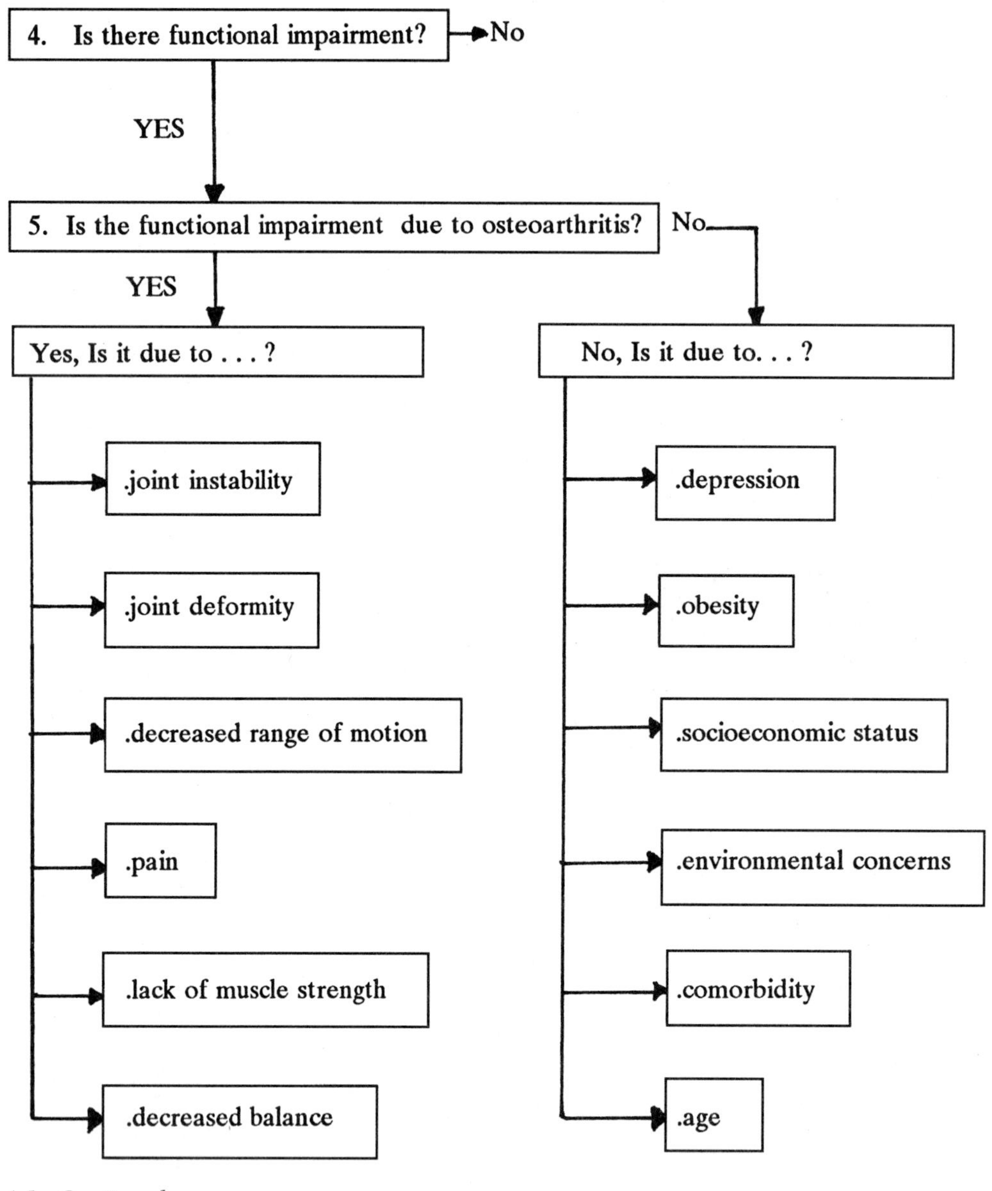

Figure 14-1. *Continued*

- decreased range of motion of the neck and right shoulder
- joint gelling and stiffness
- occasional pain in her neck and down her arms
- obesity
- age-related changes
- wears trifocal lenses
- decreased muscle strength that could be due to disuse, aging, and/or protective responses to pain stimuli
- concerns about her avocation, driving her car, and working at her computer

Given all of this information, the answer to Q.5, *Is her functional impairment due to osteoarthritis?* is Yes. To formulate the care plan the next question is: *What is Mrs. G. willing and able to do*

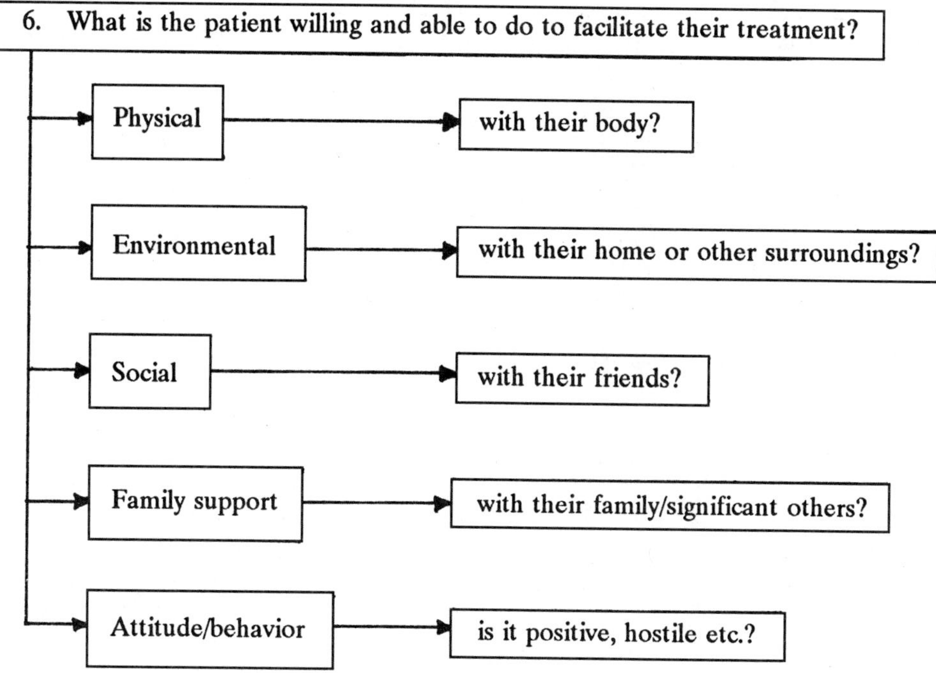

Figure 14-1. *Continued*

for her treatment? (Q.6). In the *physical area*, Mrs. G. is willing to do neck and shoulder exercises at least once daily and is willing to begin a walking program 3–5 days/week, gradually working toward a 30- to 45-minute period of steady walking. She does not believe she can be successful making significant changes in her eating habits.

In the *environmental area*, Mrs. G. is willing to modify her computer station so that her monitor screen is at eye level. She can place her typing materials to avoid always turning her head to one side. She is willing to purchase a pair of glasses that has the lenses she needs to work at the computer so that she does not have to hyperextend her neck. She also is willing to pace her work so that she does not sit in front of the computer for long periods of time without standing and moving her head.

In the *social area*, Mrs. G. is a socially active woman with her friends and family. She has agreed, however, to take better control of her time so that she intersperses periods of rest with her social activities.

In the *family support* area, Mrs. G. has excellent family support. She has four grown children, their spouses, and children who are responsive to her needs. Her need for approval from all of them does place increased stress and demand on her as a baby sitter, confidante, and visitor. She notes she has more problems with her neck when she has had "a lot of company."

In *attitude and behavior*, Mrs. G. is a self-assured elder in many respects. She appears to be determined to stay independent and not become a burden on her family. She needs to have honest answers and a rationale for why she should follow your advice.

Having determined what Mrs. G. is willing to do about her care, question 7 is: *What are you willing and able to do to facilitate Mrs. G.'s treatment plan in terms of prevention, soft tissue care, handling techniques, and exercises?*

Treatment Implementation: Using the Paradigm

The four categories of prevention, soft tissue care, handling techniques, and exercises derive from the art of PT practice and making observations about what occurs in patient care. Therefore, for this discussion, the categories will be defined as follows.

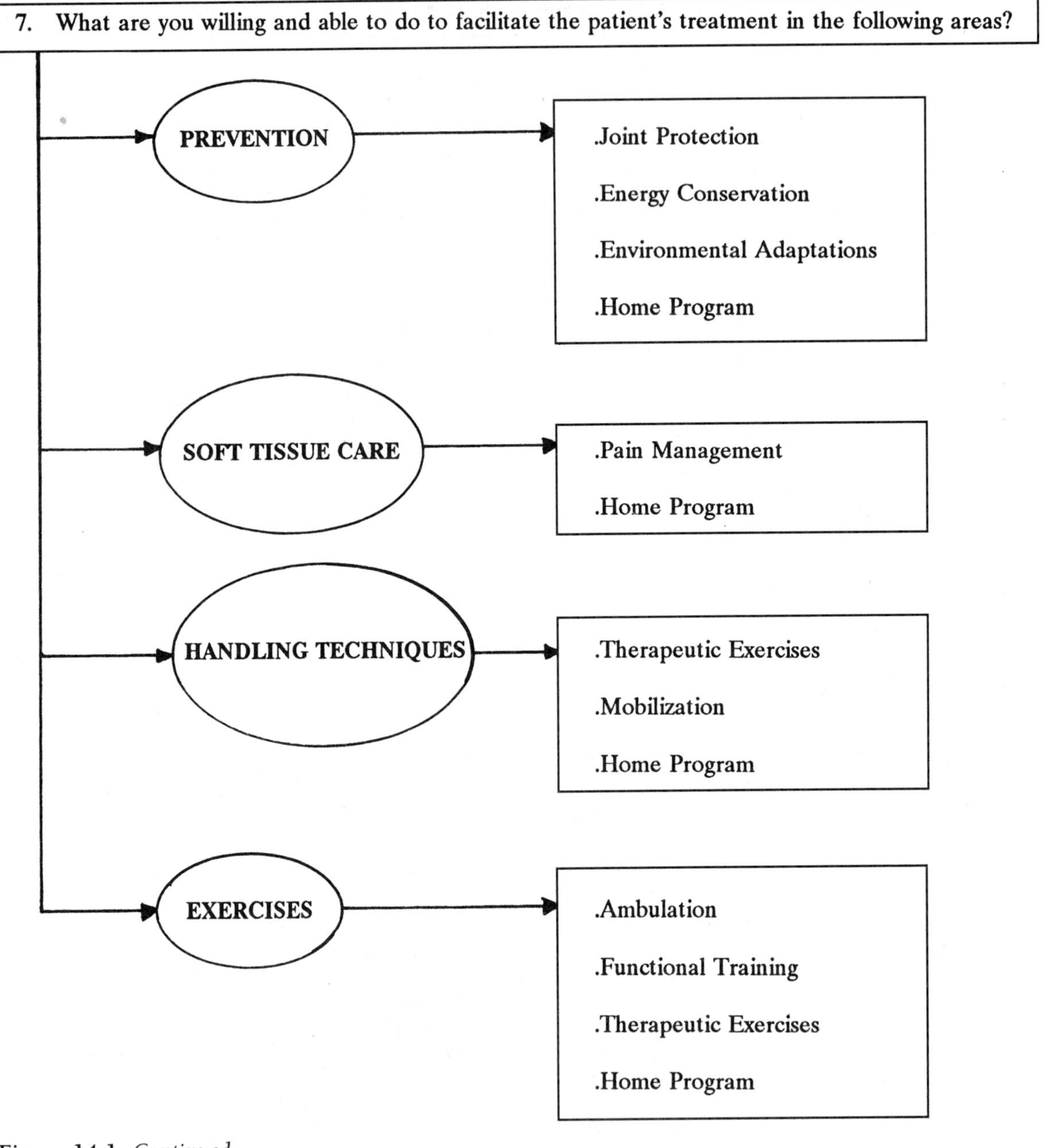

Figure 14-1. *Continued*

Prevention

Prevention is the component of the plan of care that addresses how the person with arthritis might prevent further injury to the joints and further decreases in mobility and activities of daily living (ADL).

Soft Tissue Care

Soft tissue care is the component of the plan of care that focuses on relieving symptoms, such as muscle tightness, pain, trigger points, tenderness, and swelling. This is not an all-inclusive listing, as other soft tissue problems might be identified.

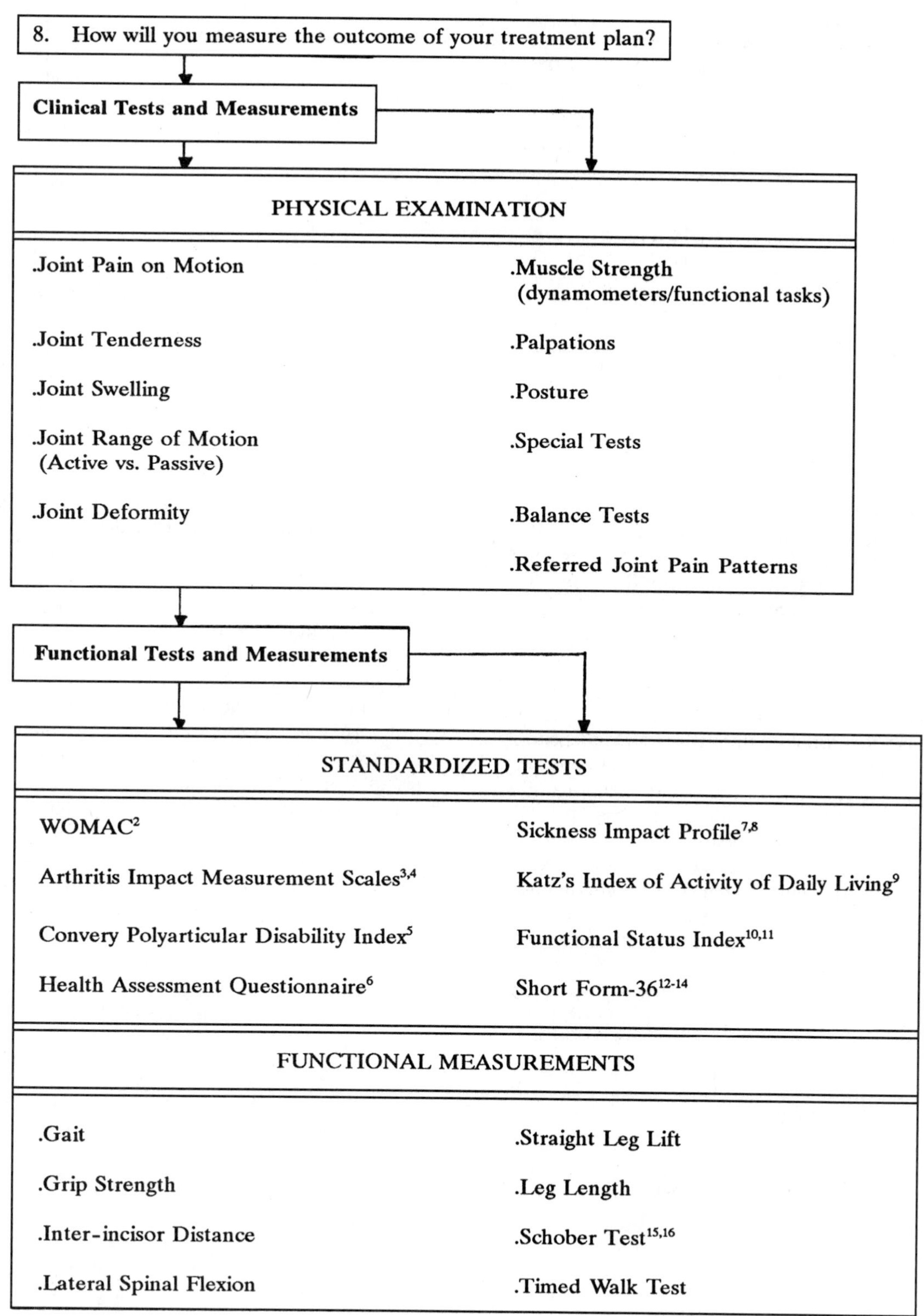

Figure 14-1. *Continued*

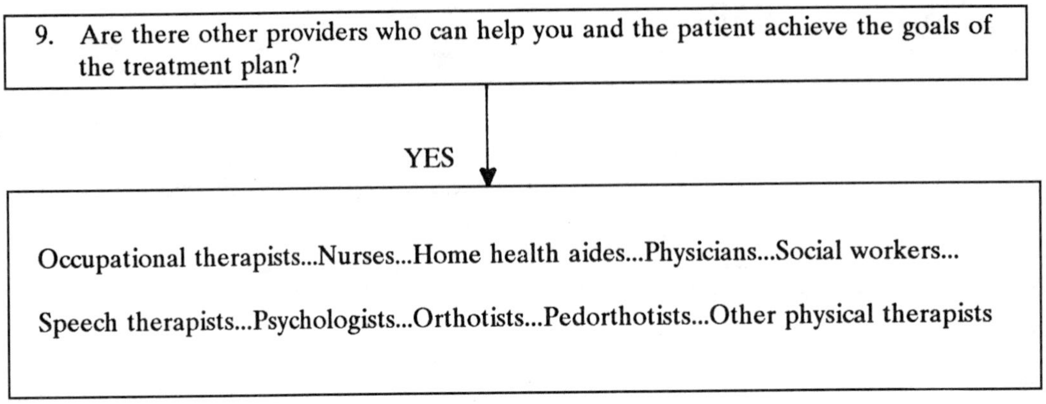

9. Are there other providers who can help you and the patient achieve the goals of the treatment plan?

YES

Occupational therapists...Nurses...Home health aides...Physicians...Social workers...

Speech therapists...Psychologists...Orthotists...Pedorthotists...Other physical therapists

Figure 14-1. *Continued*

Handling Techniques

Handling techniques are those measures therapists do by direct hand contact with the patient, such as posture training, joint mobilization, facilitation techniques, therapeutic exercises.

Exercise

This component of the plan is comprised of those activities that require the patient to perform exercises to improve their quality of life, mobility, and general health. Initial guidance from the therapist may be given; however, it is the responsibility of the patient to accomplish the exercise program as prescribed.

Accepting the rationale that most of the plan of care will fall into one or more of these categories, the plan of care for Mrs. G. will become more specific. As seen in Figure 14-1, there are various activities assigned to each category. In order to implement the plan of care, let us give consideration by category and activity to what Mrs. G. might do for her cervical spondylosis. Each category is presented in tabular form. Table 14-1 depicts activities and choices that might be used in the category of prevention. Table 14-2 outlines some alternatives for soft tissue care. Table 14-3 presents options for handling techniques, and Table 14-4 describes activities that might fall under exercises accomplished by the patient. The activities suggested are not meant to be the only alternatives to treat Mrs. G., but rather to demonstrate a way of planning. Some activities overlap categories. The purpose for that is to demonstrate the importance of addressing Mrs. G.'s plan of care more completely.

Having established the PT measures, it then becomes important to ensure that Mrs. G. complies with her program. While it is outside the scope of this chapter to discuss techniques that enhance compliance, there is ample literature from which to obtain ideas.[18–25] First and foremost, the therapist must focus on Mrs. G.'s most important goal and see it through. In Mrs. G.'s case, she wants to

Table 14-1. Treatment Implementation: Prevention Component

Joint Protection	Energy Conservation	Environmental Adaptations	Home Program
Cervical collar Cervical pillow for sleep High-backed chair for head rest	Short rest periods Pace activities Relaxation techniques	Modify computer station Change glasses Modify telephone use	Relaxation techniques Gentle exercise program Modify sitting and sleeping postures

Table 14-2. Treatment Implementation: Soft Tissue Care Component

Pain Management	Home Program
Heat or ice as tolerated Ultrasound? TENS Acupressure Gentle stretching Isometric exercises Resting/relaxation techniques Cervical collar Intermittent gentle traction in supine position Massage techniques	Moist heating pad Cervical pillow for night TENS Resting/relaxation techniques Isometric exercises progressing to strengthening exercises Gentle range of motion exercises

TENS, transcutaneous electrical nerve stimulation.

be able to continue driving her car and to continue with her genealogy work on the computer.

Suppose Mrs. G. is cooperative in most respects and is achieving the mutual goals established early in the treatment planning phase of her care. Question 8 then becomes: *How will you measure the outcome of Mrs. G.'s treatment?* For a capsule view of the answer to this question, another table (Table 14-5) is appropriate to depict the options. Suppose the goals mutually agreed upon directly related to PT have been achieved but Mrs. G. does not seem to understand the importance of relaxation techniques as a method of stress management. Although you were trained to use these methods, teaching relaxation techniques was never a strength of yours and might be better done by another provider. That brings us to the last question (Q.9) in the paradigm.

Are there other providers who can help Mrs. G. with relaxation techniques? If the answer is yes, is such a provider accessible to Mrs. G.? This requires consultation with more experienced colleagues, including the patient's physician, to find a suitable individual, such as a clinical psychologist or health educator. The Arthritis Society or Arthritis Foundation might provide the patient with a listing of individuals who specialize in biofeedback or relaxation technique instruction.

Literature Review Related to the Plan of Care

The foregoing process of creating a plan of care has been based on both anecdotal information and literature pertinent to OA. There are some treatment issues that have been investigated and reported in the literature related to PT in OA, some issues that have been decided based entirely on clinical experience, and there are some issues that need to be investigated. In keeping with the treatment algorithm addressed earlier, I will review the literature with the patient as a treatment team member (cooperation and adherence issues), prevention measures, soft tissue care, handling techniques, exercise, and outcome measures that could be utilized to assess patient progress and the plan of care. Since exercise is addressed elsewhere in the text, the discussion regarding exercise will be a selective review.

The Patient as a Worker

Wiener[26] has suggested that the patient is the central worker in his or her care and that as such

Table 14-3. Treatment Implementation: Handling Techniques

Therapeutic Exercises	Mobilization	Home Program
Range of motion exercises for neck and shoulders Stretching exercises Strengthening exercises Aerobic exercises for general body conditioning Posture training	Gentle distraction and stretching	Short version of range of motion, stretching, and strengthening exercises Walking program 3 times a week for 30 minutes for 10 weeks

Table 14-4. Treatment Implementation: Exercise Component

Ambulation	Functional Training	Therapeutic Exercises	Home Program
Suggest good walking shoes and changes in gait deviations Discuss falls prevention	Brisk walking Rest periods	Gentle range of motion, isometric, and strengthening exercises on a daily basis	Exercises for neck and shoulders Relaxation techniques Walking program

presents to the physical therapist (PT), or any other provider, untrained, unpaid, and often unacknowledged for the important role ahead of them. When a chronic illness like OA intrudes upon the life of an untrained patient, it demarcates quickly what the person might perceive they were in the past from what they perceive themselves to be now that they have OA. The change in perception of the body's ability to perform activities, its appearance, and physiological function can change the inner core of beliefs the person possesses. Accommodating to these changes is *work* for the patient, along with all the other day-to-day complexities that could arise from having OA. Living, coping with OA, and everyday work must be integrated by the patient, as well as completing the *work* of cooperating with a treatment regimen.[26] These are important concepts to appreciate during treatment planning and implementation.

Unfortunately, in our Western society, we equate the worth of work with the amount of pay received or vice versa. Our patient, as a worker, is unpaid. As therapists it is important that we value and dignify the effort the patient is making to complete the work that goes with their having OA, such as emotional work, living life, balancing treatment options, pacing their activities, and coping with disability if it is present. Recall that just because we are unable to see the work the patient is doing does not mean they are not making an honest effort.[27,28] The patient is the one who does the bulk of the work to manage a chronic illness, not the PT. An important professional role the PT can play is to acknowledge and honestly praise the patient for the work they are doing to contribute to their care.

Table 14-5. Two Main Categories of Outcome Measures: Clinical Tests and Functional Tests and Measurements

Clinical Tests and Measurements	Functional Tests and Measurements
Range of motion in degrees or percent of gain or loss Muscle test scores Visual analogue scales Decreased use of TENS Scores on standardized functional assessment tools (AIMS,[3,4] Convery,[5] HAQ,[6] SIP,[7,8] Katz,[9] FSI,[10,11] SF-36[12–14])	Pain-free range of motion in rotation while backing car out of driveway Increased length of walking time Increased tolerance for sitting at the computer measured in time or self-report Decreased fatigue as measured by self-report

In their article on the role of expectations and preferences in health care satisfaction of persons with arthritis, Ross et al stated that expectations are what people *expect* from care and preferences are what people *want* from care.[29] These authors suggest that expectations and preferences are different constructs and have different mechanisms for influencing patient satisfaction with care. It has been demonstrated that there is an association between arthritis experience, as measured by duration of joint discomfort, number of affected joints, and number of treatments or procedures; physical functioning and depression; and expectations.[29] Lower expectations of care occurred in those patients with greater disease experience, lower physical functioning, and greater depression. The implication of these findings for PT is that patients who have longstanding arthritis and low expectations from treatment may experience dissatisfaction with physical therapy regardless of the quality of care given. Thus, it is important for the therapist to try and ascertain what the expectations of the patient might be.

No studies have been completed to examine the preferences of patients with arthritis regarding patient care.[29] Persons with arthritis may represent a distinct subgroup of individuals seeking care that differs in important ways in the value they place on health care.[29] While patients with arthritis may not differ in their ultimate satisfaction with care, they could differ in their preferences for different attributes of care.[29] For example: the person with OA may come to realize that there are certain limits to the success that might be achieved from care and shift their priority to having a valuable relationship with the provider. The intent is to maintain a good relationship with the provider and to have support and advice through the variable course sometimes experienced with OA.[29] In other words, the person with OA may come to value the interaction with the PT in preference to emphasis on efficiency and access to care, although these are indeed important. The conclusion to draw from this information is that the patient's expectations and preferences are important considerations to know when planning and implementing a plan of care.

The patient's expectations and preferences are important considerations to know when planning and implementing care.

Prevention

It has been reported that the incidence of OA is higher in persons who consistently overuse certain joints,[30] who are obese,[1] and who sustain a traumatic injury to the joint.[31] This information is useful during treatment planning in relation to joint protection and energy conservation techniques. Brown et al investigated the energy required to walk with OA of the hip before and after a total hip arthroplasty.[32] The difference in energy consumption before surgery was 56% of their predicted maximum capacity. One year following total hip arthroplasty the customary walking speed increased from 41 m/min (50% of normal) to 55 m/min (67% of normal) and the oxygen cost decreased, although not within limits established for equivalent persons without OA. Gussoni et al measured the energy costs of walking in 12 patients with hip joint impairments. Their data revealed that during level treadmill walking the energy costs increased up to 50% above normal and up to 70% while walking a 5% incline.[33]

The addition of assistive devices, such as a cane or crutches, can impact the energy requirements dramatically, provided the upper extremities can tolerate their use.[34] Data have been reported on the use of crutches, canes, or walkers in persons with rheumatoid arthritis (RA) that demonstrate how the use of these devices might influence gait parameters, heart rate, and oxygen uptake.[34] Individuals who did not require assistive devices had the highest velocity of 45 m/min and had the highest oxygen uptake of 11.0 ml/kg/min. Those requiring bilateral crutches or a walker had the slowest velocities of 26 m/min and 21 m/min, respectively. Oxygen consumption was the lowest in those requiring a walker. Considering the slow velocity of gait with a walker, the oxygen costs were considered high by the researchers. The highest heart rate was in patients using both arms with bilateral crutches or a walker and lowest in patients using one cane or a crutch. Caution must be exercised when applying these results to persons with OA. We do not know from these data the extent of involvement of the upper extremities of the patient with RA, which could influence the weight-bearing ability of the patient with the assistive devices. These were preoperative total joint candidates and likely only surgery would make a difference in their functional capacity. No mention was made about how the initial use of the assistive device contributed to lessening the pain the patient experienced. The foregoing example is offered in order to appreciate the fact that when an assistive device is added to help a person walk, the energy costs may increase, although pain decreases.

Patients with unilateral hip disease should use a cane on the opposite side and carry loads on the same side.

Joint protection principles originated as intuitive thought; however, recent work by Neumann[35] addressed scientifically the use of a cane as a method of hip joint protection. While therapists have routinely suggested that patients place the cane in the hand opposite to the hip with arthritis, the results from this study explain biomechanically why use of the cane in this way is important. In addition, the results of this study suggest that patients with unilateral hip disease should carry loads *on the side* of the hip arthritis so a cane can be used on the opposite side.[35]

Cervical collars are commonly suggested for use in OA of the cervical spine. Rationale for their use is to immobilize and rest the joints of the neck, provide protection, and heat and provide weight release.[36,37] Spondylosis causes pain and occasionally radicular symptoms into the neck and arm. Selection of a collar will be made based upon the goals to be achieved by use of the collar. A comparative study of the effectiveness of cervical collars in limiting neck motion by Johnson et al[38] compared the effectiveness of a soft cervical collar, a Philadelphia collar, a four-poster brace, a cervicothoracic brace, a Somi brace, and a halo device with a plastic body vest in limiting neck motion in healthy subjects.[38] The results of their investigation indicated what might be expected. The halo device limited the greatest amount of motion (96% of flexion and extension of the neck) and the soft cervical collar limited the least amount (26% of flexion and extension). Rotation was poorly controlled by all of the collars with the exception of the halo device.

What this suggests is that the PT and the patient must be realistic about the use of a cervical collar. If the goal is to provide an analgesic effect on the painful joints of the neck by resting them or assisting them biomechanically, then a soft collar may be a suitable choice. If, on the other hand, there are neurological warnings of an active destructive process, a more rigid collar, such as a Philadelphia or cervicothoracic brace may be indicated. Use of a neck support should offer support and immobilization to protect damaged joints, rather than as a corrective measure for a postural deviation in the neck. Biomechanical derangement of facet joints due to OA may be aggravated by the use of an externally applied corrective force from a brace or collar through contact on the mandible, occiput, and thorax.

Other joint protection and energy conservation techniques might include taking elevators rather than stairs, riding in a golf cart rather than walking, limiting the number of times stairs are used, using high stools rather than standing at work stations, and pacing activities so that light tasks are mixed with heavy tasks.[39]

Additional measures are given in Chapter 10. Often, patients fail to realize that the more physically fit they are, the more efficient the body becomes in terms of joint protection and energy conservation. Various authors have demonstrated that individuals with OA can improve their fitness level without worsening their arthritis.[40–47]

Soft Tissue Care

Use of thermal agents in treating OA is common; however, deciding which thermal agent to use is not always straightforward. Michlovitz has suggested several guidelines that may be used to reach a decision.[48] These are depicted in Table 14-6. The author makes the recommendation that acute symptoms in OA might be treated with cold, electrical stimulation, or superficial heat, while chronic manifestations are better suited to respond to conversion heat, such as ultrasound or diathermy, superficial heat, or cold application.

The literature on the efficacy of ultrasound in treatment of OA contains mixed reviews. Lehman et al reported an increase of range of motion of the shoulder with ultrasound and exercise.[49] Other researchers suggest that there is no statistically significant difference in the range of motion achieved in persons with OA of the knee who received sham versus actual treatment with ultrasound and exercise.[50] Falconer et al published a thorough review of the literature on the use of ultrasound and pain relief and concluded that while persons with OA may experience pain relief, we cannot be confident as clinicians that ultrasound caused this improvement. Placebo effects and experimenter expectancy bias may be contaminating the results.[51] Further well-designed clinical trials on the use of ultrasound in OA must be completed.

Sheon et al suggested that the use of medications may be least important in treatment of soft tissue disorders accompanying OA.[52] Gentle stretching exercises, joint distraction in the form of manual or mechanical traction, and avoidance of aggravating factors on the joint often provide more sustained benefit. Soft tissue techniques are particularly useful in painful musculoskeletal conditions and impaired function.[53] Danneskiold-Samsoe et al investigated the effects of massage on myofascial pain and determined that 21 of 26 patients improved symptomatically with a concurrent decline in muscle tension.[54] Using measurable biochemical parameters, they determined that gradual decline occurred in plasma myoglobin concentration after each massage session.

Selected physical agents, suggested in the literature for treatment of OA, have been described in Chapter 13. The principal rationale for use of

Table 14-6. Factors to Consider in the Use of Thermal Agents in Osteoarthritis

Factors	Treatment Maneuver
1. Inflammatory versus noninflammatory polyarthritis	*Osteoarthrosis*: use a deeper heating technique
2. Acute versus chronic inflammation	*Inflamed*: use cold and/or electrical stimulation to reduce pain and inflammation
3. Loss of range of motion	*Joint capsule shortening or musculotendinous contracture*: use deep heat with slow, gentle stretch; use cold applications cautiously
4. Position for treatment	*Joints should be positioned to decrease pain or to decrease the chance of pain occurring during treatment*
5. Joints involved	*Multiple joints involved*: Use hydrotherapy in the form of Hubbard tank or swimming pool
6. Clinic versus home care	Select *practical methods* the patient can easily employ at home safely
7. Precautions/ contraindications	Some *medical conditions or comorbidity* existing with the OA may preclude the use of thermal agents
8. Preconceived notions	Some *patients have varied experiences* with the use of heat, cold, or home remedies; they may need to be reeducated about the use of these modalities

these modalities is to decrease pain, relax musculature, and increase mobility in joints. Borrell concluded that fluidotherapy delivered more heat than did paraffin baths or hydrotherapy; however, only two joints were studied in four healthy young men.[55]

Several investigators have reported their results from studies regarding the effects of heat and exercise versus exercise alone for increasing range of motion in arthritis.[56–59] The results of these studies suggest that heat and exercise together produce no more range of motion in a patient with RA, OA of the hips and knees, or following total knee arthroplasty (TKA), than exercise alone. Hecht et al[60] noted that cold and exercise produced no greater increase in the range of motion of patients following a TKA than exercise alone. Chamberlain et al indicated that shortwave diathermy and exercise produced no difference in muscular endurance in patients with OA of the knee when compared to a group receiving exercise alone.[56] Before coming to the conclusion, however, that heat and cold add little to exercise regimens for improving strength, pain, range of motion, and endurance, it is important to ask at least one crucial question. Are there other variables that are affected by use of heat and cold? Swezey[61] noted that the placebo phenomenon cannot be discounted when using therapeutic modalities for arthritis management. Little is known about the action of these agents in OA; hence, there exists a need for clinical investigations to demonstrate their efficacy.

Handling Techniques

Placing the hands upon a patient to guide their exercises, reeducate muscle, direct body movements, or mobilize soft tissues is a characteristic essential to the profession of PT. The extent to which sophisticated mobilization techniques may be used depends upon the interest and ability of the therapist and the status of the patient to receive these techniques. It is not the purpose of this chapter to teach the basics of manual therapy, but rather to suggest that the person with OA who experiences hypomobility, pain, disability and decreased range of motion might benefit from the proper use of mobilization to reverse these conditions. Barak et al have described joint mobilization as an attempt to improve joint mobility or decrease pain by using selected grades of accessory movements.[62] The rationale they provide for the use of accessory movements suggests that these techniques could be useful in persons with OA (Table 14-7). Gentle distraction of the joint and stretching of the cap-

Table 14-7. Accessory Movement Techniques for Joint Mobilization

1. Used when primary resistance is encountered from the ligament and capsule of the joint and there is minimal muscular resistance
2. Can be done in any part of the physiological range of motion
3. Can be done in any direction (posteriorly, caudally, or anteriorly)
4. Causes less pain per degree of range of motion gained
5. Used for tight articular structures
6. Safe method because it employs short lever arm techniques

sular tissues can be useful to increase mobility. Other authors also have described the guidelines for manual techniques that could be used in the treatment of OA.[63–68]

Connective tissue massage,[69] proprioceptive neuromuscular facilitation techniques, resisted exercises, and stretching exercises should be applied with a complete understanding of the status of the joint, the musculature, and the tolerance of the patient for any of these measures. Nothing will turn the patient away from care quicker than the use of excessive force on painful joints. The application of therapeutic techniques used judiciously will enhance the ability to reach established treatment goals.

General Exercise

Considerable progress has been made in understanding of the effects of exercise on OA, particularly that of aerobic conditioning.[40–47,70–72] It is important to monitor how the patient does their exercise program. There are some individuals who believe that more exercise may be better; therefore, the patient should be cautioned to avoid doing too much or too little of their home program. Unfortunately, the patient is often the only person who can determine what their level of tolerance for exercise will be. A walking program might be given to a person with OA, provided the lower extremity joints will tolerate walking. The same program could be done in a swimming pool. The reader is referred to Chapter 11 for in-depth guidelines and scientific rationale for proceeding with an exercise program for people with OA.

How the patient exercises is critical in terms of protecting the joint from further damage. Consideration should be given to such mechanical factors as moments produced around the joint, the duration of the exercise, and the status of joint structures. In a healthy knee, these forces may be easily tolerated; however, in an eburnated, painful knee joint, loading with excessive resistance will only exacerbate the problem. In an elderly, sedentary individual, lifting the weight of the leg when the knee is painful may be a maximum effort. Nothing will interfere with patient compliance more than providing treatment that causes more harm than good. Thus, it is important to have the patient begin joint protection activities early in the course of treatment in the form of carefully planned exercise, taking into account the age and physical status of the patient. Low intensity exercises of short duration with minimal repetitions and frequent sessions per day may be the only way to achieve initial success.[73] Intensity is defined as the percentage of the maximal capacity a person should exercise, duration as the length of time the person can do continuous exercise, and frequency is the number of workout periods per day or week.

While minimal guidelines have been described for increasing the capacity of the patient to exercise, these are simply that—guidelines.[74] Consideration should be given to the patient's aerobic capacity; however, age, medication taken, physical status, and willingness to adhere to the program are important factors. Low intensity for a 60-year-old person who has been inactive, may be 50–60% of the maximal heart rate. Short duration may be 5–10 minutes of continuous work. Minimal repetitions may be from five to ten repetitions completed two to three times daily.

Physical Therapy Considerations for the Surgical Patient

While PT measures may be employed to provide relief of pain and restoration of function, there may come a time when the patient will need surgical intervention to restore joint function. The single major advance in the relief of pain and restoration of a severely damaged knee or hip from OA has been total joint replacement. While there are surgical options other than joint replacement, particularly in younger patients, older patients may be encouraged to have an arthroplasty when their quality of life is being measurably impacted and severe deterioration of the joint surfaces has occurred. Although many surgeons and PTs consider that rehabilitation is imperative following a total joint arthroplasty, there are few published studies that describe the ideal PT program for the patient.[75] Scientific evidence aside, surgeons in the field of joint replacement surgery usually refer their patients to PT based upon experience that active participation of the patient with a PT in a postoperative exercise program will improve muscle strength, increase motion, and educate the patient in proper protection of the operated joint. Physical therapy following total joint arthroplasty appears to be based largely on local custom and surgeon preference. Figgie[76] suggests that a patient with a hip arthroplasty should not be discharged from the hospital until they are ambulatory with a walking aid and can manage stairs independently. After a total knee replacement (TKR), the patient should be able to bend the knee to 90 degrees and able to maneuver up and down stairs prior to leaving the hospital. Little information has been published describing the rehabilitation process undertaken by a PT; however, there seems to be some consistent aspects of a plan of care that the therapist should consider. For example, if there is an opportunity to conduct a preoperative evaluation of the joint slated for surgery, some of the elements that should be determined are range of motion, muscle strength, muscular imbalances, gait deviations, age, mental status, living arrangements, and family and social support networks. The patient should be made aware of the goals of PT management and what he or she might expect following surgery.

Kampa et al[77] and others[78,79] have suggested guidelines for postoperative rehabilitation that are important for a PT to consider. A summary of these customary programs are depicted in Tables 14-8 and 14-9. Postoperative rehabilitation will be influenced by the age, cognitive status, muscular strength, general health, type of prosthesis used (cemented versus cementless), the surgical approach done, and the cooperative behavior of the patient. Weight-bearing status of the patient also will be influenced by the foregoing parameters as well as the surgeon's preference for bearing weight on the prosthesis.

In recent years, several authors have completed studies on patients with total joint arthroplasty that is enhancing our understanding of rehabilitation practices for these patients. Barrett et al[80] and Stauffer et al[81] have reported that patients with OA of the knee demonstrate diminished position sense when compared to normal subjects of various ages. Furthermore, Barrett et al[80] determined that patients with TKRs exhibit greater accuracy in position sense when compared with subjects who have OA in their knees ($p<.02$). These authors compared position sense accuracy in patients having semiconstrained knee replacements with those who received constrained prostheses. Test results favored the patients with the semiconstrained knee, although statistical significance was not achieved. It was concluded that the total knee replacement likely restores joint alignment and "joint space height," contributing to improved position sense; however, recovery did not reach the accuracy of age-matched subjects with normal knees. These data are important to consider when planning a PT regimen both pre- and postoperatively. The therapist could reasonably expect that postoperative joint position sense will improve in patients with a knee arthroplasty.

Jevsevar and others compared locomotor activities in 15 subjects (19 knees) with knee arthroplasties (KA), and 11 control subjects (22 knees).[82] All subjects were analyzed kinematically and kinetically while walking barefoot, climbing and descending stairs, and rising from a chair. Using sophisticated gait analysis equipment, the investigators showed that although the KA group had an excellent result when assessed clinically, the KA group demonstrated functional performance decrements, particularly in knee torque and angular velocity during locomotion, when compared to the healthy controls.

A combination of factors could account for these results, such as severity of preoperative OA, scar tissue formation following surgery, and concurrent hip OA. Since patients with a KA will need to compensate any loss of range of motion in the knee by increasing hip motion, severe OA of the hip should be addressed before a KA is done. The investigators recommended that exercise programs for rehabilitation should be selected to address knee angular velocity and torque during gait and ADL. They further concluded that locomotor activities of daily living demand relatively slow loaded angular velocities and low knee torques, also important when planning exercise protocols.[82]

Strickland et al[83] and Givens-Heiss et al[84] have reported data derived from a patient who underwent the implantation of a right instrumented hip endoprosthesis designed to quantify contact pressures on the acetabular cartilage. The prosthesis instrumentation has been described elsewhere.[85,86] The prosthesis was designed to transmit acetabular cartilage pressure data via ten different transducers to a computer where it could be stored and analyzed. Although data are reported only for a single

Table 14-8. Physical Therapy Protocol for Total Hip Arthroplasty

Status	Time	Activity
Preoperative	1 month prior to admission	1. Attend class on total hip arthroplasty 2. Evaluate range of motion, strength, limb length, pain, gait patterns 3. Review precautions and postoperative exercise plan 4. Fit walker and instruct in use
Postoperative	Day 1	1. Supine bed exercises 2. Bed to chair transfers
	Day 2	1. Supine bed exercises: isometric and ankle pumping exercises 2. Active-assistive range of motion 3. Assisted walker/crutch ambulation dependent upon weight-bearing status
	Days 3–5	1. Supine bed exercises 2. Sitting bed exercises 3. Bathroom transfers 4. Gait training on level surfaces
Postoperative	Day 6 to discharge	1. Progressive strengthening program 2. Ambulation training with walker 3. Discharge planning 4. Home program instruction and future precautions
	4–6 weeks	1. Home exercise program 2. Crutch walking: full weight bearing with cemented prosthesis 3. Crutch walking: partial weight bearing with cementless prosthesis 4. Stationary bicycle with no resistance
	7–12 weeks	1. Continue exercises: strengthening, balance, proprioception activities 2. Gradually begin walking without use of crutches if local custom permits 3. Increase time on the stationary bicycle with slight resistance
	12–24 weeks	1. Continue exercises 2. Maintain flexion of knee at 110 degrees and extension to 0 degrees 3. Walking program for 15–20 minutes 4. Stationary bicycle for 20–30 minutes with slight resistance

Table 14-9. Physical Therapy Protocol for Total Knee Arthroplasty

Status	Time	Activity
Preoperative	1–2 months	1. Instruct in range of motion exercises 2. Restore or improve functional strength of the knee 3. Instruct and/or fit with continuous passive motion machine to acquaint patient 4. Instruct in deep breathing exercises
Postoperative	24 hours	1. Check on continuous passive motion machine or complete manual passive motion 2. Deep breathing and coughing exercises 3. Exercises for circulation and range of motion within a pain-free range
	Day 2	1. Gentle mobility of patella 2. Bed to chair transfers 3. Ambulation with walker with assistance if this is local custom
	Days 3–5	1. Range of motion exercises 2. Gentle strengthening exercises 3. Ambulation training with walker
Postoperative	Day 6 to discharge	1. Reinforce bed exercises 2. Reinforce postoperative precautions 3. Gait training 4. Stair climbing 5. Discharge planning 6. Home exercise and ADL program
First clinic visit	2–3 weeks after surgery	1. Review home program 2. Add standing hip abductor exercises 3. Supine IT band stretches 4. Walker/crutch ambulation review
Second clinic visit	At 6 weeks	1. Review exercise program 2. Hip abduction side lying 3. Supine IT band stretches 4. Cane ambulation (cemented prosthesis) 5. Progressive weight bearing with walker/crutches (uncemented prosthesis)
Third clinic visit	At 12 weeks	1. Review entire exercise program 2. Begin cane ambulation with noncemented prosthesis

IT, iliotibial.

patient, the results are revealing about the effect of various exercises and activities upon the hip joint. During the period immediately following surgery, the patient was asked to complete several non-weight-bearing activities, as it is a common belief these activities require reduced contact on the joint surfaces while lying supine, namely: isometric quadriceps setting, isometric gluteus maximus setting, active hip flexion, and active hip abduction. Measured in megapascals (MPa), active hip flexion produced the greatest amount of acetabular pressure (4.79 MPa), while isometric quadriceps contraction with the knee in extension produced the lowest. The next highest peak pressure on the acetabular cartilage was during isometric gluteus maximus contraction (4.65 MPa).

Research has shown that *touchdown weight bearing*, when performed correctly, generates less acetabular stress than partial weight bearing, full weight bearing, or non–weight bearing with the knee extended.

Weight-bearing activities included stepping exercises with both right and left leg (weight shifting), and standing up from a chair. When all activities were placed in order of pressure produced, the pressures on the acetabulum occurred in the following ascending order: isometric quadriceps setting (3.44 MPa), stepping right, active abduction exercise, stepping left, standing up, isometric gluteus maximus exercises, and active hip flexion (4.79 MPa). While these results cannot be extrapolated to other patients with an endoprosthesis, they do point out that exercises we ask patients to do are not benign activities. We could be asking the patient to complete exercises that are producing higher femoroacetabular pressures than those required by weight shifting and standing up activities. More studies must be completed before these results are generalizable to all patients with total hip replacements.

In a subsequent study of the postacute phase of this same patient,[84] other rehabilitation parameters were measured including full weight-bearing free speed walking, partial weight bearing (13.6 kg) with crutches, touchdown weight bearing (4.5 kg) with crutches, non–weight bearing with crutches (swing to or through gait), maximal voluntary isometric abduction exercise with resistance, and straight leg raising. These were evaluated to determine in vivo pressures on the acetabular cartilage. Study results showed that aided gait can reduce the stress on the acetabular cartilage. Partial weight-bearing, touchdown weight-bearing, and non–weight-bearing ambulation, however, did not always follow a hierarchical relationship based on the degree of prescribed weight bearing. The authors suggested that exercises such as straight leg raising and gravity-reduced abduction that do not produce high muscle forces could be favored over resisted isometric exercise to reduce acetabular contact pressures. There might be, however, lower muscle strength gains than expected from resisted exercises. Touchdown weight bearing, when performed correctly, generated less acetabular stress than partial weight bearing, full weight bearing or non–weight bearing with the knee extended. In order to generalize these findings, further research is needed on a larger sample of patients. These studies are a good start in what actually happens when a person with an endoprosthesis exercises and ambulates.

Outcome Measures

Objective treatment outcomes are needed in all spheres of PT, as regulators and health services payees demand more cost-effective services. You will recall from Figure 14-1 that outcome measures were divided into two major categories: "clinical tests and measurements," and "functional tests and measurements" (see Appendix III).

Clinical Tests and Measurements

These tests are not necessarily unique to the assessment of a patient with arthritis, but are generic measures used in other orthopedic entities. Unique to these tests is the rheumatologic slant in their interpretation. For example, in the rheumatology literature, scores related to joint pain on motion, joint tenderness, or joint swelling are usually reported on a scale from 0–3, with 3 being the most severe situation.[87] The score may appear as an examiner's score or as a self-report score by the patient. The Visual Analog Scale (VAS) is commonly used to determine by patient report how well she or he is doing in terms of pain, tolerance for the disease, fatigue, sleep, and any other factors known only by the patient. It is important to ask the patient for their assessment in terms of "today," since memory of past experiences can be deceiving.

Manual or any other form of muscle testing can have spurious results when there is joint pain, instability, or deformity. Having the patient demonstrate functional tests, such as the "Get-up-and-Go-Test"[88] and timing how long it takes the patient to do this activity will give more realistic information regarding the status of the involved lower extremity. Balance tests while standing on the lower extremity, in the absence of central nervous system disease, will inform the therapist about the status of the ligaments, muscles, and mechanoreceptors of the joints in the kinetic chain. Special tests used when evaluating the patient can be completed periodically throughout treatment to determine if progress has been made, such as: Ober's test, Faber's test, valgus/varus stress tests.

In OA, pain can be referred to other sites that may or may not be involved with the disease. OA of the hip can cause referred pain to the groin and to the knee; OA of the lumbar spine can cause pain referred to the hip and knee; and shoulder OA may refer pain to the lateral humerus. These referral patterns identified during the initial evaluation and throughout the course of treatment, may diminish as the patient improves.

Functional Tests and Measurements

Several standardized assessment questionnaires have been developed to assess the abilities of the patient with OA (for specific tests see Appendix III). Each of these instruments has strengths and weaknesses.

The Western Ontario and McMaster Universities (WOMAC)[2] Index has been validated by Bellamy et al for specific measurement of OA patients in clinical trials. All of the measurement scales mentioned hereafter were validated on rheumatoid arthritis patients; therefore, the generalizability of the results of these tests to the measurement of disease in OA is not optimum. The WOMAC Index asks the patient to report information in three dimensions: pain, stiffness, and physical function. It is a useful measurement tool to use before and after treatment to measure the perception of the patient regarding their treatment.

The Arthritis Impact Measurement Scale (AIMS) was developed for use as a research tool to collect a wide variety of information from the patient about their arthritis, general health, and socioeconomic well-being. While it is an invaluable data collecting instrument, it is not easily administered in a busy clinic.[3] The authors of this instrument have created a shorter version of this instrument called the AIMS2,[4] which could be used by clinicians.

The Convery Polyarticular Disability Index[5] requires the therapist to observe the patient performing various tasks. It takes about 15 minutes to administer and is excellent for obtaining baseline data, provided time is available to observe patients perform the tasks. Periodically throughout treatment the patient could be asked to repeat their performance of a given task to determine whether progress is occurring.

The Health Assessment Questionnaire (HAQ)[6] is a widely used self-report tool given to the patient for their opinion of their functional abilities. It is easily filled out and could be used as a pre- and post-treatment test if patient report is what is wanted. Another functional assessment tool is the Functional Status Index.[10,11] This tool is available in both an interview and self-report form. While the title of the Katz Index of Activities of Daily Living suggests it would be useful for assessing function, in actuality it only considers basic ADLs and one aspect of physical mobility—transfers.[9] The Sickness Impact Profile is well known for assessing the patient's perception of how their illness impacts on their life.[7,8]

A generic health-related quality-of-life measure, the Short Form-36 (SF-36), has been reported by various authors[12–14] for use as a measure of disease-specific pain, physical function, quality of life, mobility, and so forth before and after a total knee or hip replacement. Comparisons made between the AIMS2 and the SF-36 suggests that the two should be used together to gain important information regarding the status of the patient, as these two instruments complement each other.[12]

A considerable body of literature published on PT demonstrates the importance and use of measurement scales that are reliable and valid. For example, testing at the same time of the day, by the same observer, will enhance the reliability of the measurement. Careful selection of the instrument to be used to measure the patient is critical if the test is to be valid. As therapists, if we are to make any statement about treatment efficacy, the validity and reliability of instruments and testing environments must be carefully considered.

Future Challenges and Implications

It is well known that the prevalence of OA increases with age. Physical therapists are expected to be treating more elders as we approach the year 2000. A major challenge for therapists, when creating a treatment plan, will be to understand and distinguish between changes that are due to the aging musculoskeletal system from the changes produced by OA proper or the problems that may be due to comorbid conditions, such as osteoporosis. Patients that maintain an appropriate weight, engage in a moderate exercise program, and adopt other healthy life styles often do well. Physical therapists must resist the temptation to tell patients that they will have to live with their arthritis. A third challenge will be to create a mutually agreed upon plan of care wherein the patient will cooperate and be a willing worker to take care of themselves.

Research Questions

A challenge to PT researchers will be to validate treatment methods and suggest improved ways of delivery of care. For example, to what extent do the modalities we use to treat OA make a difference on the outcomes of treatment? What are the most effective ways to deliver PT services to persons with OA? How do we measure outcomes that indicate PT has increased the quality of life of the patient? To what extent does physical therapy intervention deter disability and enhance a return to the work force by persons with OA?

Since a cure for OA is not imminent, our attitudes and practices as therapists should maximize the quality of life experienced by our patients. The question remains: What are our preconceived notions about persons with OA and do these attitudes influence treatment and outcome measures? These are some challenges that current and future researchers might investigate.

References

1. Felson DT, Anderson JJ, Naimark A, et al: Obesity and knee osteoarthritis: the Framingham Study. Ann Intern Med 1988; 109:18–24.
2. Bellamy N, Buchanan WW, Goldsmith CH, et al: Validation study of WOMAC: a health status instrument for measuring clinically important patients relevant, outcomes to antirheumatic drug therapy in patients with OA of the hip or knee. J Rheumatol 1988; 15:1833–1840.
3. Meenan RF: The AIMS approach in health status measurement: conceptual background and measurement properties. J Rheumatol 1982; 9:785–788.
4. Meenan RF, Mason JH, Anderson JJ, et al: AIMS2: the content and properties of a revised and expanded Arthritis Impact Measurement Health Status Questionnaire. Arthritis Rheum 1992; 35:1–10.
5. Convery FR, Minteer MA, Amiel D, et al: Polyarticular disability: a functional assessment. Arch Phys Med Rehabil 1977; 58:494–499.
6. Fries JF, Spitz P, Kraines RG, et al: Measurement of patient outcome in arthritis. Arthritis Rheum 1980; 23:137–145.
7. Bergner M, Bobbitt RA, Pollard WE, et al: The Sickness Impact Profile: validation of a health status measure. Med Care 1976; 14:56–67.
8. Pollard WE, Bobbitt RA, Bergner M, et al: The Sickness Impact Profile: reliability of a health status measure. Med Care 1976; 14:146–155.
9. Katz S, Ford AB, Roland W, et al: Studies of illness in the aged. The index ADL: a standardized measure of biological and psychosocial function. JAMA 1963; 185:914–919.
10. Jette AM: Functional capacity evaluation: an empirical approach. Arch Phys Med Rehabil 1980; 61:85–89.
11. Jette AM: Functional Status Index: reliability of a chronic disease evaluation instrument. Arch Phys Med Rehabil 1980; 61:395–401.
12. Chewning B, Bell C, Nowlin N, et al: A comparison of AIMS 2 and SF-36 health quality of life measures. Arthritis Rheum 1994; 37(Suppl):S225.
13. Bombardier C, Melfi CA, Paul J, et al: Comparison of a generic and a disease-specific measure of pain and physical function after knee replacement surgery. Arthritis Rheum 1994; 37(Suppl):S225.
14. Stucki G, Daltroy L, Liang MH, et al: The Short Form-36 is superior to the Sickness Impact Profile as a generic health status measure in patients undergoing total hip arthroplasty. Arthritis Rheum 1994; 37(Suppl):S227.
15. Macrae IF, Wright V: Measurement of back movement. Ann Rheum Dis 1969; 28:584–589.
16. Moll JMH, Wright V: Normal range of spinal mobility: an objective clinical study. Ann Rheum Dis 1971; 30:381–386.
17. Mathews JA: Neck pain. In Klippel JH, Dieppe PA (eds): Rheumatology, pp 5.1–5.14. St Louis, Mosby Yearbook, 1994.
18. Dunbar J, Dunning EJ, Dwyer K: Compliance measurement with arthritis regimen. Arthritis Care Res 1989; 2:S8–S16.
19. Ross FM: Patient compliance—whose responsibility? Soc Sci Med 1991; 32:89–94.
20. Sluijs EM, Knibbe J: Patient compliance with exercise: Different theoretical approaches to short-term and long-term compliance. Patient Educ Couns 1991; 17:191–204.
21. Sluijs EM, Kok GJ, van der Zee J: Correlates of exercise compliance in physical therapy. Phys Ther 1993; 73:771–782.
22. Carpenter JD, Davis LJ: Medical recommendations followed or ignored? Factors influencing compliance

in arthritis. Arch Phys Med Rehabil 1976; 57:241–246.
23. Parker JC, Bradley LA, DeVellis R, et al: Biopsychosocial contributions to the management of arthritis disability. Arthritis Rheum 1993; 36:885–889.
24. Jensen GM, Lorish C: Physical therapists' approach to home exercise programs: identification of routine beliefs and behaviors. Phys Ther 1992; 72:S72.
25. Dexter PA: Joint exercises in elderly persons with symptomatic osteoarthritis of the hip or knee: performance patterns, medical support patterns, and the relationship between exercising and medical care. Arthritis Care Res 1992; 5:36–41.
26. Wiener C: Untrained, unpaid, and unacknowledged: the patient as a worker. Arthritis Care Res 1989; 2: 16–21.
27. Corbin J, Strauss A: Unending Work and Care: Managing Chronic Illness at Home, 358 pp. San Francisco, CA, Jossey Bass Publishers, 1988.
28. Daniels A: Invisible work. Soc Probl 1987; 34:403–415.
29. Ross CK, Sinacore JM, Stiers W, et al: The role and expectations and preferences in health care satisfaction of patients with arthritis. Arthritis Care Res 1990; 3:92–98.
30. Lawrence JS: Generalized osteoarthrosis in a population sample. Am J Epidemiol 1969; 90:381–389.
31. Mankin HJ: The reaction of articular cartilage to injury and osteoarthritis. N Engl J Med 1974; 291(24): 1285–1340.
32. Brown MB, Hislop HJ, Waters RL, et al: Walking efficiency before and after total hip replacement. Phys Ther 1980; 60:1259–1263.
33. Gussoni M, Margonato V, Ventura R, et al: Energy cost of walking with hip joint impairment. Phys Ther 1990; 70:295–301.
34. Waters RL: Energy expenditure. In Perry J (ed): Gait Analysis: Normal and Pathological Function, pp 444–481. Thorofare, Slack Publishers Inc, 1992.
35. Neumann DA: Biomechanical analysis of selected principles of hip joint protection. Arthritis Care Res 1989; 2:146–155.
36. Hart DL: Spinal mobility: Braces and corsets. In Gould JA (ed): Orthopedic and Sports Physical Therapy, 2nd edition, pp 272–280. St Louis, CV Mosby Co, 1990.
37. Krämer J: The treatment of cervical syndrome. In Krämer J (ed): Intervertebral Disc Diseases: Causes, Diagnosis, Treatment and Prophylaxis, pp 85–102. Chicago, Year Book Publishers, 1981.
38. Johnson RM, Hart DL, Simmons EF, et al: Cervical orthoses: a study comparing their effectiveness in restricting cervical motion in normal subjects. J Bone Joint Surg 1977; 59(Am):332–339.
39. Melvin JL: Osteoarthritis (degenerative joint disease). In Melvin JL (ed): Rheumatic Disease in the Adult and Child: Occupational Therapy and Rehabilitation, 3rd edition, pp 49–61. Philadelphia, FA Davis Co, 1989.
40. Peterson MGE, Kovar-Toledano PA, Otis JC, et al: Effects of a walking program on gait characteristics in patients with osteoarthritis. Arthritis Care Res 1993; 6:11–16.
41. Kovar PA, Allegrante JP, MacKenzie CR, et al: Supervised fitness walking in patients with osteoarthritis of the knee: a randomized, controlled trial. Ann Intern Med 1992; 116:529–534.
42. Perlman SG, Connell KJ, Clark A, et al: Dance-based aerobic exercise for rheumatoid arthritis. Arthritis Care Res 1990; 3:29–35.
43. Minor MA, Hewett JE, Webel RR, et al: Efficacy of physical conditioning exercise in patients with rheumatoid arthritis and osteoarthritis. Arthritis Rheum 1989; 32:1396–1405.
44. Tork SC, Douglas V: Arthritis water exercise program evaluation: a self-assessment survey. Arthritis Care Res 1989; 2:28–30.
45. Price LG, Hewett JE, Kay DR, et al: Five-minute walking test of aerobic fitness for people with arthritis. Arthritis Care Res 1988; 1:33–37.
46. Minor MA, Hewett JE, Webel RR, et al: Exercise tolerance and disease related measures in patients with rheumatoid arthritis and osteoarthritis. J Rheumatol 1988; 15:905–911.
47. Beals CA, Lampman RM, Banwell BF, et al: Measurement of exercise tolerance in patients with rheumatoid arthritis and osteoarthritis. J Rheumatol 1985; 12:458–461.
48. Michlovitz SL: Use of heat and cold in the management of rheumatic diseases. In Michlovitz SL (ed): Thermal Agents in Rehabilitation, vol I, pp 277–294. Philadelphia, FA Davis Co, 1986.
49. Lehman JF: Therapeutic hot and cold. In Lehman JF (ed): Therapeutic Heat and Cold, pp 404–602. Baltimore, Williams & Wilkins, 1982.
50. Mueller EE, Mead S, Schulz BF, et al: A placebo-controlled trial study of ultrasound treatment for periarthritis. Am J Phys Med 1954; 33:31–35.
51. Falconer J, Hayes KW, Chang RW: Therapeutic ultrasound in the treatment of musculoskeletal conditions. Arthritis Care Res 1990; 3:85–91.
52. Sheon RP, Moskowitz RW, Goldberg VM: An overview of diagnosis and management. In Sheon RP, Moskowitz RW, Goldberg VM (eds): Soft Tissue Rheumatic Pain: Recognition, Management, Prevention, 2nd edition, pp 1–15. Philadelphia, Lea & Febiger, 1987.
53. Wells PE, Frampton V, Bowsher D: Manipulative procedures. In Wells PE, Frampton V, Bowsher D (eds): Pain Management in Physical Therapy, pp 182–217. Norwalk, CT, Appleton & Lange, 1988.
54. Danneskiold-Samsoe B, Christiansen E, Andersen RB: Myofascial pain and the role of myoglobin. Scand J Rheumatol 1986; 15:174–178.
55. Borrell RM, Parker R, Henley EJ, et al: Comparison in-vivo temperatures produced by hydrotherapy, paraffin wax treatment, and Fluidotherapy[R]. Phys Ther 1980; 60:1273–1276.

56. Chamberlain MA, Care G, Harfield B: Physiotherapy in osteoarthrosis of the knee: a controlled trial of hospital versus home exercises. Int Rehabil Med 1982; 4:104–106.
57. Dellhag B, Wollersjö I, Bjelle A: Effect of active hand exercise and wax bath treatment in rheumatoid arthritis patients. Arthritis Care Res 1992; 5:87–92.
58. Falconer J, Hayes KW, Chang RW: Effect of ultrasound on mobility in osteoarthritis of the knee: a randomized clinical trial. Arthritis Care Res 1992; 5: 29–35.
59. Green J, McKenna F, Redfern EJ, et al: Home exercises are as effective as outpatient hydrotherapy for osteoarthritis of the hip. Br J Rheumatol 1993; 32: 812–815.
60. Hecht PJ, Bachmann S, Booth RE, et al: Effects of thermal therapy on rehabilitation after total knee arthroplasty. Clin Orthop 1983; 178:198–201.
61. Swezey RL: Therapeutic modalities for pain relief. In Swezey RL (ed): Arthritis: Rational Therapy and Rehabilitation, pp 133–148. Philadelphia, WB Saunders Co, 1978.
62. Barak T, Rosen ER, Sofer R: Basic concepts of orthopedic manual therapy. In Gould JA (ed): Orthopedic and Sports Physical Therapy, 2nd edition, pp 195–211. St Louis, CV Mosby Company, 1990.
63. Cyriax J: Textbook of Orthopedic Medicine. Treatment by Manipulation, Massage and Injection, vol 2. Baltimore, Williams & Wilkins, 1974.
64. Grimsby O: Fundamentals of Manual Therapy: A Course Workbook. Vagsbydgd, Norway, Sørlandets Fysikalske Institute, 1984.
65. Kaltenborn F: Mobilization of the Extremity Joints: Examination and Basic Treatment Techniques. Universitetsgaten, Olaf Norlis Bokhandel, 1980.
66. McKenzie RA: Mechanical Diagnosis and Therapy. Waikanae, New Zealand, Spinal Publications Ltd, 1981.
67. Mennell J: Joint Pain Diagnosis and Treatment Using Manipulative Techniques, 178 pp. New York, Little, Brown & Co, 1964.
68. Kessler RM: Arthrology. In Hertling D, Kessler RM (eds): Management of Common Musculoskeletal Disorders: Physical Therapy Principles and Methods, 2nd edition, pp 33–38. Philadelphia, Harper & Row, 1983.
69. Travell JG, Simons DG: Apropos of all muscles. In Travell JG, Simons DG (eds): Myofascial Pain and Dysfunction: The Trigger Point Manual, vol I, pp 86–88. Baltimore, Williams & Wilkins, 1983.
70. Burckhardt CS, Clark SR, Nelson DL: Assessing physical fitness of women with rheumatic disease. Arthritis Care Res 1988; 1:38–44.
71. Lankhorst GJ, Van de Stadt RJ, von der Korst JK, et al: Relationship of isometric knee extension torque and functional variables in osteoarthrosis of the knee. Scand J Rehab Med 1982; 14:7–10.
72. Liberson WT: Brief isometric exercises. In Basmajian J (ed): Therapeutic Exercise, 4th edition, pp 236–256. Baltimore, Williams & Wilkins, 1984.
73. Kirkendall DT: Mobility: conditioning programs. In Gould JA (ed): Orthopedic and Sports Physical Therapy, 2nd edition, pp 227–252. St Louis, CV Mosby Co, 1990.
74. American College of Sports Medicine: Guidelines for Graded Exercise Testing and Exercise Prescription, 2nd edition, 151 pp. Philadelphia, Lea & Febiger, 1980.
75. Sledge CB: Introduction to surgical management. In Kelley WN, Harris ED, Ruddy S, et al (eds): Textbook of Rheumatology, 4th edition, volume 2, pp 1745–1751. Philadelphia, WB Saunders Co, 1993.
76. Figgie MP: Introduction to the surgical treatment of rheumatic diseases. In Klippel JH, Dieppe JA (eds): Rheumatology, pp 8.20.1–8.20.6. St Louis, CV Mosby Co, 1994.
77. Kampa K: Hip injuries: a rehabilitation perspective. In Lewis CB, Knortz KA (eds): Orthopedic Assessment and Treatment of the Geriatric Patient, pp 243–262. St Louis, CV Mosby Co, 1993.
78. Knortz KA: Knee injuries: a rehabilitation perspective. In Lewis CB, Knortz KA (eds): Orthopedic Assessment and Treatment of the Geriatric Patient, pp 301–322. St Louis, CV Mosby Co, 1993.
79. Nelson KA, Rasmussen T: Total Knee Replacement, pp 1–20. Salt Lake City, UT, Intermountain Health Care, 1985.
80. Barrett DS, Cobb AG, Bentley G: Joint proprioception in normal, osteoarthritic and replaced knees. J Bone Joint Surg Br 1991; 73-B:53–56.
81. Stauffer RN, Chao EYS, Gryöry AN: Biomechanical gait analysis of the diseased knee joint. Clin Orthop 1977; 126:246–255.
82. Jevsevar DS, Riley PO, Hodge AW, et al: Knee kinematics and kinetics during locomotor activities of daily living in subjects with knee arthroplasty and in healthy control subjects. Phys Ther 1993; 73: 229–239.
83. Strickland EM, Fares M, Krebs DE, et al: In vivo acetabular contact pressures during rehabilitation. Part I. Acute phase. Phys Ther 1992; 72:691–699.
84. Givens-Heiss DL, Krebs DE, Riley PO, et al: In vivo acetabular contact pressures during rehabilitation. Part II. Postacute phase. Phys Ther 1992; 72:700–710.
85. Mann RW, Burgess RG: An instrumented endoprosthesis for measuring pressure on acetabular cartilage in vivo. In Proceedings of the Workshop on Implantable Telemetry in Orthopaedics, pp 1–13. Berlin, Federal Republic of Germany, 1990.
86. Krebs DE, Elbaum L, Riley PO, et al: Exercise and gait effects on in vivo hip contact pressures. Phys Ther 1991; 71:301–309.
87. American Rheumatism Association: Joint Examination. Dictionary of the Rheumatic Diseases, pp 75–80. New York, Contact Associates International Ltd, 1982.
88. Mathias S, Nayak USL, Isaacs B: Balance in elderly patients: The "get up and go" test. Arch Phys Med Rehabil 1986; 67:387–389.

CHAPTER 15

Physical Therapy Management of Ankylosing Spondylitis

Barbara Stokes, PT

This chapter will emphasize the role of physical therapy (PT) in the management of ankylosing spondylitis (AS), a condition that is unpredictable in its course, but which usually has a favorable outcome with appropriate management.

The etiology, diagnostic criteria, disease characteristics, and medical management are discussed in Chapter 4. Physical therapy can be an important adjunct to anti-inflammatory medication.

In a randomized, controlled trial of home PT, 26 experimental subjects had significant improvement of spinal mobility and function. Subjects were able to maintain this improvement in the following 4 months, with minimal PT intervention.[1,2] In both studies, patients reported a high degree of satisfaction with the programs provided. A subsequent trial comparing individual and group physiotherapy demonstrated that group PT was superior to individualized therapy in improving thoracolumbar mobility and fitness.[3] It is therefore not surprising that many physical therapists (PTs) find it gratifying to treat people with AS. The patient population is usually young, otherwise healthy, and generally acknowledge that they feel better following exercise. AS also can be a challenge due to the slowly progressive nature of the condition. This may require ongoing monitoring and treatment to prevent or reduce the postural changes and slow loss of function that can occur. The responsibility for monitoring posture and for exercising regularly must rest with the patient. The PT has a major role to play as an educator and motivator.

Assessment

History of the Disorder

In contrast to common low back disorders, AS distinguishes itself clinically by a history of insidious

PHYSICAL THERAPY IN ARTHRITIS, Joan M. Walker, PhD, PT, and Antoine Helewa, MSc(Clin Epid), PT, W.B. Saunders Company © 1996.

onset of low back pain and stiffness lasting more than 3 months, unrelieved by rest, and improved by exercise. It is not unusual in clinical practice for the PT to receive a referral that states simply, "low back pain." Given such an inadequate diagnosis, the PT needs to obtain a detailed history of the complaint from the patient and to be alert to the possibility of a missed diagnosis, especially in relatively young adults, age 20–40 years. Table 15-1 highlights the differences between AS and other low back disorders.

Physical Assessment

Physical examination of the spine is covered in detail in Chapter 8. Of particular note in the patient with AS is the characteristic posture seen due to loss of lumbar lordosis, increased thoracic kyphosis, and the compensatory extension of the cervical spine (see Fig. 4-14). These changes, however, are not always obvious, especially in the early stages of the disease, and a slight flattening of the lumbar spine may be overlooked. Therefore, it is important to carry out specific measurements of spinal mobility, to establish a baseline, and to monitor treatment effect or disease progression.

There are a number of valid techniques available for measuring spinal mobility.[4–6] Of these, perhaps the simplest overall measure of spinal mobility is the finger-to-floor technique, which is valid, reliable, and reproducible. In a validation study carried out prior to the trial on home PT reported earlier, a portable spinal mobility scale (Figs. 15-1 and 15-2) was found to be superior to a flexible measuring tape in terms of reliability and reproducibility. This was recommended for clinical practice.[7] The device was also useful for measuring occiput-to-wall distance. Range of motion of the cervical spine can be measured with a flexible tape and the distances recorded as follows:

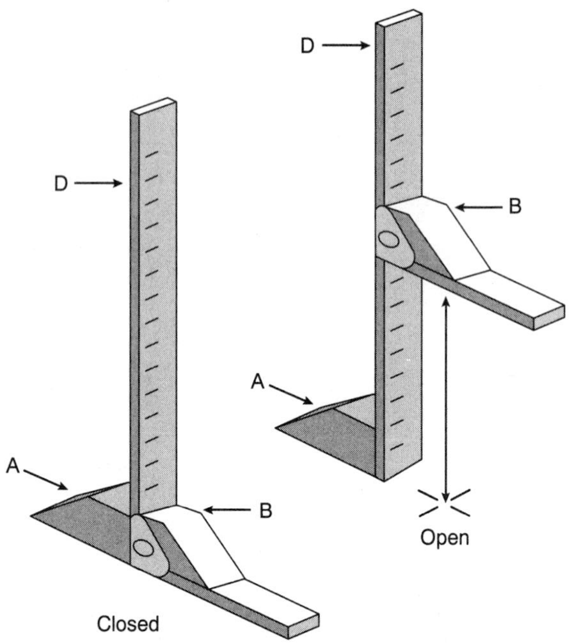

Figure 15-1. Portable spinal mobility scale in open and closed position. *A*, Fixed stop; *B*, spring loaded, sliding stop; *C*, extension to sliding stop; *D*, fixed scale.

- flexion-extension—base of chin to sternal notch in full flexion, then full extension
- rotation—cleft of chin to lateral edge of acromion process in full rotation to right and left
- lateral flexion—tragus to lateral edge of acromion process in full lateral flexion to right and left
- occiput-to-wall—base of occiput to wall with patient in standing, heels, buttocks, and shoulders against the wall (use of the portable spinal mobility scale for occiput-to-wall distance is recommended)

The Smythe test described in Chapter 8 is useful for establishing baseline measures and for follow-up, but may be difficult to do with patients

Table 15-1. Differential Diagnosis Between Ankylosing Spondylitis and Low Back Pain

Ankylosing Spondylitis	Other Low Back Disorders
Slow onset	Sudden onset
Worse with rest, improves with exercise	Better with rest, worse with activity
Sacroiliitis on radiograph	Negative radiograph
Positive family history (B27-positive)	Negative family history (B27-negative)

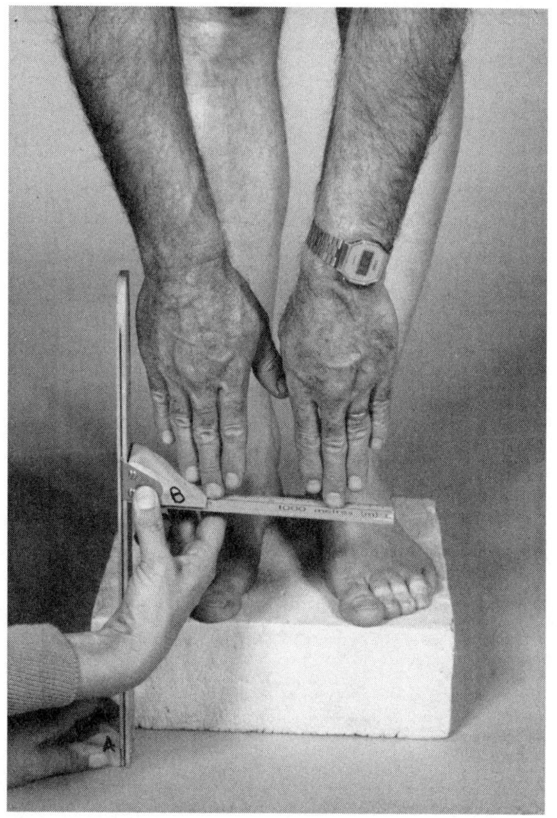
A

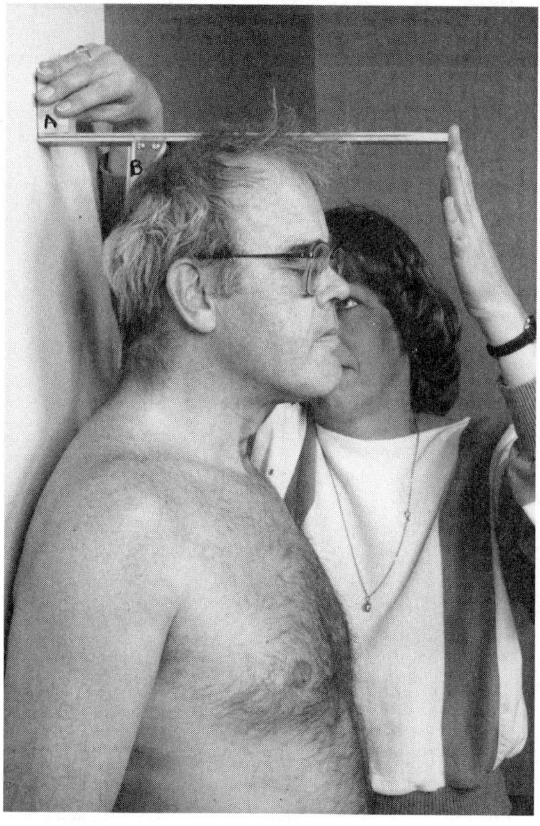
B

Figure 15-2. *A*, Portable spinal mobility scale used to measure standing, finger-to-floor distance. *B*, Portable spinal mobility scale used to measure occiput to wall distance. (From Stokes BA, Helewa A, Goldsmith CH, et al: Reliability of spinal mobility measurements in ankylosing spondylitis patients. Physiother Can 1988; 40:340. With permission.)

who have established limitation of hip flexion or who are unable to lie prone.

Chest expansion also should be monitored because of the potential for diminished movement in costovertebral joints and the effect on vital capacity. This is easily done by placing the measuring tape around the chest at the level of the xiphisternum, asking the patient to exhale completely and breathe in deeply, and recording the difference in the measurements.

Some patients may have peripheral joint involvement, and for this reason an active joint count (see Chapter 8) is appropriate, as well as measurement of range of motion in any affected peripheral joints. Particular attention should be paid to the shoulders and to the hip joints, as these joints may be involved, either due to active synovitis or to soft tissue contractures.

Some patients may have pain and tenderness at the entheses (sites where tendon attaches to bone). The attachment of the Tendo Achilles to the calcaneus, where the patellar tendon attaches to the tibial tubercle and the upper medial and lateral borders of the patella are common sites, as well as costochondral junctions. Isometric muscle strength can be measured using the modified sphygmomanometer where there is evidence of muscle weakness (see Chapter 8). An example of a single-page physical assessment form is illustrated in Figure 15-3.

The PT's major role is as an educator and motivator.

Patient's Name: ______________________ Date: ____________

Posture (as observed in standing) | Yes | No

hyperextension of cervical spine ___ ___
thoracic kyphosis ___ ___
diminished lumbar curve ___ ___

A.M. Stiffness

_____ Hr _____ Min

Chest expansion

_________ cm

RANGE OF MOTION (in cm)
CERVICAL SPINE

	R	L
Flex. (chin-sternal notch)	___	___
Ext.. (chin-sternal notch)	___	___
Rot.. (chin-acromion process)	___	___
Lat. flex. (tragus-acromion process	___	___
Occiput to wall	________	

THORACOLUMBAR SPINE

Flex. (fingertip-floor) ________

Smythe Test
- upper ________
- mid ________
- lower ________

Side flex. (stride sitting fingertip to floor) R ___ L ___

ACTIVE JOINTS

● = active joints
If range is limited, indicate loss in degrees adjacent to affected joint.

MUSCLE TESTING*

Muscle Group	R	L	Muscle Group	R	L
________	___	___	________	___	___
________	___	___	________	___	___
________	___	___	________	___	___
________	___	___	________	___	___

ADDITIONAL COMMENTS ______________________

* using modified sphygmomanometer

Figure 15-3. Physical assessment form for AS.

Functional Assessment

The functional losses associated with AS differ from those of patients with arthritis affecting mainly peripheral joints. It is therefore important to recognize these differences when assessing function. Some functional assessment questionnaires have been reported that are specific to AS.[8,9] They are fast and simple to administer, and can be useful for clinicians in monitoring treatment outcomes. The common functional activities with which the patient with AS may have problems are listed below.

- body transfers
- dressing
- ambulation
- work activities
- bending/lifting/carrying
- endurance
- sleeping
- driving

Functional assessment questionnaires specific to AS are available and can be useful in monitoring treatment outcome.

Difficulty with body transfers usually relates to problems with rolling in the lying position, or when rising from the floor. Other activities involving rotational movements of the spine may be difficult to perform. Inability to reach the feet may result in dressing difficulties. Ambulation may be affected by loss of rotational movements, armswing, or hip involvement. Work activities involving static positions or bending/lifting/carrying can pose problems due to pain or stiffness. Loss of respiratory function, pain, and limitation of movement all result in diminished endurance.

Psychosocial Issues

Because this disorder commonly affects young people, it is often important to explore, with the patient, their current work situation and any difficulties that they are experiencing.

Patients in the younger age groups may have needs relating to career and family planning, as well as fears about future functional losses. Early identification will allow these to be addressed either through provision of disease education or through appropriate counseling.

Aims of Management

The aims of treatment involve at least some of the following:

- provide disease education
- decrease pain
- increase mobility
- maintain/increase respiratory function
- improve posture
- increase strength and endurance
- adapt/improve activities of daily living
- improve function and quality of life

Physical Therapist's Approach

Education

An understanding of the disease process, the importance of self-monitoring and regular exercise, and the role of drug therapy should form the basis of any proposed management program. This should be tailored to the specific needs of each patient.

Since the disease and its effects on posture and spinal mobility tend to be insidious, emphasis should be placed on teaching the patient to self-monitor any losses of range of motion or postural changes. Most patients should be taught the principles of proper posture in standing, sitting, and lying. It is useful to demonstrate the normal curves of the spine using a model or good illustrations.

Self-help groups in Canada and the United States provide good educational materials that explain the disease process and medical treatment, and outline strategies to manage the condition. Audio and video tapes, as well as printed materials are available from these organizations at low cost. These resources are useful adjuncts to the individualized education provided by the PT (see Appendix I).

Pain Management

In the active or uncontrolled phase of AS, patients may experience acute pain that affects sleep, function, mobility, and emotions. The cause of the pain may be due to inflammation in the sacroiliac joints, the apophyseal joints, or in the surrounding soft tissues. Acute muscle spasm may be present.

Pain relief may be obtained through the use of anti-inflammatory drugs to control the inflammation. Analgesic medications, as well as the application of simple modalities such as hot or cold packs, may provide sufficient short-term relief to improve sleep and function. When applied preceding therapeutic exercise, they can relieve pain and spasm, therefore improving exercise outcomes. Use of ultrasound or other electrotherapeutic modalities is not warranted due to cost and lack of studies reporting their use in AS. Relief of acute muscle spasm can be achieved through the use of modified proprioceptive neuromuscular facilitation (PNF) techniques as outlined in Table 15-2.

Mobility

Reduced spinal mobility may be due to a number of factors. Acute pain and muscle spasm may be the primary cause, as may soft tissue contracture and ankylosis of certain areas of the spine. Large peripheral joints may be affected by enthesopathy, soft tissue contracture, or ankylosis. The exercise techniques selected should be based on the assessed causes of the limitation. While there is no scientific evidence that exercise prevents ankylosis, there are data to show that exercise improves mobility, posture, and function.[1–3,10–14] Emphasis should be placed on maintenance or improvement of mobility, as it is related both to the relief of pain and stiffness, as well as to improvements in function. Because the disease is progressive in nature, it is critical for patients to be able to monitor their mobility and to carry out regularly a self-administered program of stretching and free active exercise.

Patients should be taught to have at least 5 minutes of "warm-up" prior to exercising, by applying a hot pack, or preferably taking a warm shower followed by light arm movement or brisk walking to prepare the muscles for exercise. It also is advisable for patients to perform the exercises at the time of day when they are least stiff or tired.

Target areas for stretching are the short neck muscles, pectoral girdle muscles, hamstrings and hip flexors, as well as the spinal rotators. The modified PNF techniques outlined in Table 15-2 will assist in selecting appropriate manually applied techniques. Manually applied exercises which may be employed in the hands-on component of the treatment program are given in Figure 15-4.

Patients with peripheral joint involvement may not be able to tolerate forces exerted across inflamed joints (e.g., resistance at the ankle with the knee in extension). There also may be permanent restrictions to areas of the spine. In these cases, the traditional holds involved in these techniques may need to be adapted to the patient's condition, by applying the resistance closer to the fulcrum. However, the patterns of movement and basic procedure will remain unchanged.

At the beginning of the course of treatment, these techniques are emphasized and augmented by a self-administered program of free active exercise designed to increase mobility, strength, and endurance. Gradually, the self-administered program should be increased over several weeks and the hands-on PT component correspondingly decreased.

Table 15-2. Indications for Proprioceptive Neuromuscular Facilitation Techniques

Indication	Technique
Acute pain/spasm affecting mobility	Hold-relax or rhythmic stabilizations
Chronic or no pain but limited mobility	Contract-relax or slow reversals followed by free active exercise
Decreased rib cage expansion	Slow reversals resisting rib cage expansion with or without the stretch reflex
Poor postural habits	Rhythmic stabilizations
Limitations of strength	Resisted maximal slow reversals; repeated contractions using stretch, traction, and approximation
Decreased endurance	Low-resistance slow reversals

Respiratory Function

Pain due to inflammation of the costochondral joints or costovertebral joints may inhibit deep breathing. Patients may find applications of heat or the use of pain medication helpful. They should be encouraged to practice deep breathing, with emphasis on full rib cage expansion. Use of a towel or the hands helps to provide resistance to expan-

Region	Starting	Patterns	Technique
1. Neck	Sitting, head in desired range. Back supported.	Flexion and rotation to right and extension and rotation to left. Same for contralateral side. 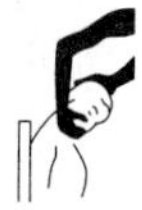 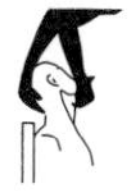	Rhythmic stabilization & hold relax
2. Neck and upper trunk	Sitting, head and upper trunk in desired range.	Flexion and rotation to right of neck & upper trunk. Same for contralateral side.	Rhythmic stabilization Slow reversal
3. Trunk	Stride standing.	Upper trunk rotation to right, lower trunk rotation to left. Same for contralateral side. Also side to side. 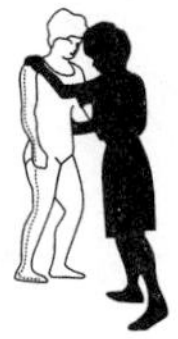	Rhythmic stabilization
4. Lower trunk	Crook lying to bridging.	Lower trunk rotation left to right and right to left. Same for contralateral sides. Also side to side. 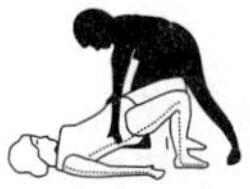	Rhythmic stabilization
	Crook lying.	Anterior to posterior pelvic tilting.	Slow reversals

Figure 15-4. Recommended neck and trunk patterns and techniques using proprioceptive neuromuscular facilitation. (Adapted from Voss DE, Ionta MK, Myers BJ: Proprioceptive Neuromuscular Facilitation, 3rd edition, pp 33, 163, 188. Philadelphia, JB Lippincott, 1985. With permission.)

sion and can assist in pulling the lower ribs down and towards the midline on expiration (Fig. 15-5). Patients should be educated about the increased risks of respiratory infections, and encouraged to cease smoking and to maintain their respiratory function through regular exercise.

Patients should be encouraged to practice deep breathing, with emphasis on full rib cage expansion.

Strength and Endurance

Improvement of strength and endurance may be addressed through both the therapist-applied exercise techniques and the self-administered exercise program, by increasing resistance as tolerated, increasing repetitions or speed. Major muscle groups to which strengthening exercise should be directed include back extensors, shoulder retractors, hip extensors, and other postural muscles.

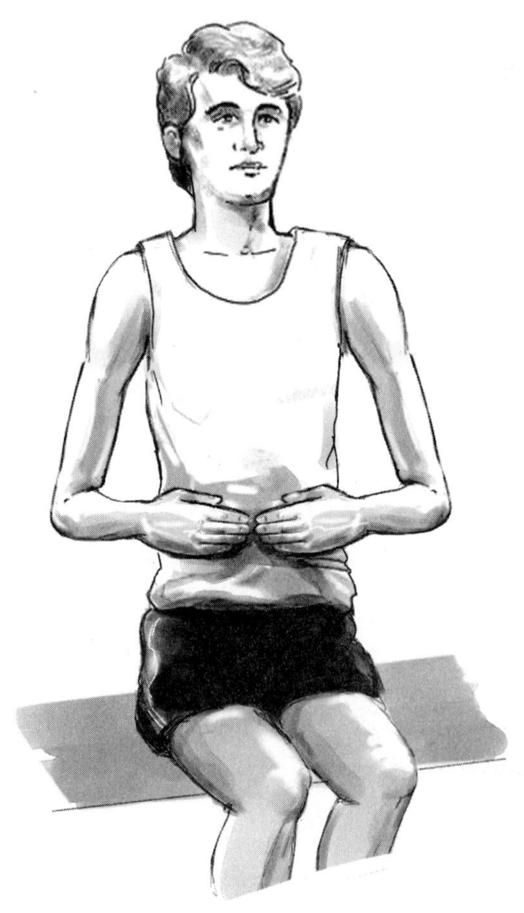

Figure 15-5. Rib cage expansion, manual resistance.

Posture

As mentioned earlier in this chapter, education plays an important role in the management of AS. Patients who are well educated about the importance of maintaining correct posture and about the functions of the spine will be able to monitor the changes that may take place as a result of the disease process or the treatment program.

Patients can be instructed in basic assessment techniques such as checking postural alignment by attempting to touch occipital protuberance to the wall while standing with the heels, buttocks, and shoulders against the wall, and maintaining their chin parallel to the floor. A simple means of monitoring postural change is for patients to measure their height on a regular basis. They should be taught to avoid positions that encourage a stooped posture, such as slouching in chairs, and cautioned against maintaining a fixed position that encourages spinal flexion for prolonged periods. While working at a desk, patients should stop and check their posture from time to time or perform some simple stretching exercises. Working at a drafting table may facilitate movement and help to maintain an upright posture for some patients.

Attention should be given to sleeping positions and advice given about the use of pillows or neck supports during sleep. In some instructional materials patients are advised to sleep on a firm mattress with one small flat pillow. For a patient with established neck deformities, this is extremely difficult. The important thing is to have the patient achieve as much extension as possible by providing adequate support to the painful or restricted areas. This may require the addition of pillows or rolled towels to gain adequate support. If the patient can gain some relaxation, the amount of support may be decreased.

AS is progressive. It is critical that patients learn to monitor their mobility and regularly self-administer their exercise program.

Prone lying for a period of 15 minutes or more, performed on a daily basis, is frequently required. Again, if the patient can tolerate this position, this may be helpful in maintaining hip extension, but if the patient cannot lie flat in the prone position, adaptations may be necessary. These may be in the form of a pillow placed under the abdomen, or to accommodate for inability to turn the head to the side, a rolled towel under the forehead allows the patient to be more comfortable (Fig. 15-6). Lying supine at the end of a bed with the buttocks on the edge and the hips extended can be substituted when the patient is unable to lie prone.

Maintaining normal, reciprocal arm swing while walking and encouragement of rotational movements of the lower spine and pelvis should be taught, as many patients tend to lose the reciprocal patterns of normal gait.

Rotation of the spine and pelvis should be encouraged.

Assistive Devices

Assistive devices are infrequently required by this group of patients, since they usually maintain good function of the distal extremities. Some patients, however, having difficulty with activities involving reaching the floor or the feet may find reaching implements, such as grabbers, dressing sticks, or long-handled shoehorns helpful.

Another area of concern is inability to turn the head to back up a car or safely make a lane change. Many automotive supply stores carry a range of wider rear view mirrors, which not only make driving simpler for the patient but also safer. Chapter 10 contains other suggestions that may apply to this patient population.

Work/Leisure Activities

Some patients may benefit from a workplace assessment, particularly if they report difficulty with seating, desk height, or angle of work surfaces. Many patients find it difficult to maintain a static posture and some simply cannot meet the physical demands of their job. An on-site visit may lead to identification of opportunities for changes in the physical environment or adaptations of tasks to accommodate the patient's disability/dysfunction. In some instances, vocational counseling may be indicated and job retraining may be facilitated with the PT's input and recommendations.

PT intervention can result in patients reporting a decrease in pain and stiffness, and a corresponding increase in their functional ability and in their sense of general well-being. It is appropriate at this stage to explore with the patient those perhaps previously enjoyed recreational activities that they may have abandoned due to pain, restriction, or fear of injury.

Some of the educational materials designed for patients contain excellent suggestions and guidelines, tailored to patients with varying degrees of involvement and severity (see Appendix I). Advice should be given to avoid rough contact sports. Encouragement should be given to those activities that involve free active movement, contain rotational movements, and increase cardiovascular fitness, such as archery, walking, swimming (especially the backstroke or breaststroke), and cross-country skiing. These activities do not replace the therapeutic exercise program but provide a recreational and social benefit to overall well-being.

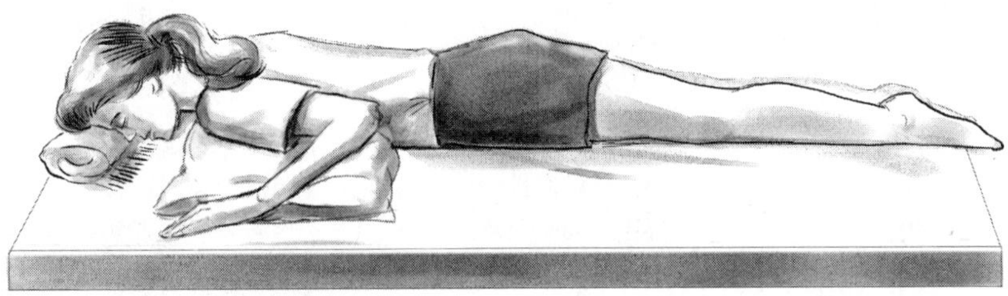

Figure 15-6. Positioning in prone lying. Note pillow under the chest and abdomen and the rolled towel under the forehead.

By following the formal exercise program and improving posture and fitness levels, many patients are able to remain active. Once convinced that they feel better following exercise, they are encouraged to participate in recreational activities and to maintain their fitness level.

Discharge Planning

For patients with chronic, progressive diseases that may require many life style changes and that place demands upon the individual, it is vital that the overall plan of management is acceptable to the patient. The treatment program must be realistic and relevant to the individual. The exercise scheme should be short and simple, and while it may cause discomfort, this discomfort should not result in an increase in pain. If these criteria are not met, patients will become discouraged and disinterested, and will discontinue this important aspect of the management of their condition.

It is vital that the overall plan of management is acceptable, and the treatment program is realistic and relevant to the individual.

The overall goal in the provision of PT to patients with AS is to enable the individual to manage their disease through a variable, usually progressive course, maintaining their independence and function. This is facilitated by a thorough understanding of the disease and its effects and of the options for treatment that exist. Most patients are able to adhere to the management program for short periods, but some may require a "refresher course" or they may experience exacerbations and new symptoms requiring modification of the management program.

Prior to discharge, patients should be made aware of community resources for pool programs and fitness classes. They also should be told what symptoms require medical intervention and when to seek other kinds of assistance, such as information on transportation or job retraining. Encouragement should be given to continue self-monitoring and to request regular physical therapy checks in order to avoid future problems. They may wish to establish a series of regular assessments with the PT, on an ongoing basis (e.g., every 3 months).

In summary, the overall prognosis for these patients is favorable and key to the successful management is the intelligent application of therapeutic exercise.

Case History #1

The first case history illustrates the success of physical therapy intervention in AS.

Mr. D.C. is a 46-year-old married man, with a family of two, who works as a human resources officer. His symptoms began at age 15 with low back pain onset and stiffness following a session of gymnastics. He did not see a physician at that time, and over the next 10 years he noticed a decrease in his ability to do gymnastics and experienced episodic stiffness of his lower back. He attended fitness classes and felt better following exercise, but after 6 months, he noticed pain in his mid back and a decreased ability to do the fitness exercises. He occasionally took aspirin or pain relievers for his symptoms. At age 30, he went to a sports medicine clinic where his symptoms were diagnosed as mechanical strain. He was referred to PT for strengthening of his abdominal muscles and given some postural training.

Over the next 3 years the back pain progressed and he eventually had radiographs taken that showed evidence of sacroiliitis. A referral to a rheumatologist was made and a diagnosis of AS was established. He was treated with Indocid and naproxen, which provided good relief of pain, but he stated that he was always aware of stiffness in his mid and low back that prevented him from gardening and recreational sailing.

Mr. D.C. was referred to The Arthritis Society, Consultation and Therapy Service for home PT when he complained to his rheumatologist about his increasing stiffness and reduced function. When the PT visited, he stated that he had no other history of illness, but the family history indicated that both his mother and an aunt had low back pain.

Functional Assessment Enquiry revealed that his sleep was disturbed by back discomfort, he tired easily, and noticed shortness of breath on exertion. He had difficulty with dressing activities, such as tying shoelaces and bending to put on shorts or trousers. He had difficulty getting in and out of the car and difficulty turning his head while driving. He reported increased pain and stiffness after sitting at his desk to read or write for anything more than a brief period. His ability to sail his boat had decreased due to lack of mobility and agility. He was feeling depressed about his loss of energy and inability to carry out recreational activities with his family. His wife stated that he was irritable and tired at the end of each day, and that they were discouraged and worried about the future.

Physical assessment revealed:

- slight thoracic kyphosis and flattening of the lumbar curve
- decreased cervical rotation to R and L
- decreased lateral cervical flexion to R and L
- fingertip to floor distance was 23.5 cm
- decreased side flexion in stride sitting of 13 cm R, 14.5 cm L
- pain and spasm in the thoracolumbar region

Mr. D.C.'s **management goals** were to reduce the level of pain he was experiencing, and to improve his ability to perform dressing activities, body transfers, and tolerance for working at his desk. He also wanted information about the disease and managing fatigue. The PT spent time with Mr. D.C. and his wife, explaining the nature of AS, its treatment, and the value of exercise in this condition.

The agreed-upon **management program** consisted of the following:

- provision of educational materials, booklets, and an audio tape
- heat to the affected areas, neck, and back in the form of either hot packs for severe back pain or warm shower preceding his exercise routine
- a daily exercise program was set up to include modified PNF techniques followed by free active exercise designed to improve mobility of the spine
- the PT visited twice weekly for the first 3 weeks to monitor and progress the exercise routine
- his wife was instructed in the application of resistance to various patterns of movement
- Mr. D.C. was instructed in the use of rhythmic stabilizations and how to self-administer these techniques in his work setting to relieve the muscle spasm in his mid to low back.
- posture correction and advice provided with respect to positioning of his work surface and the value of taking regular breaks in order to stretch and relieve stiffness.

The frequency of the PT's visits was decreased from twice weekly to once every 2 weeks over 4 months. **After 4 months**, the client and his wife reported high satisfaction with the program. His functional ability had improved. He dressed with no difficulty, found body transfers much easier, and was able to tolerate working at his desk for longer periods by performing the rhythmic stabilizations and by taking periodic exercise breaks. He had resumed his gardening and sailing activities.

The **physical assessment** revealed:

- less thoracic kyphosis
- improved cervical rotation
- improved lateral cervical flexion
- finger to floor distance: 11 cm
- improved side flexion in stride sitting, he was able to touch the floor
- reported only occasional mild pain and stiffness in thoracolumbar region

The client was **discharged** from active treatment, having provided assurance that he would be seen again should the need arise. Six weeks following discharge, he telephoned to inquire about joining the local AS self-help group to enhance his compliance with exercise and to provide encouragement to others.

Case History #2:

Ms. A.K. is a divorced, 34-year-old mother of an 11-year-old boy. She works as a social worker for a children's agency. She has a 15-year history of low back pain and stiffness and an 11-year history of intermittent neck pain and stiffness associated with a gradual loss of mobility of her lower spine and cervical spine.

Initially, her low back pain was diagnosed as mechanical low back strain and treated with rest and analgesics. Over the next 4 years, she noticed difficulty turning her head when driving, and had difficulty with bending to put on shoes or pick up objects from the floor. She remained relatively active, working part time and cycling and swimming regularly. Following the birth of her son, she experienced increasing low back pain and stiffness, pain in her neck, and occasional pain in her shoulders. She related this to increased physical demands of caring for an infant and took analgesics and hot baths for relief. In 1986, she was divorced and went back to work on a fulltime basis. She saw her family physician regularly and was advised that her back pain was probably chronic and that she should get more rest and take aspirin as necessary.

One year later, her low back pain flared, her neck became very painful and stiff, and she had difficulty sleeping as a result of the pain. Her family physician referred her to a rheumatologist. Radiographs showed bilateral sacroiliitis and she was found to have a positive HLA-B27 antigen. The diagnosis of AS was confirmed, naproxen 500 mg/day was prescribed, and the client was referred to The Arthritis Society, Consultation and Therapy Service for home PT.

Physical assessment revealed:

- morning stiffness of 45 minutes
- posture in standing: increased cervical lordosis, thoracic kyphosis, flattened lumbar curve
- occiput to wall distance: 6 cm
- cervical rotation reduced to R and L
- fingertip to floor distance: 12 cm
- side flexion in stride sitting: 8 cm R, 7 cm L

Functional Assessment Ms. A.K. had difficulty with household activities, such as vacuuming, reaching into low cupboards, cleaning the bathroom, and hanging laundry. Her work involved driving and she was experiencing difficulty with backing the car and with lane changes. Getting in and out of the car was difficult and she found sitting for long periods increased her pain.

Management Program

- disease education with emphasis on the importance of exercise and posture training
- advice regarding sleeping position, positioning of the car seat, use of a back support in the car and at work, and purchase of a wide rear view mirror
- an exercise program designed to relieve muscle spasm and improve mobility of her lower spine and her neck using modified PNF techniques
- stretching and mobilizing exercises for the shoulder girdle and hip flexors
- a self-administered exercise routine for upper and lower spine, hips, and shoulders to be performed daily

Because of the client's reluctance to take time off from work, it was not possible for her to receive the hands-on component of the treatment program, as she was able to see the PT only once every 2 weeks. Over the next year, she performed the exercises "when she had time and when she wasn't too tired." **At the end of that year**, she experienced another flare, saw the rheumatologist, and agreed to taking 1 month off work. Her medication was changed to Indocid 150 mg/day with good effect. She was referred again to The Arthritis Society.

Physical assessment revealed:

- morning stiffness: 60 minutes
- increased postural changes
- occiput to wall distance: 8 cm
- less cervical rotation to R and L
- fingertip to floor distance: 16 cm
- side flexion in stride sitting: 8 cm R, 7.5 cm L

She was seen by the PT, who visited twice weekly over the next month. It was agreed that Ms. A.K. would perform her exercise routine daily following a warm shower and that she would give thought to how exercise could be incorporated into her schedule when she returned to work.

Ms. A.K. was alarmed by the results of the physical assessment and concerned about the deterioration of the spinal mobility measures, but also very worried about the loss of function that was occurring. She reported increasing difficulty with activities that required stooping or bending, difficulty with dressing activities, and her inability to participate in recreational activities. One incident that frightened her significantly occurred when she was returning home one evening and dropped the keys to her house. She was unable to pick them up, and after many tries, resorted to waking a neighbor. The threatened loss of independence had an influence on her willingness to incorporate an exercise routine into her life.

After the month off work, and increased PT visits, Ms. A.K. had improved in all measures of spinal mobility and had regained some of her dressing skills. The improvement was sufficient that she was willing to rise earlier in the morning to do her exercises before work and join the local pool exercise program. She negotiated with her employer for some space where she could lie down for breaks twice a day. On these breaks, she could do a few exercises and could spend some time lying prone. The PT visited Ms. A.K. monthly to monitor progress and increase the scope of the exercise program.

After 6 months the physical assessment revealed the following improvement:

- morning stiffness: 20 minutes
- improved posture in standing
- occiput to wall distance: 4 cm
- cervical rotation was improved by 3 cm bilaterally
- fingertip to floor distance: 9 cm
- side flexion in stride sitting: 6 cm R, 7 cm L

Functionally, Ms. A.K. still found heavy household activity such as vacuuming very difficult, but she was able to do dressing activities with greater ease. She could reach into cupboards and had little difficulty with stockings or shoes. She had purchased a folding reacher that she kept in her handbag. She then could retrieve her house keys and had no worry about returning home from the pool program and being unable to enter her home!

Comment Often, young and busy people will ignore the insidious onset of the limitations of spinal mobility with unfortunate consequences. This client learned after a setback the value of exercise. Today, 3 years after the last PT visit, she still attends the pool program and continues to work and care for her son. *The moral of this case history is "do your exercises"!*

References

1. Kraag G, Stokes B, Groh J, et al: The effects of comprehensive home physiotherapy and supervision on patients with ankylosing spondylitis—a randomized controlled trial. J Rheumatol 1990; 17:228–233.
2. Kraag G, Stokes B, Groh J, et al: The effects of comprehensive home physiotherapy and supervision on patients with ankylosing spondylitis—an 8-month followup. J Rheumatol 1994; 21:261–263.
3. Hidding A, van der Linden S, Boers M, et al: Is group physical therapy superior to individualized therapy in ankylosing spondylitis? Arthritis Care Res 1993; 6:117–125.
4. Frost M, Stuckey S, Smalley LA, et al: Reliability of measuring trunk motions in centimeters. Phys Ther 1982; 62:1431–1437.
5. Miller M, Lee P, Smythe HA, et al: Measurement of spinal mobility in the sagittal plane: new skin contraction technique compared with established methods. J Rheumatol 1984; 11:507–511.
6. Pile KD, Laurent MR, Salmond CE, et al: Clinical assessment of ankylosing spondylitis: a study of observer variation in spinal measurements. Br J Rheumatol 1991; 30:29–34.
7. Stokes BA, Helewa A, Goldsmith CH, et al: Reliability of spinal mobility measurements in ankylosing spondylitis patients. Physiother Can 1988; 40:338–344.
8. Dougados M, Gueguen A, Nakache JP, et al: Evaluation of a functional index and an articular index in ankylosing spondylitis. J Rheumatol 1988; 15:302–307.
9. Nemeth R, Smith F, Elswood J, et al: Ankylosing spondylitis (AS)—an approach to measurement of severity and outcome: Ankylosing Spondylitis Assessment Questionnaire (ASAQ)—a controlled study. Br J Rheumatol 1987; 26:69–70.
10. O'Driscoll SL, Jayson MIV, Baddeley H: Neck movements in ankylosing spondylitis and their responses to physiotherapy. Ann Rheum Dis 1978; 37:64–66.
11. Tomlinson MJ, Barefoot J, Dixon A St J: Intensive inpatient physiotherapy courses improve movement and posture in ankylosing spondylitis. Physiotherapy 1986; 72:238–240.
12. Viitanen JV, Suni J, Kautiainen M, et al: Effect of physiotherapy on spinal mobility in ankylosing spondylitis. Scand J Rheumatol 1992; 21:38–41.
13. Hidding A, Van der Linden S, De Witte L: Individual physical therapy in ankylosing spondylitis related to duration of disease. Clin Rheumatol 1993; 12(3): 334–340.
14. Calin A: Can we define the outcome of ankylosing spondylitis and the effect of physiotherapy management. J Rheumatol 1994; 21:184–185.

CHAPTER 16

Community-Based Physical Therapy Management of Arthritis

Barbara Stokes, PT

Background and Philosophy

Current trends in the provision of health services are towards more community-based programs with an emphasis on a "wellness" model, with the client assuming responsibility for disease self-management.

A diagnosis of arthritis carries with it an uncertain prognosis. The onset may vary from slow and insidious to sudden and severe. The course of the disease may be characterized by periods of exacerbation and remission, or may be slowly progressive over many years. The implications on the individual's ability to function may be significant and will vary with age, occupation, and life style. Most often, it is within the community that the client will experience the impact of the disease on their life style. It is, therefore, important that physical therapists (PTs) offer more community-based management in the overall management of clients with arthritis.

What would be an ideal community delivery system for people with arthritis? The service that approximates the ideal may be the community-based program in Ontario, Canada.

For over 40 years, The Arthritis Society in Ontario, Canada, has provided physical therapy (PT),

PHYSICAL THERAPY IN ARTHRITIS, Joan M. Walker, PhD, PT, and Antoine Helewa, MSc(Clin Epid), PT, W.B. Saunders Company © 1996.

occupational therapy (OT), and social work (SW) services to clients with complex forms of arthritis in the home, school, and workplace. The philosophy of this program has been based on the premise that the individual with a long-term chronic illness, pain, and limitation can become immobilized physically and psychologically within his/her own community.

Hospitalization in a rheumatic diseases unit has, in many cases, been shown to control arthritis.[1-3] However, these units, which traditionally provided a multidisciplinary and specialized approach to disease education and management, are faced with cost constraints, reduction in numbers of beds, and shortened hospital stays. These constraints on hospital services increased the demand for community-based services and focused attention on the importance and relevance of this form of management.

Early intervention, disease education, and self-management are critical to arthritis control. These cannot always be adequately provided in traditional health care facilities. Cost of hospitalization, volume of clients in outpatient departments, waiting periods in clinics or doctors' offices, and the unsuitability of these settings in the provision of disease education and self-management strategies may lead to delays that will impact negatively on outcomes.[2,4]

The PT in the community is uniquely positioned to reinforce, adapt, or expand a disease management program that may have been initiated in a physician's office, a clinic, or an inpatient setting, or by the client. In many cases, the community-based PT (CPT) is the primary contact professional who monitors disease activity, response to drug therapy, and changes resulting from the natural history of the disease or its treatment.

The use of a multidisciplinary approach to disease management in any setting is important. This is especially relevant within the community to minimize the numbers of health care providers to the client's home, lend consistency to the management plan, and reduce costs. Team members may be the family physician, the rheumatologist, PT, OT, social worker, nurse, and pharmacist; all can contribute importantly either as primary contacts or consultants at any point in the continuum of care. Other support services within the community may include homemaking, meals on wheels, transport services, pool programs, and various self-help groups. The community-based PT must be familiar with the support services available to a particular client and must encourage their appropriate use (Fig. 16-1).

Home Assessment

The total assessment of the client with arthritis, with its major components, the history, physical assessment, and functional assessment, has been well detailed in Chapter 8 and the principles apply whatever the setting. However, the importance of a detailed health history cannot be overestimated in the community setting. The client may be referred with simply a diagnosis of "arthritis," and on that basis, with no other relevant information, the PT enters the client's home. The conventional history contained in a hospital chart is often inaccessible. It therefore is the responsibility of the PT to obtain, from the client, sufficient information about the disease, its course, and its effects to begin to formulate a problem list and establish with the client's management goals. Supplementary information (laboratory or radiographic findings) may be available later, but the health history sets the stage for whatever interventions may be initiated.

Advantages of Home Assessments

- **observe the client in own environment**
- **interact with the family**
- **determine the impact of the disease**
- **observe performance of activities of daily living (ADL)**
- **comfort and convenience for client**

Among the advantages of providing community-based care are those of being able to observe the client in their own environment, to interact with other family members, and to determine the impact of the disease, not only on the client but also upon those with whom they live and work. Frequently, it is easier for the client to recall significant clinical events and to divulge sensitive or personal information when they are within the privacy of their own home. Family members may assist in recalling relevant events or changes in the client's functional status. The home is the ideal place to inquire about medication use, including over-the-counter medication, and monitor compliance and side effects. The community-based PT must become familiar with the drugs used in the management of arthritis, their dosages, expected response time, and be alert to the possible side ef-

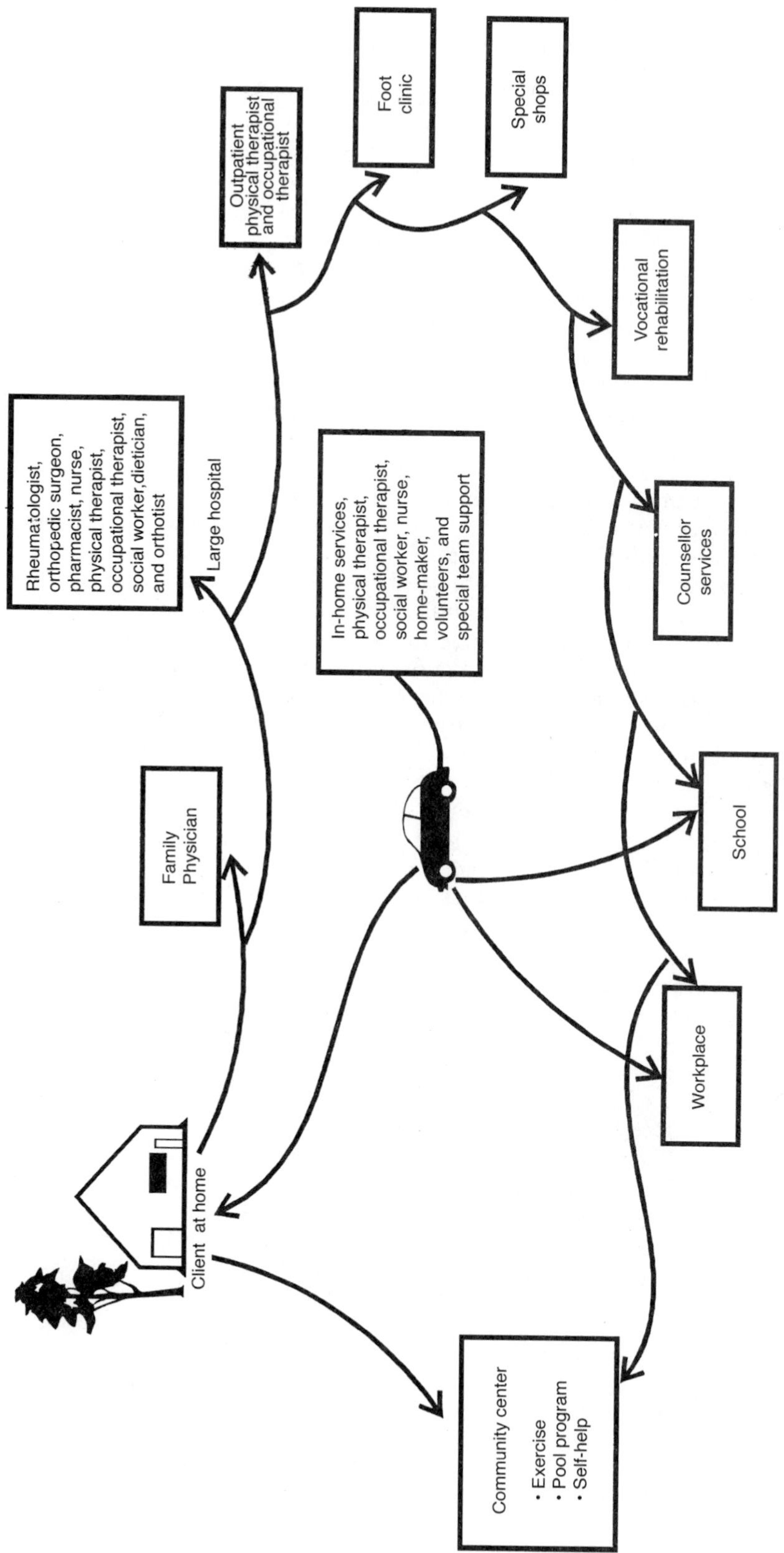

Figure 16-1. Community-based services. Availability of all services shown will vary by community.

fects or interactions. Information on drug therapy is contained in Chapter 9.

PTs trained in the standardized assessment techniques, described in Chapter 8, can be as effective as rheumatology fellows in quantifying the effects of joint inflammation and damage in clients with inflammatory arthritis.[5] The active joint count, combined with the duration of morning stiffness, grip strength, and extra-articular features, provides the PT with invaluable information in planning treatment interventions, monitoring progress, and modifying treatment plans. This information can be conveyed to other treatment team members in a standardized, easily communicated manner (Fig. 16-2).

Training in these techniques has been provided by the Ontario Division of The Arthritis Society, Canada, annually since 1976, to over 250 PTs and OTs. An unpublished survey, in 1992, of 212 PTs and OTs who completed the program showed that of the 61% who responded, all reported that they used these skills regularly. Most found the course to be very valuable. Therapists reported it produced significant changes in their assessment and management of arthritis. This training also enhanced their ability to communicate and interact with other health professionals.

Assessment Equipment

The equipment used in assessing clients with arthritis is minimal. It usually consists of small easily portable items, such as a goniometer, a tape measure, and the modified sphygmomanometer to measure grip strength and strength in affected muscle groups.

Basic Equipment for Home Assessment

- goniometer
- tape measure
- modified sphygmomanometer

The physical assessment can be easily conducted within the home setting. It is important to be cognizant of the client's tolerance and schedule. Sometimes it is necessary to conduct the total assessment over two or three visits. If this is the case, the client should be provided with some kind of intervention at the first visit, whether it be demonstration of the use of ice packs for an inflamed joint, or the provision of educational materials. In this way, the client may be reassured that their concerns are being addressed.

The active joint count and damaged joint count can usually be accomplished quickly with the client on the bed or couch. Privacy may be a problem in a household of several small children, dogs, cats, well-meaning neighbors, and ringing telephones! When making appointments, it is helpful to explain clearly the length of the visit, what the client should wear, what activities will take place, and where in the home the assessment will take place.

Education about the disease and its treatment begins while the PT is carrying out the assessment by explaining the purpose of the techniques. Physical findings should be explained, in terms that the client can understand.

Another distinct advantage to assessing clients at the home or work environment is the ability to observe how they perform activities of daily living, a difficult if not impossible task in the clinical setting. In the home, the PT can gather a tremendous amount of information regarding physical barriers to the performance of many activities, observing everything from the weight and storage of pots and pans to the height of seating, numbers of stairs, and the terrain within the home and outside the home. The actual functional assessment may be as simple as administering a standardized questionnaire with the client identifying those activities that pose difficulties. Certain impairments such as muscle weakness, loss of range of motion (ROM), or joint instability may be the underlying reason for the difficulty; each of these will require different interventions. Examples are provided in Table 16-1. Determination also can be made as to the safety or efficiency of particular activities, such as stair climbing, use of a bathtub, and furniture placement.

The psychosocial effects of the disease upon clients are more easily observed in the home setting. The PT has the opportunity to watch family interactions, to ask family members about the impact of the illness upon the family, and to determine the roles and expectations of each member in the household. The PT also has the opportunity to identify the level of understanding about the disease and its management within the family unit, and to determine what level of involvement of family members may be appropriate for education.

The four components of the assessment—detailed history, physical assessment, functional assessment, and the psychosocial factors—assist in the identification and the setting of realistic treat-

PHYSICAL ASSESSMENT

Patient's Name: ______

Observations:

Gait:

A.M. Stiffness ______ Hrs. ______ Mins. Grip Strength: R ______ /20 L ______ /20

Active Joints and Extra-articular Features

(Definite localized tenderness, stress pain, effusions, not just pain during arc of movement)

No. of active joints ______

(E) Effusion

(X) Tenderness or stress pain

Damaged Joints and Limitations of ROM

(Including lax collaterals, subluxation, bone-on-bone crepitus, malalignment, loss of more than 20% passive ROM. Excluding Heberden's nodes)

No. of damaged joints ______ ● Damage

Indicate adjacent to respective fingers the composite range of flexion in centimeters.

WEAK MUSCLE GROUPS

Region \ Ms.	Flex		Ext		Abd		Add		E.R.		I.R.	
	R	L	R	L	R	L	R	L	R	L	R	
Should.												
Elbow *												
Wrist												
Hip												
Knee												
Ankle **												

RANGE OF MOVEMENT (SPINE)

Cervical Spine

LSF RSF FLEX LL RR EXT

Th. Lumbar Spine

Fingertip to Floor ______ cms.

Side Flexion: Fingertip to Fib: R cm. L cms.

10 cm. Segments:
Upper — ______ cms.
Middle — ______ cms.
Lower — ______ cms.

* Forearm supination and pronation should be recorded under elbow region E.R. and I.R., respectively.
** Foot inversion and eversion should be recorded under ankle E.R. and I.R., respectively.

OF-52A

Figure 16-2. Example of a physical assessment form for use in the community. (From The Arthritis Society, Ottawa, Canada. With permission.)

Table 16-1. Examples of Activities Clients May Have Difficulty Performing, the Possible Causes, and Solutions

Functional Difficulty	Possible Causes	Possible Solutions
Rising from chair	Decreased ROM Muscle weakness Joint instability	↑ ROM Raised cushion Strengthen quadriceps Surgery
Brushing hair	Limited grasp Muscle weakness Decreased ROM, wrist, elbow, shoulder	Pad handle Strengthening exercises Lower head, ↑ ROM Long handle
Lifting pots	Weakness, hand, wrist Instability, wrist, elbow Pain	Strengthening exercises Splint wrist Lighter pots Slide pots
Carrying files	Pain, wrists Weakness, fingers, wrists ↓ ROM, elbow, wrist	Work splint Strengthening exercises Joint protection Wheeled cart Fewer files

ment goals, specific to that client and their own environment.

Identification of Management Goals

It is vitally important in this age of consumer awareness and escalating health care costs to determine at the outset what the client wishes or expects from the physical therapy, what their treatment goals are, and whether these goals are realistic or achievable. The client needs sufficient information about the disease, implications, and management to make an informed decision about which interventions are realistic and acceptable. Physical therapy in the home is an expensive service. Although most of the management of the disease must be the client's responsibility, regular monitoring of disease activity and treatment response by the PT will be required.

Modification or progression of the treatment goals should be based on periodic reassessments. The client and the PT can negotiate a mutually agreeable "contract" based on a list of treatment goals, strategies and, wherever possible, outcome measures to determine if these goals have been met. Planning for discharge from active treatment must start on the first visit with the client actively participating in this process.

Family members and other caregivers can take part in the goal-setting process and must become aware of the proposed management plan. They may assist with the application of various modalities, taking on some household tasks or learning about the level of emotional support the client may need. At this point, referral to other support services such as homemaking or social work may be necessary.

Management Plan

Only when the total assessment (history, physical and functional assessment) is completed, psychosocial issues addressed, and the client goals identified can the treatment program be established. It is particularly important in the home setting to develop a treatment program that is simple, that responds to the client's goals, and that is relevant to the individual. A program that requires a great deal of equipment can be complicated and time consuming, and may be cast aside as other family or household demands take precedence. Inappropriate equipment also can increase pain and the level of discomfort.

The disease itself may be very active at the time of referral. The client may be exhausted, experiencing significant pain, and be unable to actively participate in a full exercise program. PT has a limited but important role to play at this point. Service provision in the home setting allows the client to conserve energy by eliminating the need to dress, arrange transport, and travel to and from an outpatient setting. It is critical that the first steps of medical management are underway, but response to medications may not yet have occurred. During this interval, the CPT must provide emotional support and educate the client and the caregivers about the nature of the disease and its management. The importance of rest, the value of joint protection, and energy conservation techniques can be introduced at this time. There are a number of useful booklets detailing these principles that can be left with the client to provide reinforcement and to inform other household members (Appendix I).

Disease Education

One of the primary treatment goals is disease education, in relation to the natural history, prognosis, medical and PT management, and the range of therapeutic interventions that may be available. This includes information about the role of PT modalities, exercise, and use of assistive devices. Clients will have varied needs for information. It is important to recognize the readiness of the recipient to comprehend the vast amount of information that may be required to adjust to the demands of the disease, and to accept the diagnosis of a chronic and progressive illness. Some individuals may be able to assimilate only very basic information due to anxiety or depression; others may demand very technical and sophisticated reading materials. Others may be vulnerable to well-meaning but possibly misguided friends and family who will bombard them with materials on alternative therapies or "quack" remedies.

A great deal of client educational material has been published, by The Arthritis Society in Canada and by The Arthritis Foundation in the United States, relating to specific conditions and to treatment methods. Appendix I contains information on obtaining these materials. This is usually in the form of easily understood pamphlets or brochures. In recent years, a number of audiocassettes and videotapes have been produced that can be loaned to or purchased by the client.

There also are many books published and widely distributed about arthritis and its management. These are of variable content and quality. Clients may require some guidance in selecting reading materials. Two recent companion books (Appendix I), *Arthritis: A Comprehensive Guide to Understanding Your Arthritis* and *The Arthritis Helpbook* are recommended by The Arthritis Foundation and The Arthritis Society for use in an arthritis self-management program. These provide an excellent resource to the PT, who should be thoroughly familiar with the content of any material provided. These can be left with the client to read and discussed at a subsequent visit. This material is not a substitute for one-on-one, or even group education sessions but is used to reinforce the information provided by the PT.

It is generally helpful to educate the client with respect to the disease process, in terms that they can understand. Using the illustrations in the pamphlets may be helpful in explaining the effects of the inflammatory process on the joints and on other body systems. Explaining the processes that can cause joint damage, limit motion and the meaning of certain symptoms enhances the client's ability to self-monitor their disease and to understand the rationale behind the proposed treatment strategies.

Rest, both general and local, has been shown to reduce joint inflammation.[3,6] In the early stages of the disease, the importance of rest should be emphasized as an item over which the client can take direct control, and a means by which they can participate in the overall management of the disease. In the home setting, the PT can assist in teaching the client to break up their daily activities into manageable components and to schedule rest into the daily timetable.

Often, when the PT sees clients in the workplace, it is useful to meet with the employer or the occupational health nurse; education about arthritis can be provided and their cooperation gained in accommodating the special needs of the employee. For example, modification of the workspace, or scheduled rest periods, may be required.

Incorporated into the education package, and useful in the early stages of the intervention, is the teaching of joint protection and energy conservation techniques. The principles, which are addressed in Chapter 10, can be introduced early to a client whose disease activity is still very limiting. These principles can be reinforced and reviewed throughout the treatment process.

Observation of the client in their own environment and the use of concrete examples within the home or work setting is an advantage of the community-based therapist. In summary, excellent printed materials, as well as audiocassettes and videotapes, are available to reinforce one-on-one client education.

Medication Usage

Working in the community places additional responsibility on the PT, as they are frequently the only health care professional with regular, ongoing contact with the client. Physician appointments may be several months apart, and when they do occur, the client's anxiety or the physician's schedule may not provide opportunity to clarify issues or address concerns with respect to medication dosage, side effects, or response. Many clients do not understand the difference between analgesics and anti-inflammatories. This is particularly true of aspirin in its many forms. Clients often will not take their aspirin in the therapeutic range because, "I don't like to take a lot of pills." A client also may not understand the use of the slower acting disease remitting agents and may be extremely disappointed, for example, when they notice no change in their status after 2 weeks of taking methotrexate.

The PT must be aware of the actions and interactions of the various drugs prescribed, alert to the potential side effects, and must educate the client in this regard. It is important to encourage compliance with the medication scheme and to report, to the physician, any changes, adverse or beneficial, that may be occurring as a result of medication use.

Modalities in the Home

In most cases, the presence of active synovitis makes it difficult to achieve analgesia through the use of thermal modalities or electrical stimulation. Pain relief is usually the result of adequate response to anti-inflammatory therapy; however, the application of pain-relieving PT agents may provide some short-term relief and are particularly useful before or after therapeutic exercise or engaging in ADL.

The choice of thermal modalities is influenced by client preference. Clients often are reluctant to apply ice to painful joints, but with an adequate explanation resistance to the idea can be overcome. The use of ice applications to acutely inflamed joints can be beneficial by reducing pain sensation and decreasing muscle spasm,[7,8] as well as having an anti-inflammatory effect.[9] In addition, ice massage applied briefly to muscles that are in spasm can facilitate movement (see Chapter 13).

Applications of heat can be local or general and are usually preferred to relieve stiffness and to prepare for exercise. Often, clients report that a warm shower assists with relief of morning stiffness and that they can more easily do their exercises following the application of heat.

Safety

The use of modalities in the home setting must be governed by practical considerations, with a particular emphasis on safety issues. Careful explanation must be given to the client about the indications for the use of any of the range of modalities available for home use and potential risks that can result from overuse or misuse. It is not unusual when first visiting clients in the home to discover that they already are inappropriately applying various forms of heat, such as electric heating pads. For example, some elderly clients may wrap a heating pad around a knee and sleep with it on at low heat; this practice causes tissue damage. Other misuses that are potentially hazardous are the use of analgesic rubs in conjunction with heating pads or hot water bottles, insufficient layers of towelling between the source of heat and the client's skin, and the application of heat or cold to areas that may have impaired circulation or sensation. It is therefore critical that clients are well educated with respect to the use of these modalities, particularly since they are generally applying them without supervision.

Alternative to Wax Baths

One popular form of treatment in the home setting for many years was the use of wax baths for the relief of stiffness and pain in the hands. Wax application, still used in the clinical setting, is potentially hazardous due to the risk of fire from improper heating procedures and the risk of burns if the temperature is not well controlled. It also is time consuming and cumbersome to the client. An alternative that is safer and easier is the use of *rubber gloves and oil*. A generous application of mineral oil or baby oil to the hands followed by putting on ordinary rubber gloves then immersing the hands in hot tap water for 5–10 minutes is a more practical solution. Clients report that it eases morning stiffness.

Pain-Relieving Modalities

These are widely available commercially and can be costly. Clients should be advised of the availability of these items. Some may be loaned for evaluation, but generally it is preferable to use simple, inexpensive items found in most households.

A 1-lb package of frozen peas or corn makes an effective and reusable *ice pack* when wrapped in a damp towel, molding well to the joint, light and easy to handle. Clients should be advised against applying ice directly to the skin, as they may sustain a burn, particularly if they rest the weight of the body part on top of the ice.

The use of *moist heat* is advisable, since it allows for more even distribution of heat over the affected area and reduces the risk of burns, since moist applications cool down gradually. A hot water bottle wrapped in a damp towel molds well to the affected joint, as does a wet facecloth placed in a plastic bag and heated for 1 minute in a microwave oven and then wrapped in a damp towel.

Clients with Raynaud's phenomenon must be cautioned against the use of either heat or ice for peripheral joints, since the risk of tissue damage is always present.

The Use of Electrical Modalities

Modalities such as ultrasound or interferential currents are impractical in the home setting. Ultrasound (US) units tend to lose their calibration when carried in cars and in and out of homes. Furthermore, the frequency with which US can be used is problematic and there is a lack of evidence of its efficacy in treating inflammatory polyarthritis.[10] Effects of interferential current on clients with arthritis has not been studied and the equipment is simply not available for home use.

Many studies on the effects of *transcutaneous electrical nerve stimulation (TENS)* have been carried out; however, those that were conducted on clients with RA were flawed.[11–14] The portability and relatively low cost of the units make TENS suitable for home use. In many cases, however, clients with limited hand function find TENS difficult to apply. Also, with the multiple sites involved in inflammatory arthritis, TENS becomes impractical. Some community-based programs stock a few TENS units to lend to clients to evaluate, and in some situations, such as refractory shoulder or neck pain, clients report relief from the use of these units. Purchase or rental for home use may be possible.

In summary, many thermal modalities can be applied simply and inexpensively in the home. In some situations, where one or two joints remain problematic, a trial of some therapy in an outpatient setting or referral to another facility may be appropriate in the short term.

Rest

Local Rest

Relief of pain may be achieved through the use of support to the affected joints, and training in proper rest positions. Devices such as resting splints for the hands, wrists, and knees may reduce inflammation through local rest of the affected joints and relieve associated muscle spasm (see Chapter 10 for details of orthotics).

Hand Splints

Morning stiffness of more than an hour is considered an indication for hand resting splints, as is persistent wrist and metacarpophalangeal (MCP) joint effusion or tenosynovitis. Many clients, however, find a full hand splint too restrictive for independent use at home. The PT must be aware of the limitations that such splints impose and recognize the importance of maintaining client independence in applying the splints, turning light switches on and off, pulling up bedclothes, or even scratching their nose! Because of the considerable limitations, the full hand splint, particularly with the thumb incorporated, is usually unsatisfactory for home use. A more acceptable alternative is a splint that leaves the thumb and web space between the thumb and index finger free, but supports the MCPs and allows opposition of the thumb and little finger for minimal light hand function. Some clients are advised to wear the right hand splint on one night and the left on the next night, until they accommodate to the splints, and manage to rest undisturbed by these appliances.

Knee Splints

Support for inflamed knees with associated spasm of the hamstrings and lack of extension may be provided by means of commercially available knee splints or by molded thermoplastic splints. These are easily applied by the client and fastened with Velcro. They should maintain the knee in as much extension as possible, without exerting an uncomfortable force.

Home Manufacture

There are many thermoplastic materials available that are suitable for fabrication of splints in the client's home. The materials can be pre-cut and easily heated in a standard oven or an electric frying pan. A simple portable kit containing scissors, splinting materials, Velcro, stockinette, and a heat gun for spot molding is all that is needed for home use. Printed instructions on the use and care of splints should be provided. Clients should be cautioned against applying analgesic rubs prior to wearing splints, as this can produce skin rash or even burns. At every visit, the PT should check splints for fit and pressure points and modify the splints if necessary.

For *general rest*, client education materials often describe proper resting positions. Illustrations show the client resting supine, with one small, flat pillow under the neck, arms at the sides, and knees out absolutely straight. These instructions are totally unrealistic, as few if any clients can relax or are able to sleep in this posture. To relax, *the joints must be adequately supported*. The presence of effusion in the knees or hamstring spasm will render a client unable to straighten the knees completely in supine. While traditionally clients are told not to use pillows under the knees, unless there is some support, relaxation will be impossible and pain may increase. If splinting is not possible or practical, the client can be instructed to use a towel folded several times to support the knees *in as much extension as possible*. Resting the forearm on a pillow laid lengthwise beside the client may assist in alleviating pain in shoulders and elbows. Bedclothes should be lightweight and should not restrict movement of the feet and ankles. If needed, a cardboard carton can be used to lift the bedclothes from the feet, and sheepskin elbow or heel protectors are sometimes helpful.

Neck Care

The neck deserves special attention to relieve pain and to maintain correct postural alignment. Use of too many pillows under the head should be avoided. Frequently, neck and shoulder pain can be attributed to inadequate neck support during rest. Therefore, the client should be taught to support the cervical spine by means of specially shaped pillows, neck rolls, or cervical ruffs. These can be fabricated from stockinette stuffed with dressing roll or fiberfill batting. Usually two small ruffs fit better and are more comfortable than one large ruff. The advantage of using ruffs is that they stay in place during sleep and also can be helpful when the client is in the upright position. Advice should be given to the client to be alert to neurological signs, such as dizziness, blurred vision, or numbness and tingling in the extremities, which could develop due to atlantoaxial subluxation. While such occurrences are infrequent and the PT should avoid alarming the client unduly, these symptoms should be promptly reported and investigated.

Working with the client in their own setting provides the opportunity to identify those postures or habits that help or hinder, to problem solve, to demonstrate the use of appropriate support, and to demonstrate alternative positioning using the client's own furnishings.

General Relaxation

Relaxation techniques may be helpful for clients with intractable pain, who are unable to control the pain with analgesics and other modalities. These techniques may be used in combination with modalities and medication to maximize their effectiveness. Clients also may choose from the array of available relaxation audiocassettes, selected music, or guided imagery to assist in managing their pain.

Whatever the client chooses as the most beneficial form of pain control, they need to be assured that their pain is real. Each client needs to recognize which types of pain respond to which interventions, and when to seek assistance from health professionals.

Therapeutic Exercise

Perhaps the most challenging aspect of providing home PT is that of delivering therapeutic exercise, which is, after all, the very essence of what is unique to physical therapy. (See Chapter 13 for principles of exercise therapy in inflammatory conditions, and Chapter 11 for cardiovascular fitness in clients with arthritis.) This section deals with exercise prescription within the community setting.

In the acute stage clients are often fatigued, depressed, and in pain, with an understandable apprehension about moving the affected joints. They may be deconditioned, due to the effects of the disease, or they may have been placed on a program of rest and told to avoid exercise. Clients require considerable education with respect to the purpose and different types of therapeutic exercise, and encouragement to participate in designing an acceptable, custom-tailored exercise program.

Compliance

To enhance compliance, the exercise program must be relevant, pain-free, and short in duration. A program that is time consuming, complicated, or which causes increased pain very quickly will be stopped. Careful explanation should be given with regard to the purpose of the three types of exercises prescribed: mobilizing, strengthening, and conditioning.

The time of day at which the exercise program is carried out will depend on many factors. Ideally, exercise should be done at a time when the client has the least pain and is not fatigued. However, this may not be possible due to other competing life style factors. The PT should work with the client to identify the means by which the exercises can be incorporated into everyday activity.

The PT should design a short, simple exercise program for certain target areas, especially if the client has identified a specific functional problem, such as inability to rise unassisted from a chair. If this is due to muscle weakness, the exercise program can be directed at quadriceps strengthening. Difficulty reaching objects on shelves may be addressed by increasing shoulder ROM. Pointing out the improvements in function as a result of the exercise can provide the client with incentive to comply.

Morning stiffness affecting the hands may interfere with dressing activities. A few minutes of gentle hand exercises in warm water may relieve the stiffness and make dressing easier. Mid morning may be the most pain-free period of the day and therefore a good time to perform other ROM and strengthening exercise. Some clients take their morning medication and return to bed until it takes effect and then carry out their exercises.

Factors Enhancing Exercise Compliance

- purpose of the exercise
- length of program
- comfort of client
- functional gains

Mobilizing Exercises

Mobilizing exercises are indicated to increase ROM in affected joints, increase flexibility, and relieve stiffness.

Actively inflamed joints should be moved gently through the available range, once or twice daily for no more than three repetitions. This may require assistance from a family member or other caregiver if the client is weak or has difficulty moving a shoulder, for example. The assistant should merely support the affected limb and allow the client to carry out the actual movement. As the inflammation decreases, the client can be taught to move through the available range and then attempt to go a little farther in order to begin to stretch tight joint structures. For example, with forward flexion of the shoulder, the client can be taught to use a doorway, slide the hand up the door frame as far as possible, hold for a few seconds, and then attempt to reach up a little farther. Pulleys can be useful for regaining ROM in the shoulders and are easily mounted in a doorway, for example, using a single pulley, sash cord, and pipe insulation for handles, all inexpensive and available in hardware stores.

Hold-relax techniques can be of great value in regaining lost ROM and relieving stiffness in periarticular structures. These techniques can be taught to the client or to an assistant and modified in the home setting very easily. Clients should be warned that it is inadvisable to apply a force across more than one affected joint. The client may use the side of the bed or front of an upholstered chair to provide isometric resistance to the hamstrings followed by voluntary relaxation of these muscles and then active extension of the knee.

Exercise Considerations

- physical assessment
- inflammatory activity
- joint damage
- muscle strength
- general condition/age

The pain and limitation of movement caused by inflammatory arthritis frequently results in reflex inhibition and disuse atrophy. Muscle weakness, combined with ROM and endurance losses, can result in difficulties with ADL. Daily exercise designed to improve ROM, build strength and endurance is an important feature of disease management.

Strengthening Exercises

When joints are actively inflamed, the client should be advised not to perform many repetitions, not to exercise to the point of fatigue, and to avoid resisted movements. The muscles acting on inflamed joints should be exercised isometrically, to maintain and increase strength and endurance. These exercises are easily performed in the home setting and require only minimal equipment. For example, the knee can be positioned over a large juice can wrapped in a towel to perform isometric quadriceps exercises in mid range.

Once joint inflammation has subsided and muscle strength improved, the exercise program can be increased to include isotonic movement, beginning gradually and using low resistance. The exercises should be performed once daily.

While clients can be taught to self-resist various muscle groups, clients with hand/wrist involvement may find this difficult. The PT then can instruct other household members to apply resistance, or teach the client to use belts, resistive rubber bands, tubing, or other elastic materials. Since clients will be expected to carry out the exercise program unsupervised, it is important to remind them to monitor the number of repetitions and that the strengthening exercises should be pain free. Exercises that cause increased joint pain or swelling should be discontinued until the PT can reassess and modify the program.

It is important to custom tailor the program to the specific needs of the individual client, bearing in mind the need to incorporate this aspect of disease management into the life style of the client. The PT should determine, with the client, how the program can fit into their daily schedule and should emphasize that ADL are not a substitute for therapeutic exercise.

Conditioning Exercise

In recent years, the importance of maintaining physical fitness has replaced the emphasis previously placed on rest and avoidance of strenuous activity. People with arthritis experiencing pain, fatigue, or disability may abandon previously enjoyed activities such as gardening, skiing, or cycling. They may have a sense of loss, depression, and further deconditioning as a result of inactivity.

Exercise/Recreation in the Community

The CPT can encourage the client to resume conditioning exercise by exploring alternatives or adapting activities. In many communities, there are recreational programs designed for people with physical limitations, such as low-impact aerobic classes, walking groups, and pool exercise programs. These activities may be appropriate for clients, but due to fear of pain, lack of self-confidence, and depression, some clients may be reluctant to participate. The PT can be of great assistance in providing reassurance and encouragement to use appropriate resources.

Pool exercise programs for people with arthritis are becoming increasingly popular and available. Frequently, water-fitness instructors consult PTs about exercises that are suitable for people with arthritis. It is preferable that the pool be accessible by graduated steps or ramp and that the temperature is warm, ideally about 85°F (29°C). Pool exercise can confer benefits for clients, since the warmth of the water promotes relaxation, buoyancy of the water assists with ROM, and water offers controlled resistance for strengthening activities. A pool program can be recreational and enhances social interaction among participants.

The PT may accompany the client to a designated pool program or exercise group to determine if the program offered is suitable or the facility is safe and accessible. The CPT may consult with the instructor and provide reassurance to the client about the potentially new experience of a pool/exercise program.

Other clients may wish to pursue more self-directed activities, such as cycling or cross-country skiing. Advice should be provided to the client with respect to suitable types of activities and to the equipment used. Ski pole handles can be padded and bicycle seats and handlebars adjusted to allow the client to carry out the activity in a safe and pain-free manner. Again, the client must learn to pace themselves by starting slowly and building up their tolerance levels and watching for signs of increased joint pain or swelling.

The management of arthritis demands a great deal of the client, physically and emotionally. To improve the client's overall sense of well-being, attention must be paid to those pursuits the client finds pleasurable and rewarding. If the activity can be suitably adapted and increases the client's strength, tolerance, and sense of well-being, it is well worth the therapist's effort.

Audiovisual Aids to Exercise

Since at home the client will not be receiving direct supervision, the exercises must be carefully taught, and the provision of written exercise materials can be helpful. The language should be very clear and specific. Sometimes it is helpful to develop an exercise chart so that the client can check off which exercises they have performed on a daily basis and which they have found difficult by keeping a diary that can be seen by the CPT on subsequent visits. There are many pamphlets and exercise sheets available, some produced by pharmaceutical companies, others by hospital departments. Some of these have excellent and very clear illustrations that can serve as good reminders for starting positions and desired movements. There also are many audiocassettes and videotapes available that vary in content and quality. Some of these can be useful as a resource to clients but should be reviewed with the PT and custom tailored to the individual.

Otherwise, there is a risk of harm to the client in performing an exercise incorrectly or doing too many repetitions, resulting in unnecessary or inappropriate exercise. Therefore, while these materials are a useful adjunct to treatment, they must be accompanied with specific instructions relating to their purpose, frequency, number of repetitions, and progression or modification.

With the increasing availability of computer-based exercise programs that enable individual item selection, exercise pamphlets can be tailor made for specific clients.

Ambulation

The importance of supportive and comfortable footwear cannot be overestimated (see Chapter 10). In the home, the PT can examine the footwear habitually worn around the house, look at the shoes the client may have tried or prefers, and encourage adaptation or replacement of footwear. Basic footwear modifications are easy to perform in the home. Insoles can be fabricated with thermoplastics, or metatarsal and longitudinal arch supports can be put in existing shoes. The PT should have available a list of recommended brands of shoes and the sources for shoes and other modifications, such as names of orthotic suppliers or retail outlets. It also is helpful to provide a handout on the recommended features of shoes.

On occasion the PT may accompany the client to the shoe store or orthotist to ensure that proper fit and adaptation is obtained. It may be difficult to convince the client of the value of good, supportive, and often expensive footwear. By pointing out the number of uncomfortable shoes the client may have tried and discarded, and the associated expense of continually purchasing unsuitable shoes, the PT may convince the client to accept the recommended footwear and to absorb the cost. Once properly fitted and comfortable, the client frequently adheres to the suggestions and finds they are better able to tolerate walking and standing.

In some communities, there are special footwear outlets, occasionally with orthotists who have special knowledge of foot pathology and who can work with the client and the PT to find acceptable solutions to foot problems. A region may have access to mobile, visiting services where the supplier will see a client at home to provide fitting and adaptation services. Referral to an OT is appropriate in many circumstances when the foot problems are complex and require specialized modification. Similarly, referral to chiropodists or special outpatient foot clinics for management of problem nails, calluses, bunions, or skin breakdown may be indicated.

Clients should be carefully taught about foot care and instructed in the importance of monitoring skin condition and care of pressure areas that may occur. Clients with limited mobility may have difficulty reaching and seeing these areas. The use of a hand-held mirror may help, as well as having family members check on foot conditions.

Caution should be given *not* to attempt foot care if it cannot be done properly, as this can be a cause of infection.

Ambulatory Aids

Ambulatory aids can be of great value whether a client has a single knee or hip involvement, as in OA, or multiple inflamed joints, such as in rheumatoid arthritis (RA). Properly used, they afford joint protection and an element of pain relief, allowing a client more mobility in the home and in the community. Used inappropriately, they can put a client at risk of falls and may reinforce poor posture.

Some clients "borrow" canes from relatives or friends that are too long or too short. Many misguidedly use the cane in the wrong hand. It is, therefore, important to assess clients carefully for the prescription of canes, crutches, or walkers. Clients should be educated about the dangers inherent in holding on to furniture or leaning against walls in order to get about the home. Caution should be given about the risks of loose carpets or slippery floors.

Adjustable canes are easily available and can be lent to a client for a trial. Some clients may have difficulty with the conventional rounded handle of a cane. There are some types of canes on the market with specially molded hand grips. The PT may modify a cane handle with wide rubber bands or some other material to make it easier to grasp. Instruction in measurement for the correct length of a walking aid may be required.

Clients with arthritis of the upper limbs usually have great difficulty managing conventional axillary crutches because of the need to transfer weight through the elbows and wrists. If crutches are necessary, either postsurgically or when joints are painful or unstable, then forearm support crutches are recommended. These permit the weight to be distributed over the forearm and therefore avoid pressure on inflamed hand joints and wrists. They can be cumbersome for some clients, a nuisance for indoor use or use on stairs, and the Velcro straps securing the forearm can be problematic. Forearm crutches, however, are helpful outdoors or in shopping malls.

Whether canes or crutches are used, clients should be taught to go up and down stairs safely, to use special tips with ice picks in winter, and to check the tips regularly for wear.

Many types of walkers are available, some very simple and lightweight, some with features such as a carrying basket that converts to a seat, and some with various types of wheels. When prescribing a walker, it is helpful to assess the specific needs of the client, particularly within the home, as many factors must be taken into consideration. These include the ability of the client to lift and move the walker safely, the layout of the rooms and furniture, and the requirement to use stairs.

Often a walker supplied in an outpatient or rehabilitation center appears suitable but may be unsafe or unsuitable at home. This is exemplified in the case of an elderly, frail lady with advanced RA who, following total knee arthroplasty, moved well in the corridors and gymnasium of the rehabilitation center using a high delta walker. She was discharged to her small bungalow with this walker, which proved to be too cumbersome and unwieldy. In attempting to move the walker through a doorway and around a corner, the client fell, pulling the walker down on top of herself and sustaining a fractured femur. For this client, a home assessment by a PT immediately following discharge may have prevented this unfortunate occurrence.

Motorized scooters have become popular and are in widespread use, but should be prescribed only when the disabled client is likely to become homebound without such assistance. These vehicles are very expensive, although some insurance schemes will partially cover the cost, and they are cumbersome in the ordinary home. The client may require assistance to be able to transfer safely. They may, nevertheless, permit freedom of movement for very limited clients who otherwise might not be able to get out in the community. These vehicles are sometimes very helpful to those clients who can use them at work. In some instances, these permit clients to continue their employment.

When assessing clients for any type of ambulatory aid, careful consideration must be given, not only to the client's physical ability to use such aids but also to the environment in which they are to be utilized.

Activities of Daily Living

The goal common to most clients with arthritis is to maintain their independence within their home and community. This goal is achieved in a variety of ways. The provision of aids and adaptations may, in many cases, provide the solution to problems with ADL. Aids and adaptations, however, should be provided judiciously.

They should be used in the acute phase of the disease to protect inflamed joints or to allow the performance of an activity that would otherwise not be possible due to pain and weakness. For example, the use of a raised toilet seat for a client with painful, effused knees and weak quadriceps would be appropriate but is in no way a substitute for the exercise program necessary to preserve or increase ROM and strengthen the quadriceps. With proper management and disease control, the client will not require this aid. Similarly, the provision of a reaching device may be indicated for a client who cannot bend because of limitation of joint movement. Again, an exercise program may restore joint mobility and eliminate the need for the device. Should the disease progress and joint damage occur precluding improvement of ROM or joint stability, such devices become necessary.

Facilitating a client's ability to carry out ADL is a very tangible means of gaining a client's confidence as she or he can immediately perceive the impact of using a tap turner or a raised cushion. It is important, however, not to load up a client with equipment that is neither needed nor wanted and will not therefore be used. It is frequently more appropriate to lend a piece of equipment for the client to evaluate over a period of time than it is to ask them to purchase an expensive item they may not use.

When working in the home setting, it is easy to determine if a client is not using the cane or the raised cushion, as these items may not be visible or may be hidden deep in a closet. Working with the client to achieve maximum function and independence can be greatly enhanced by first-hand observation, and the principles of joint protection and energy conservation can be reinforced by using concrete examples.

Safety Concerns

One of the primary considerations when working with a client to achieve increased function and independence is the issue of safety. Many times, clients will adapt to altered functional status by using poor body mechanics, leaning on unstable pieces of furniture, or grabbing at towel bars or the sink. The PT should carefully observe such activities as transfers from beds, chairs, and the bathtub or shower, movement about the kitchen; and use of stairs, and educate the client about the inherent hazards within the home setting. Any piece of equipment that is supplied should be checked for safe installation and use. The PT should identify, to the client, potentially unsafe activities such as lifting and reaching and hazards such as loose scatter mats, stairs without rails, and slippery surfaces.

Safety Concerns

- **poor body mechanics**
- **unstable furniture**
- **loose scatter mats**
- **inappropriate equipment**
- **stairs and railings**
- **slippery surfaces**

Within the household, many simple adjustments can be made with little expense or effort, such as raising the height of chairs, changing faucet handles to levers, reorganizing kitchen shelves, and teaching the client easier ways to perform certain tasks. Simply by watching a client move about the home or carrying out a few kitchen activities, the PT can be of great assistance in identifying and helping to correct poor body mechanics or work habits. An occupational therapy (OT) referral is appropriate if extensive modification to the household appears indicated. The OT has skills and resources that will enhance the client's function and independence. Costs of home modifications are sometimes covered by private insurance schemes, and in some states/provinces, government grants may be available.

Visiting the Workplace

Visiting a client in the workplace provides the opportunity for the PT to directly observe work habits, posture, tools involved, organization of the workspace, and to demonstrate alternatives or modify existing equipment or furnishings. The PT has an important role to play in determining the client's level of disease activity and physical capability of carrying out their job responsibilities.

Consultation with an OT can be very helpful in making modifications for a specific client in the workplace. In many communities, OTs with rheumatology experience are actively working in this field. Currently, businesses are becoming more aware of the importance of ergonomics. Modifications and updating of furnishings and equipment are being made, not only to prevent injury in the workplace but also to facilitate employment for people with physical limitations. Often, with appropriate information and explanation, employers are able to provide rest breaks or adapted equipment in order to facilitate the individual's return to work. In large organizations, there may be facilities available to allow the client to lie down for a break, or to carry out the prescribed exercise routine. There may be nursing staff available to assist in monitoring the client's condition and, in some instances, the provision of educational presentations or printed materials is welcomed by the organization. A meeting with the client, employer, fellow workers, and other treatment team members, as appropriate, can result in a satisfactory return to the workplace and exemplifies the concept of a team approach within the community.

Other Resources

In the institutional setting, the roles of various team members may be strictly defined, but in the community, a multiskilled approach is essential in order to provide more efficient and cost-effective service. For example, in Ontario, Arthritis Society social workers operating from regional offices are well poised to provide consultation services to the Society's PTs, OTs, and clients.

Social work services can be invaluable in helping a client make the transition from home to the workplace. The client may require an advocate to assist with the formalities of benefits, disability pensions, financial assistance in the purchase of special equipment, or returning to work on a part-time basis. Family or personal counseling may be needed to help clients and families to cope with the impact of arthritis.

At various stages throughout the course of the disease, the client may require modification of the drug regimen; consultation with a pharmacist, chiropodist, or orthopedic surgeon; or referral to vocational rehabilitation services. The PT providing care in the community should ensure that appropriate communication takes place between the service providers, and that the client can recognize when to seek advice or services.

Discharge Planning

Discharge planning ideally begins at the time of the first visit of the PT to the client. This is the time when the relationship between the PT and the client begins. It should be clear, especially with a client who has a long-term, chronic disease, that resources are available to assist the client in achieving realistic goals. The major responsibility, however, rests with the client, who must assume an active role in the selection and implementation of treatment strategies. It is easy for clients seen at home to establish a dependency either on the service or on the care provider. While this may be gratifying to the provider, the therapist must remember that the purpose of the intervention is to allow the client to remain active and independent within the community. The ultimate aim of the PT will be to provide disease education and self-management methods with information on resources.

Because the course of the disease is unpredictable and the severity is variable, the needs of individual clients will differ. Coping strategies unique to each person often will determine how much is required. Discharge planning should be coordinated with other treatment team members, so that the client is not left feeling abandoned. It is useful to communicate to the client, on reassessment, what progress has been made, what outcomes of the treatment program are expected, and what indicators are being used to recognize achievement of the goals related to treatment.

When planning for discharge, it is sometimes helpful to taper off the frequency of visits, spacing them out from weekly, for example, to every 2 weeks or once monthly, so that the therapist may reassure the client of their ability to manage independently. Another strategy is to arrange a monthly telephone check. On discharge, clients are advised to call the CPT if new problems arise or when they have specific concerns.

Summary

The advantages of service provision in the home are obvious for clients with a chronic condition that results in energy depletion and can cause significant functional and psychological problems. Bridging the gap between the hospital or outpatient department, the CPT can assist the patient in applying the principles of self-management and treatment strategies that may have been initiated in a clinical setting but must be incorporated into an individual's life style.

As part of a team that may have few or many members, the CPT has the opportunity and obligation to mobilize community resources, advocate on behalf of the client, and to work in a variety of settings, creatively employing multidisciplinary skills to enable the client to adapt and to maintain function and independence within their own community.

The following two case reports provide examples of the value of community-based care to individuals with arthritis.

Case History #1

Mrs. K., a 39-year-old married woman with three sons, worked as a retail buyer and had an active life style until she developed progressive, symmetrical, seropositive RA. She was referred to The Arthritis Society for physical and occupational therapy following a 10-day stay in a rheumatic diseases unit, 18 months after onset of RA. She had been started on naproxen and gold injections, a program of rest, disease education, heat, ice, and exercise, and was provided with hand resting splints.

At the first home visit, Mrs. K.'s own treatment goals were relief of both pain and motion restriction that would allow her to return to work, manage her household activities, and resume cross-country skiing and tennis.

Assessment

Physical Assessment showed

- morning stiffness—2 hours
- grip strength—84/20, R; 92/20, L
- 18 active joints (6 with effusions)
- 12 damaged joints
- decreased ROM in L knee, both wrists, both shoulders, and in PIPs of both hands
- decreased muscle strength affecting shoulder girdle, quadriceps, and both wrists

Functional Assessment showed

- walking difficulties due to foot and knee pain
- difficulty climbing stairs and rising from sitting
- problems in self-care and household chores due to hand, wrist, and shoulder pain and weakness
- inability to work caused by fatigue, lack of endurance, and upper extremity involvement
- decreased social and recreational activities

Additionally, Mrs. K. was experiencing depression and family difficulties.

Treatment Plan Mrs. K.'s goals were to learn more about the disease and how to manage the pain and stiffness, and to regain ROM and strength in order to return to her previous active life style and return to work. A treatment plan was negotiated between the PT and the client to include:

- reinforcement of disease education provided in hospital with additional reading materials provided for client and family
- instruction in the application of heat for shoulders and hands and the application of ice to swollen joints
- exercise to maintain and increase ROM in affected joints and isometric exercise for major muscle groups
- provision of a raised toilet seat, tap turners, and jar opener
- fabrication of polyethylene work splints
- referral to OT for footwear modifications and reinforcement of joint protection and energy conservation techniques
- A meeting between the PT, husband, and sons to answer questions and suggest redistribution of household chores to reduce stress on the client

Progress The PT visited weekly over the next 6 weeks to monitor progress and adjust therapy as required. On assessment at 6 weeks, the client reported reduction of morning stiffness to 1 hour, an increase in her energy, and increased ability to carry out activities of daily living. The active joint count was 12 with 2 effusions, ROM had improved in shoulders and wrists, but the left knee remained hot, swollen, and lacked 10 degrees of extension. Grip strength had improved to 130/20 (R) and 142/20 (L).

Mrs. K. felt that she was beginning to respond to gold therapy and was making good use of the joint protection and energy conservation techniques she had been shown. Work splints enabled her to carry out light kitchen duties and the footwear modifications had reduced her foot pain. She also reported that her husband was becoming angry and frustrated at her inability to go to work, cost of medications, and the increased workload on family members. The client was considering returning to work and discontinuing her medication because of cost.

The PT reported the client's status to the rheumatologist who injected the left knee with good result. Referral was made to a homemaking service. At that point, both the therapist and client felt that the exercise program could be increased moderately in scope and intensity and that a referral to social work was indicated due to the increased financial and family stresses.

The social worker was able to secure financial assistance to pay for the medications and to work with the patient and her husband towards resolving the family problems.

Over the next 4 months, the PT decreased the frequency of her visits, as Mrs. K. was able to carry out the treatment program independently and was learning to monitor her disease activity. In consultation with the OT and the social worker, it was felt that Mrs. K., while responding well to the overall treatment program, was becoming socially isolated and withdrawn. Physically, she was ready to begin a more active exercise program and could benefit from a recreational activity. She agreed to attend weekly hydrotherapy sessions at a warm pool, which she enjoyed and which allowed her to interact socially with others. At this point, the PT and OT discontinued regular visits, agreeing to revisit should this be desired by the client.

Nine Months after Referral A visit to Mrs. K.'s workplace by the OT to provide consultation on the need for modifications enabled the client to return to work on a part-time basis. The PT visited the client at home, once more, to reassess and determine whether the treatment goals had been achieved. Mrs. K. had 20 minutes of morning stiffness, six active joints, grip strength of 192/20 (R) and 212/20 (L), ROM was full in both shoulders and the left knee, 75% in both wrists, and she was largely independent in ADL but still required assistance with cleaning and laundry. Although unable to play tennis, she was able to resume cross-country skiing on gentle terrain, limiting herself to brief periods. On discharge the client felt she had, at least partially, fulfilled her treatment goals. Although some of the family stresses remained, the treatment program had resulted in Mrs. K. becoming an informed and active participant in the management of her disease. She was able to integrate the treatment strategies into her life style, appropriately utilizing professional services and community resources.

Case History #2

Mrs. H. was a 76-year-old widow with widespread osteoarthritis (OA) affecting both hands, knees, and hips. She relocated from another city to share a small apartment with her son. Because of increasing functional limitations, she was referred to The Arthritis Society by her family physician for physical therapy. The PT met with Mrs. H. and her son in their home. Both were concerned with Mrs. H.'s increasing difficulty with ambulation, transfers, and bathing, as well as her social isolation and depression.

Assessment

Physical Assessment findings

- bony enlargement, limitation of motion of DIPs, PIPs bilaterally, CMC involvement of both thumbs, muscle wasting, loss of dexterity
- pain, crepitus on movement of right knee, 20-degree flexion contracture, 75-degrees of flexion, quadriceps wasting and weakness
- left knee which had undergone an arthroplasty was pain free with ROM 0–95 degrees
- hips, limited to 50% of full ROM, pain on lateral rotation and flexion

Functional Assessment findings

- ambulation was limited to 20 ft, was slow and painful; she held onto furniture
- difficulty with transfers
- difficulty with self-care due to decreased dexterity and difficulty with meal preparation due to limited mobility and strength

Treatment Plan The client's goals were relief of pain, and increased independence in ambulation, self-care, and meal preparation. She also wanted to be able to go shopping and to socialize. Her son was anxious about her depression and her physical condition. The treatment plan included:

- discussion with family physician, prescription of analgesics, and referral to a rheumatologist regarding potential surgical intervention
- application of oil and rubber glove routine, provision of tap turners, jar opener, padding handles of utensils
- addressing safety issues (chair height, use of raised toilet seat, bath bench and bars, instruction in use of walker, removal of loose carpets)
- son instructed in application of moist heat to hips and right knee, positioning at rest
- instruction in ROM exercises for knees and hips within tolerance and isometric exercises for quadriceps, hamstrings, hip extensors
- referral to Friendly Visitors

Mrs H. was referred by the rheumatologist to an orthopedic surgeon who recommended a total knee arthroplasty. Prior to surgery she required reassurance and encouragement to strengthen her lower extremities. She was able to move about the apartment using a walker, but her tolerance was low and she was unable to go outdoors independently.

Following surgery and a brief period in a rehabilitation center, she was discharged to her son's home. The Arthritis Society PT again visited to assess client safety and to follow-up on the exercise program. Mrs. H. was able to carry out her exercise program unsupervised, was ambulating well with a walker within the apartment, but was afraid to try outdoors or even to go to the mailroom alone. The treatment program was to:

- increase scope and intensity of exercises
- progress to ambulation indoors with one cane
- commence hydrotherapy to increase strength, endurance, and social contacts

Mrs. H. was reluctant to attempt ambulation outside of the apartment, even with her son. With the PT accompanying her, she gradually increased her confidence and was able to walk to the nearest street corner within a few weeks. She was fearful of attending hydrotherapy sessions on her own, so the PT arranged for her son to accompany her for the first few sessions, after which she met another participant who offered to drive her to and from the pool.

Three months following her hospitalization, Mrs. H. was able, with the use of aids, to prepare meals independently, perform self-care, and ambulate. On discharge from The Arthritis Society, she was planning a move into her own apartment and had arranged for a homemaker to assist with housework. She was attending a seniors' group, as well as the hydrotherapy program. The community-based PT, working with other team members, was effective in assisting this client to achieve independence within the community.

References

1. Helewa A, Bombardier C, Goldsmith CH, et al: Cost-effectiveness of inpatient and intensive outpatient treatment of rheumatoid arthritis. Arthritis Rheum 1989; 32(12):1505–1514.
2. Anderson RB, Needleman RD, Gatter RH, et al: Patient outcome following inpatient vs outpatient treatment of rheumatoid arthritis. J Rheumatol 1988; 15:556–560.
3. Swezey RL: Rheumatoid arthritis: the role of the kinder and gentler therapies. J Rheumatol 1990; 17(Suppl 25):8–13.
4. Katz S, Vignos PJ, Moskowitz W, et al: Comprehensive outpatient care in rheumatoid arthritis. A controlled study. JAMA 1968; 206(6):1249–1254.
5. Helewa A, Smythe HA, Goldsmith CH, et al: The total assessment of rheumatoid polyarthritis—evaluation of a training program for physiotherapists and occupational therapists. J Rheumatol 1987; 14: 87–92.
6. Banwell BF: Physical therapy in arthritis management. In Ehrlich GE (ed): Rehabilitation Management of Rheumatic Conditions, 2nd edition, pp 264–284. Baltimore, Williams & Wilkins, 1986.
7. Kirk JA, Kersley GD: Heat and cold in the physical treatment of rheumatoid arthritis of the knee. A controlled trial. Ann Phys Med 1968; 9:270–274.
8. Williams J, Harvey J, Tannebaum H: Use of superficial heat versus ice for the rheumatoid arthritic shoulder. A pilot study. Physiother Can 1986; 38: 8–13.
9. Oosterveld FGJ, Rasker JJ, Jacobs JWG, et al: The effect of local heat and cold therapy on the intraarticular and skin surface temperature of the knee. Arthritis Rheum 1992; 35:146–151.
10. Falconer J, Hayes KW, Chang RW: Therapeutic ultrasound in the treatment of musculoskeletal conditions. Arthritis Care Res 1990; 3:85–91.
11. Simmonds MJ, Kumar S: Pain and the placebo in rehabilitation using TENS and laser. Disabil Rehabil 1994; 16(1):13–20.
12. Kumar VN, Redford JB: Transcutaneous nerve stimulation in rheumatoid arthritis. Arch Phys Med Rehabil 1982; 63:595–596.
13. Langley GB, Sheppeard H, Johnson M, et al: The analgesic effects of transcutaneous electrical nerve stimulation and placebo in chronic pain patients. A double-blind non-crossover comparison. Rheumatol Int 1984; 4:119–123.
14. Abelson K, Langley GB, Sheppeard H, et al: Transcutaneous electrical nerve stimulation in rheumatoid arthritis. NZ Med J 1983; 96:156–158.

CHAPTER 17

Methodological Principles for Physical Therapy Research in Arthritis—How to Critically Appraise the Literature

Charles H. Goldsmith, MSc, PhD
Antoine Helewa, MSc(Clin Epid), PT
Joan M. Walker, PhD, PT

This chapter is concerned with the principles needed for reading the clinical literature critically, scoring the literature to decide what is the best thing to do for patients with arthritis, choosing measurements that reflect what is important to the care of patients, and applying the principles of evidence-based care to choose amongst the different research designs that are used in the literature, and identifying research questions. The chapter is directed to the clinician as much as to the researcher.

Physical therapists (PTs) in clinical settings need to rely less on clinical experience, physiological principles, traditional principles, and common sense, and rely more on becoming familiar with systematic observation and applying the rules of evidence to the literature that they read. Current clinical journals are using the structured abstract[1] to present evidence in a systematic way to allow the clinician-reader to judge whether the methods used to generate the results justify their adoption for use in the care of patients. Moncur[2] has identified that an entry-level PT frequently needs to be able to interpret the results of a research project. Also, it would be useful, but not essential, to be able to apply the results of the research to patient care, participate in an ongoing project designed by another investigator, and be able to design and

PHYSICAL THERAPY IN ARTHRITIS, Joan M. Walker, PhD, PT, and Antoine Helewa, MSc(Clin Epid), PT, W.B. Saunders Company © 1996.

conduct an independent clinical investigation to answer frequently asked questions in the physical therapy management of rheumatic disease. To cope with these new realities, a new set of principles need to become part of the toolkit used by PTs.

PTs should become more familiar with systematic observation and applying the rules of evidence to the literature that they read.

The purpose of this chapter is to provide some of these tools for the PT with an interest in keeping up with these developments.

Critical Appraisal of the Literature

A basic principle of research in any discipline is to start with the literature search to find out what others have done before you. Once the literature search is complete, the PT researcher needs to appraise the literature critically to see what is relevant and how sound the methodology was before starting a new research project.

Flaws in the literature that detract from the credibility of the evidence is one justification for conducting another study. Another reason is to ensure that the research question has not already been answered adequately. It is hoped the proposed study would avoid the flaws identified in the work of others and extend the understanding of the principles of PT. Whether reading to judge the efficacy of a therapy, the validity of a diagnostic test, or the quality of an economic analysis for a policy application, determining the quality of the evidence that is derived from a critical appraisal is a necessary step.

Critical appraisal principles are outlined in the first CMAJ series,[3–5] later compiled into a text by Sackett et al,[6] and simplified for clinical use in the JAMA series.[7–15] Those with an interest in evidence-based care may wish to consult a more recent series in CMAJ.[16–22] For example, if a researcher or clinician were to critically appraise a series of PT modality articles selected from the literature, then the six questions about therapy efficacy or effectiveness could be answered Yes or No (or Can't tell), with a 1 for a Yes.[4,6]

1. Was the assignment of patients to treatments really randomized?
2. Were clinically relevant outcomes reported?
3. Were the study patients recognizably similar to your own?
4. Were both statistical significance and clinical importance considered?
5. Is the therapeutic maneuver feasible in your practice?
6. Were all the patients who entered the study accounted for at its conclusion?

The first and sixth questions are listed as the most important in the JAMA series.[10] They could serve as two screening questions for quickly scanning articles. Each question has from one to four additional subquestions to help focus the answer to the main question. A quality score for a therapy efficacy article could vary from a low of 0 to high of 6. High-quality articles may lead to the direct application of the therapy to the patient, while low-quality articles should encourage the search for better evidence or to stimulate research to improve the evidence.

Similarly, for critically appraising a diagnostic test, there are eight questions.[3] These questions help a reader to focus on the relevant issues to judge the evidence prior to using the test to diagnose or assess a patient with arthritis.

1. Was there an independent blind comparison with a gold standard of diagnosis?
2. Was the setting for the study, as well as the filter through which study patients passed, adequately described?
3. Did the patient sample include an appropriate spectrum of mild and severe, treated and untreated, plus individuals with different but commonly confused disorders?
4. Were the tactics for carrying out the test described in sufficient detail to permit their exact replication?
5. Was the reproducibility of the test (precision) and its interpretation (observer variation) determined?
6. Was the term "normal" defined sensibly?
7. If the test is advocated as part of a cluster or sequence of tests, was its contribution to the overall validity of the cluster or sequence determined?
8. Was the utility of the test determined?

Again, if Yes responses are scored 1 while the other responses are scored 0, then a diagnostic test quality score can vary from a low of 0 to high of

8. Applications of these criteria to primary care based on evidence have been published.[16–22]

For example, in Chapter 4, Jones has suggested using an HLA-B27 test to diagnose a patient with ankylosing spondylitis. What is the quality of this diagnostic test from a critical appraisal viewpoint? For the proposed nonsteroidal anti-inflammatory drugs (NSAIDs) listed to manage patients with rheumatoid arthritis (RA), also in Chapter 4, which of them have had a critical appraisal of their efficacy? Was evidence presented to allow you, the reader, to decide whether the six efficacy questions were supported?

Likewise, there are eight questions for critically appraising an economic analysis article.[23] The questions permit a reader or reviewer to become more critical about an economic analysis. As a future manager of a health care facility or advocate for your patients, you may wish to decide whether the therapy was cost-effective for your patients.

1. Was the economic question properly posed?
2. Were alternative programs adequately described?
3. Have the programs' effectiveness been validated?
4. Were all important and relevant costs and effects identified?
5. Were credible measures for the costs and effects selected?
6. Was an appropriate analysis carried out?
7. Were comparisons between programs properly adjusted for time?
8. Were the presence and magnitude of bias identified?

Again, if a 1 is assigned to a Yes response, and 0 to all other responses, then an economic critical appraisal score could vary from a low of 0 to high of 8. In this text, how many authors have given answers to these eight questions for you to decide whether the therapies advocated by these experts are indeed chosen with cost-benefit methods to help the patients with arthritis you treat? Similar questions and guides are available for critically appraising articles on causation, meta-analysis, and prognosis.[6]

Scoring the Physical Therapy Literature

To evaluate the literature, criteria should be established to apply to each study for their selection, scoring and combining to evaluate what new evidence is being sought. While many scoring criteria are published, their ease of use needs to be considered. The criteria for critical appraisal can be used in this way. Tugwell and Goldsmith[24] have shown a set of criteria to score the statistical content of the rheumatology literature of interest to PTs working with patients with arthritis. These criteria contain ten questions that can be answered with a Yes or No (or uncertain), with 1 being assigned to a Yes. The best papers could score as high as 10 while the worst papers would score near 0. The process of creating these criteria, as well as reliability and validity testing, have been conducted on this scale.[25] These biostatistical criteria help a reader or reviewer to determine the quality of the statistical reporting in the article.

1. Was the patient *population* reproducibly described?
2. Was the method of *sampling* the population reproducibly described?
3. Was the *study design* described in sufficient detail to reproduce it?
4. Was the *sample size* justified?
5. Was the *significance level* specified?
6. Was there a description of all *statistical procedures* utilized?
7. Were *at least 80%* of the patients who started the study reported as outcomes in the analysis?
8. Were the statistical *test results* supported by: test value, df, tails and *p* value? **OR** Was a *confidence interval* and its *confidence coefficient* provided?
9. Was a *power* analysis reported for a no-difference conclusion?
10. Were possible *biases* discussed?

Tugwell and Goldsmith[24] applied these criteria to three rheumatology journals: *Journal of Rheumatology, Arthritis and Rheumatism*, and *Scandinavain Journal of Rheumatology*. They showed that 38% of the criteria were satisfied in a sample of 52 articles from the 1982 editions and 40% were satisfied in a sample from the 1991 editions, indicating very little improvement with time. Would the physical therapy (PT) literature be any better?

A clinician/researcher also could use one of the critical appraisal guides discussed earlier to evaluate a sample of papers from the relevant literature. This would help to select the best quality evidence to apply to patients with arthritis.

Measurement Issues in PT

Before conducting a research study in PT, the researcher should decide which outcomes will be collected in the study to measure the responses of interest. Clinicians also should be concerned with the properties of the measurement tools they use to monitor the response of their patients with arthritis, to the care provided. While these measurement issues may be standardized by the previous literature, the researcher has to decide the important issues to build into the measurement system, to provide adequate justification of reliability, validity, and responsiveness appropriate to the study design or clinical setting. The purpose of the exercise is to sort the factors into the *important few* that need to be considered in the design of the study and caring for patients, from the *trivial many* that can be ignored. Figure 17-1 shows the issues needed to generate the components of the measurement process that may be important for the study. The concepts are listed as beginning with the letter **E** to illustrate their importance: Environment, Examinee (patient), Examiner (researcher/clinician), Examination (instrumentation).

In deciding which concepts are important, the factors that may lead to variation from each source by itself should be listed, along with the factors where one component affects the other by looking at each direction (letters A to F on Fig. 17-1); that is, from examiner to examinee (C), as well as, examinee to examiner (D), etc. The concepts then are listed in priority order for the proposed study, and evidence is sought from the literature about whether the effect is important to the measurement. If no information can be found in the literature, then an investigator/clinician will need to conduct a pilot study to decide whether the factors are important. Important factors ("important few") have to be considered in the design of the project or in monitoring patients, while unimportant factors ("trivial many"[26]) can be left as noise in the measurement process.

Use of questions about therapy efficacy or effectiveness, cost-effectiveness, and benefit will help you critically appraise the literature.

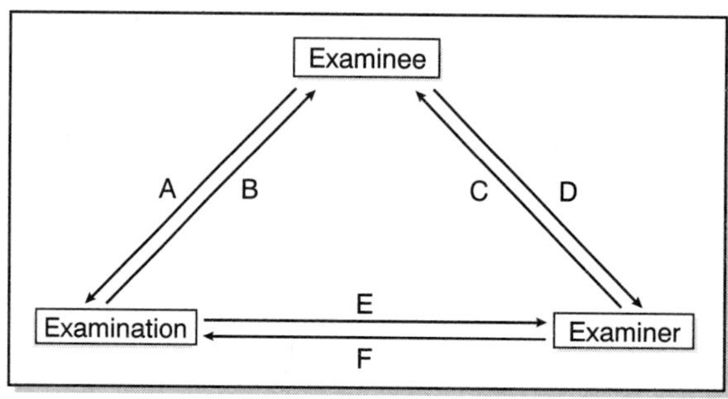

Figure 17-1. The three key ingredients of a measurement situation are enclosed in small boxes inside the larger box representing the Environment. The environment may be an outpatient clinic, a private office, the patient's home, or a public setting. The Examinee is usually a patient or a subject; the Examination is a procedure, instrument or a questionnaire; and the Examiner is generally a physical therapist (PT), but could be the patient or some other blinded observer of the phenomena being measured. The patient (examinee) is at the top of the measurement pyramid, since the patient is the prime focus of care.

When enumerating possible sources of variation, the properties of each boxed **E** need to be enumerated singly, in pairs denoted by the letters **A** to **F**, or all three together by the setting or environment. For example, when measuring RA patients, their disease duration, age, sex, and socioeconomic status may be important; while the tender joint count may be the examination where the number of tender joints is being counted, the scale being used may influence the measurements; while if the Examiner is a PT, the years of experience treating and measuring RA patients, sex, and age may be important to measurement. Considering the ingredients in pairs, such as how the Examinee affects the Examination (**A**) might be the degree of joint destruction, position of patient, or deformities. The letters **B** to **F** are labels to suggest the consideration of the other pairs.

If more than one outcome is chosen to measure the response to therapy, consideration should be given to combining the outcomes in an index with a method such as the pooled index.[23] An index is generally a more sensitive measure of change to detect improvements in patients in the clinical setting, as well as in a research study. This sensitivity leads to detection of clinically important effects on patients with smaller sample sizes.

For example, in Chapter 10, Hanes has discussed various ways of using orthotics to benefit patients. In an evaluation trial of an orthotic device, say a hand splint, on a patient with RA, the measurements might include: (1) patient's perception of pain, (2) wrist range of motion, (3) patient's assessment of fatigue, and (4) grip strength with a modified sphygmomanometer. Each of these measurements would need to be investigated for their measurement properties, to assess which features need to be considered in the study design. For example, after choosing a 10-cm Visual Analogue Scale (VAS) for the patient to mark after the therapy, the researcher should consider whether anchors, such as "pain as bad as it could be" to "pain free," might be used on each end of the VAS.

Will giving the patient the baseline assessment before the therapy began reduce the variation due to measurement, and should baseline assessment be used in the design?

The multiplicity of measurements may be handled by making one measurement the primary outcome. Another way is to combine each of the measures with an index, such as with a pooled index.[23] A pooled index also is more efficient for combining standardized benefits to the patient over the therapy time, provided each measure of benefit with a low correlation outcome is included. Here, a pooled index is an arithmetic mean of standardized component changes that make a pooled index. Helewa et al[27] found that a pooled index using five measures of patient benefit was more efficient than any one measure of the benefit of PT in patients with rheumatoid arthritis.

Strengths and Weaknesses of Designs for PT Studies

Case series can give an alert clinician/researcher an idea worth pursuing for a study. A case series is relatively easy to gather, particularly if the clinical setting keeps good records. However, without a protocol or a comparison group, a group treated with a therapy cannot give an estimate of the effect of treatment unless no effect is the norm with all other therapies.

A better design is the ***case-control design*** where a group of cases is compared with a group of noncases (controls) to determine whether various etiologic factors including therapy played a role in the formation of the particular case group. Where it does, the case-control study is quickly done, provided the spectrum of etiologic factors is measured in the data base being studied. However, record systems are usually designed for managing patients, and not for studies, so the attention to measurement issues, such as consistency of recorder, standardization of measurements, and other details that are controlled in prospective studies, are often lacking in a case-control study.

Most often, however, a prospective creation of groups that are followed along from inception to outcome is a preferred design, the ***cohort design***. When the allocation of patients to experimental or control groups is done by ***randomization*** to balance known and unknown factors that may be confounded with the experimental/control outcome difference, the design is a ***randomized controlled trial*** (**RCT**). Without the benefit of randomization, the cohort design is open to allocation biases that may be confounded with the experimental/control outcome difference; while the RCT does not have this defect. The prospective collection of data under the control of the investigator also ensures more complete data and more standardized recording.

> ***Randomization*** **of patients or subjects to groups is important to balance known and unknown factors that may be confounded with the experimental/control outcome difference.**

It is sometimes possible to run an entire experiment within a single patient with an *N-of-1* design. Again, randomization is important with this design as it would be with a group of patients in an RCT.[28]

For example, in Chapter 4, were the results suggested for the therapies to manage patients with osteoarthritis tested with RCTs, or did the evidence come from a case series or a cohort design? Indeed no, only the opinion of the authors. Were the results from the therapies for patients with RA using the outcomes suggested by the ACR[29] for evaluating therapies for patients with RA? If so, did multiple outcomes get reported, or were the results from the seven or eight outcomes combined to some form of an index? Indeed, no, the results were reported separately.

Research Questions

A *research question* should clearly state five things: What is the maneuver being evaluated, the type of evaluation, in which patients, the minimum criterion for success, and be answerable with a Yes or No. For example, "Does heat applied for 20 minutes to the neck of a patient with RA improve range of motion by at least 20 degrees?" Here, heat is the maneuver, range of motion is the evaluation, the patient has rheumatoid arthritis, and the criterion for success is at least 20 degrees. If a study shows these results, then the answer is Yes, while if the study does not, the answer is No. Another question is: "Does isometric exercise applied to the quadriceps of patients with RA improve isometric muscle strength by at least 60 mm Hg?" This also has the ingredients to be a good question. However, "Are patients better off with physical therapy?" is not a good research question, since we do not know which maneuver is included in physical therapy, the outcome being evaluated is not specified, the type of patients is not specified, and the minimum criterion for success is not specified.

Conclusion

The focus of this chapter has been to cover the basic principles needed for a PT, either clinician or researcher, to keep abreast with current and new therapy, assess the current literature, recognize common designs of research studies, and formulate research questions. The principles can be applied in typical clinical settings and by the researcher who is faced with selecting a sound research question and reviewing the literature to obtain research funding from a granting agency.

References

1. Ad Hoc Working Group for Critical Appraisal of the Medical Literature: A proposal for more informative abstracts of clinical articles. Ann Intern Med 1987; 106:598–604.
2. Moncur C: Physical therapy competencies in rheumatology. Phys Ther 1985; 65:1365–1372.

First CMAJ Series.

3. Department of Clinical Epidemiology & Biostatistics: How to read clinical journals: II. To learn about a diagnostic test. Can Med Assoc J 1981; 124:703–710.
4. Department of Clinical Epidemiology & Biostatistics: How to read clinical journals: V. To distinguish useful from useless or even harmful therapy. Can Med Assoc J 1981; 124:1156–1162.
5. Department of Clinical Epidemiology and Biostatistics: How to read clinical journals: VII. To understand an economic evaluation. Can Med Assoc J 1984; 130:1428–1433(part A), 1542–1549(part B).

6. Sackett DL, Haynes RB, Guyatt GH, et al (eds): Clinical Epidemiology. A Basic Science for Clinical Medicine, 2nd edition. Boston, Little, Brown & Co, 1991.

JAMA Series

7. Evidence-Based Medicine Working Group: Evidence-based medicine: a new approach to teaching the practice of medicine. JAMA 1992; 268: 2420–2425.
8. Guyatt GH, Rennie D: Users' guides to the medical literature. JAMA 1993; 270(17):2096–2097.
9. Oxman AD, Sackett DL, Guyatt GH, for the Evidence-Based Medicine Working Group: Users' guides to the medical literature: I. How to get started. JAMA 1993; 270(17):2093–2095.
10. Guyatt GH, Sackett DL, Cook DJ, for the Evidence-Based Medicine Working Group: Users' guides to the medical literature: II. How to use an article about therapy or prevention. A. Are the results of the study valid? JAMA 1993; 270(21):2598–2601.
11. Guyatt GH, Sackett DL, Cook DJ, for the Evidence-Based Medicine Working Group: Users' guides to the medical literature: II. How to use an article about therapy or prevention. B. What were the results and will they help me in caring for my patients? JAMA 1994; 271(1):59–63.
12. Jaeschke R, Guyatt GH, Sackett DL, for the Evidence-Based Medicine Working Group: Users' guides to the medical literature: III. How to use an article about a diagnostic test. A. Are the results of the study valid? JAMA 1994; 271(5):389–391.
13. Jaeschke R, Guyatt GH, Sackett DL, for the Evidence-Based Medicine Working Group: Users' guides to the medical literature: III. How to use an article about a diagnostic test. B. What were the results and will they help me in caring for my patients? JAMA 1994; 271(9):703–707.
14. Levine MAH, Walter SD, Lee H, et al, for the Evidence-Based Working Group: Users' guides to the medical literature: IV. How to use an article about harm. JAMA 1994; 271(20):1615–1619.

15. Laupacis A, Wells G, Richardson WS, Tugwell P, for the Evidence-Based Medicine Working Group: Users' guides to the medical literature: V. How to use an article about prognosis. JAMA 1994; 272(3): 234–237.

Second CMAJ Series

16. Squires BP: Evidence-based care. Can Med Assoc J 1994; 150(8):1191.
17. For the Evidence-Based Care Group: Evidence-Based Care: 1. Setting priorities: how important is the problem? Can Med Assoc J 1994; 150(8):1249–1254.
18. For the Evidence-Based Care Group: Evidence-Based Care: 2. Setting guidelines: how should we manage this problem? Can Med Assoc J 1994; 150(9): 1417–1423.
19. For the Evidence-Based Care Group: Evidence-Based Care: 3. Measuring performance: how are we managing this problem? Can Med Assoc J 1994; 150(10): 1575–1579.
20. For the Evidence-Based Care Group: Evidence-Based Care: 4. Improving performance: how can we improve the way we manage this problem? Can Med Assoc J 1994; 150(11):1793–1796.
21. For the Evidence-Based Care Group: Evidence-Based Care: 5. Lifelong learning: how can we learn to be more effective? Can Med Assoc J 1994; 150(12): 1971–1973.
22. Rafuse J: Evidence-based medicine means MDs must develop new skills, attitudes, CMA conference told. Can Med Assoc J 1994; 150(9):1479–1481.

Other References

23. Goldsmith CH, Smythe HA, Helewa A: Interpretation and power of a pooled index. J Rheumatol 1993; 20:575–578.
24. Tugwell PSL, Goldsmith CH: Science of rheumatic disease management. In Klippel JH, Dieppe PA (eds): Rheumatology, pp 2.1–8. London, Mosby-Year Book Europe Ltd, 1994.
25. Goldsmith CH, Russell DR: Biostatistical critical appraisal: how to read the rheumatology literature critically. Unpublished Manuscript. McMaster University 1983–12–19. [Copies available on request].
26. Juran JM: Juran on Quality by Design: The New Steps for Planning Quality into Goods and Services. Toronto, Maxwell Macmillan Canada, 1992.
27. Helewa A, Smythe HA, Goldsmith CH: Can specially trained physiotherapists improve the care of patients with rheumatoid arthritis? A randomized health care trial. J Rheumatol 1994; 21:70–79.
28. Guyatt GH, Sackett DL, Taylor DW, et al: Determining optimal therapy—randomized trials in individual patients. N Engl J Med 1986; 314:889–892.
29. Felson DT, Anderson JJ, Boers M, et al: The American College of Rheumatology preliminary core set of disease activity measures for use in rheumatoid arthritis clinical trials. Arthritis Rheum 1993; 36(6): 729–740.

APPENDIX I

Resources

Educational Materials

A. For Children

Fun workbooks that can help children understand.

1. Falco JL, Block DV, Vostrejs MD, et al: *JRA and Me—A Fun Workbook*. Atlanta, GA, Rocky Mountain Juvenile Arthritis Center, Arthritis Foundation, 1987.
   For school aged children, contains puzzles, games, worksheets (US$6.73).
2. Isenberg B, Jaffe M: *Albert the Running Bear's Exercise Book*. New York, Clarion Books, 1984.
3. Labelle M, Racine N, St-Cyr C: *Arthritis and Me—JRA Coloring Book*. Quebec, Hopital Saint-Justine Occupational Therapy Services, 1992.
4. Reichbecker L, et al: *The Arthritis Coloring Book: A Guide for Children and Their Families*. Houston, TX, Texas Children's Hospital, 1981.

B. For Parents and Teachers

Materials with a self-help focus.

1. Arthritis Foundation: *We Can: A Guide for Parents of Children with Arthritis*, Atlanta, GA, The Arthritis Foundation, 1992 (US$3.55).
2. Arthritis Foundation: *Arthritis and Children*, 40 pp. Atlanta, GA, The Arthritis Foundation, AJAO, 1993 (single copies free).
3. Arthritis Foundation: *When Your Student has Arthritis, Guide for Teachers*, 18 pp. Atlanta, GA, The Arthritis Foundation, AJAO, 1992.
4. Brewer EJ, Angel KC: *Parenting a Child with Arthritis*, Los Angeles, CA, Lowell House, 1990.
5. Erson T: *Courageous Pacers—The Complete Guide to Running, Walking and Fitness for Kids*. Corpus Christi, TX, Pro-Activ Publications, 1993.
6. Featherstone H: *A Difference in the Family—Living with a Disabled Child*. England, Penguin Books, 1980.
7. Lazzarotto L, O'Brien C: *Children with Arthritis in Your Classrooms*. The Hugh MacMillan Rehabilitation Center, 350 Rumsey Rd, Toronto, Ontario, Canada M4G 1R8.
8. NASA: *Juvenile AS Booklet*. Los Angeles, CA, National Ankylosing Spondylitis Association.
   An overview for parents on AS in persons under 17.
9. Parker EH: *A Parent's Guide to Better Understanding of JRA. A Guidebook*. Southern California Chapter, Medical Dept, 4311 Wilshire Blvd Suite 350, Los Angeles, CA 90010, 81 pp (US$4).
10. Ziebell B: *As Normal as Possible*. Atlanta, GA, The Arthritis Foundation.
11. Southern Arizona Chapter, "*A Child's View of the World*," 6464 East Grant Rd, Tucson, AZ 85715, 60 pp. 1976.

C. For Health Professionals on Juvenile Arthritis

Kovalesky A, et al: *Understanding Juvenile Arthritis. A Health Professional's Guide to Teaching Children*

PHYSICAL THERAPY IN ARTHRITIS, Joan M. Walker, PhD, PT, and Antoine Helewa, MSc(Clin Epid), PT, W.B. Saunders Company © 1996.

and Parents. Atlanta, GA, Arthritis Foundation, 1988 (US$61.20).
Large binder covering all aspects of care, designed so material can be copied and given to parents.

D. For Adults

1. Aladjem H: *Understanding Lupus.* New York, Macmillan Publishing Co, 1985.
"Extremely comprehensive and authoritative; some information only relevant to Americans . . . possibly of more interest to health professionals," Arthritis Foundation.
2. Alexander D: *Arthritis and Common Sense.* New York, Simon & Schuster, Inc, 1954/1981.
"Best example of all that is wrong with information available to patients . . . in general, the text could lead to erroneous ideas and actions," Arthritis Foundation.
3. American Physical Therapy Association, Department of Information Services: *Arthritis Education Resource Guide,* 1111 North Fairfax St, Alexandria, VA 22314-1488, Phone: 800-999-2782 EXT 3219. Quinn P: Bibliography on Arthritis, 1993.
Contains addresses of organizations, publishers' addresses of arthritis materials and articles previously in published in Physical Therapy *and* Clinical Management. *Lists of Grants for Patients and Organizations dealing with arthritis.*
4. Blau S, Schultz D: *Lupus: The Body Against Itself.* New York, Doubleday Co, Inc, 1984.
"Well written and informed," Arthritis Foundation.
5. Brown TM, Scammell H: *The Road Back,* New York, M Evan Co, Inc, 1988.
The Arthritis Foundation considers it "does not give a balanced view of knowledge about rheumatoid arthritis . . . may be confusing to the patient."
6. Davidson P: *Chronic Muscle Pain Syndrome,* Ontario, Villard Books Inc, Random House of Canada, 1990.
Written by an M.D. generally useful with some concerns about authors' theories and opinions, Arthritis Foundation.
7. Ediger B: *Coping with Fibromyalgia,* Toronto, FM Facts, 1991.
Generally clear and useful.
8. Ellert G: *Arthritis and Exercise: A User's Guide to Fitness and Independence.* Vancouver, Trelle Enterprises Inc, 1985.
Written in consultation with G Parker, PT; a practical guide covering most types of exercises.
9. Fries JF: *Arthritis: A Comprehensive Guide to Understanding Your Arthritis.* Ontario, Addison-Wesley Publishing, 1986.
Factual information for readers with average education.
10. Gairdner J: *Fitness for People with Rheumatoid Arthritis.* Markham, Ontario, Fitzhenry & Whiteside Ltd, 1986.
Not in depth but generally "information is accurate and advice appropriate," Arthritis Foundation.
11. Lorig K, Fries JF: *The Arthritis Helpbook.* Don Mills, Ontario, Addison-Wesley Publishing, 1990.
Text used in arthritis self-management programs offered in USA, Australia, New Zealand, Canada. Six-week program with sessions 2 hours a week, taught in classes of 10–14 people. Sessions are led by trained volunteers. Teaches individuals to become an arthritis self manager.
12. Phillips RH: *Coping with Rheumatoid Arthritis.* New York, Avery Publishing Group, Inc, 1988.
General reading, comprehensive.
13. Pitzele SK: *We Are Not Alone: Learning to Live with Chronic Illness.* New York, Workman Publishing, 1986.
"Written by a lupus sufferer . . . comprehensive and inspirational," Arthritis Foundation.
14. Sayce V, Fraser I: *Exercise Beats Arthritis.* An Easy-to-Follow Programme of Exercises, 2nd edition. London, Thorsons, 1991.
15. Sayce V, Fraser I: *Exercise Can Beat Your Arthritis: A Guide to Overcoming Arthritis.* New York, Avery Publishing Group, Inc, 1988.
16. Sobel D: *Arthritis: What Works.* New York, St. Martin's Press, 1991.
Based on a survey not true research.

Exercise

1. ARRTC: *Good Moves for Everybody.* Exercise videotape. Arthritis Rehabilitation Research & Training Center, Columbia, University of Missouri. (Order from: Arthritis Center ATTN: Exercise Video, MA 427 Health Sciences Center, University of Mis-

souri, Columbia, MO 65212 [US$30.00 ppd]).

2. Arthritis Society / Foundation Recreational Exercise programs Aquatics Programs (AFYAP/AFAP and Plus), *PACE*—land-based program, Joint Efforts.
3. Arthritis Foundation: *Arthritis Self-management Course.*
   Contact your local Arthritis Foundation or Society Chapter office for local programs and training opportunities.
4. Arthritis Foundation: *Pool Exercise Program (PEP)*. Exercise video. (Order from: Cox Entertainment, PO Box 23451, Pleasant Hill, CA 94523 [US$33.95 ppd].)
5. Ellert G: *Arthritis and Exercise: A User's Guide to Fitness and Independence*, Vancouver, Trelle Enterprises Inc, 1985.
6. Erson T: *Courageous Pacers—The Complete Guide to Running, Walking and Fitness for Kids*. Corpus Christi, TX, Pro-Activ Publications, 1993.
7. Francis L, Francis P: *A Pre-aerobic Exercise Program*. San Diego State University, supported by Reebok International, Avon, MA 02322.
8. Francis PR, Francis L: *If it Hurts Don't Do It: Tune Up Your Body for Pain-Free, Injury-Free Life Long Fitness*, 161 pp. Rocklin, CA, Prima Publishing and Communications, 1988.
9. Jetter J, Kadlec N: *The Arthritis Book of Water Exercise*. London, Granada, 1985.
10. Krasevec JA, Grimes DC: *HydroRobics®: A Water Exercise Program for Individuals of all Ages and Fitness Levels*, 2nd edition, 224 pp. West Point, NY, Leisure Press, 1985.
11. Lorig K, Fries JF: *The Arthritis Helpbook*, 3rd edition, Don Mills, Ontario, Addison-Wesley Publishing, 1990.
12. Rockport Walking Institute: *The Rockport Fitness Walking Test*. Rockport Walking Institute, 72 Howe Street, Marlboro, MA 01752.
13. ROM Institute: *ROM Dance: A Range of Motion Exercise and Relaxation Program*. Instructional materials and training available. ROM Institute, New Ventures of Wisconsin Inc, 3601 Memorial Drive, Madison, WI 53704.
14. Sayce V, Fraser I: *Exercise Can Beat Your Arthritis: A Guide to Overcoming Arthritis*. New York, Avery Publishing Group, Inc, 1988.
15. Sayce V, Fraser I: *Exercise Beats Arthritis. An Easy-to-Follow Programme of Exercises*, 2nd edition. London, Thorsons, 1991.
16. Sobel D, Klein AC: *What Exercises Work*. New York, St. Martin's Press, 1993.

Periodicals

1. *Arthritis To-day*. Bimonthly magazine available from the Arthritis Foundation and its chapters with $20(US) or more membership donation.
2. *Arthritis News*. Quarterly publication of The Arthritis Society, 250 Bloor St E, Suite 901, Toronto, ON M4W 3P2; annual subscription $10(CAN).
3. *AS NEWS*. Quarterly publication of the Ankylosing Spondylitis Association (USA). Ankylosing Spondylitis Association, 511 N La Cienega #216, Los Angeles, CA 90048.
4. *Living with Arthritis*. Monthly newsletter published by the Association for People with Arthritis, PO Box 954, 6 Commercial Street, Hicksville, NY 11802 (1-800-323-2243).

Peer-Reviewed Journals

Annals of Rheumatic Diseases
Arthritis and Rheumatism (Arthritis Foundation)
Bulletin on Rheumatic Diseases (ARF, New York)
Current Therapy in Allergy, Immunology (formerly *Current Therapy in Allergy, Immunology and Rheumatology*)
Journal of Rheumatology
Reports on Rheumatic Diseases. Topical Reviews. "Series 2" (ARC for Research, Great Britain)
Reports on Rheumatic Diseases. Practical Problems. "Series 2" (ARC for Research, Great Britain)
Rheumatic Diseases/Reports on Rheumatic Diseases (ARF, London)
Scandinavian Journal of Rheumatology. Supplement/Acta Rheumatologica Scandinavica. Supplement (Sweden)
Scandinavian Journal of Rheumatology/Acta Rheumatologica Scandinavica
British Journal of Rheumatology; Experimental Rheumatology; Arthritis Care and Research (AHPA); *Rheumatology International; Seminars in Arthritis*

Organizations

1. **The Arthritis Foundation**
   1314 Spring Street NW, Atlanta, GA 30309
   Phone: 404-872-7100 FAX: 404-872-0457
   For Publications: PO Box 19000-Drawer A1, Atlanta, GA 30326
   Phone: 1-800-283-7800
   Offers a rich variety of resources of general information, advocacy, children, services, treatments, types of arthritis. Single copies available from state chapters, bulk orders to the Foundation, some items at lower cost to members, some materials in other languages.
2. **American Juvenile Arthritis Organization**
   1314 Spring Street NW, Atlanta, GA 30309, Contact: Linda Wetherbee.
   Advocacy group for all interested in JRA.
3. **American Lupus Society**
   East 2617 Columbia Ave, Spokane, WA 99207
4. **Arthritis Health Professions Association**
   1314 Spring Street NW, Atlanta, GA 30309
   Phone: 404-872-7100
   Multidisciplinary professional organization concerned with all issues related to arthritis, conducts national and regional meetings.
5. **Arthritis Society**
   National office, 250 Bloor Street East, Suite 901, Toronto, Ontario, M4W 3P2
   FAX: 416-967-7171
   Phone: 1-800-361-1112 (Ontario only)
   Phone (Ontario Division: 416-967-5679)
   Addresses of provincial offices may be obtained from the National Office.
6. **Arthritis Foundation of Australia**
   National Office, P.O. Box 121, Sydney, NSW 2001, Australia
   Phone: (02) 221-2456.
7. **Arthritis Foundation of New Zealand**
   National Office, P.O. Box 10-020, Wellington, New Zealand
   Phone: (04) 721-427.
8. **Lupus Canada**
   040-635 6th Ave SW, Calgary, Alberta T2P 0T5
   Phone: 1-800-265-4613.
   Branches in ten provinces providing information and support.
9. **Lupus Foundation of America**
   1717 Massachusetts Ave NW, Suite 203, Washington, DC 20036
   Phone: 202-328-4550
10. **National Osteoporosis Association**
    2100 M Street NW, Suite 602, Washington, DC 20037
    Phone: 202-223-2226
11. **Osteoporosis Society of Canada**
    Box 280, Station Q, Toronto, ON M4T 2M1
12. **Silver Ring Splint Company**
    P.O. Box 2856, Charlottesville, VA 22902
    Phone: (804) 971-4052, FAX: (804) 971-8828
    Contact local occupational therapists who may have the measuring kit.

Spondylitis Associations

Canada: Ontario Spondylitis Association (five chapters), Ankylosing Spondylitis Association of British Columbia, Manitoba Ankylosing Spondylitis Association.
For addresses contact The Arthritis Society (see above).
United States of America: Ankylosing Spondylitis Association, 511 N La Cienega #216, Los Angeles, CA 90048. Phone (310) 652–0609.
Contact for addresses of state support groups (29 states). Supplies educational materials, patient guidebook, videos, publishes a quarterly AS NEWS.

United Kingdom offices of Arthritis & Rheumatism Council for Research (ARC)

ARC, Copeman House, St. Mary's Gate, Chesterfield, Derbys, England, S41 7TD Phone (44) (011) 246-558033
ARC, 17 Cleland Park South, Bangor, County Down, N Ireland BT20 3EW
ARC, P.O. Box 304, Swanea, Wales SA1 1W2
ARC, 140 High Street, Lochee, Dundee, Scotland DD2 3BZ

Audiovisual Materials

1. AHPA Arthritis Teaching Slide Collection. The Arthritis Foundation, 294 slides and instruction guide (US$250, $150 members).
2. ARRTC: Good Moves for Everybody. Exercise videotape. Arthritis Rehabilitation Research & Training Center, Columbia,

University of Missouri (see **Exercise** section).

3. Arthritis Foundation: Pool Exercise Program (PEP) (see **Exercise** section)
4. Arthritis Foundation: PACE People with Arthritis Can Exercise. 2 videocassetes, Parts 1 & 11. Order: 1-800-PACE-236, in Virginia 1-703-391-7896.
5. Arthritis Foundation: In Control (#9035). 68-minute videotape with optional book and audiocassetes. Arthritis Foundation.
6. Arthritis Foundation: Living with Arthritis (#9037). 60-minute videotape.
7. Jassom: Age-Related Physical Therapy Programs. Atlanta, GA, Arthritis Foundation, 1984.
8. NASA: The Water Workout-Exercise Video, 1/2″ VHS, National Ankylosing Spondylitis Association, Los Angeles, CA.
9. NASA: Fight Back Exercise Video, 35 min VHS, National Ankylosing Spondylitis Association, Los Angeles, CA.
10. Vostrejs, MD: Aquonastics. Denver, CO, National Jewish Center for Immunology and Respiratory Medicine, 1986.

APPENDIX II

Competency Statements for Physical Therapy Management of Arthritis

(From Moncur C: Physical Therapy Competencies. In Banwell BF, Gall V [eds]: Physical Therapy Management of Arthritis, pp 34–39. New York, Churchill Livingstone Inc, 1988. With permission.)

Table 1. Competency Statements

Basic Knowledge

The entry-level physical therapist (PT) should be able to make decisions regarding screening and the need for specific evaluation techniques based on a basic knowledge of the following:

1. Pathophysiology of the common forms of rheumatic disease
2. Progression of the common forms of rheumatic disease
3. Medication regimen, side effects, and speed of efficacy
4. Impact of rheumatic disease on all phases of the patient's life
5. Common types of surgery, precautions for treatment, and the process of tissue healing

Patient Evaluation

The entry-level PT should be able to perform physical therapy assessment procedures on the patient with arthritis including an evaluation of the patient as follows:

1. Ambulation and transfer status
2. Skin and vascular condition
3. Neurologic signs
4. Knowledge of the disease and the treatment regimen
5. Ability to cope with the chronicity of the illness
6. Pain status
7. Swelling and/or synovitis of joints
8. Muscle strength
9. Deformity and joint stability
10. Respiratory function
11. Fatigue and endurance levels
12. Morning stiffness and joint gelling
13. Dexterity
14. Personal care
15. Home conditions
16. Ability to participate in recreational activities
17. Ability to fulfill an occupational role
18. Workplace conditions

Designing a Physical Therapy Plan of Care

The entry-level PT should be able to design a plan of care based upon the results of the physical therapy evaluation including the following patient information:

1. History
2. Goals, expectations, and motivation
3. Pain and/or tolerance for activity
4. Deficits in muscle strength
5. Status of joint deformities (fixed versus correctable)
6. Deficits in functional activities
7. Activity of the disease (flare versus remission)
8. Potential problems which could develop due to the disease or the patient's life style
9. Ambulation status
10. Ability to rest
11. Tolerance for physical therapy modalities
12. Need for adaptive and orthotic equipment

The entry-level physical therapist also should be able to do the following:

1. Recognize and respond to changes in the patient's physiologic status
2. Recognize and respond to changes in the patient's ability to cope with the disease
3. Continue, modify, or discontinue physical therapy and/or goals when necessary
4. Design a discharge plan of care and home program based upon the results of periodic physical therapy reassessment

Implementing a Physical Therapy Plan of Care

The entry-level PT should be able to implement these programs:

1. A therapeutic exercise program for the patient with arthritis-related problems
2. An ambulation program for the patient with arthritis-related problems
3. A pain management program
4. An activities for daily living program for the patient with arthritis-related problems
5. A joint protection and energy conservation training program
6. Relate the hospital and/or clinic treatment program to a home management program
7. Recommend solutions for adapting the patient's home and work environment

Patient Compliance

The entry-level PT should be able to enhance the patient's compliance to the physical therapy regimen as follows:

Table 1. (*Continued*)

1. Determine the patient's expectations about the physical therapy
2. Determine treatment goals of the patient and physical therapist
3. Design a treatment program that has simplicity in terms of numbers of exercises/tasks the patient must do and that transfers to the patient's life situation
4. Establish that the patient knows what is expected by having him or her repeat or demonstrate what has been instructed
5. Provide written instructions for home programs
6. Interpret and respond appropriately to the nonverbal message of patients

Patient, Family, and Community Education

The entry-level PT should be able to design and implement patient education strategies including the following:

1. Lectures
2. Leading discussions
3. Individualizing instruction
4. Programmed learning programs
5. Leading practice skills and activities
6. Role-playing techniques
7. Imitating correct behavior

The entry-level PT should be able to instruct the patient and family in the proper use of the following:

1. Therapeutic exercise and activity
2. Joint protection
3. Energy conservation
4. Therapeutic electrical equipment (transcutaneous electrical nerve stimulation [TENS], biofeedback, etc)
5. Traction
6. Therapeutic massage
7. Therapeutic heat and cold
8. Orthotic devices and supports

The therapist should be able to instruct the patient:

1. And the family about the nature and progression of the type of arthritis the patient has
2. And the family about community resources available to them
3. And the family about the hazards of unproven remedies
4. Appropriately about physical/sexual problems related to contractures, deformities, and postoperative joint replacement.

The entry-level PT should be able to:

1. Design and implement a community education program about physical therapy and arthritis
2. Select and refer the patient to other health professionals for treatment, education, and/or utilization of community resources

Research Activities

The entry-level PT should be able to:

1. Interpret the results of a research project
2. Apply the results of the research to patient care
3. Participate in an ongoing project designed by another investigator
4. Design and carry out an independent clinical investigation to answer a frequently arising question in physical therapy management of rheumatic disease

Table 2. Domain 1. Basic Knowledge

Competency Statement	Decision
The entry-level PT should be able to make decisions regarding screening and the need for specific evaluation techniques based on a *basic* knowledge of the following:	
1. Impact of rheumatic disease on all phases of the patient's life	Absolutely essential
2. Pathophysiology of the common forms of rheumatic disease	Frequently essential
3. Medication regimen, side effects, and speed of efficacy	Frequently essential
4. Progression of the common forms of rheumatic disease	Frequently essential
5. Common types of surgery, precautions for treatment, and the process of tissue healing	Frequently essential

Table 3. Domain 2. Patient Evaluation

Competency Statement	Decision
The entry-level PT should be able to perform physical therapy assessment procedures on the patient with arthritis including an evaluation of the patient's:	
1. Ambulation and/or transfer status	Absolutely essential
2. Knowledge of the disease and treatment regimen	Absolutely essential
3. Pain status	Absolutely essential
4. Swelling/synovitis	Absolutely essential
5. Muscle strength	Absolutely essential
6. Deformity/joint instability	Absolutely essential
7. Joint range of motion	Absolutely essential
8. Fatigue/endurance	Absolutely essential
9. Skin and vascular conditions	Frequently essential
10. Neurologic signs	Frequently essential
11. Ability to cope with chronic disease	Frequently essential
12. Respiratory function	Frequently essential
13. Morning stiffness/joint gelling	Frequently essential
14. Dexterity	Frequently essential
15. Personal care	Frequently essential
16. Home conditions	Frequently essential
17. Recreational activities	Frequently essential
18. Ability to fulfill occupational role	Frequently essential
19. Workplace	Frequently essential

Table 4. Domain 3. Designing a Plan of Care

Competency Statement	Decision
The entry-level PT should be able to design a plan of care based on the results of the physical therapy evaluation. The plan should include a data base of the patient's:	
1. History	Absolutely essential
2. Goals, expectations, and motivation	Absolutely essential
3. Pain and/or tolerance level	Absolutely essential
4. Deficits in muscle strength	Absolutely essential
5. Status of joint deformities (fixed versus correctable)	Absolutely essential
6. Deficits in functional abilities	Absolutely essential
7. Activity of the disease (flare versus remission)	Absolutely essential
8. Ambulation status	Absolutely essential
9. Ability to rest	Absolutely essential
10. Tolerance for physical therapy modalities	Absolutely essential
11. Need for adaptive and orthotic equipment	Absolutely essential
The entry-level PT should be able to:	
1. Recognize and respond to changes in the patient's physiologic status	Absolutely essential
2. Continue, modify, or discontinue the physical therapy goals and/or treatment when necessary	Absolutely essential
3. Design a plan of care and home program based upon the results of periodic physical therapy reassessment	Absolutely essential
4. Recognize and respond to changes in the patient's abilities to cope with the disease	Frequently essential
5. Include in the data base for the plan of care any potential problems which could develop due to the disease or the patient's life style.	Frequently essential

Table 5. Domain 4. Implementing a Plan of Care

Competency Statement	Decision
The entry-level PT should be able to implement:	
1. A therapeutic exercise program for the patient with arthritis-related problems	Absolutely essential
2. An ambulation program for the patient with arthritis-related problems	Absolutely essential
3. A pain management program	Frequently essential
4. An activities for daily living for the patient with arthritis-related problems	Frequently essential
5. Identify and recommend solutions for adapting the patient's home and work environment	Frequently essential
6. Relate the hospital and/or clinic treatment program to a home management problem	Frequently essential
7. Select and refer the patient to other health professionals for treatment, education, and/or utilization of community resources	Frequently essential

Table 6. Domain 5. Patient Compliance

Competency Statement	Decision
The entry-level PT should be able to enhance the patient's compliance to the physical therapy regimen by:	
1. Determining the patient's expectations about the physical therapy plan of care	Absolutely essential
2. Determining a treatment program based on the mutual goals of the patient and the therapist	Absolutely essential
3. Designing a treatment program that has simplicity in terms of the numbers of exercises/tasks the patient must do and that transfers to the patient's life situation	Absolutely essential
4. Establishing that patients know what is expected to be done by having them repeat or demonstrate what was instructed	Absolutely essential
5. Providing written instructions for home programs	Absolutely essential
6. Interpreting & responding appropriately to the nonverbal messages of the patient	Frequently essential

Table 7. Domain 6. Patient, Family, and Community Education

Competency Statement	Decision
The entry-level PT should be able to:	
1. Design and implement patient education strategies	Absolutely essential
2. Individualize instruction	Absolutely essential
3. Instruct the patient in the proper use of: Therapeutic exercises and activity Joint protection Energy conservation Therapeutic heat and cold	Absolutely essential
4. Lecture	Frequently essential
5. Lead discussions	Frequently essential
6. Imitate correct behavior	Frequently essential
7. Do programmed learning	Frequently essential
8. Lead practice skills and activities	Frequently essential
9. Instruct the patient and family in the proper use of: Therapeutic electrical equipment (TENS), biofeedback, etc Traction Therapeutic massage Orthotic devices and supports	Frequently essential
10. Instruct the patient and the family about the nature and progression of the type of arthritis the patient has	Frequently essential
11. Instruct the patient and the family about community resources available to them	Frequently essential
12. Instruct the patient and the family about the hazards of unproven remedies	Frequently essential
13. Instruct the patient appropriately about physical sexual problems related to contractures, deformities, and postoperative joint replacements	Frequently essential
14. Lead peer-group discussions	Useful, but not essential
15. Use role-play techniques	Useful, but not essential
16. Design and implement a community education program about physical therapy and arthritis	Useful, but not essential

Table 8. Domain 7. Research Activities

Competency Statement	Decision
Given a patient with a diagnosis of one of the common forms of arthritis, such as rheumatoid or osteoarthritis, the entry-level physical therapist should be able to:	
1. Apply the results of the research to patient care	Frequently essential
2. Interpret the results of a research project	Useful, but not essential
3. Participate in an ongoing project designed by another investigator	Useful, but not essential
4. Design and carry out an independent clinical investigation to answer a frequently arising question in PT management of arthritis	Useful, but not essential

APPENDIX III

Assessment Instruments and Outcome Measures

1. **Independent Measure of Functional Capacity (IMFC).** From Helewa A, Goldsmith CH, Smythe HA: Independent measurement of functional capacity in rheumatoid arthritis. J Rheumatol 1982; 9(5):794–797. With permission.
2. **Fibromyalgia Impact Questionnaire (FIQ).** From Burckhardt CS, Clark SR, Bennett RM: The Fibromyalgia Impact Questionnaire: development and validation. J Rheumatol 1991; 18:728–733. With permission.
3. **McMaster Toronto Arthritis Patient Preference Disability Questionnaire (MACTAR).** From Tugwell P, Bombardier C, Buchanan WW, Goldsmith CH, Grace E, Hanna B: The MACTAR Patient Preference Disability Questionnaire—an individualized functional priority approach for assessing improvement in physical disability in clinical trials in rheumatoid arthritis. J Rheumatol 1987; 14:446–451. With permission.
4. **Western Ontario and McMaster Universities Osteoarthritis Index (WOMAC)-VA3.0.** From Bellamy N, Buchanan WW, Goldsmith CH, Campbell J, Stitt LW: Validation study of WOMAC: a health status instrument for measuring clinically important patient relevant outcomes to anti-rheumatic drug therapy in patients with osteoarthritis of the hip or knee. J Rheumatol 1988; 15: 1833–1840. With permission.
5. **Health Assessment Questionnaire for Spondyloarthropathies (HAQ-S).** From Daltroy LH, Larson MG, Roberts WN, Liang MH: A modification of the Health Assessment Questionnaire for the spondyloarthropathies. J Rheumatol 1990; 17(7): 946–950. With permission.
6. **Health Assessment Questionnaire (HAQ) Disability and Discomfort Scales (revision 1994).** From Fries JF, Spitz P, Kraines RG, Holman HR: Measurement of patient outcome in arthritis. Arthritis Rheum 1980; 23: 137–145. With permission.
7. **Arthritis Impact Measurement Scales 2 (AIMS2).** From Meenan RF, Mason JH, Anderson JJ, Guccione AA, Kazis LE: AIMS2. The content and properties of a revised and expanded arthritis impact measurement scales health status questionnaire. Arthritis Rheum 1992; 35:1–10. With permission.
8. **Functional Status Index (FSI).** From Jette AM, Deniston OL: Inter-observer reliability of a functional status assessment instrument. J Chronic Dis 1978; 31:573–580. With permission.
9. **Foot Assessment.** The Arthritis Society, Ontario Division, Consultation and Therapy Service, Ottawa, Canada. With permission.

PHYSICAL THERAPY IN ARTHRITIS, Joan M. Walker, PhD, PT, and Antoine Helewa, MSc(Clin Epid), PT, W.B. Saunders Company © 1996.

INDEPENDENT MEASURE OF FUNCTIONAL CAPACITY

Courtesy of the authors.

Source: *J Rheumatol* 1982; 9:794–797.

Contact Address: Professor Antoine Helewa
Department of Physical Therapy
Elborn College
The University of Western Ontario
London, Ontario
Canada N6G 1H1
Telephone: 519-661-3357

ID # [ ][ ][ ][ ][ ] [ ][ ]

SECTION [0][5][1]

TIME [ ][ ]:[ ][ ]

1–14

15–19

V. TORONTO ACTIVITIES OF DAILY LIVING

PRERECORD "CHANGE" QUESTIONS 2, 4, 6, 8, 10, 12, 14, 17, 19A, 19B, 21. REFER TO INTERVIEWER'S MANUAL.

Now, I have a few more questions I would like to ask you about your daily activities.

1. WALKING

A. Are you able to walk at all either with or without help?

YES 1
YES, WITH DIFFICULTY 2
NO .... 3 → (SKIP TO Q2) [ ]

Ba. When you walk, do you walk by yourself, without any assistance whatsoever?

YES .... 1 } → (SKIP TO C)
YES, WITH DIFFICULTY .... 2 }
NO .... 3 [ ]

IF NO, ASK:
Bb. What kind of aid or assistance do you require?

(SPECIFY) ______________________ [ ]

C. Are you able to walk within your home?

YES 1
YES, WITH DIFFICULTY 2
NO .... 3 → (SKIP TO Q2) [ ]

D. Are you able to walk outside your home?

YES 1
YES, WITH DIFFICULTY 2
NO .... 3 → (SKIP TO Q2) [ ]

IMF Continued

E. Are you able to walk a distance of one block?

YES 1
YES, WITH DIFFICULTY 2
NO .... 3 ⟶ (SKIP TO Q2)

F. Are you able to walk four blocks or more?

YES 1
YES, WITH DIFFICULTY 2
NO .... 3 ⟶ (SKIP TO Q2)

G. Are you able to walk one mile?

YES 1
YES, WITH DIFFICULTY 2
NO .... 3 ⟶ (SKIP TO Q2)

H. Are you able to run several hundred yards?

YES 1
NO 3

20–28

IMF Continued

2. Since (MEDICATION DAY) ____________ would you say your ability to walk has changed to become: (SHOW CARD V AND TELL R WE WILL BE REFERRING TO IT AGAIN.)

   a lot better 1
   somewhat better 2
   somewhat worse 3
   a lot worse 4
   or has there been no change at all 5

   ☐

3. USE OF TRANSPORT

   A. If you had to, at present, are you able to travel in a bus, street car, or train?

      YES 1
      YES, WITH DIFFICULTY 2
      NO 3

      ☐

   B. If you had to, at present, are you able to travel by car or taxi?

      YES 1
      YES, WITH DIFFICULTY 2
      NO 3

      ☐

4. Since (MEDICATION DAY) ____________ would you say your ability to use transport has changed to become: REFER TO CARD V.

   a lot better 1
   somewhat better 2
   somewhat worse 3
   a lot worse 4
   or has there been no change at all 5

   ☐

5. CLIMBING

   A. Are you able, at present, to manage stairs with or without help?

      YES 1
      YES, WITH DIFFICULTY 2
      NO .... 3 → (SKIP TO Q6)

      ☐

   B. At present, are you able to manage two flights of stairs (16 steps)?

      YES .... 1 } → (SKIP TO Q6)
      YES, WITH DIFFICULTY .... 2 }
      NO 3

      ☐

   C. At present, are you able to manage one flight of stairs (8 steps)?

      YES .... 1 } → (SKIP TO Q6)
      YES, WITH DIFFICULTY .... 2 }
      NO 3

      ☐

   D. Are you able to manage two to four steps?

      YES 1
      YES, WITH DIFFICULTY 2
      NO 3

      ☐
      29–36

IMF Continued

6. Since (MEDICATION DAY) ________ would you say your ability to manage stairs has changed to become: REFER TO CARD V.

   a lot better 1
   somewhat better 2
   somewhat worse 3
   a lot worse 4
   or has there been no change at all 5

   ☐

7. CHAIRS AND TRANSFERS

   A. Are you able to get from bed to (chair/wheelchair) and back again at the present time?

      YES 1
      YES, WITH DIFFICULTY 2
      NO 3

      ☐

   B. Are you able, at present, to get up from an ordinary chair, i.e., a chair without arms?

      YES 1
      YES, WITH DIFFICULTY 2
      NO 3

      ☐

   C. If you had to, are you able, at present, to get up from the floor by yourself?

      YES 1
      YES, WITH DIFFICULTY 2
      NO 3

      ☐

   Since (MEDICATION DAY) ________ would you say your ability to move out of bed, out of a chair, or get up from the floor has changed to become: REFER TO CARD V.

   a lot better 1
   somewhat better 2
   somewhat worse 3
   a lot worse 4
   or has there been no change at all 5

   ☐

8. EATING

   A. At present, are you able to eat without the use of special utensils?

      YES 1
      YES, WITH DIFFICULTY 2
      NO 3

      ☐

   B. At present, are you able to cut meat by yourself?

      YES 1
      YES, WITH DIFFICULTY 2
      NO 3

      ☐ 37–43

IMF Continued

C. At present, are you able to eat without the assistance of another person?

YES 1
YES, WITH DIFFICULTY 2
NO 3

D. At present, are you able to grip and lift full glasses or cups?

YES 1
YES, WITH DIFFICULTY 2
NO 3

E. At present, are you able to pour tea or coffee from a pot?

YES 1
YES, WITH DIFFICULTY 2
NO 3

10. Since (MEDICATION DAY) ____________ would you say your ability to feed yourself has changed to become: REFER TO CARD V.

a lot better 1
somewhat better 2
somewhat worse 3
a lot worse 4
or has there been no change at all 5

11. DRESSING

Aa. At present, are you able to dress and undress completely for your usual daily activities?

YES 1
YES, WITH DIFFICULTY 2
NO 3

IF NO, ASK:
Ab. What kinds of aids or assistance do you require?

(SPECIFY) ____

B. Are you able to manage all your buttons, zippers, and fasteners, at present?

YES 1
YES, WITH DIFFICULTY 2
NO 3

C. Are you able to manage all other activities related to dressing and undressing, at present?

YES .... 1 → (SKIP TO Q12)
YES, DIFFICULTY WITH SOME 2
YES, DIFFICULTY WITH MOST 3
NO 4

44–51

IMF Continued

D. Could you tell me which dressing activities are difficult for you, at present? (For example, managing shoes, shoelaces, socks, stockings, neckties, scarves, undergarments, over-the-head clothing, etc.)

1. ____________________ ☐
2. ____________________ ☐
3. ____________________ ☐
4. ____________________ ☐
5. ____________________ ☐

E. Could you tell me which dressing activities you are unable to manage by yourself, at present?

1. ____________________ ☐
2. ____________________ ☐
3. ____________________ ☐
4. ____________________ ☐
5. ____________________ ☐

12. Since (MEDICATION DAY) __________ would you say your ability to dress or undress has changed to become: REFER TO CARD V.

a lot better 1
somewhat better 2
somewhat worse .... 3 ☐
a lot worse 4
or has there been no change at all 5

13. WASHING AND GROOMING

A. Are you able, at present, to turn taps and faucets off tightly?

YES 1
YES, WITH DIFFICULTY .... 2 ☐
NO 3

B. Are you able, at present, to wash your face and hands?

YES 1
YES, WITH DIFFICULTY .... 2 ☐
NO 3

C. Are you able, at present, to brush your teeth?

YES 1
YES, WITH DIFFICULTY .... 2 ☐ 52–65
NO 3

IMF Continued

D. Are you able, at present, to shave or apply cosmetics?

YES 1
YES, WITH DIFFICULTY 2
NO 3

E. Are you able, at present, to wash your hair?

YES 1
YES, WITH DIFFICULTY 2
NO 3

F. Are you able, at present, to comb your hair?

YES 1
YES, WITH DIFFICULTY 2
NO 3

G. Are you able, at present, to bathe in a bathtub?

YES 1
YES, WITH DIFFICULTY 2
NO .... 3 → (SKIP TO QI)

H. Are you able, at present, to bathe without relying on a bath stool or tub board?

YES .... 1 } → (SKIP TO QJ)
YES, WITH DIFFICULTY .... 2 }
NO 3

I. Do you have difficulty getting in and out of a bathtub at present?

YES 1
NO 2

J. Are you able, at present, to scrub <u>all</u> parts of your body?

YES 1
YES, WITH DIFFICULTY 2
NO 3

14. Since (MEDICATION DAY) ________ would you say your ability to wash and groom yourself has changed to become: REFER TO CARD V.

a lot better 1
somewhat better 2
somewhat worse 3
a lot worse 4
or has there been no change at all 5

15. <u>TOILET</u>

Are you able to use the toilet, at present?

YES 1
YES, WITH DIFFICULTY (INCLUDES RAISED TOILET SEAT OR COMMODE) 2
NO (RELIES ON BEDPAN OR OTHER MEANS) 3

66–74

IMF Continued

WORK/PLAY ACTIVITIES

16. SPECIAL HAND AND ARM FUNCTIONS

A. Are you able to grip and turn a doorknob or handle, at present?

YES 1
YES, WITH DIFFICULTY 2
NO 3

B. Are you able to grip and turn a key, at present?

YES 1
YES, WITH DIFFICULTY 2
NO 3

C. Are you able to use your fingers for fine work such as picking up change, at present?

YES 1
YES, WITH DIFFICULTY 2
NO 3

D. Are you able to open jars with screw tops, at present?

YES 1
YES, WITH DIFFICULTY 2
NO 3

E. Are you able to use a pen or pencil to write with, at present?

YES 1
YES, WITH DIFFICULTY 2
NO 3

F. Are you able to use scissors or clippers for cutting or grooming your fingernails, at present?

YES 1
YES, WITH DIFFICULTY 2
NO 3

G. Are you able to use scissors or clippers for cutting or grooming your toenails, at present?

YES 1
YES, WITH DIFFICULTY 2
NO 3

17. Since (MEDICATION DAY) ____________ would you say your ability to perform these hand and arm functions has changed to become: REFER TO CARD V.

a lot better 1
somewhat better 2
somewhat worse 3
a lot worse 4
or has there been no change at all 5

75–82

IMF Continued

18. WORK OUTSIDE THE HOME

Now, I will ask you some questions about your general ability to participate in activities outside your home.

A. Did you, in the past, work for pay or participate in a volunteer activity outside your home?

YES 1
NO 2

B. Do you now work for pay or participate in a volunteer activity outside your home?

YES ....1 → (SKIP TO QE)
NO 2

IF RESPONDENT ANSWERED YES TO (A) AND NO TO (B), ASK THE FOLLOWING QUESTION. OTHERWISE SKIP TO QUESTION (D).

C. Has this changed:

1. because of arthritis?
2. due to retirement?
3. due to other reasons? (SPECIFY) ____________

YES 1
NO 2

D. If you had to, are you able, at present, to perform in either volunteer or paid employment outside your home?

YES 1
NO 2

E. Have you ever tried to obtain employment since your arthritis started?

YES 1
NO 2

F. In the last 2 weeks, how many days were you confined to your home because of arthritis? (RECORD VERBATIM)

____
NUMBER OF DAYS

DAYS
83–91

IMF Continued

WORK AT HOME

G. Are you able, at present, to work around the house doing such things as:

YES 1
NO 2

1. carrying light objects, such as books? ______ ☐
2. dusting? ______ ☐
3. washing clothes by hand? ______ ☐
4. washing windows? ______ ☐
5. sweeping floors? ______ ☐
6. moving furniture? ______ ☐
7. carrying heavy objects, such as a full shopping bag? ______ ☐
8. digging in the garden? ______ ☐
9. pulling weeds? ______ ☐
10. mowing the lawn either by hand or power? ______ ☐

REST PERIODS

H. How long can you do light work before you must take at least a few minutes' break?

______ OR ______
MINUTES HOURS

MINUTES ☐☐☐

I. How long can you do heavy work before you must take at least a few minutes' break?

______ OR ______
MINUTES HOURS

MINUTES ☐☐☐

19A. Since (MEDICATION DAY) ______ would you say your ability to do light housework has changed to become: REFER TO CARD V.

a lot better 1
somewhat better 2
somewhat worse 3
a lot worse 4
or has there been no change at all 5

☐

B. Since (MEDICATION DAY) ______ would you say your ability to do heavy housework has changed to become: REFER TO CARD V.

a lot better 1
somewhat better 2
somewhat worse 3
a lot worse 4
or has there been no change at all 5

☐
92–109

IMF Continued

20. PLAY

A. Do you, at present, participate in any recreational activity or hobby?

YES 1
NO .... 2 → (SKIP TO Q21)

B. What activities or hobbies do you participate in?

YES 1
NO 2

1. Skiing ______
2. Tennis ______
3. Golf ______
4. Swimming ______
5. Walking ______
6. Activities, hobbies in the home only (SPECIFY) ______
7. Other (SPECIFY) ______

21. Since (MEDICATION DAY) ______ would you say your ability to participate in recreational activities or hobbies has changed to become: REFER TO CARD V.

a lot better 1
somewhat better 2
somewhat worse 3
a lot worse 4
or has there been no change at all 5

TIME ☐☐:☐☐
110–122

FIBROMYALGIA IMPACT QUESTIONNAIRE (FIQ)

Courtesy of the authors and the Editor, *J Rheumatol* 1991; 18:728–733.

Contact Address: Dr. R. M. Bennett
Division of Arthritis and Rheumatic Diseases
Department of Medicine-L329A
Oregon Health Sciences University
3181 SW Sam Jackson Park Road
Portland, OR
U.S.A. 97201-3098
Telephone: 503-494-8963
Fax: 503-494-4348

	Always	Most times	Occasionally	Never
1. Were you able to:				
a. Do shopping	0	1	2	3
b. Do laundry with a washer and dryer	0	1	2	3
c. Prepare meals	0	1	2	3
d. Wash dishes/cooking utensils by hand	0	1	2	3
e. Vacuum a rug	0	1	2	3
f. Make beds	0	1	2	3
g. Walk several blocks	0	1	2	3
h. Visit friends/relatives	0	1	2	3
i. Do yard work	0	1	2	3
j. Drive a car	0	1	2	3

2. Of the 7 days in the past week, how many days did you feel good?

   1 2 3 4 5 6 7

3. How many days in the past week did you miss work because of your fibromyalgia? (If you don't have a job outside the home leave this item blank.) 1 2 3 4 5

4. When you did go to work, how much did pain or other symptoms of your fibromyalgia interfere with your ability to do your job?

   No problem ________________________________ Great difficulty

5. How bad has your pain been?

   No pain ________________________________ Very severe pain

6. How tired have you been?

   No tiredness ________________________________ Very tired

7. How have you felt when you got up in the morning?

   Awoke well rested ________________________________ Awoke very tired

8. How bad has your stiffness been?

   No stiffness ________________________________ Very stiff

9. How tense, nervous, or anxious have you felt?

   Not tense ________________________________ Very tense

10. How depressed or blue have you felt?

    Not depressed ________________________________ Very depressed

McMASTER TORONTO ARTHRITIS PATIENT PREFERENCE DISABILITY QUESTIONNAIRE (MACTAR)

Courtesy of Dr. Peter Tugwell and the Editor, *J Rheumatol* 1987: 14:446–451.

Contact Address: Dr. Peter Tugwell
Department of Medicine
Ottawa General Hospital
501 Smyth Road
Ottawa, Ontario
Canada
Telephone: 613-737-8900
Fax: 613-737-8851

Baseline

1. Do you think your arthritis limits your ability to carry out any of your activities? i.e., Are there activities that you used to have no problems with before you had arthritis that you now find painful or have difficulty with because of arthritis?

   (Interviewer lists disabilities)

2. Does your arthritis limit:
   (a) Any (other) activities around the house such as getting around, cooking, housework, dressing, etc.

   (b) Any (other) activities at your work/outside the home/driving, etc.

   (c) Any (other) activities such as athletic (e.g., bowling, swimming, golf), or nonathletic (e.g., needlework, wood work, etc.)

   (d) Any (other) social activities such as visiting, playing cards, going to church, etc.

3. Which of these activities would you most like to be able to do without the pain or discomfort of your arthritis?

4. Which of these activities would you *next* most like to be able to do without the pain or discomfort of your arthritis?

   (The rest of the activities are rank ordered in the same way)

Follow-up

Each of the disabilities identified at baseline is reviewed as follows:

Since the first interview 8 weeks ago have you noticed any change in your ability to (Name of Disability) ☐ No ☐ Yes

If yes, has your ability to _____ Improved ☐ or become Worse ☐

MACTAR Continued

In the past 2 weeks, were you able to do the following tasks without the use of splints and/or mechanical aids?

	Yes, Without Difficulty	Yes, With Some Difficulty	No, Too Difficult To Do
(a) Turn your head from side to side?	____	____	____
(b) Comb your hair (at back of head)?	____	____	____
(c) Close your drawers (with arms only)?	____	____	____
(d) Open drawers?	____	____	____
(e) Lift a full teapot?	____	____	____
(f) Lift a cup with one hand to drink from it?	____	____	____
(g) Turn a key in a lock?	____	____	____
(h) Cut meat with a knife?	____	____	____
(i) Butter bread?	____	____	____
(j) Wind a watch?	____	____	____
(k) Walk?	____	____	____
(l) Walk without:			
1. Someone's help	____	____	____
2. Crutches	____	____	____
3. A walking stick	____	____	____
(m) Stand up with your knees straight?	____	____	____
(n) Stand up on your toes?	____	____	____
(o) Bend down to pick something off the floor?	____	____	____
(p) Walk up a flight of stairs?	____	____	____
(q) Walk down a flight of stairs?	____	____	____
(r) Wash your face and hands?	____	____	____
(s) Prepare meals?	____	____	____
(t) Dress/undress yourself?	____	____	____
(u) Stand up from a chair?	____	____	____
(v) Do light housework?	____	____	____
(w) Get on or off the toilet?	____	____	____
(x) Shave yourself?	____	____	____
(y) Go shopping?	____	____	____

WESTERN ONTARIO AND McMASTER UNIVERSITIES OSTEOARTHRITIS INDEX (WOMAC)-VA3.0

Courtesy of the originator.

Source: *J Rheumatol* 1988; 15:1833–1840.

Contact Address: Dr. Nicholas Bellamy
Division of Rheumatology
Victoria Hospital
P.O. Box 5375
London, Ontario
Canada N6A 4G5
Telephone: 519-667-6815
Fax: 519-667-6687

INSTRUCTIONS TO PATIENTS

In Sections A, B, and C questions will be asked in the following format and you should give your answers by putting an "X" on the horizontal line.

NOTE:

1. If you put your "X" at the left-hand end of the line, i.e.,

   NO PAIN |—X———————————————| EXTREME PAIN

   then you are indicating that you have no pain.

2. If you place your "X" at the right-hand end of the line, i.e.,

   NO PAIN |———————————————X—| EXTREME PAIN

   then you are indicating that your pain is extreme.

3. Please Note:

   a) that the further to the right-hand end you place your "X" the **more** pain you are experiencing.

   b) that the further to the left-hand end you place your "X" the **less** pain you are experiencing.

   c) **Please do not** place your "X" outside the end markers.

You will be asked to indicate on this type of scale the amount of pain, stiffness, or disability you are experiencing. Please remember the further you place your "X" to the right, the more pain, stiffness, or disability you are indicating that you experience.

WOMAC Continued

Section A

INSTRUCTIONS TO PATIENTS

The following questions concern the amount of pain you are currently experiencing due to arthritis in your hips and/or knees. For each situation please enter the amount of pain recently experienced (please mark your answers with an "X").

QUESTION: How much pain do you have?

1. Walking on a flat surface.

NO PAIN |————————————————————| EXTREME PAIN

2. Going up or down stairs.

NO PAIN |————————————————————| EXTREME PAIN

3. At night while in bed.

NO PAIN |————————————————————| EXTREME PAIN

4. Sitting or lying.

NO PAIN |————————————————————| EXTREME PAIN

5. Standing upright.

NO PAIN |————————————————————| EXTREME PAIN

Section B

INSTRUCTIONS TO PATIENTS

The following questions concern the amount of joint stiffness (not pain) you are currently experiencing in your hips and/or knees. Stiffness is a sensation of restriction or slowness in the ease with which you move your joints (please mark your answers with an "X").

1. How **severe** is your stiffness **after first wakening** in the morning?

NO STIFFNESS |————————————————————| EXTREME STIFFNESS

2. How **severe** is your stiffness after sitting, lying or resting **later in the day**?

NO STIFFNESS |————————————————————| EXTREME STIFFNESS

WOMAC Continued

Section C

INSTRUCTIONS TO PATIENTS

The following questions concern your physical function. By this we mean your ability to move around and to look after yourself. For each of the following activities, please indicate the degree of difficulty you are currently experiencing due to arthritis in your hips and/or knees (please mark your answers with an "X").

QUESTION: **What degree of difficulty do you have with:**

1. Descending stairs.

   NO DIFFICULTY |———| EXTREME DIFFICULTY

2. Ascending stairs.

   NO DIFFICULTY |———| EXTREME DIFFICULTY

3. Rising from sitting.

   NO DIFFICULTY |———| EXTREME DIFFICULTY

4. Standing.

   NO DIFFICULTY |———| EXTREME DIFFICULTY

5. Bending to floor.

   NO DIFFICULTY |———| EXTREME DIFFICULTY

6. Walking on flat.

   NO DIFFICULTY |———| EXTREME DIFFICULTY

7. Getting in/out of car.

   NO DIFFICULTY |———| EXTREME DIFFICULTY

8. Going shopping.

   NO DIFFICULTY |———| EXTREME DIFFICULTY

9. Putting on socks/stockings.

   NO DIFFICULTY |———| EXTREME DIFFICULTY

10. Rising from bed.

    NO DIFFICULTY |———| EXTREME DIFFICULTY

11. Taking off socks/stockings.

    NO DIFFICULTY |———| EXTREME DIFFICULTY

12. Lying in bed.

    NO DIFFICULTY |———| EXTREME DIFFICULTY

WOMAC Continued

13. Getting in/out of bath.

NO DIFFICULTY |————————————————| EXTREME DIFFICULTY

14. Sitting.

NO DIFFICULTY |————————————————| EXTREME DIFFICULTY

15. Getting on/off toilet.

NO DIFFICULTY |————————————————| EXTREME DIFFICULTY

16. Heavy domestic duties.

NO DIFFICULTY |————————————————| EXTREME DIFFICULTY

17. Light domestic duties.

NO DIFFICULTY |————————————————| EXTREME DIFFICULTY

HEALTH ASSESSMENT QUESTIONNAIRE FOR THE SPONDYLOARTHROPATHIES (HAQ-S)

Courtesy of the authors and the Editor, *J Rheumatol* 1990; 17:946–950.

Contact Address: Dr. Lawren H. Daltroy
Robert B. Brigham Multipurpose Arthritis Center
Brigham and Women's Hospital
75 Francis Street
Boston, MA
U.S.A. 02115
Telephone: 617-732-5149
Fax: 617-731-9032

How much stiffness have you had because of your illness in the past week? Place a mark on the line to indicate the severity of the stiffness

No stiffness — Very severe stiffness

0 ____ 100

Please check the *one* response that best describes your usual abilities over the past week:

Activities	(0) Without ANY Difficulty	(1) With SOME Difficulty	(2) With MUCH Difficulty	(3) UNABLE To Do
Are you able to carry heavy packages such as grocery bags?	______	______	______	______
Are you able to sit for long periods of time, such as at work?	______	______	______	______
Are you able to work at a flat-topped table or desk?	______	______	______	______
Driving a car (Check here ____ if you DO NOT have a driver's license or a car).				
Are you able to look in the rear view mirror?	______	______	______	______
Are you able to turn your head to drive in reverse?	______	______	______	______

HAQ-S Continued

HEALTH ASSESSMENT QUESTIONNAIRE

Name____________________ Date________________

In this section we are interested in learning how your illness affects your ability to function in daily life. Please feel free to add any comments on the back of this page.

Please check the response which best describes your usual abilities OVER THE PAST WEEK:

	Without ANY Difficulty	With SOME Difficulty	With MUCH Difficulty	UNABLE To Do	
DRESSING & GROOMING Are you able to:					
Dress yourself, including tying shoelaces and doing buttons?	____	____	____	____	
Shampoo your hair?	____	____	____	____	DRESSNEW____
ARISING Are you able to:					
Stand up from a straight chair?	____	____	____	____	
Get in and out of bed?	____	____	____	____	RISENEW____
EATING Are you able to:					
Cut your meat?	____	____	____	____	
Lift a full cup or glass to your mouth?	____	____	____	____	
Open a new milk carton?	____	____	____	____	EATNEW____
WALKING Are you able to:					
Walk outdoors on flat ground?	____	____	____	____	
Climb up five steps?	____	____	____	____	WALKNEW____

Please check any AIDS OR DEVICES that you usually use for any of these activities:

____Cane
____Walker
____Crutches
____Wheelchair
____Devices used for dressing (button hook, zipper pull, long-handled shoe horn, etc.)
____Built-up or special utensils
____Special or built-up chair
____Other (Specify:________)

Please check any categories for which you usually need HELP FROM ANOTHER PERSON:

____Dressing and Grooming
____Arising
____Eating
____Walking

PATKEY#____
QUESTDAT____
HAQADMIN____
QUESTYPE 2
PMSVIS 1
RASTUDY____
QUESTNUM____

DRSGASST____
RISEASST____
EATASST____
WALKASST____

HAQ-S Continued

Please check the response which best describes your usual abilities OVER THE PAST WEEK:

	Without ANY Difficulty	With SOME Difficulty	With MUCH Difficulty	UNABLE To Do	
HYGIENE					
Are you able to:					
Wash and dry your body?	____	____	____	____	
Take a tub bath?	____	____	____	____	
Get on and off the toilet?	____	____	____	____	HYGNNEW ____
REACH					
Are you able to:					
Reach and get down a 5-lb object (such as a bag of sugar) from just above your head?	____	____	____	____	
Bend down to pick up clothing from the floor?	____	____	____	____	REACHNEW ____
GRIP					
Are you able to:					
Open car doors?	____	____	____	____	
Open jars which have been previously opened?	____	____	____	____	
Turn faucets on and off?	____	____	____	____	GRIPNEW ____
ACTIVITIES					
Are you able to:					
Run errands and shop?	____	____	____	____	
Get in and out of a car?	____	____	____	____	
Do chores such as vacuuming or yardwork?	____	____	____	____	ACTIVNEW ____

Please check any AIDS OR DEVICES that you usually use for any of these activities:

____Raised toilet seat
____Bathtub seat
____Jar opener (for jars previously opened)
____Bathtub bar
____Long-handled appliances for reach
____Long-handled appliances in bathroom
____Other (Specify: ____________)

Please check any categories for which you usually need HELP FROM ANOTHER PERSON:

____Hygiene
____Reach
____Gripping and opening things
____Errands and chores

HYGNASST ____
RCHASST ____
GRIPASST ____
ACTVASST ____

We are also interested in learning whether or not you are affected by pain because of your illness.
How much pain have you had because of your illness IN THE PAST WEEK:

PLACE A VERTICAL (|) MARK ON THE LINE TO INDICATE THE SEVERITY OF THE PAIN

NO PAIN ____ SEVERE PAIN

0 100

PAINSCAL ____

HAS-Q Continued

SYMPTOMS

Please check any items which apply to your health during the **PAST 7 DAYS**. If "none", check here:______

HEAD, EYES, EARS, NOSE, MOUTH, AND THROAT:

______Blurred vision
______Dry eyes
______Ringing in ears
______Hearing difficulties
______Mouth sores
______Dry mouth
______Loss, change in taste
______Headache
______Dizziness
______Fever
______Night sweats

CHEST, LUNGS, AND HEART:

______Chest pain on taking a deep breath
______Shortness of breath
______Wheezing (asthma)

GASTROINTESTINAL TRACT:

______Loss of appetite
______Difficulty swallowing or feeling of food getting stuck?
______Nausea
______Heartburn, indigestion, or belching
______Vomiting
______Pain or discomfort in upper abdomen (stomach)
______Jaundice
______Liver problems, kind ______________________________
______Pain or cramps in lower abdomen (colon)
______Diarrhea (frequent, explosive watery bowel movements, severe)
______Constipation
______Black or tarry stools (not from iron)

GENITOURINARY:

______Protein in urine (confirmed by a doctor)
______Frequency or burning on urination
______Kidney problems, kind ______________________________

FEMALES ONLY:

______Are you pregnant?

OTHER:

______Any others, (specify)______________________________

MUSCULOSKELETAL:

______Joint pain
______Joint swelling
______Low back pain
______Muscle pain
______Neck pain
______Numbness/tingling in hands or feet
______Swelling of legs
______Weakness of muscles

______If you are stiff in the morning, about (hr/min) how long does the stiffness last?

NEUROLOGIC AND PSYCHOLOGIC:

______Depression
______Insomnia
______Nervousness
______Seizures or convulsions
______Tiredness (fatigue)
______Trouble thinking or remembering

SKIN:

______Easy bruising
______Facial skin tightening
______Hives or welts
______Loss of hair
______Itching
______Rash
______Rash over cheeks
______Red, white, and blue skin color change in fingers on exposure to cold or with emotional upset
______Sun sensitivity (unusual skin reaction, not sunburn)

BLOOD:
(Please check only if doctor confirmed results)

______Low white blood count
______Low platelets
______Low red blood count (anemia)

MALES ONLY:

______Discharge from penis
______Impotence
______Rash or ulcers on penis

HAS-Q Continued

MEDICATIONS

In the **PAST 6 MONTHS (JANUARY 1, 1994 through JUNE 30, 1994)** have you taken any medications? ______Yes ______No

PLEASE COMPLETE ALL THE BLANKS ON THE LINE FOR ANY MEDICATIONS THAT YOU HAVE TAKEN.

MEDICATIONS FOR YOUR ARTHRITIS

(For example: prednisone, methotrexate, Plaquenil, and anti-inflammatory drugs such as aspirin, Naprosyn, voltaren, ibuprofen, and Feldene.)

ORAL MEDICATIONS

Medication Name	Months out of Last 6 Months on Drug	Number of Tablets Per Day	Milligrams Per Tablet	Still Taking Circle Yes or No	Month Stopped
				Yes No	
				Yes No	
				Yes No	
				Yes No	
				Yes No	
				Yes No	
				Yes No	
				Yes No	

INJECTIONS and/or INTRAVENOUS (IV) MEDICATIONS (Pulse Therapy)

Medication Name	Months Out of Last 6 Months on Drug	Total Number of Treatments in the Last 6 Months	Still Taking Circle Yes or No	Month Stopped
			Yes No	
			Yes No	

Please list all other medications (both prescription and over-the-counter) you have taken in the **PAST 6 MONTHS (JANUARY 1, 1994 through JUNE 30, 1994)** for any other medical condition. Please complete all the blanks on the line for each medication.

OTHER MEDICATIONS

Medication Name	Months out of Last 6 Months on Drug	Number of Tablets Per Day	Milligrams Per Tablet	Still Taking Circle Yes or No	Month Stopped
				Yes No	
				Yes No	
				Yes No	
				Yes No	
				Yes No	
				Yes No	

HAS-Q Continued

DRUG SIDE EFFECTS

Have you had any side effect(s) from your medication in the **PAST 6 MONTHS (JANUARY 1, 1994 through JUNE 30, 1994)?** ______Yes ______No

COMPLETE THE REST OF THIS PAGE ONLY IF YOU HAVE SAID "YES."

DIRECTIONS:

1. Write in the name of the drug causing the side effect(s).
2. Indicate whether you stopped the drug.
3. List side effect(s) for each drug. You may want to refer back to "Symptoms." Please list any abnormal laboratory findings such as:

low white blood count	protein in urine
low platelets	kidney problems
anemia	liver problems

4. Check the severity of each side effect.
5. If you need more room, please use the back of this page.

SE6MO

A. (1)______________ DRUG NAME

(2) Did you STOP the drug because of a side effect? ______Yes ______No

(3) LIST SIDE EFFECT(S)

(4) SEVERITY of each side effect:

______________	______mild	______moderate	______severe
______________	______mild	______moderate	______severe
______________	______mild	______moderate	______severe

DRUG1______
STOP1______
SE1DRG1______
SEVSE1D1______
SE2DRG1______
SEVSE2D1______
SE3DRG1______
SEVSE3D1______

B. (1)______________ DRUG NAME

(2) Did you STOP the drug because of a side effect? ______Yes ______No

(3) LIST SIDE EFFECT(S)

(4) SEVERITY of each side effect:

______________	______mild	______moderate	______severe
______________	______mild	______moderate	______severe
______________	______mild	______moderate	______severe

DRUG2______
STOP2______
SE1DRG2______
SEVSE1D2______
SE2DRG2______
SEVSE2D2______
SE3DRG2______
SEVSE3D2______

C. (1)______________ DRUG NAME

(2) Did you STOP the drug because of a side effect? ______Yes ______No

(3) LIST SIDE EFFECT(S)

(4) SEVERITY of each side effect:

______________	______mild	______moderate	______severe
______________	______mild	______moderate	______severe
______________	______mild	______moderate	______severe

DRUG3______
STOP3______
SE1DRG3______
SEVSE1D3______
SE2DRG3______
SEVSE2D3______
SE3DRG3______
SEVSE3D3______

HAS-Q Continued

MEDICAL HISTORY

We are interested in your use of health care providers in the **PAST 6 MONTHS (JANUARY 1, 1994 through JUNE 30, 1994)**. Please include **ALL** visits.

1. In the **PAST 6 MONTHS (JANUARY 1, 1994 through JUNE 30, 1994)** did you stay in the hospital overnight or visit an emergency room for any reason? _____Yes _____No

   If "Yes," please describe each hospitalization or emergency room visit:

Reason	Hospital (City, State)	Admission Date (Month, Year)	Number Of Days in Hospital
______	______	______	______
______	______	______	______
______	______	______	______
______	______	______	______

HOSPAUDT_______

ERVISIT_______

2. Were any of these hospitalizations related to a side effect from any of your medications? If "Yes," which hospitalization(s) and which medication(s):_______________

3. Did you develop any complications or secondary problems during any of the hospitalizations? If "Yes," list hospitalization and problem:_______________

4. In the **PAST 6 MONTHS (JANUARY 1, 1994 through JUNE 30, 1994)** have you had any outpatient surgery or procedures? _____Yes _____No

   If "Yes," please list:

Surgery/Procedure	Doctor's Name	Location and Address (Hospital, Doctor's Office)	Date (Month, Year)
______	______	______	______
______	______	______	______

5. In the **PAST 6 MONTHS (JANUARY 1, 1994 through JUNE 30, 1994)** were you a patient in a nursing or convalescent home or live-in rehabilitation center? _____Yes _____No

   If "Yes," for how many days? __________Days

NURHOMDY_______

6. In the **PAST 6 MONTHS (JANUARY 1, 1994 through JUNE 30, 1994)** have you received care from a doctor, nurse, or other health professional in your home? _____Yes _____No

   If "Yes," how many visits in the PAST 6 MONTHS? __________Visits

HOMEVSTS_______

HAS-Q Continued

7. In the **PAST 6 MONTHS (JANUARY 1, 1994 through JUNE 30, 1994)** have you been told that you have any kind of tumor or cancer? _____Yes _____No

   If "Yes," was it malignant or benign? (circle one)

   What kind? (for example: leukemia, lymphoma, lung)

   ____

   What treatment was given? (for example: surgery, chemotherapy, radiation therapy)

   ____

CANCER__________
BENIGN__________
CANCTYPE__________
CANCSURG__________
CANCCHEM__________
CANCRAD__________

8. Have you had any infections in the **PAST 6 MONTHS (JANUARY 1, 1994 through JUNE 30, 1994)**? DO NOT INCLUDE COLDS OR FLU. _____Yes _____No

   PLEASE INCLUDE EMERGENCY ROOM AND OUTPATIENT VISITS

   If "Yes," please answer the following:

	Number of Infections	Number of Emergency Room or Outpatient Visits	Number of Times Admitted to the Hospital	
_____Septicemia (sepsis, bloodstream infection)	_____	_____	_____	BLOODINF__________
_____Pneumonia	_____	_____	_____	PULMINF__________
_____Shingles (herpes zoster)	_____	_____	_____	HERPEINF__________
_____Bone/joint infection (osteomyelitis, septic joint, infected artificial joint)	_____	_____	_____	SKELINF__________
_____Skin infections (infected skin ulcer, cellulitis, infected nodules)	_____	_____	_____	SKULCINF__________
_____Urinary tract infection/kidney infection/bladder infection	_____	_____	_____	RENALINF__________
_____Other, please specify: ______________________	_____	_____	_____	OTHERINF__________

HAS-Q Continued

9. Have you seen any doctors or any other health workers in the **PAST 6 MONTHS (JANUARY 1, 1994 through JUNE 30, 1994)**? DO NOT INCLUDE ANY WHILE YOU WERE A PATIENT IN THE HOSPITAL. _____Yes _____No

If "Yes," please complete:

	NUMBER of Visits in Last 6 Months	
Rheumatologist	_____	**RHEUMVST** _____
Internist	_____	**INTERNVT** _____
Family physician (general practitioner)	_____	**GPVST** _____
General or orthopedic surgeon	_____	**SURGNVT** _____
Podiatrist (foot doctor)	_____	**PODVST** _____
Chiropractor	_____	**CHIROVT** _____
Physical or occupational therapist	_____	**PTOTVST** _____
Other doctors (dermatologist or others)		
_____	_____	
_____	_____	**MISCVST** _____
Other health workers (social worker, or others)		
_____	_____	
_____	_____	**MISCHWVT** _____

Diagnostic Procedures

10. Have you had any diagnostic tests or treatments in the **PAST 6 MONTHS (JANUARY 1, 1994 through JUNE 30, 1994)**? DO NOT INCLUDE ANY THAT WERE DONE WHILE YOU WERE A PATIENT IN THE HOSPITAL. _____Yes _____No

If "Yes," please complete the following:

Test	**Number of Tests**	**Part of Body**	
			HDWTXRAY _____
X-Rays (chest, stomach or bowels, joints, etc.)	_____	_____	**SHLDXY** _____
			HIPXRAY _____
	_____	_____	**KNEEXRAY** _____
			FEETXRAY _____
	_____	_____	**NECKXY** _____
			LOBKXY _____
	_____	_____	**SPINXY** _____
			CHTXY _____
			GIXRAY _____
			MISCXRAY _____
Nuclear medicine scans (NMR) or magnetic resonance imaging (MRI)	_____	_____	**NMR** _____
CT scan	_____	_____	**CTSCAN** _____
Blood tests (number of times blood was drawn)	_____		**VENPUNCT** _____
Urine tests	_____		**URINALYS** _____
Endoscopy (gastroscopy)	_____		**ENDOSCOP** _____
Colonoscopy	_____		**COLONOSC** _____
Other tests, please specify	_____	_____	

HAS-Q Continued

11. In the **PAST 6 MONTHS (JANUARY 1, 1994 through JUNE 30, 1994)**, have you had any nontraditional treatments? ______Yes ______No

If "Yes," please complete:

	Number of Visits	
Acupuncturist	______	ACUPUNNT______
Acupressurist	______	ACUPRENT______
Massage therapist	______	MASSAGNT______
Herbalist	______	HERBALNT______
Homeopathic practitioner	______	HOPATHNT______
Other, please specify:		
______________	______	OTHERNT______

12. In the **PAST 6 MONTHS (JANUARY 1, 1994 through JUNE 30, 1994)** have you had to pay someone to help in the house or for personal care, or paid for help in business matters that you are normally able to handle yourself, but could not do because of your health? ______Yes ______No

If "Yes," please list:

Type of Care	Hours per Month	Number of Months	
______________	______________	______________	
______________	______________	______________	MISCUNIT______

HEALTH STATUS

1. Considering all the ways that your arthritis affects you, rate how you are doing on the following scale by placing a mark on the line.

| - - - - | - - - - | - - - - | - - - - | - - - - | - - - - | - - - - | - - - - | - - - - | - - - - |

0 very well — 20 — well — 40 — fair — 60 — poor — 80 — 100 very poor

GLOBAL______

2. Are any of your joints tender? ______Yes ______No

If "Yes," please circle the tender joints.

Knuckles Wrists Elbows Shoulders Hips Knees Ankles Toes

PTTENJTN______

3. Are any of your joints swollen? ______Yes ______No

If "Yes," please circle the swollen joints.

Knuckles Wrists Elbows Shoulders Hips Knees Ankles Toes

PTSWOJTN______

HAS-Q Continued

4. For each of the following questions, please circle the number for the one answer that best describes how you have been feeling in the **PAST 4 WEEKS**.

How much of the time did you:	All of the Time	Most of the Time	Some of the Time	Almost Never	Never	
a. Feel full of pep?	1	2	3	4	5	**PEPPY**______
b. Feel worn out?	1	2	3	4	5	**WORNOUT**______
c. Feel calm and peaceful?	1	2	3	4	5	**ATPEACE**______
d. Have enough energy to do the things you want to do?	1	2	3	4	5	**ENRGETIC**______
e. Feel downhearted and blue?	1	2	3	4	5	**FEELBLUE**______
f. Feel very happy?	1	2	3	4	5	**HAPPY**______
g. Feel very nervous?	1	2	3	4	5	**NERVOUS**______
h. Feel tired?	1	2	3	4	5	**TIRED**______
i. Feel so down in the dumps nothing could cheer you up?	1	2	3	4	5	**DOWN**______

5. How much of the time, during the **PAST 4 WEEKS**, has your health limited your social activities (like visiting with friends or close relatives)?

______All of the time
______Most of the time
______A good bit of the time
______Some of the time
______A little of the time
______None of the time

SOCLCHG______

6. In general, would you say your current health is:

______Excellent
______Very good
______Good
______Fair
______Poor

GLOBALGN______

7. How satisfied are you with your HEALTH NOW?

______Very satisfied
______Somewhat satisfied
______Neither satisfied nor dissatisfied
______Somewhat dissatisfied
______Very dissatisfied

GLOBALNW______

HAS-Q Continued

8. Do you participate in exercise for your arthritis on a regular basis? ____Yes ____No — EXERWEEK________

   If "Yes," how many times per week? __________Times
   How many minutes per time? __________Minutes

9. Do you participate in exercise for aerobic conditioning on a regular basis? ____Yes ____No — AEROWEEK________

   If "Yes," how many times per week? __________Times
   How many minutes per time? __________Minutes

We would like to know how your arthritis pain affects you. Please **circle** the number which corresponds to your certainty that you can now perform the following task.

1. How certain are you that you can make a small-to-moderate reduction in your arthritis pain by using methods other than taking extra medication? — SEPS4__________

1	2	3	4	5	6	7	8	9	10
Very Uncertain									Very Certain

In the following questions, we'd like to know how you feel about your ability to control your arthritis. For each of the following questions, please **circle** the number on the scale which corresponds to the certainty that you can now perform the following activities or tasks.

2. How certain are you that you can manage your arthritis symptoms so that you can do the things you enjoy doing? — SESS5__________

1	2	3	4	5	6	7	8	9	10
Very Uncertain									Very Certain

3. How certain are you that you can deal with the frustrations of arthritis? — SESS6__________

1	2	3	4	5	6	7	8	9	10
Very Uncertain									Very Certain

STANFORD-RA (PHASE 27)

HAS-Q Continued

EMPLOYMENT STATUS

1. Which one of the following categories best describes you at this time? EMPLOY________

________Working for pay: Occupation____________________ OCCUPA________
Job duties____________________
Hours/week__________ WORKHRS________
Personal yearly earnings—nearest thousand (optional)________
(NOT TOTAL HOUSEHOLD INCOME) PERINCOM________

________Retired

________Homemaker

________Student

________Disabled

________Looking for work

________On sick leave: Occupation____________________

________On vacation: Occupation____________________

________Other (Specify):____________________

2. If you retired or became disabled in **1994**, what was your prior occupation?

Occupation____________________

3. In the **PAST 6 MONTHS (JANUARY 1, 1994 through JUNE 30, 1994)** have there been days when you have had to **CUT DOWN** or **LIMIT** your usual activities (including housework, school)? _____Yes _____No CUTDOWN________

If "Yes," how many days?________

IF YOU ARE NOT EMPLOYED, PLEASE ANSWER QUESTION #4.
IF YOU ARE EMPLOYED, PLEASE GO TO QUESTION #5.

4. IN THE **PAST 6 MONTHS**, have there been days when you have been COMPLETELY UNABLE to carry out your usual activities BECAUSE OF YOUR HEALTH? _____Yes _____No DAYSLOST________

If "Yes," how many days?________

IF YOU ARE NOT EMPLOYED, PLEASE GO TO THE PATIENT SATISFACTION SECTION ON THE NEXT PAGE.

IF YOU ARE EMPLOYED, PLEASE ANSWER THE FOLLOWING QUESTIONS:

5. IN THE **PAST 6 MONTHS**, have you been unable to work any days BECAUSE OF YOUR HEALTH? _____Yes _____No UNABLE________

If "Yes," how many days?________

HAS-Q Continued

6. IN THE **PAST 6 MONTHS**, have you stopped or started working BECAUSE OF YOUR HEALTH? (Include early retirement) ______Yes ______No CHGWORK________

   If "Yes," please explain?

7. IN THE **PAST 6 MONTHS**, have you changed your HOURS of work BECAUSE OF YOUR HEALTH? ______Yes ______No CHGAMT________

   If "Yes," please explain?

8. In the **PAST 6 MONTHS (JANUARY 1, 1994 through JUNE 30, 1994)**, have you taken unpaid time off from work to visit your doctor, a psychologist, or other health professional? ______Yes ______No

   If "Yes," how many hours have you taken off? ________hours/past 6 months HRSLOST________

PATIENT SATISFACTION

Here are some questions about your own health care. Please rate the following by circling one number on each line:

	Poor	Fair	Good	Very Good	Excellent	
1. Overall, how would you evaluate your health care	1	2	3	4	5	PSOVER________
2. Access to specialty care if you need it	1	2	3	4	5	PSSACCS________
3. Access to medical care in an emergency	1	2	3	4	5	PSMACCS________
4. Arrangements for making appointments for medical care by phone	1	2	3	4	5	PSAPPT________
5. Skill, experience, and training of doctors	1	2	3	4	5	PSSKILL________
6. Attention given to what you have to say	1	2	3	4	5	PSSAY________
7. Friendliness and courtesy shown to you by staff	1	2	3	4	5	PSFRND________
8. Amount of time you have with doctors and staff during a visit	1	2	3	4	5	PSTIME________

HAS-Q Continued

BACKGROUND INFORMATION

1. What type(s) of health insurance do you have? Check all that apply.

    ______None
    ______Health maintenance organization (HMO) Name:______________________
    ______Medicaid/Medi-Cal
    ______Private insurance company, including self-insured employers (e.g., Aetna, Guardian) Name:______________________
    ______Medicare
    ______Medicare disability
    ______Blue Cross/Blue Shield
    ______Champus/VA
    ______Cobra coverage
    ______Preferred provider organization (PPO) Name:______________________
    ______Other Name:______________________

HLTHCARE______

2. If you have health insurance, is your insurance:

    ______Provided through your employer or your spouse's or partner's employer
    ______Purchased by you directly from the insurer or from an insurance agent

HLTHINSR______

3. Where do you regularly receive your medical care? Please check one.

    ______At a hospital outpatient clinic
    ______At a private physician's office
    ______At a physician's office in a large clinic, not at a hospital
    ______At a community-based, publicly financed clinic

MEDCARE______

COMMENTS:

____
____
____
____
____
____
____
____
____
____
____
____
____

HAS-Q Continued

This page asks you for permission to allow us to review medical records pertaining to your involvement in this research program. This information will be kept strictly confidential and used for research purposes only.

RELEASE OF MEDICAL INFORMATION

I give permission for the release of information pertaining to my medical care to the Outcome in Rheumatic Disease Study.

PLEASE USE INK

PLEASE PRINT

Name: ______________________________

Address: ______________________________

______________________________ ______________
Postal/Zip Code

Date of Birth: ______________________________

Signature: ______________________________ ______________
Date

ARTHRITIS IMPACT MEASUREMENT SCALES 2 (AIMS2)

Courtesy of the originator

Source: *Arthritis Rheum* 1992; 35:1–10.

Contact Address: Robert F. Meenan MD, MPH
The Arthritis Center
Boston University School of Medicine
Conte Building
80 East Concord Street
Boston, MA
U.S.A. 02118-2394
Telephone: 617-638-4310
Fax: 617-638-5226

Please check (X) the most appropriate answer for each question.

These questions refer to MOBILITY LEVEL.

DURING THE PAST MONTH . . .	All Days (1)	Most Days (2)	Some Days (3)	Few Days (4)	No Days (5)	
1. How often were you physically able to drive a car or use public transportation?	____	____	____	____	____	8/
2. How often were you out of the house for at least part of the day?	____	____	____	____	____	9/
3. How often were you able to do errands in the neighborhood?	____	____	____	____	____	10/
4. How often did someone have to assist you to get around outside your home?	____	____	____	____	____	11/
5. How often were you in a bed or chair for most or all of the day?	____	____	____	____	____	12/

AIMS

These questions refer to WALKING AND BENDING.

DURING THE PAST MONTH . . .	All Days (1)	Most Days (2)	Some Days (3)	Few Days (4)	No Days (5)	
6. Did you have trouble doing vigorous activities such as running, lifting heavy objects, or participating in strenuous sports?	____	____	____	____	____	13/
7. Did you have trouble either walking several blocks or climbing a few flights of stairs?	____	____	____	____	____	14/
8. Did you have trouble bending, lifting or stooping?	____	____	____	____	____	15/
9. Did you have trouble either walking one block or climbing one flight of stairs?	____	____	____	____	____	16/
10. Were you unable to walk unless assisted by another person or by a cane, crutches, or walker?	____	____	____	____	____	17/

AIMS2 Continued

AIMS

Please check (X) the most appropriate answer for each question.

These questions refer to HAND AND FINGER FUNCTION.

DURING THE PAST MONTH . . .	All Days (1)	Most Days (2)	Some Days (3)	Few Days (4)	No Days (5)	
11. Could you easily write with a pen or pencil?	_____	_____	_____	_____	_____	18/
12. Could you easily button a shirt or blouse?	_____	_____	_____	_____	_____	19/
13. Could you easily turn a key in a lock?	_____	_____	_____	_____	_____	20/
14. Could you easily tie a knot or a bow?	_____	_____	_____	_____	_____	21/
15. Could you easily open a new jar of food?	_____	_____	_____	_____	_____	22/

AIMS

These questions refer to ARM FUNCTION.

DURING THE PAST MONTH . . .	All Days (1)	Most Days (2)	Some Days (3)	Few Days (4)	No Days (5)	
16. Could you easily wipe your mouth with a napkin?	_____	_____	_____	_____	_____	23/
17. Could you easily put on a pullover sweater?	_____	_____	_____	_____	_____	24/
18. Could you easily comb or brush your hair?	_____	_____	_____	_____	_____	25/
19. Could you easily scratch your low back with your hand?	_____	_____	_____	_____	_____	26/
20. Could you easily reach shelves that were above your head?	_____	_____	_____	_____	_____	27/

AIMS2 Continued

AIMS

Please check (X) the most appropriate answer for each question.

These questions refer to SELF-CARE TASKS.

DURING THE PAST MONTH . . .	Always (1)	Very Often (2)	Sometimes (3)	Almost Never (4)	Never (5)	
21. Did you need help to take a bath or shower?	____	____	____	____	____	28/
22. Did you need help to get dressed?	____	____	____	____	____	29/
23. Did you need help to use the toilet?	____	____	____	____	____	30/
24. Did you need help to get in or out of bed?	____	____	____	____	____	31/

AIMS

These questions refer to HOUSEHOLD TASKS.

DURING THE PAST MONTH . . .	Always (1)	Very Often (2)	Sometimes (3)	Almost Never (4)	Never (5)	
25. If you had the necessary transportation, could you go shopping for groceries without help?	____	____	____	____	____	32/
26. If you had kitchen facilities, could you prepare your own meals without help?	____	____	____	____	____	33/
27. If you had household tools and appliances, could you do your own housework without help?	____	____	____	____	____	34/
28. If you had laundry facilities, could you do your own laundry without help?	____	____	____	____	____	35/

AIMS2 Continued

AIMS

Please check (X) the most appropriate answer for each question.

These questions refer to SOCIAL ACTIVITY.

DURING THE PAST MONTH . . .	All Days (1)	Most Days (2)	Some Days (3)	Few Days (4)	No Days (5)	
29. How often did you get together with friends or relatives?	____	____	____	____	____	36/
30. How often did you have friends or relatives over to your home?	____	____	____	____	____	37/
31. How often did you visit friends or relatives at their homes?	____	____	____	____	____	38/
32. How often were you on the telephone with close friends or relatives?	____	____	____	____	____	39/
33. How often did you go to a meeting of a church, club, team, or other group?	____	____	____	____	____	40/

AIMS

These questions refer to SUPPORT FROM FAMILY AND FRIENDS.

DURING THE PAST MONTH . . .	Always (1)	Very Often (2)	Sometimes (3)	Almost Never (4)	Never (5)	
34. Did you feel that your family or friends would be around if you needed assistance?	____	____	____	____	____	41/
35. Did you feel that your family or friends were sensitive to your personal needs?	____	____	____	____	____	42/
36. Did you feel that your family or friends were interested in helping you solve problems?	____	____	____	____	____	43/
37. Did you feel that your family or friends understood the effects of your arthritis?	____	____	____	____	____	44/

AIMS2 Continued

AIMS

Please check (X) the most appropriate answer for each question.

These questions refer to ARTHRITIS PAIN.

DURING THE PAST MONTH . . .	Severe (1)	Moderate (2)	Mild (3)	Very Mild (4)	None (5)	
38. How would you describe the arthritis pain you usually had?	_____	_____	_____	_____	_____	45/

	All Days (1)	Most Days (2)	Some Days (3)	Few Days (4)	No Days (5)	
39. How often did you have severe pain from your arthritis?	_____	_____	_____	_____	_____	46/
40. How often did you have pain in two or more joints at the same time?	_____	_____	_____	_____	_____	47/
41. How often did your morning stiffness last more than 1 hour from the time you woke up?	_____	_____	_____	_____	_____	48/
42. How often did your pain make it difficult for you to sleep?	_____	_____	_____	_____	_____	49/

AIMS

These questions refer to WORK.

DURING THE PAST MONTH . . .	Paid work (1)	House work (2)	School work (3)	Unemployed (4)	Disabled (5)	Retired (6)	
43. What has been your main form of work?	_____	_____	_____	_____	_____	_____	50/

If you answered unemployed, disabled, or retired, please skip the next four questions and go to the next page.

DURING THE PAST MONTH . . .	All Days (1)	Most Days (2)	Some Days (3)	Few Days (4)	No Days (5)	
44. How often were you unable to do any paid work, house work, or school work?	_____	_____	_____	_____	_____	51/
45. On the days that you did work, how often did you have to work a shorter day?	_____	_____	_____	_____	_____	52/
46. On the days that you did work, how often were you unable to do your work as carefully and accurately as you would like?	_____	_____	_____	_____	_____	53/
47. On the days that you did work, how often did you have to change the way your paid work, house work, or school work is usually done?	_____	_____	_____	_____	_____	54/

AIMS2 Continued

AIMS

Please check (X) the most appropriate answer for each question.

These questions refer to LEVEL OF TENSION.

DURING THE PAST MONTH . . .	Always (1)	Very Often (2)	Sometimes (3)	Almost Never (4)	Never (5)	
48. How often have you felt tense or high strung?	_____	_____	_____	_____	_____	55/
49. How often have you been bothered by nervousness or your nerves?	_____	_____	_____	_____	_____	56/
50. How often were you able to relax without difficulty?	_____	_____	_____	_____	_____	57/
51. How often have you felt relaxed and free of tension?	_____	_____	_____	_____	_____	58/
52. How often have you felt calm and peaceful?	_____	_____	_____	_____	_____	59/

AIMS

These questions refer to MOOD.

DURING THE PAST MONTH . . .	Always (1)	Very Often (2)	Sometimes (3)	Almost Never (4)	Never (5)	
53. How often have you enjoyed the things you do?	_____	_____	_____	_____	_____	60/
54. How often have you been in low or very low spirits?	_____	_____	_____	_____	_____	61/
55. How often did you feel that nothing turned out the way you wanted it to?	_____	_____	_____	_____	_____	62/
56. How often did you feel that others would be better off if you were dead?	_____	_____	_____	_____	_____	63/
57. How often did you feel so down in the dumps that nothing would cheer you up?	_____	_____	_____	_____	_____	64/

AIMS2 Continued

AIMS

Please check (X) the most appropriate answer for each question.

These questions refer to satisfaction with each health area.

DURING THE PAST MONTH . . .	Very Satisfied (1)	Somewhat Satisfied (2)	Neither Satisfied Nor Dissatisfied (3)	Somewhat Dissatisfied (4)	Very Dissatisfied (5)	
58. How satisfied have you been with each of these areas of your health?						
MOBILITY LEVEL (example: do errands)	_____	_____	_____	_____	_____	65/
WALKING AND BENDING (example: climb stairs)	_____	_____	_____	_____	_____	66/
HAND AND FINGER FUNCTION (example: tie a bow)	_____	_____	_____	_____	_____	67/
ARM FUNCTION (example: comb hair)	_____	_____	_____	_____	_____	68/
SELF-CARE (example: take bath)	_____	_____	_____	_____	_____	69/
HOUSEHOLD TASKS (example: housework)	_____	_____	_____	_____	_____	70/
SOCIAL ACTIVITY (example: visit friends)	_____	_____	_____	_____	_____	71/
SUPPORT FROM FAMILY (example: help with problems)	_____	_____	_____	_____	_____	72/
ARTHRITIS PAIN (example: joint pain)	_____	_____	_____	_____	_____	73/
WORK (example: reduce hours)	_____	_____	_____	_____	_____	74/
LEVEL OF TENSION (example: felt tense)	_____	_____	_____	_____	_____	75/
MOOD (example: down in dumps)	_____	_____	_____	_____	_____	76/

AIMS2 Continued

ID 1-4/
ADM# 5-6/
CARD #2 7/
AIMS

Please check (X) the most appropriate answer for each question.

These questions refer to arthritis impact on each area of health.

DURING THE PAST MONTH . . .	Not a Problem for Me (0)	Due Entirely to Other Causes (1)	Due Largely to Other Causes (2)	Due Partly to Arthritis and Partly to Other Causes (3)	Due Largely to My Arthritis (4)	Due Entirely to My Arthritis (5)	
59. How much of your problem in each area of health was due to your arthritis?							
MOBILITY LEVEL (example: do errands)	____	____	____	____	____	____	8/
WALKING AND BENDING (example: climb stairs)	____	____	____	____	____	____	9/
HAND AND FINGER FUNCTION (example: tie a bow)	____	____	____	____	____	____	10/
ARM FUNCTION (example: comb hair)	____	____	____	____	____	____	11/
SELF-CARE (example: take bath)	____	____	____	____	____	____	12/
HOUSEHOLD TASKS (example: housework)	____	____	____	____	____	____	13/
SOCIAL ACTIVITY (example: visit friends)	____	____	____	____	____	____	14/
SUPPORT FROM FAMILY (example: help with problems)	____	____	____	____	____	____	15/
ARTHRITIS PAIN (example: joint pain)	____	____	____	____	____	____	16/
WORK (example: reduce hours)	____	____	____	____	____	____	17/
LEVEL OF TENSION (example: felt tense)	____	____	____	____	____	____	18/
MOOD (example: down in dumps)	____	____	____	____	____	____	19/

AIMS2 Continued

AIMS

You have now answered questions about different AREAS OF YOUR HEALTH. These areas are listed below. Please check (X) up to THREE AREAS in which you would MOST LIKE TO SEE IMPROVEMENT. Please read all 12 areas of health choices before making your decision:

check = 1
blank = 0

60. AREAS OF HEALTH	THREE AREAS FOR IMPROVEMENT	
MOBILITY LEVEL (example: do errands)	________	20/
WALKING AND BENDING (example: climb stairs)	________	21/
HAND AND FINGER FUNCTION (example: tie a bow)	________	22/
ARM FUNCTION (example: comb hair)	________	23/
SELF-CARE (example: take bath)	________	24/
HOUSEHOLD TASKS (example: housework)	________	25/
SOCIAL ACTIVITY (example: visit friends)	________	26/
SUPPORT FROM FAMILY (example: help with problems)	________	27/
ARTHRITIS PAIN (example: joint pain)	________	28/
WORK (example: reduce hours)	________	29/
LEVEL OF TENSION (example: felt tense)	________	30/
MOOD (example: down in dumps)	________	31/

Please make sure that you have checked no more than THREE AREAS for improvement.

AIMS2 Continued

AIMS

Please check (X) the most appropriate answer for each question.

These questions refer to CURRENT and FUTURE HEALTH.

	Excellent (1)	Good (2)	Fair (3)	Poor (4)	
61. In general would you say that your HEALTH NOW is excellent, good, fair or poor?	____	____	____	____	32/

	Very Satisfied (1)	Somewhat Satisfied (2)	Neither Satisfied Nor Dissatisfied (3)	Somewhat Dissatisfied (4)	Very Dissatisfied (5)	
62. How satisfied are you with your HEALTH NOW?	____	____	____	____	____	33/

	Not a Problem for Me (0)	Due Entirely to Other Causes (1)	Due Largely to Other Causes (2)	Due Partly to Arthritis and Partly to Other Causes (3)	Due Largely to My Arthritis (4)	Due Entirely to My Arthritis (5)	
63. How much of your problem with your HEALTH NOW is due to your arthritis?	____	____	____	____	____	____	34/

	Excellent (1)	Good (2)	Fair (3)	Poor (4)	
64. In general do you expect that your HEALTH 10 YEARS FROM NOW will be excellent, good, fair, or poor?	____	____	____	____	35/

	No Problem at All (1)	Minor Problem (2)	Moderate Problem (3)	Major Problem (4)	
65. How big a problem do you expect your arthritis to be 10 YEARS FROM NOW?	____	____	____	____	36/

AIMS2 Continued

AIMS

Please check (X) the most appropriate answer for each question.

This question refers to OVERALL ARTHRITIS IMPACT.

	Very Well (1)	Well (2)	Fair (3)	Poor (4)	Very Poorly (5)	
66. CONSIDERING ALL THE WAYS THAT YOUR ARTHRITIS AFFECTS YOU, how well are you doing compared to other people your age?	_____	_____	_____	_____	_____	37/

AIMS

67. What is the main kind of arthritis that you have?

check = 1
blank = 0

Rheumatoid arthritis	_______	38/
Osteoarthritis/degenerative arthritis	_______	39/
Systemic lupus erythematosus	_______	40/
Fibromyalgia	_______	41/
Scleroderma	_______	42/
Psoriatic arthritis	_______	43/
Reiter's syndrome	_______	44/
Gout	_______	45/
Low back pain	_______	46/
Tendonitis/bursitis	_______	47/
Osteoporosis	_______	48/
Other	_______	49/

68. How many years have you had arthritis? _______ 50–51/

DURING THE PAST MONTH . . .	All Days (1)	Most Days (2)	Some Days (3)	Few Days (4)	No Days (5)	
69. How often have you had to take MEDICATION for your arthritis?	_____	_____	_____	_____	_____	52/

AIMS2 Continued

AIMS

Please check (X) yes or no for each question.

70. Is your health currently affected by any of the following medical problems?

	Yes (1)	No (2)	
High blood pressure	______	______	53/
Heart disease	______	______	54/
Mental illness	______	______	55/
Diabetes	______	______	56/
Cancer	______	______	57/
Alcohol or drug use	______	______	58/
Lung disease	______	______	59/
Kidney disease	______	______	60/
Liver disease	______	______	61/
Ulcer or other stomach disease	______	______	62/
Anemia or other blood disease	______	______	63/

	Yes (1)	No (2)	
71. Do you take medicine every day for any problem other than your arthritis?	______	______	64/

	Yes (1)	No (2)	
72. Did you see a doctor more than three times last year for any problem other than your arthritis?	______	______	65/

AIMS2 Continued

AIMS

Please provide the following information about yourself:

73. What is your age at this time? ______ 66–67/

74. What is your sex?

Male (1) ______ 68/
Female (2) ______

75. What is your racial background?

White (1) ______ 69/
Black (2) ______
Hispanic (3) ______
Asian or Pacific Islander (4) ______
American Indian or Alaskan Native (5) ______
Other (6)

76. What is your current marital status?

Married (1) ______ 70/
Separated (2) ______
Divorced (3) ______
Widowed (4) ______
Never married (5) ______

77. What is the highest level of education you received.

Less than seven years of school (1) ______ 71/
Grades seven through nine (2) ______
Grades ten through eleven (3) ______
High school graduate (4) ______
One to four years of college (5) ______
College graduate (6) ______
Professional or graduate school (7) ______

78. What is your approximate family income including wages, disability payment, retirement income, and welfare?

Less than \$10,000 (1) ______ 72/
\$10,000–\$19,999 (2) ______
\$20,000–\$29,999 (3) ______
\$30,000–\$39,999 (4) ______
\$40,000–\$49,999 (5) ______
\$50,000–\$59,999 (6) ______
\$60,000–\$69,999 (7) ______
More than \$70,000 (8) ______

Thank you for completing this questionnaire.

FUNCTIONAL STATUS INDEX (FSI)

Contact Address: Alan M. Jette PT, PhD
Senior Research Scientist
New England Research Institute, Inc.,
9 Galen Street
Watertown, MA
U.S.A. 02172
Telephone: 617-923-7747
Fax: 617-926-8246

KEY: ASSISTANCE: 1 = independent; 2 = uses devices; 3 = uses human assistance; 4 = uses devices and human assistance; 5 = unable or unsafe to do the activity

PAIN: 1 = no pain; 2 = mild pain; 3 = moderate pain; 4 = severe pain

DIFFICULTY: 1 = no difficulty; 2 = mild difficulty; 3 = moderate difficulty; 4 = severe difficulty

Time Frame—on the average during the past (7) days

Activity	Assistance (1–5)	Pain (1–4)	Difficulty (1–4)	Comments
Mobility				
Walking inside	_____	_____	_____	
Climbing up stairs	_____	_____	_____	
Rising from a chair	_____	_____	_____	
Personal Care				
Putting on pants	_____	_____	_____	
Buttoning a shirt/blouse	_____	_____	_____	
Washing all parts of the body	_____	_____	_____	
Putting on a shirt/blouse	_____	_____	_____	
Home Chores				
Vacuuming a rug	_____	_____	_____	
Reaching into low cupboards	_____	_____	_____	
Doing laundry	_____	_____	_____	
Doing yardwork	_____	_____	_____	
Hand Activities				
Writing	_____	_____	_____	
Opening container	_____	_____	_____	
Dialing a phone	_____	_____	_____	
Social/Role Activities				
Performing your job	_____	_____	_____	
Driving a car	_____	_____	_____	
Attending meetings/appointments	_____	_____	_____	
Visiting with friends and relatives	_____	_____	_____	

FSI Continued

THE ARTHRITIS SOCIETY
ONTARIO DIVISION
CONSULTATION AND THERAPY SERVICE

See also
OF 52 ☐ or
OF-4-92 ☐

FOOT ASSESSMENT

Client Name: ______________________ Date: ______________

Therapist: ______________________ Duration of foot involvement: ________ years

Reason for assessment: ____

____

____

The pain in my ____________ over the past __________ is best described as:

____

No pain severe pain

PREVIOUS MANAGEMENT:

Conservative - Shoes: ____

Orthotics: ____

Other: ____

Surgical - ____

FUNCTIONAL MOBILITY REQUIRED: ____

____

Assessment continues on reverse . . .

CLIENT/THERAPIST GOALS:

(Pain): ____

(Gait): ____

(Footwear:) ____

(Hygiene/cosmesis) ____

(Education) ____

(Other) ____

TREATMENT PLAN:

Education:
- ☐ Hygiene
- ☐ Footwear
- ☐ Use of mobility aids
- ☐ Related disease process
- ☐ Range of Motion X's
- ☐ Calf Stretches
- ☐ Gait Training
- ☐ Modalities ______________

Shoe Modifications: ☐ Spot Stretching ☐ Tongue Pads ☐ Heel Counter ☐ Other __________

☐ Insole ☐ 3/4 ☐ Full Material Used: ______________

☐ Components ☐ long arch ☐ met. splay ☐ met. cookie ☐ met. bar Material used: __________

☐ lat. wedge ☐ med. wedge ☐ heel pad ☐ heel cup

Referred for: ☐ lift _____ cms. R/L ☐ rocker ☐ med./lat. wedge R/L ☐ med./lat. flare R/L

☐ Other ____

Review Date: ______________ Change (+) (−) ______________mm.

The pain in my ______________ over the past __________ is best described as:

|——————————————————————————|

No pain severe

OBSERVATIONS AND ASSESSMENT

R	L	LEGEND
		Active Effused Blister .... B Callus .... Cock-up toes .... C Corn .... C Fungus .... F Hallux valgus .... H Hammer toes .... H Nodule .... N Tenosynovitis .... T Ulcer .... U Wart .... W

R		L
Toe in / Toe out / Normal	Stance	Toe in / Toe out / Normal
↓ / Normal	One foot balance	↓ / Normal
Invert / Evert / Normal	Hindfoot	Invert / Evert / Normal
↑ / ↓ / Normal Mobile / Rigid	Longitudinal	↑ / ↓ / Normal Mobile / Rigid
↓ / Normal Mobile / Rigid	Metatarsal	↓ / Normal Mobile / Rigid
Mobile / Rigid	Forefoot	Mobile / Rigid
↑ / ↓ / Normal	Toe Off	↑ / ↓ / Normal
Mobile / Rigid	1st MTP	Mobile / Rigid

Bibliography

Akeson WH, Amiel D, Abel MF, et al: Effects of immobilization on joints. Clin Orthop 1987; 219:28–37.

Akeson WH, Amiel D, Woo SL-Y: Physiology and therapeutic value of passive motion. In Helminen HJ, et al (eds): Joint Loading, pp 375–394. Bristol, Wright, 1987.

Ansell BM, Rudge S, Schaller JG: Color Atlas of Pediatric Rheumatology. London, Wolfe Publishing Limited, 1992.

Badley EM, Rasooly I, Webster GK: Relative importance of musculoskeletal disorders as a cause of chronic health problems, disability and health care utilization: findings from the 1990 Ontario Health Survey. J Rheumatol 1994; 21:505–514.

Badley EM, Ibanez D: Socioeconomic risk factors and musculoskeletal disability. J Rheumatol 1994; 21:515–522.

Banwell BF: Physical therapy in arthritis management. In Ehrlich GE (ed): Rehabilitation Management of Rheumatic Conditions, 2nd edition, pp 264–284. Baltimore, Williams & Wilkins, 1986.

Cassidy JT (ed): Textbook of Rheumatology. New York, Churchill Livingstone Inc, 1990.

Conference on outcome measures in rheumatoid arthritis clinical trials. Maastrich, the Netherlands April 29–May 3, 1992. J Rheumatol 1993; 20:525–603.

Creed F: Psychological disorders in rheumatoid arthritis: a growing consensus? Ann Rheum Dis 1990; 49: 808–812.

Deyo RA: Compliance with therapeutic regimens in arthritis: issues, current status, and a future agenda. Semin Arthritis Rheum 1982; 12(2):233–244.

Falconer J: Hand splinting in rheumatoid arthritis. A perspective on current knowledge and directions for research. Arthritis Care Res 1991; 4:81–86.

Felson DT, Anderson JJ, Boers M, et al: The American College of Rheumatology preliminary core set of disease activity measures for rheumatoid arthritis trials. Arthritis Rheum 1993; 36:729–740.

PHYSICAL THERAPY IN ARTHRITIS, Joan M. Walker, PhD, PT, and Antoine Helewa, MSc(Clin Epid), PT, W.B. Saunders Company © 1996.

Gallin JI, Goldstein IM, Snyderman R (eds): Inflammation: Basic Principles and Clinical Correlates, 2nd edition. New York, Raven Press, 1992.

Goldsmith CH, Smythe HA, Helewa A: Interpretation and power of a pooled index. J Rheumatol 1993; 20: 575–578.

Gordon NF, Kohl HW, Scott CB, et al: Reassessment of the guidelines for exercise testing. Sports Med 1992; 13(5):293–302.

Hawley DJ, Wolfe F: Depression is not more common in rheumatoid arthritis: a 10 year longitudinal study of 6,608 rheumatic disease patients. J Rheumatol 1993; 20:2025–2031.

Helewa H, Goldsmith CH, Smythe HA: Patient, observer and instrument variation in the measurement of strength of shoulder abductor muscles in patients with rheumatoid arthritis using a modified sphygmomanometer. J Rheumatol 1986; 13:1044–1049.

Helewa A, Smythe HA, Goldsmith CH: Can specially trained physiotherapists improve the care of patients with rheumatoid arthritis? A randomized health care trial. J Rheumatol 1994; 21:70–79.

Helewa A, Bombardier C, Goldsmith CH, et al: Cost-effectiveness of inpatient and intensive outpatient treatment of rheumatoid arthritis. A randomized, controlled trial. Arthritis Rheum 1989; 32:1505–1514.

Helewa A, Smythe HA, Goldsmith CH, et al: The total assessment of rheumatoid polyarthritis—evaluation of a training program for physiotherapists and occupational therapists. J Rheumatol 1987; 14:87–92.

Jamison L, Ogden D: Aquatic therapy using PNF patterns. Tucson, AZ, Therapy Skill Builders, 1994

Kelley WN, Harris ED, Ruddy S, et al (eds): Textbook of Rheumatology, 4th edition, vols 1 and 2. Philadelphia, WB Saunders Co, 1993.

Kelsey JL: Epidemiology of Musculoskeletal Disorders. New York, Oxford University Press, 1982.

Klippel JH, Dieppe PA (eds): Rheumatology. St. Louis, Mosby Yearbook, 1994.

Koda-Kimble MA, Young LY (eds): Applied Therapeutics, The Clinical Use of Drugs, 5th edition. Vancouver, Applied Therapeutics Inc, 1992.

Kovar PA, Allegrante JP, Mackenzie CR, et al: Supervised

fitness walking in patients with osteoarthritis of the knee: a randomized, controlled trial. Ann Intern Med 1992; 116:529–534.

Kraag G, Stokes B, Groh J, et al: The effects of comprehensive home physiotherapy and supervision on patients with ankylosing spondylitis—an 8-month followup. J Rheumatol 1994; 21:261–263.

Krogh CME (ed): CPS, 29th edition. Ottawa, Canadian Pharmaceutical Association, 1994.

Kuettner K, et al (eds): Articular Cartilage and Osteoarthritis. New York, Raven Press Ltd, 1992.

Lanza AF, Revenson TA: Social support interventions for rheumatoid arthritis patients: the cart before the horse? Health Educ Q 1993; 20:97–117.

Leadbeater WB, Buckwalter JA, Gordon SL (eds): Sports-Induced Inflammation: Clinical and Basic Science Concepts, pp 23–54. Park Ridge, IL, American Academy of Orthopedic Surgeons, 1990.

Lee P, Helewa A, Smythe HA, et al: Epidemiology of musculoskeletal disorders (complaints) and related disability in Canada. J Rheumatol 1985; 12:1169–1173.

Levy AS, Marmar E: The role of cold compression dressings in the postoperative treatment of total knee arthroplasty. Clin Orthop 1993; 297:174–178.

Logigian MK, Ward JD (eds): A Team Approach for Therapists—Pediatric Rehabilitation. Boston, Little, Brown & Co, 1989.

McCain GA, Bell DA, Mai FM, et al: A controlled study of the effects of a supervised cardiovascular fitness training program on the manifestations of primary fibromyalgia. Arthritis Rheum 1988; 31:1135–1141.

McCarty DJ, Koopman WJ (eds): Arthritis and Allied Conditions, 12th edition, vols 1 and 2. Philadelphia, Lea & Febiger, 1993.

McCormick MC, Stemmler MM, Athreya BH: The impact of childhood rheumatic diseases on the family. Arthritis Rheum 1986; 29:872–879.

Melvin J (ed): Rheumatic Disease in Adult and Child: Occupational Therapy and Rehabilitation, 3rd edition. Philadelphia, FA Davis Co, 1989.

Minor MA, Hewett JE, Webel RR, et al: Efficacy of physical conditioning exercise in patients with rheumatoid arthritis or osteoarthritis. Arthritis Rheum 1989; 32:1397–1405.

Moncur C: Perceptions of physical therapy competencies in rheumatology. Physical therapists versus rheumatologists. Phys Ther 1987; 67(3):331–339.

Moncur C: Physical therapy competencies in rheumatology. Phys Ther 1985; 65:1365–1372.

Mullen PD, Laville EA, Biddle AK, Lorig K: Efficacy of psychoeducational interventions on pain, depression, and disability in people with arthritis: a meta-analysis. J Rheumatol 1987; 14:33–39.

Murphy S, Creed F, Jayson MIV: Psychiatric disorder and illness behaviour in rheumatoid arthritis. Br J Rheumatol 1988; 27:357–363.

National Arthritis Data Workgroup: Arthritis prevalence and activity limitations. US Morbidity and Mortality Weekly Report 1994; 4:433–438.

Nickel VL, Botte MJ (eds): Orthopaedic Rehabilitation, 2nd edition. New York, Churchill Livingstone, 1992.

Pincus T, Callahan LF: Taking mortality in rheumatoid arthritis seriously—predictive markers, socioeconomic status and comorbidity. J Rheumatol 1986; 13: 841–845.

Pollack ML, Wilmore JH: Exercise in Health and Disease, 2nd edition. Philadelphia, WB Saunders Co, 1990.

Price LG, Hewett JE, Kay DR, et al: Five-minute walking test of aerobic fitness for people with arthritis. Arthritis Care Res 1988; 1:33–37.

Salter RB: Continuous Passive Motion (CPM): A Biological Concept for the Healing and the Generation of Articular Cartilage, Ligaments, and Tendons: From its Origination to Research to Clinical Applications. Baltimore, Williams & Wilkins, 1993.

Schlapbach P, Gerber NJ (eds): Physiotherapy: Controlled Trials and Facts, Rheumatology, vol 14. Basel, Karger, 1991.

Schumacher HR Jr (ed): The Primer on the Rheumatic Diseases, 10th edition. Atlanta, Arthritis Foundation, 1993.

Semble EL, Loeser RF, Wise CM: Therapeutic exercise for rheumatoid arthritis and osteoarthritis. Semin Arthritis Rheum 1990; 20:32–40.

Sheon RP, Moskowitz RW, Goldberg VM (eds): Soft Tissue Rheumatic Pain: Recognition, Management, Prevention, 2nd edition. Philadelphia, Lea & Febiger, 1987.

Smythe HA, Buskila D, Gladman DD: Performance of scored palpation, a point count, and dolorimetry in assessing unsuspected nonarticular tenderness. J Rheumatol 1993; 20:352–357.

Spilker B (ed): Quality of Life: Assessments in Clinical Trials. New York, Raven Press, 1990.

Stokes BA, Helewa A, Goldsmith CH, et al: Reliability of spinal mobility measurements in ankylosing spondylitis patients. Physiother Can 1988; 40:338–344.

Uveges JM, Parker JC, Smarr KL, et al: Psychological symptoms in primary fibromyalgia syndrome: relationship to pain, life stress, and sleep disturbance. Arthritis Rheum 1990; 33:1279–1283.

Walker SR, Rosser SR (eds): Quality of Life: Assessment and Application. Lancaster, MTP Press Limited, 1988.

Wells C: Bones, Bodies, and Disease: Evidence of Disease and Abnormality in Early Man. London, Thomas & Hudson, 1964.

Woessner JF, Howell DS (eds): Joint Cartilage Degradation. New York, Marcel Dekker, 1993.

Wolfe F, Pincus T (eds): Rheumatoid Arthritis, Pathogenesis, Assessment, Outcome and Treatment. New York, Marcel Dekker, 1994.

Wright V, Radin EL (eds): Mechanics of Human Joints. New York, Marcel Dekker, 1993.

Wynn KS, Eckel EM: Juvenile rheumatoid arthritis and home physical therapy program compliance. Phys Occup Ther Pediatr 1986; 6:55–63.

Ziegler E: Current Concepts in Orthotics: A Diagnosis-Related Approach to Splinting. Rolyan Medical Products, 1984.

Glossary

active joint A joint considered to have active inflammation when any of three conditions are present: effusion, tenderness, or stress pain

ACR American College of Rheumatology

aggrecan Groupings of collagen protein monomers in articular cartilage

AIMS Arthritis Impact Measurement Scales (*Not to be confused with Piper's AIMS for infants*)

angiogenesis Formation of new blood vessels (neovascularization)

ARA American Rheumatism Association, *former* name of the American College of Rheumatology

arteritis Inflammation of arteries

arthrodesis Surgical fusion of a joint

arthroplasty The operative procedure of reconstruction of a diseased joint

ASA Acetylsalicylic acid or aspirin

ASMC The Arthritis Self-Management Course (Arthritis Foundation, USA)

avascular necrosis Cell/tissue death due to loss of blood supply

Baker's cyst Leakage of joint synovial fluid into an adjacent bursa, commonly seen at the knee due to increased intra-articular pressure

Bouchard's nodes Osteophytes on the proximal interphalangeal joints

boutonnière "Button hole" deformity of digit due to erosion of the extensor mechanism over the proximal interphalangeal joint

case control design A group of cases is compared with a group of noncases (controls) to determine whether various factors played a role in caseness formation

CES-D The Center for Epidemiological Studies—Depression Scale

COF Coefficient of friction, the shear force needed to make one surface slide on another divided by the normal force pressing them together

cohort study Prospective (forward-in-time) study with two groups, one with the risk factor(s) and a matched control group without the risk factor(s); used to compare between the two groups rates of disease occurrence or incidence

complement system A group of 20 plasma proteins involved in the body's defense and immune systems

CPPD Calcium pyrophosphate dihydrate—crystal deposition disease

CRP C-reactive protein, a nonspecific indicator of the presence of inflammation

CTAP-III A connective tissue activating protein

cytokines Extracellular messenger proteins, peptide growth factors secreted by a variety of inflammatory cells with multiple biological activities (examples are transforming growth factor [TGF], platelet-derived growth factor [PDGF])

cytotoxic Adverse effects on cells, associated with drug therapy

CPT Community physical therapy

Damage-Duration Index Index of rate of destruction; number of "damaged" joints divided by disease duration, in years

débridement Surgical cleaning of debris in a joint

DMARDs Disease modifying antirheumatic drugs (also slow-acting antirheumatic drugs [SAARDs])

enthesis Ligament-bone junction

epidemiology The study of the distribution and determinants of health-related states and events in populations and the application of this study to the control of health problems

ESR Erythrocyte sedimentation rate, a nonspecific indicator of the presence of inflammation

fibromyalgia tender points Characteristic "active" sites that are tender and can be distinguished from equally characteristic "control" points that are nontender

fibromyalgia (FM) Widespread pain and tenderness at 11 or more of 18 defined sites

FSI Functional Status Index

hemarthrosis Joint effusion containing blood products, forms rapidly

HAQ Health Assessment Questionnaire

Heberden's nodes Excessive bone formation (osteophytes) at joint margins, seen in digits of patients with OA

hemosiderin An iron blood corpuscle pigment

HLA-B27 Histocompatibility antigen demonstrated in patients with ankylosing spondylitis, indicator of relative risk when present (positive)

PHYSICAL THERAPY IN ARTHRITIS, Joan M. Walker, PhD, PT, and Antoine Helewa, MSc(Clin Epid), PT, W.B. Saunders Company © 1996.

hydroxyapatites Crystals of calcium salts
hyperplasia Increase in cell number
hypertrophy Increase in size
hyperuricemia Supersaturation of urate in serum, seen in gout
IAP Intra-articular pressure within intact joint cavity, normally negative
seronegative arthritis Inflammatory arthritic conditions in which the serological test for the rheumatoid factor is characteristically negative
IGF-I, IGF-II Insulin-like growth factors
IL-1 Interleukin-1, a proinflammatory mediator
incidence The rate of occurrence of new cases of a disease during a given period, in a defined population at risk
inflammatory arthritis Damage to a joint characterized by a process of inflammation
intra-articular therapy Injection of drugs directly into a joint
iontophoresis Topical administration of active drug ions that can be driven through the skin by a continuous direct current
JA Juvenile arthritis, also know as juvenile rheumatoid arthritis
JAFAR Juvenile Arthritis Functional Assessment Report
JAQQ Juvenile Arthritis Quality of Life Questionnaire
JASI Juvenile Arthritis Functional Status Index
JRA Juvenile rheumatoid arthritis, also known as juvenile arthritis
N of 1 Entire experiment within a single patient including randomization of intervention(s)
NSAIDs Nonsteroidal anti-inflammatory drugs
orthotic (splints) Externally applied devices that support a joint or enhance its function
osteoarthritis (degenerative joint disease, osteoarthrosis) Process characterized by thinning and destruction of articular cartilage, remodeling of bony surfaces
osteopenia Radiologic term for thinning or deficiency of bone (not synonymous with osteoporosis)
osteophyte Formation of new bone at joint margins (bony spur)
paleopathology The study of disease and trauma in extinct societies
pannus Inflammatory fibrinous exudate, highly vascular, contains several cell types, spreads over joint surfaces and destroys articular cartilage; characteristic of rheumatoid arthritis
PAR-Q Physical Activity Readiness Questionnaire
pauciarticular Arthritis involving four or fewer joints
photophobia Intolerance of light
polyarticular Arthritis involving five or more joints
prevalence The proportion of cases identified in a population at a given point in time (*point prevalence*) or during a specified interval (*period prevalence*), or at any time (*lifetime prevalence*)
PT Physical therapy, physiotherapy, physical therapist, physiotherapist
randomized clinical trial (RCT) An experiment in which subjects are allocated at random to two or more groups to receive different interventions or a placebo
reactive arthritis Nonsuppurative inflammatory process due to an infectious process at a distance from the primary process
reliability (consistency) The degree of stability in a measurement, when repeated under identical conditions; the degree to which a measure is free of random error
responsiveness Ability of a measures to detect *clinically important change,* after application of a treatment maneuver
rheumatoid factor Antibody (usually of IgM isotype) that reacts with antigenic determinants on the immunoglobin molecule, an anti-antibody
RIL Repetitive impulsive loading, excessive mechanical loading
Romanus lesions Bone erosions at anterior margin vertebral bodies
Schöber test 10-cm segment measure from S_1 of spinal flexion—extension range of motion
scleroderma (systemic sclerosis) Generalized disorder of collagen
sclerosis Thickening
sensitivity Ability to detect true positives in diagnostic tests
septic arthritis Secondary to a bacterial infection
SLE Systemic lupus erythematosus, an inflammatory disease affecting many organs
specificity Ability to detect true negatives in diagnostic tests; having a defined and limited effect/outcome (i.e., drug therapy, exercise)
reproducibility Ability to achieve the same response/outcome in repeated trials (test-retest reliability or stability over time)
spondylitis Arthritis of the vertebral column
Still's disease JRA with a systemic onset
Swan-neck Deformity of digit due to "bow-stringing" of the collateral ligaments
syndesmophytes Bony bridges between vertebral bodies due to calcification then ossification of outer fibers of the annulus
synovectomy Removal of synovial tissues by surgery
synovial lining tissue (SLT) Term that has replaced the former inappropriate "synovial membrane"; covers most intra-articular structures
tidemark Junction between the uncalcified and calcified layers of articular cartilage
TNF Tumor necrosis factor, a proinflammatory mediator
tophi Deposits of urate crystals in and around joints in gouty arthritis
validity Degree to which a test measures what it purports to measure
VAS Visual Analogue Scale, a line of known length on which patients score their symptoms
vasculitis Inflammation of blood vessels
WOMAC Western Ontario and McMaster Universities Osteoarthritis Index
xerophthalmia Dry eyes due to chronic inflammation of lacrimal and salivary glands

AUTHOR INDEX

Note: Page numbers in *italics* indicate the page on which the complete reference appears.

SUBJECT INDEX

Note: Page numbers in *italics* indicate figures; page numbers followed by t indicate tables.

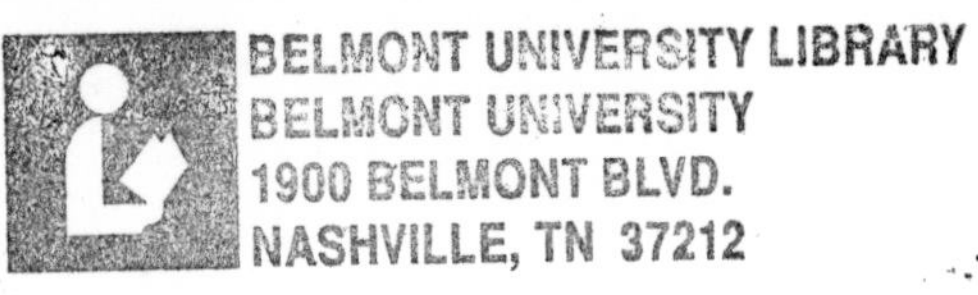